CELLULAR AND MOLECULAR MECHANISMS OF DRUGS OF ABUSE II

Cocaine, Substituted Amphetamines, GHB, and Opiates

ANNALS OF THE NEW YORK ACADEMY OF SCIENCES
Volume 965

CELLULAR AND MOLECULAR MECHANISMS OF DRUGS OF ABUSE II

Cocaine, Substituted Amphetamines, GHB, and Opiates

Edited by Syed F. Ali

The New York Academy of Sciences
New York, New York
2002

Library of Congress Cataloging-in-Publication Data

Cellular and molecular mechanisms of drugs of abuse II: cocaine, substituted amphetamines, GHB, and opiates / edited by Syed F. Ali
    p. ; cm. — (Annals of the New York Academy of Sciences ; v. 965)
    Includes bibliographical references and index.
    ISBN 1-57331-408-0 (cloth : alk. paper) — ISBN 1-57331-409-9 (pbk : alk. paper)
    1. Drugs of abuse—Physiological effect—Congresses. 2. Drug abuse—Pathophysiology—Congresses. 3. Neurotoxicology—Congresses.
I. Ali, Syed F. II. Series.
    [DNLM: 1. Substance-Related Disorders—physiopathology
—Congresses. 2. Amphetamines—pharmacokinetics—Congresses.
3. Benzalkonium Compounds—pharmacokinetics—Congresses.
5. Narcotics—pharmacokinetics—Congresses. W1 AN626YL
v. 965 2002/WM 270 C3932 2002]
    Q11 .N5 vol. 965
    [RB316]
    500 s—dc21
    [616.86'407]   2002007658

GYAT/PCP
Printed in the United States of America
ISBN 1-57331-408-0 (cloth)
ISBN 1-57331-409-9 (paper)
ISSN 0077-8923

ANNALS OF THE NEW YORK ACADEMY OF SCIENCES

Volume 965
June 2002

CELLULAR AND MOLECULAR MECHANISMS OF DRUGS OF ABUSE II

Cocaine, Substituted Amphetamines, GHB, and Opiates

Editor
SYED F. ALI

Conference Organizers
SYED F. ALI, RICARDO DUFFARD, ANA MARÍA EVANGELISTA,
YASUO TAKAHASHI, KUNIO YUI, AND M. AMELIA FERREIRA

[This volume comprises the proceedings of a conference entitled **Cellular and Molecular Mechanisms of Drugs of Abuse: Cocaine, GHB, Ibogaine, and Substituted Amphetamines,** held August 22–24, 2001, at Mar del Plata, Argentina.]

CONTENTS

Financial assistance was received from:

- INTERNATIONAL SOCIETY FOR NEUROCHEMISTRY
- NATIONAL INSTITUTE ON DRUG ABUSE
- ARGENTINIAN SECRETARY OF STATE FOR PREVENTION OF DRUG
  ADDICTION AND NARCOTRAFFIC (SEDRONAR)
- SCHOOL OF BIOMEDICAL AND PHARMACEUTICAL SCIENCES,
  NATIONAL UNIVERSITY OF ROSARIO, ARGENTINA
- SIGMA-TAU HEALTH SCIENCES
- NATIONAL CENTER FOR TOXICOLOGICAL RESEARCH,
  U.S. FOOD AND DRUG ADMINISTRATION

Preface

SYED F. ALI

Neurochemistry Laboratory, Division of Neurotoxicology,
National Center for Toxicological Research/FDA, 3900 NCTR Road,
Jefferson, Arkansas 72079-9501, USA

This volume contains papers presented at the satellite meeting of the 18th biennial meeting of the International Society for Neurochemistry and the American Society for Neurochemistry. The satellite meeting, entitled **Cellular and Molecular Mechanisms of Drugs of Abuse: Cocaine, GHB, Ibogaine, and Substituted Amphetamines,** was held August 22–24, 2001 at the Torres de Manantiales, Mar del Plata, Argentina. The overall atmosphere of the meeting—especially the surroundings—was very pleasant. Because of the relatively small number of participants, each was able to enjoy the scientific exchange in a relaxing and informal atmosphere.

The major goal of the conference was to understand the cellular and molecular mechanisms of drugs of abuse such as cocaine, GHB, ibogaine, and substituted amphetamines (*d*-amphetamine, methamphetamine, and MDMA), as well as drugs that have been proposed for the treatment of drug addiction such as ibogaine, noribogaine, and GBR. Researchers from the Food and Drug Administration presented the clinical aspect in the development of medications designed to treat drug addiction. Although a tremendous body of data has been gathered on the neurochemical changes engendered by exposure to drugs of abuse, the cellular and molecular mechanisms responsible for these changes remain unclear. Separate sessions were devoted to the underlying mechanisms of drug addiction such as gene expression/ molecular mechanisms, medication development, free radical–induced neurotoxicity, neurodegeneration, neuroprotection and neuroadaptation, specific neuronal markers, neurotoxicity of toluene, alcohol and nicotine, MDMA neurotoxicity, drugs of abuse and imaging brain structure and function, heroin and opiates. At the end of the meeting, there was a panel discussion and open forum, in which overall content of the meeting was summarized and future recommendations made. The goal of the conference was to bring together clinical and basic scientists in a multinational, multidisciplinary forum to exchange ideas and data related to this expanding field of research.

We express our gratitude to the organizations and the U.S. government agencies who supported this meeting. All papers included in this volume were reviewed by at least one referee, and we want to thank the referees for their valuable time and effort. We also thank the New York Academy of Sciences for their efficiency and professionalism in seeing this volume through the press. Last, but not least, we want to thank many of our colleagues who helped in the organization of this meeting. The next ISN/APSN–sponsored satellite meeting dealing with the same topic will be held from July 30–August 1, 2003, in Nagoya, Japan.

Ann. N.Y. Acad. Sci. 965: xi (2002). © 2002 New York Academy of Sciences.

Identification of Chronic Cocaine-Induced Gene Expression Through Dopamine D1 Receptors by Using cDNA Microarrays

JIANHUA ZHANG, DONGSHENG ZHANG, AND MING XU

Department of Cell Biology, Neurobiology and Anatomy, University of Cincinnati College of Medicine, Cincinnati, Ohio 45267-0521, USA

ABSTRACT: A major goal of drug abuse research is to understand the molecular mechanisms underlying the behavioral changes caused by repeated exposure to cocaine. Enduring behavioral changes, such as behavioral sensitization, can be induced in rodents by repeated cocaine administration. The neurobiological mechanisms underlying such behavioral changes are associated with the brain mesocorticolimbic dopamine (DA) pathway. Moreover, the DA D1 receptors are involved in mediating the long-term behavioral effects of cocaine. The long-lasting behavioral effects of repeated cocaine exposure are highly likely to be associated with underlying changes in gene expression. To examine this possibility, we have started to combine the use of D1 receptor mutant mice with cDNA microarrays to identify gene expression changes mediated through the D1 receptors induced by repeated cocaine administration. Our initial experiments focused on a target of the mesocorticolimbic DA pathway, the nucleus accumbens (NAc), which is the primary neural substrate for mediating the long-term effects of cocaine. We found that multiple genes are differentially expressed in wild-type and D1 receptor mutant mice after chronic cocaine treatment. Further studies are in progress to determine the physiological significance of the differential expression of these genes in chronic cocaine-induced behaviors.

KEYWORDS: drugs of abuse; cocaine; dopamine; gene expression; mesocorticolimbic DA; Fos; microarray technology

INTRODUCTION

Drugs of abuse, such as cocaine, can elicit compulsive drug-taking behaviors in humans upon repeated exposure, and widespread cocaine abuse creates one of the foremost public health problems in this country. Repeated cocaine exposure can also lead to striking behavioral changes in rodents, such as sensitization.[1–6] This enduring alteration in behavioral response to cocaine is thought to be similar to the intensification of drug craving after repeated exposure, and has been used as a model to study contributing factors involved in compulsive drug-taking behaviors in humans.[5,6]

Address for correspondence: Ming Xu, Ph.D., Department of Cell Biology, Neurobiology and Anatomy, University of Cincinnati College of Medicine, Cincinnati, Ohio 45267-0521. Voice: 513-558-2922; fax: 513-558-4454.

ming.xu@uc.edu

Ann. N.Y. Acad. Sci. 965: 1–9 (2002). © 2002 New York Academy of Sciences.

The neurobiological mechanisms underlying the actions of cocaine are primarily associated with the mesocorticolimbic DA pathway which consists of DA neurons that originate in the midbrain ventral tegmental area and project to the NAc, amygdala (AMG), olfactory tubercle, and frontal cortex.[7,8] DA binds to DA receptors expressed by both target neurons and DA-containing neurons upon release from nerve terminals. Binding of DA to cell-surface receptors initiates a variety of neuronal and ultimately behavioral responses. The DA D1 receptor is widely expressed in the brain, including the NAc, AMG, and frontal cortex,[9] brain regions that are critical for mediating the effects of cocaine and other drugs of abuse.[3,4] Pharmacological studies have shown that D1 receptor agonists and antagonists can influence locomotor and stereotyped responses to cocaine and cocaine self-administration.[10–14] Moreover, D1 receptor antagonists can prevent or attenuate the development of behavioral sensitization induced by cocaine.[15] Repeated cocaine administration also leads to persistent increases in D1 receptor sensitivity within the NAc.[16,17] These behavioral and electrophysiological studies strongly suggest that the D1 receptors may play critical roles in mediating the effects of cocaine.

The time course for the acquisition and the relative stability for the expression of behavioral responses suggest the involvement of enduring neuroadaptations in response to repeated cocaine exposure.[3,4,18] Changes in gene expression through the D1 receptors may mediate some of the neuroadaptations to chronic cocaine exposure.[19] Much evidence suggests an involvement of the Fos family proteins in the acute and chronic effects of cocaine. Fos expression is induced through D1 receptors upon acute cocaine injections.[20] Bilateral delivery of an antisense oligonucleotide to c-fos in the NAc can block the acute locomotor-stimulating effects of cocaine without affecting spontaneous exploratory activity.[21] Repeated injections of cocaine induce long-lasting AP-1 transcription complexes consisting of ΔFosB.[22] Expression of ΔFosB in mice can increase the rewarding and locomotor-stimulating effects of cocaine.[23] Chronic cocaine treatments also lead to network-level changes in immediate early gene expression.[24] c-Fos expression can also be induced in the NAc, AMG, striatum, and medial prefrontal cortex by cocaine self-administration.[25] These observations argue that Fos-regulated gene expression may be an important component in mediating responses to chronic cocaine exposure.[6,27]

In spite of extensive studies, the underlying changes in gene expression that occur in drug addiction are still only poorly understood. Part of this is due to a lack, until recently, of means to effectively examine the effects of drug treatment on more than dozens of genes within an experiment. The development of cDNA microarray technology provides a powerful new tool for high throughput analysis of gene expression patterns.[28–30] It is clearly established that with this approach, one can determine relative levels of gene expression under specific physiological conditions.[31–36] This technology currently enables the simultaneous analysis of gene expression patterns of tens of thousands of genes. The cDNA microarray technology will have a profound impact in understanding changes in gene expression patterns in biological systems in response to environmental stimuli.[37,38] It provides new opportunities to efficiently capture neuroadaptations involving complex changes in gene expression in the brain that accompany the development of drug addiction.

A better understanding of the global gene expression profile induced by cocaine through DA D1 receptors may help to elucidate how cocaine induces addictive behaviors through this receptor. To examine this possibility, we have started to use cDNA microarray analysis to compare gene expression patterns induced by repeated cocaine injections in the brains of D1 receptor mutant and wild-type mice.[39,40] We initially focused on a target of the mesocorticolimbic DA pathway, the NAc, which is the primary neural substrate for mediating the long-term effects of cocaine. To date, we made three comparisons. First, to identify cocaine-regulated genes and to control for stress-induced genes, we compared gene expression patterns in cocaine- and saline-treated wild-type mice. Second, to specifically identify target genes regulated by cocaine through the D1 receptors, we compared gene expression patterns in cocaine-treated wild-type and D1 receptor mutant mice. Third, to control for stress-induced genes and to a certain extent, to control for baseline differences between the wild-type and D1 receptor mutant mice, we compared gene expression patterns in saline-treated wild-type and mutant mice.

MATERIALS AND METHODS

Mice

Two groups each of D1 receptor mutant mice and four groups of wild-type mice ($n = 6$ per group) were used. All groups of mice were handled and treated intraperitoneally with either cocaine or saline . We treated one group of D1 receptor mutant and two groups of wild-type mice with saline, and one group of D1 receptor mutant and two groups of wild-type mice with 20 mg/kg of cocaine twice daily for seven consecutive days. Whereas cocaine-treated wild-type mice developed behavioral sensitization during the injection time window, D1 receptor mutant mice failed to do so, as described previously.[40]

Micropunch Dissection of NAc and Total RNA Isolation

On day eight, cocaine- and saline-treated mice were decapitated, and intact brains were carefully removed, and were frozen on dry ice. The NAc was obtained by micropunch dissection and homogenized in TRIZOL (GIBCO). RNA was isolated from NAc samples pooled from all six mice in each group. Because of the small tissue size, we did not distinguish the shell versus core of the NAc for RNA isolation. Total RNA was isolated by isopropanol precipitation. In our experience, about 20 mg of total RNA can be isolated from six pooled NAc. OD readings at 260 and 280 nm were determined, and the ratio is normally around 2.0. The Agilent method was used to examine the quality of the total RNA.

cDNA Microarray Chips

There are two major types of microarray chips currently available. A number of biotechnology companies, including Genome Systems Inc., manufacture high-density arrays of cDNA PCR products spotted on glass slides. Each cDNA sequence ranges from 500 to 5000 base pair in length. The size of the hybridization product and the ability to wash under stringent conditions can improve hybridization to array targets when probes are derived from low-abundance mRNAs. The two mRNA samples, the experimental and control, are each converted to cDNA and labeled fluorescently with either Cy5-dCTP or Cy3-dCTP, respectively. This two-color labeling method provides consistent across-the-array competitive hybridization controls. The combination of these effects help to improve signal-to-noise ratios, allowing the detection of twofold differences between mRNAs expressed at low levels. The sensitivity is sufficient to detect a gene expressed once per cell. Full internal controls are also present for determining sensitivity, differential expression, and reverse transcription quality. Affymetrix, among others, uses photolithographic synthesis of oligonucleotide arrays at very high density on silicon chip surfaces. Since the gene targets are short oligonucleotides, a key concern is that the probe concentration needs to be very high. Moreover, hybridization and washing stringency must be more tightly controlled than for longer target sequences, and intrinsic variation in efficiency for different targets is high. Although Affymetrix can generate extremely high-density base-specific arrays, we chose to use cDNA microarray chips from Genome Systems Inc.

cDNA Microarray Hybridization

Twenty microrgrams of the total RNA from each treatment group was sent to University of Cincinnati Microarray Core for hybridization. The Core printed the slides using the Genome System GEM1 gene set with 8734 mouse genes. Approximately half of the spotted sequences are known genes, and the other half are unknowns, but represent individual genes from ESTs cluster-mapped to the Unigene database. Each pair of RNA samples was converted into cDNA and labeled with either Cy5-dCTP or Cy3-dCTP. The two labeled samples were simultaneously applied to a single microarray, where they competitively reacted with the arrayed cDNA molecules. The intensity of the fluorescence at each array element should be proportional to the expression level of that gene in the sample. The ratio of the two fluorescent intensities provides a highly accurate and quantitative measurement of the relative gene expression level in the two samples. Data scanning was carried out by staff at the Mircroarray Core.

Data Analysis

Results obtained from three pairs of comparisons, that is, cocaine- versus saline-treated wild-type mice, cocaine-treated wild-type versus cocaine-treated mutant mice, and saline-treated wild-type versus saline-treated mutant mice, were used for data analysis. Hybridization results were analyzed using a GeneSpring (Silicon Genetics Inc.) software, which allows for the detection and visualization of coordinate regulatory behavior with respect to both change pattern and any grouping of genes one chooses. To identify the functional makeup of groups of genes that undergo changes as a function of repeated exposure to cocaine, we applied mathematical cluster analysis to the expression changes in the three pairs of comparison.[41–44]

RESULTS

Our overall goal is to identify chronic cocaine-induced gene expression though the D1 receptors. To identify cocaine-regulated genes and to control for stress-induced genes, we compared gene expression patterns in cocaine- and saline-treated

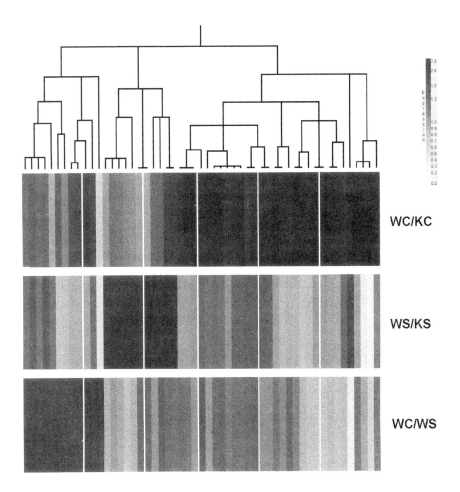

FIGURE 1. The gene tree of the 54 genes in the three experiments with ratio representation. The dark color indicates a high level of expression, the gray color represents an average expression level, and the white color indicates a low expression level. WC: wild-type
mice treated with cocaine; KC: D1 receptor mutant mice treated with cocaine; WS: wild-
type mice treated with saline; KS: D1 receptor mutant mice treated with saline.

wild-type mice. To specifically identify target genes regulated by cocaine through
the D1 receptors, we compared gene expression patterns in cocaine-treated wild-
type and D1 receptor mutant mice. To control for stress-induced genes and to a certain extent, to control for baseline differences between the wild-type and D1 receptor
mutant mice, we compared gene expression patterns in saline-treated wild-type and
mutant mice.

We used the GeneSpring software to analyze the microarray hybridization results.
Such analysis revealed that 54 genes were upregulated by at least twofold in cocaine-

treated wild-type versus cocaine-treated D1 receptor mutant pair, in saline-treated wild-type versus saline-treated D1 receptor mutant pair, or in cocaine-treated wild-type versus saline-treated wild-type pair. These 54 genes were further clustered according to their expression patterns in the three comparisons. As shown in FIGURE 1, cocaine can induce differential gene expression in wild-type and D1 receptor mutant mice. We are particularly interested in those genes that are upregulated by cocaine in wild-type mice compared to either the cocaine-treated D1 receptor mutant mice or saline-treated wild-type mice.

DISCUSSION

We performed an experiment using three pairs of RNA from pooled NAc from D1 receptor mutant and wild-type mice and found candidate genes that are differentially expressed, depending on the genotype and treatment. These initial results demonstrate that cDNA microarrays can be used to identify putative target genes regulated by repeated cocaine exposure through the D1 receptors.

One major challenge associated with microarray studies is reproducibility. Simultaneous hybridization of thousands of cDNAs to a microarray is a highly complex process. Even with RNA isolated from the same tissue samples, hybridization results can differ between experiments. This makes it difficult to judge whether a differentially expressed gene is truly physiologically relevant to cocaine actions, especially for genes whose expression levels do not vary by more than twofold. To overcome this problem, we are in the process of repeating the microarray hybridization using separate pools of RNA. We will also use RNA from the pooled NAc from mice treated with different doses of cocaine and at additional time points. If differentially expressed at several doses of cocaine and at different time points in the cocaine-treated wild-type versus mutant mouse comparison, and in the cocaine- and saline-treated wild-type mouse comparison, a candidate gene is more likely to be physiologically relevant to repeated cocaine exposure. The use of additional time points may also allow us to identify genes that are differentially involved in the initiation or maintenance of chronic cocaine-induced behaviors.

A second critical aspect of microarray studies is to validate the differential expression of candidate genes. In our case, this essential step will provide important correlative evidence for the potential relevance of these genes in behavioral changes induced by repeated cocaine exposure. Results from the expression mapping will also suggest strategies for the physiological testing of these genes in the future. To map and compare the expression levels of the potential target genes, we will perform quantitative reverse transcriptase-polymerase-chain reaction (RT-PCR) analysis using mRNA isolated from the NAc of both cocaine- and saline-treated D1 receptor mutant and wild-type mice. Quantitative RT-PCR is a sensitive technique suitable for analysis of rare mRNA from very small sample sizes, such as the tissues used in this study. We will only pursue further histological analyses if the expression of a putative target gene could be confirmed first by quantitative RT-PCR. To visualize more directly differential gene expression induced by cocaine, we will perform *in situ* hybridization using both D1 receptor mutant and wild-type mice that have been treated repeatedly with either cocaine or saline. Because the cellular location of protein products of the putative target genes may be different from their mRNA location, depending on the availability of the antibodies, we will also perform immunostaining using brains from the previously treated mutant and wild-type mice. Expression of D1 receptors will be performed in parallel to determine whether these receptors exhibit overlapping expression patterns with the putative target genes. These experiments will provide a foundation for future testing of the physiological relevance of these candidate genes.

Our ultimate goal is to identify genes that are physiologically relevant to cocaine actions. To achieve this goal, we will need to functionally perturb the expression of the candidate genes *in vivo* and investigate whether they affect behavioral changes in response to chronic cocaine exposure. Genetically engineered mouse models will be very useful for testing the importance of these genes in chronic cocaine-induced behaviors.

A systematic and temporal gene expression survey using the microarray technology may allow us to identify the molecular basis underlying the initiation and maintenance of drug-taking behaviors upon repeated exposure. Since the NAc is a key site for many drugs of abuse, understanding molecular changes induced by repeated exposure to cocaine may uncover a molecular basis for the actions of other abusive drugs. Because of the enduring nature of the behavioral responses to repeated cocaine exposure, changes in gene expression that are longer-lasting likely play a major role in the molecular adaptations. It should be noted, however, posttranslational modifications, such as protein phosphorylation, may be an integral part of molecular responses to repeated cocaine exposure.[45,46] The proteomics method will address this problem. The combined use of gene-targeted mice that exhibit altered responses to cocaine, with cDNA microarrays and proteomics, and proper physiological testing of the putative target genes, has tremendous potential to provide novel insights into the molecular basis of compulsive drug-taking behaviors and new strategies for the treatment of drug abuse.

ACKNOWLEDGMENTS

One of the authors (J.Z.) is supported by NIDA (DA11284). Another of the authors (M.X.) is also supported by NIDA (DA11005 and DA13786). We thank Bruce Aronow and Sarah Williams for advice on the analysis of the microarray results, University of Cincinnati Microarray Core for microarray hybridization and data scanning, Ryan Walsh and Danwen Lou for help.

REFERENCES

1. LESHNER, A.I. 1997. Addiction is a brain disease, and it matters. Science **278:** 45–47.
2. GAWIN, F.H. 1991. Cocaine addiction: psychology and neurophysiology. Science **251:** 1580–1586.
3. KOOB, G.F., P.P. SANNA & F.E. BLOOM. 1998. Neuroscience of addiction. Neuron **21:** 467–476.
4. BERKE, J.D. & S.E. HYMAN. 2000. Addiction, dopamine, and the molecular mechanisms of memory. Neuron **25:** 515–532.
5. ROBINSON, T.E. & K.C. BERRIDGE. 1993. The neural basis of drug craving: an incentive-sensitization theory of addiction. Brain Res. Brain Res. Rev. **18:** 247–291.

6. KALIVAS, P.W., R.C. PIERCE, J. CORNISH & B.A. SORG. 1998. A role for sensitization in craving and relapse in cocaine addiction. J. Psychopharmacol. **12:** 49–53.
7. KOOB, G.F. 1992. Drugs of abuse: anatomy, pharmacology and function of reward pathways. Trends Pharmacol. Sci. **13:** 177–184.
8. SELF, D.W. & E.J. NESTLER. 1995. Molecular mechanisms of drug reinforcement and addiction. Annu. Rev. Neurosci. **18:** 463–495.
9. GINGRICH, J.A. & M.G. CARON. 1993. Recent advances in the molecular biology of dopamine receptors. Annu. Rev. Neurosci. **16:** 299–321.
10. CABIB, S., et al. 1991. D_1 and D_2 receptor antagonists differently affect cocaine-induced locomotor hyperactivity in the mouse. Psychopharmacology **105:** 335–339.
11. TELLA, S.R. 1994. Differential blockade of chronic versus acute effects of intravenous cocaine by dopamine receptor antagonists. Pharmacol. Biochem. Behav. **48:** 151–159.
12. KOOB, G.F., H.T. LE & I. CREESE. 1987. The D1 dopamine receptor antagonist SCH23390 increases cocaine self-administration in the rat. Neurosci. Lett. **79:** 315–320.
13. CAINE, S.B. & G.F. KOOB. 1994. Effects of dopamine D-1 and D-2 antagonists on cocaine-self-administration under different schedules of reinforcement in the rat. J. Pharm. Exp. Ther. **270:** 209–218.
14. SELF, D.W., W.J. BARNHART, D.A. LEHMAN & E.J. NESTLER. 1996. Opposite modulation of cocaine-seeking behavior by D1- and D2-like dopamine receptor agonists. Science **271:** 1586–1589.
15. MATTINGLY, B.A., J.K. ROWLETT, T. ELLISON & K. RASE. 1996. Cocaine-induced behavioral sensitization: effects of haloperidol and SCH23390 treatments. Pharmacol. Biochem. Behav. **53:** 481–486.
16. HENRY, D.J. & F.J. WHITE. 1991. Repeated cocaine administration causes persistent enhancement of D1 dopamine receptor sensitivity within the rat nucleus accumbens. J. Pharm. Exp. Ther. **258:** 882–890.
17. HENRY, D.J. & F.J. WHITE. 1995. The persistence of behavioral sensitization to cocaine parallels enhanced inhibition of nucleus accumbens neurons. J. Neurosci. **15:** 6287–6299.
18. WHITE, F.J. & P.W. KALIVAS. 1998. Neuroadaptations involved in amphetamine and cocaine addiction. Drug Alcohol Depend. **51:** 141–153.
19. NESTLER, E.J. 2000. Genes and addiction. Nat. Genet. **26:** 277–281.
20. ROBERTSON, G.S., S.R. VINCENT & H.C. FIBIGER. 1990. Striatonigral projection neurons contain D1 dopamine receptor-activated c-fos. Brain Res. **523:** 288–290.
21. HEILIG, M., J.A. ENGEL & B. SODERPALM. 1993. C-fos antisense in the nucleus accumbens blocks the locomotor stimulant action of cocaine. Eur. J. Pharmacol. **236:** 339–340.
22. NESTLER, E.J., M.B. KELZ & J. CHEN. 1999. DeltaFosB: a molecular mediator of long-term neural and behavioral plasticity. Brain Res. **835:** 10–17.
23. KELZ, M.B. et al. 1999. Expression of the transcription factor deltaFosB in the brain controls sensitivity to cocaine. Nature **401:** 272–276.
24. MORATALLA, R., B. ELIBOL, M. VALLEJO & A.M. GRAYBIEL. 1996. Network-level changes in expression of inducible Fos-Jun proteins in the striatum during chronic cocaine treatment and withdrawal. Neuron **17:** 147–156.
25. HOWES, S.R. et al. 2000. Leftward shift in the acquisition of cocaine self-administration in isolation-reared rats: relationship to extracellular levels of dopamine, serotonin and glutamate in the nucleus accumbens and amygdala-striatal FOS expression. Psychopharmacology **151:** 55–63.
26. SHENG, M. & M. GREENBERG. 1990. The regulation and function of c-fos and other immediate early genes in the nervous system. Neuron **4:** 477–485.
27. MORGAN, J.I. & T. CURRAN. 1991. Stimulus-transcription coupling in the nervous system: involvement of the inducible proto-oncogenes fos and jun. Annu. Rev. Neurosci. **14:** 421–451.
28. LANDER, E.S. 1999. Array of hope. Nat. Genet. Suppl. **21:** 3–4.
29. Schena, M., D. Shalon, R.W. Davis & P.O. Brown. 1995. Quantitative monitoring of gene expression patterns with a complementary DNA microarray. Science **270:** 467–470.
30. FODOR, S.P. et al. 1991. Light-directed, spatially addressable parallel chemical synthesis. Science **251:** 767–773.

31. SOUTHERN, E., K. MIR & M. SHCHEPINOV. 1999. Molecular interactions on microarrays. Nat. Genet. Suppl. **21:** 5–9.
32. DUGGAN, D.J. *et al.* 1999. Expression profiling using cDNA microarrays. Nat. Genet. Suppl. **21:** 10–14.
33. CHEUNG, V.G. *et al.* 1999. Making and reading microarrays. Nat. Genet. Suppl. **21:** 15–19.
34. LIPSHUTZ, R.J., S.P. FODOR, T.R. GINGERAS & D.J. LOCKHART. 1999. High density synthetic oligonucleotide arrays. Nat. Genet. Suppl. **21:** 20–24.
35. BOWTELL, D.D. 1999. Options available—from start to finish—for obtaining expression data by microarray. Nat. Genet. Suppl. **21:** 25–32.
36. BASSETT, D.E., JR., M.B. EISEN & M.S. BOGUSKI. 1999. Gene expression informatics—it's all in your mind. Nat. Genet. Suppl. **21:** 51–55.
37. BROWN, P.O. & D. BOTSTEIN. 1999. Exploring the new world of the genome with DNA microarrays. Nat. Genet. Suppl. **21:** 33–37.
38. KHAN, J. *et al.* 1999. DNA microarray technology: the anticipated impact on the study of human disease. Biochim. Biophys. Acta **1423:** M17–M28.
39. XU, M. *et al.* 1994. Dopamine D1 receptor mutant mice are deficient in striatal expression of dynorphin and in dopamine-mediated behavioral responses. Cell **79:** 729–742.
40. XU, M., Y. GUO, C.V. VORHEES & J. ZHANG. 2000. Behavioral responses to cocaine and amphetamine in D1 dopamine receptor mutant mice. Brain Res. **852:** 198–207.
41. EISEN, M.B., P.T. SPELLMAN, P.O. BROWN & D. BOTSTEIN. 1998. Cluster analysis and display of genome-wide expression patterns. Proc. Natl. Acad. Sci. USA **95:** 14863–14868.
42. SHERLOCK, G. 2000. Analysis of large-scale gene expression data. Curr. Opin. Immunol. **12:** 201–205.
43. RAYCHAUDHURI, S., P.D. SUTPHIN, J.T. CHANG & R.B. ALTMAN. 2001. Basic microarray analysis: grouping and feature reduction. Trends Biotechnol. **19:** 189–193.
44. SCHULZE, A. & J. DOWNWARD. 2001. Navigating gene expression using microarrays—a technology review. Nat. Cell Biol. **3:** E190šE195.
45. GREENGARD, P., P.B. ALLEN & A.C. NAIRN. 1999. Beyond the dopamine receptor: the DARPP-32/protein phosphatase-1 cascade. Neuron **23:** 435–447.
46. EDGAR, P.F. *et al.* 1999. Proteome map of the human hippocampus. Hippocampus **9:** 644–650.

Gene Expression Profiles in the Brain from Phencyclidine-Treated Mouse by Using DNA Microarray

K. TOYOOKA,[a] M. USUI,[b] K. WASHIYAMA,[b] T. KUMANISHI,[b] AND Y. TAKAHASHI[b]

[a]Department of Psychiatry, Niigata University School of Medicine, Niigata, Japan

[b]Department of Molecular Neuropathology, Brain Research Institute, Niigata University, Niigata, Japan

ABSTRACT: Recently DNA microarray technology has been introduced into analyses of comprehensive biological functions. This DNA microarray is a new technology for simultaneous analysis to examine expression patterns of thousands of genes. It was thought that this technique should be very useful for examination of cellular and molecular mechanisms of drugs of abuse: cocaine, amphetamine, and others. This technology was therefore applied for the rapid analysis of gene expression in the brain from phencyclidine-treated mice. Mainly mouse DNA microarray was examined by using labeled cDNAs produced from a control mouse brain mRNA and from brain mRNA of mouse exposed to drugs as probes. Some changes in a probe from brain mRNA of drug-treated mouse could be observed, but it was necessary to examine another DNA microarray, including more samples from the brain.

KEYWORDS: DNA microarray technology; gene expression profile; drugs of abuse; cDNA; phencyclidine; amphetamine

INTRODUCTION

Phencyclidine (PCP) is classified as one of the dissociate anesthetics. About 40 years ago, PCP was shown to induce behavioral changes in humans and animals.[1,2] Because of some similarity between the symptoms of schizophrenics and PCP psychosis, and because PCP is a drug of abuse, a number of investigations have examined the molecular mechanism of the behavioral effect induced by PCP.[3–6] Although the molecular mechanism of PCP-induced behavioral changes in animals has not yet been clarified, the involvement of dopamine, serotonin, and their receptor systems in this mechanism has been considered by several investigators.[3,7] On the other hand, other investigators indicated that PCP inhibits excitatory amino acid neurotransmission at the level of the NMDA receptor and that this function could be related to PCP-induced behavioral changes.[3,8]

Address for correspondence: Y. Takahashi, Department of Molecular Neuropathology, Brain Research Institute, Niigata 951-8585, Japan. Voice: 025-227-0646; fax: 025-227-0818.

Ann. N.Y. Acad. Sci. 965: 10–20 (2002). © 2002 New York Academy of Sciences.

Recently, we examined PCP-induced locomotion and behavioral changes in mice and the effect of DCG-IV and L-CCG-1 upon these changes.[9]

In order to analyze this molecular mechanism of PCP-induced behavioral changes in animals, we considered applying the recently introduced new technology: DNA microarray technology.[10–13]

MATERIALS AND METHODS

Animals

We used male ICR mice weighing about 40 g obtained from a local breeder (Japan Charles River Co.). The care and use of the animals were carried out following the principles of Laboratory Animal Care and approved by the animal care committee of Niigata University School of Medicine. The animals were allowed free access to food and water.

Drugs

PCP was kindly provided by Taisho Pharmaceutical Company Ltd. (Saitama, Japan).

Injection Program

PCP was administered to the mice as follows. In the chronic experiments, PCP (10 mg/kg) was injected i.p. into mice once a day for 24 days. About 17 h after the last injection, mice were decapitated and the brains were isolated.

Hybridization Analysis

Total RNA was isolated from the mouse cerebral cortical tissue by using Isogen according to procedures of Nippon Gene Co. (Toyama, Japan).[14] cDNA was synthesized from RNA by the conventional reverse transcription procedure[15] and labeled by Cy3 fluorescent dye.[15] Clonteck Atlas glass array mouse 1.0 was hybridized with Cy3 fluorescent cDNA in an Atlas glass hybridization chamber for 20 h. The hybridized glass array was washed and was scanned using an image scanner to monitor the fluorescence of each probe that was successfully hybridized to the target.

Expression Analysis

The hybridized glass array profile, which was obtained as described earlier, was analyzed by using the Array Gauge analysis software (Fujifilm).[15]

RESULTS

DNA microarray technology has been recently introduced into analyses of gene expression. This technology was described in detail in a recent review[10] and briefly summarized in the Materials and Methods section of this paper.

a
SH28-1

b
SH28-2

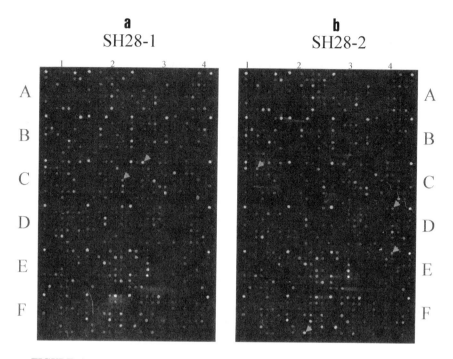

FIGURE 1. Expression pattern in Atlas DNA microarray mouse 1.0. (**a**) SH28-1: the data by cDNA from the control mouse brain; (**b**) SH28-2: the data by cDNA from the PCP-treated mouse brain. Atlas glass microarray mouse 1.0 was hybridized by Cy3 fluorescent cDNAs from the control mouse-brain total RNA and the PCP-treated mouse-brain total RNA. The microarray was scanned using an image scanner. The *arrows* show some spots with changing gene expression.

In the first step of this technique, we isolated total RNA from the brains of the control and PCP-injected mice by using Isogen. cDNAs were synthesized from RNA by the conventional reverse transcription procedure and labeled by Cy3 fluorescent dye using a Clonteck Fluorescence Labeling Kit. Clonteck Atlas glass array mouse 1.0 was hybridized with Cy3 fluorescent cDNA in an Atlas glass hybridization chamber for 20 h. The hybridized glass array was scanned using an image scanner. These data are shown in FIGURE 1. FIGURE 1a SH28-1 contains the data of control mouse, and FIGURE 1b SH28-2 contains the data from PCP-treated mouse. The electrophoretic patterns of total RNAs from the control and drug-treated mice brains were examined. These findings indicated that these RNA were not degraded (data not shown). A table containing all the data from FIGURE 1a SH28-1 and FIGURE 1b SH28-2 was made. However we cannot show it here, because of its length. TABLE 1 shows the data of the spots with high intensity ratio (>3.0) in FIGURE 1a and 1b. TABLE 2 shows the data of the spots that are mainly localized in the nervous system. The data in the table clearly indicate the influences of the drug PCP. FIGURE 2 shows the analyses of the results of the differential expression in the control and drug-treat-

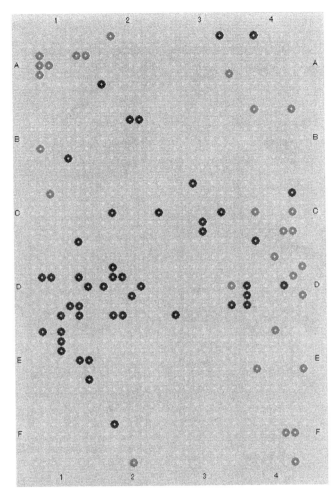

FIGURE 2. Array Gauge (Fujifilm) analysis of Atlas DNA array. The up-regulation of the spot signal in PCP-treated mouse is shown as *light*. The down-regulation of the spot signal is shown as *dark*.

ed animals using the Atlas Array Gauge (Fujifilm) analysis software. In FIGURE 2, the up-regulation of the spot signal in the PCP-treated mouse is shown as light and the down-regulation is shown as dark. There are 28 up-regulated spots and 45 down-regulated ones.

The data from FIGURE 2 were partly expressed as the numbers in TABLE 1. The evidence for up-regulation and down-regulation is very clear from the data in TABLE 1 and FIGURE 2.

We drew a figure that scatter plotted the data of the expression profile (data not shown).

TABLE 1. Gene expression profiles in the brain from the control and phencyclidine-treated mouse by DNA microarray-PCP (SH28-2)/control (SH28-1) >3.0

#	coordinate	Spot Intensity SH28-1	SH28-2	Ratio	RATIO UP	RATIO DOWN	Gene	Genbank #
52	A2a6	310	62	0.20		DOWN	TRANSCRIPTIONAL ENHANCER FACTOR TEF-3 (ETF-RELATED FACTOR-2) (ETFR-2) (TEF-1-RELATED FACTOR 1) (TEF-1-RELATED FACTOR FR-19); TEF3; TEFR1; TCF13R1	D87965
221	B1e6	288	42	0.15		DOWN	homeobox B9 protein (HOXB9); HOX2.5	M34857
264	B2e2	192	61	0.32		DOWN	U2 small nuclear ribonucleoprotein auxiliary factor 35-kDa subunit-related protein 1 (U2AF1-RS1); SP2	D17407
365	B4f1	47	164	3.46	UP		P-selectin glycoprotein ligand 1 (PSGL1; SELPLG; SELP1)	X91144
391	C1c2	372	1219	3.28	3.3		G-protein coupled purinergic receptor P2Y1 (P2RY1)	U22829
468	C2g4	857	227	0.27		3.8	MTJ1; DNAJ-like heat-shock protein from mouse tumor	L16953
484	C3c1	3841	917	0.24		4.2	ELECTOCARDIOGRAPHIC QT SYNDROME 2 POTASSIUM CHANNEL SUBUNIT	U04294
528	C4b4	115	439	3.83	UP		tyrosine 3-hydroxylase (TYH); tyrosine 3-monooxygenase isozymes	M69200
558	C4f6	44	150	3.44	UP		caspase 1 (CASP1); IL1-beta convertase (IL1BC); IL1-beta-converting enzyme (ICE)	L28095
703	D3g4	84	255	3.05	UP		epidermal growth factor (EGF)	J00380
727	D4d1	164	642	3.92	3.9		mast cell factor	U44725
799	E1g6	159	34	0.21		DOWN	mothers against dpp homolog 5 (SMAD5; MADH5)	U77638
892	E4d1	143	776	5.44	5.4		PKC-delta; protein kinase C delta type	M69042
916	E4g5	57	200	3.49	UP		guanine nucleotide-binding protein alpha stimulating activity polypeptide (GNAS)	Y00703
991	F2d7	794	3949	4.98	5.0		receptor-type protein tyrosine phosphatase (PTPRCAP); C polypeptide-associated protein; CD45-associated protein (CD45-AP); LSM	U03856
1097	F4f4	145	465	3.20	3.2		leptin (LEP); obese factor (OB)	U22421
1100	F4f7	46	158	3.42	UP		ajuba protein	U79776

TABLE 2. Gene expression profiles in the brain from the control and phencyclidine-treated mouse by DNA microarray (genes related with nervous function).

No.	Clone	3841	917	0.24	Gene description	Accession		
484	C3c1	3841	917	0.24	ELECTOCARDIOGRAPHIC QT SYNDROME 2 POTASSIUM CHANNEL SUBUNIT	U04294	4.2	
485	C3c2	123	131	1.07	potassium voltage gated channel	AF030300	ND	weak
486	C3c3	55	54	0.97	potassium channel, subfamily K, member 2	U73488		
487	C3c4	251	355	1.42	potassium inwardly-rectifying channel, subfamily J, member 12	X80417		1.4
488	C3c5	155	121	0.78	potassium large conductance calcium-activated channel, subfamily M, alpha member 1	L16912	DOWN	
489	C3c6	50	27	0.54	potassium voltage gated channel, Shab-related subf	M64228	ND	
490	C3c7	120	60	0.50	potassium voltage-gated channel, Isk-related subfamily, member 1	X60457	weak	
491	C3d1	74	83	1.11	voltage-gated potassium channel protein KQT-like 1 (KVLQT1); potassium voltage-gated channel subfamily Q member 1 (KCNQ1); KCNA9; KV1.9	U70068		weak
492	C3d2	329	348	1.06	acetylcholine receptor delta submit	K02582		1.1
493	C3d3	136	131	0.96	glutamate receptor subunit epsilon 2 (GRIN2); N-methyl D-aspartate receptor subtype 2B (NMDAR2B; NR2B)	D10651	DOWN	
494	C3d4	159	219	1.37	nicotinic acetylcholine receptor	M14537		1.4
495	C3d5	47	8	0.17	calcium-activated potassium channel beta subunit; maxi K channel beta subunit; BK channel beta subunit; SLO-beta; K(VCA)beta	AF020711	ND	
496	C3d6	43	8	0.20	voltage-gated sodium channel	L36179	ND	
497	C3d7	189	224	1.19	CCHB3; calcium channel (voltage-gated; dihydropyridine-sensitive; L-type) beta-3 subunit)	U20372		1.2
498	C3e1	47	99	2.08	sodium-dependent serotonin transporter; 5HT transporter (5HTT)	AF013604		weak
499	C3e2	63	80	1.27	sodium-dependent noradrenaline transporter; norepinephrine transporter (NET)	U76306		weak
500	C3e3	78	66	0.86	synaptic vesicle membrane protein VAT-1 homolog	X95562	weak	
501	C3e4	2466	1565	0.63	solute carrier family 6 member 9 (SLC6A9); sodium- & chloride-dependent glycine transporter 1 (GLYT1)	X67056	1.6	

—continued

TABLE 2. Gene expression profiles in the brain from the control and phencyclidine-treated mouse by DNA microarray (genes related with nervous function) —continued.

No.	Code				Call	Description	Call	Accession
502	C3e5	94	239	2.53	UP	solute carrier family 1 member 1 (SLC1A1); excitatory amino acid transporter 3 (EAAT3); excitatory amino-acid carrier 1 (EAAC1; mEAAC1)	1.0	U73521
503	C3e6	166	163	0.98	ND	gamma-aminobutyric acid transporter 1 (GABA-A transporter 1; GABT1)		M92378
504	C3e7	29	46	1.58	1.0	gamma-aminobutyric acid transporter 3 (GABA-A transporter 3; GABT3)		L04663
505	C3f1	341	349	1.02	UP	gamma-aminobutyric acid transporter 4 (GABA-A transporter 4; GABT4)		L04662
519	C4a2	106	144	1.35		prostaglandin D2 synthase (21 kDa, brain)		X89222
520	C4a3	2961	1893	0.64		prostaglandin I2 (prostacyclin) synthase	1.6	AB001607
521	C4a4	131	101	0.77		fatty acid amide hydrolase (FAAH); oleamide hydrolase	weak	U82536
522	C4a5	147	131	0.89		acetylcholinesterase (ACHE)	DOWN	X56518
523	C4a6	31	59	1.92		neuroendocrine convertase 1 (NEC 1); prohormone convertase 1 (PC1); proprotein convertase 1	ND	M58589
524	C4a7	43	27	0.63	ND	neuroendocrine convertase 2 (NEC 2); prohormone convertase 2 (PC2); proprotein convertase 2; KEX2-like endoprotease 2		M55669
525	C4b1	32	12	0.37	weak	tryptophan 5-hydroxylase (TRPH); tryptophan 5-monooxygenase		J04758
526	C4b2	38	67	1.76	weak	histidine decarboxylase (HDC)		X57437
527	C4b3	26	69	2.64		phenylalanine-4-hydroxylase (PAH); phe-4-monooxygenase		X51942
528	C4b4	115	439	3.83	UP	tyrosine 3-hydroxylase (TYH); tyrosine 3-monooxygenase isozymes		M69200
529	C4b5	31	37	1.20	ND	dopamine beta-hydroxylase (DBH); dopamine-beta-monooxygenase		S50200
530	C4b6	290	592	2.04	2.0	phenylethanolamine N-methyltransferase (PNMTase); noradrenaline N-methyltransferase		L12687

—continued

TABLE 2. Gene expression profiles in the brain from the control and phencyclidine-treated mouse by DNA microarray (genes related with nervous function) —*continued*.

No.	Symbol				UP	DOWN	Description	Accession
646	D2r1	76	76	1.00	weak		gamma-aminobutyric acid (GABA-A) receptor, subunit	U14420
647	D2r2	143	106	0.74		DOWN	gamma-aminobutyric-acid receptor beta 2 subunit (GABA(A) receptor beta 2; GABRB2)	U14419
648	D2r3	43	47	1.10	ND		gastrin releasing peptide receptor	M57922
649	D2r4	65	44	0.68		ND	ionotropic glutamate receptor delta 1 (GRID1)	D10171
650	D2r5	35	21	0.61		ND	oxytocin receptor (OXTR; OTR)	D86599
651	D2r6	461	367	0.80		1.3	ionotropic glutamate receptor AMPA 1 (GRIA1)	X57497
652	D2r7	93	88	0.94		weak	ionotropic glutamate receptor NMDA1 (GRIN1); ionotropic glutamate receptor zeta 1; N-methyl-D-aspartate receptor (NMDAR1)	D10028
653	D2g1	1779	790	0.44		2.3	5-hydroxytryptamine receptor 3A receptor (HTR3A); serotonin receptor	X72395
654	D2g2	68	79	1.17	weak		5-hydroxytryptamine receptor 1A receptor (HTR1A); serotonin receptor	U39391
655	D2g3	149	175	1.17	1.2		opioid receptor mu 1 (OPRM1)	U19380
656	D2g4	210	234	1.11	1.1		nociceptin receptor; orphanin FQ receptor; opioid receptor kappa 3 (OPRK3)	U09421
657	D2g5	59	73	1.24	weak		neuropeptide Y receptor type 1 (NPY1-R)	D63819
658	D2g6	69	101	1.46	weak		melatonin receptor type 1A (MEL-1A-R)	U52222
659	D3a2	113	79	0.70		weak	Gastrin/cholecystokinin type B receptor (CCK-B receptor) (CCK-BR)	AF019371

—continued

TABLE 2. Gene expression profiles in the brain from the control and phencyclidine-treated mouse by DNA microarray (genes related with nervous function) —*continued*.

ID	Code						Description	Accession
660	D3a3	93	55	0.59		weak	acetylcholine receptor alpha	M17640
661	D3a4	165	207	1.25	1.3		acetylcholine receptor alpha 7 neural	L37663
662	D3a5	72	51	0.71		weak	glutamate receptor 5 (GLUR5); ionotropic glutamate receptor kainate1 (GRIK1)	X66118
663	D3a6	164	108	0.66		DOWN	gamma-aminobutyric-acid receptor alpha 1 subunit (GABA(A) receptor) alpha 1; GABRA1)	M86566
664	D3a7	65	19	0.29		ND	5-hydroxytryptamine receptor 2A receptor (HTR2A); serotonin receptor	S49542
665	D3b1	65	35	0.54		ND	5-hydroxytryptamine receptor 1B receptor (HTR1B); serotonin receptor	Z11597
666	D3b2	52	38	0.73		ND	5-hydroxytryptamine receptor 1C receptor (HTR1C); serotonin receptor	X72230
667	D3b3	47	45	0.96		ND	5-hydroxytryptamine receptor 1E receptor beta (HTR1E-beta); serotonin receptor	Z14224
668	D3b4	34	33	0.97		ND	5-hydroxytryptamine receptor 2C receptor (HTR2C); serotonin receptor	Z15119
669	D3b5	35	30	0.85		ND	5-hydroxytryptamine receptor 7 receptor (HTR7); serotonin receptor	Z23107
670	D3b6	93	91	0.98		weak	cannabinoid receptor 1 (CNR1; CBR); brain cannabinoid receptor	U17985
671	D3b7	38	25	0.67		ND	macrophage cannabinoid receptor 2 (CNR2)	U21681
672	D3c1	63	67	1.06	weak		D(4) dopamine receptor; D(2C) dopamine receptor	U19880

DISCUSSION

As described in the Results section, there are some up-regulated and down-regulated spots in both the control and PCP-injected mice. However, these data may be semiquantitative. If we want to confirm these data, we have to carry out RT-PCR or Northern blot analysis of DNA from each spot. We cannot examine these spots by these methods yet.

Another limit of our methodology is the Clonteck Atlas glass array mouse 1.0. This array has the following disadvantages: Clonteck spotted the known 1000 mouse cDNA on a glass and it is very doubtful whether the selection of spots is suitable for the study of gene expression in the brain, although there are some brain-specific spots. Recently Potier *et al.*[16] examined the changes in gene expression in the knock-out mouse using the microarray containing the 200 genes involved in neurotransmission. In addition, Ngai[17] used DNA microarrays to study patterns of gene expression in selected model systems, including the developing cerebellum, olfactory system, and cortical neurons of the mouse. Our findings concerning the up-regulation and down-regulation of some spots may be related to the molecular changes in the brain caused by injection of PCP. If possible, however, we should also use the DNA microarray containing the genes involved in neurotransmission and in selected model systems, including the developing cerebellum, olfactory system, and cortical neurons of the mouse. If we use these DNA microarrays, we may be able to find more significant changes in the PCP-treated mouse brain. Shimizu *et al.*[18] reported induction of glutamate dehydrogenase in the rat brain after PCP treatment. However, our DNA microarray did not include glutamate dehydrogenase.

REFERENCES

1. ALLEN, R.M. & S.T. YOUNG. 1978. Phencyclidine-induced psychosis. Am. J. Psychiatry **135:** 1081–1084.
2. JAVITT, D.C. & S.R. ZUKIN. 1991. Recent advances in the phencyclidine model of schizophrenia. Am. J. Psychiatry **145:** 1301–1308.
3. JOHNSON, K.M. & S.M. JONES. 1990. Neuropharmacology of phencyclidine. Ann. Rev. Pharmacol. Toxicol. **30:** 707–750.
4. CASTELLANI, S. & P.M. ADAMS. 1981. Acute and chronic phencyclidine effects on locomotor activity, stereotypy and ataxia in rats. Eur. J. Pharmacol. **73:** 143–154.
5. FREED, W.J., L.A. BING & R.J. WYATT. 1984. Effects of nouroleptics on phencyclidine (PCP)-induced locomotor stimulation in mice. Nouropharmacology **23:** 175–181.
6. NABESHIMA, T., K. KITAICHI & Y. NODA. 1996. Functional changes in neuronal systems induced by phencyclidine administration. Ann. N.Y. Acad. Sci. **801:** 29–38.
7. TANII, Y., T. NISHIKAWA, A. UMINO & K. TAKAHASHI. 1990. Phencyclidine increases extracellular dopamine metabolites in rat medial frontal cortex as measured by in vivo dialysis. Neurosci. Lett. **112:** 318–323.
8. ITZHAK, Y. & S.F. ALI. 1997. Effect of ibogain on the various sites of the NMDA receptor complex and sigma binding sites in rat brain. Ann. N.Y. Acad. Sci. **844:** 245–251.
9. TOMITA, N. *et al.* 2000. The effects of DCG-IV and 1-CCG-1 upon phencyclidine (PCP)-induced locomotion and behavioral changes in mice. Ann. N.Y. Acad. Sci. **914:** 284–291.
10. MITTEL, V. 2001. DNA array technology. In Molecular Cloning, 3rd ed., J. Sambrook and D.W. Russel, Eds.: A10.1–A10.19. Cold Spring Harbor Laboratory Press. Cold Spring Harbor, NY.
11. SCHENA, M., D. SHALON, R.W. DAVIS & P.O. BROWN. 1995. Quantitative monitoring of gene expression patterns with a complementary DNA microarray. Science **270:** 467–470.

12. XU, W. *et al.* 2001. Microarray-based analysis of gene expression in very large gene families: the cytochrome P450 gene superfamily of arabidopsis thaliana. Gene **272:** 61–74.
13. WINZELER, E., M. SCHEMA & R.W. DAVIS. 1999. Fluorescence-based expression monitoring using microarray. Methods Enzymol. **306:** 3–18.
14. NIPPON GENE CO. 1999. Manual: Isogen: 349–358.
15. CLONTECK CO. 1999. Atlas cDNA Expression Arrays User Manual: 1–43.
16. POTIER, M.-C. *et al.* 2001. Differential gene expression in brain from knock-out mice using DNA microarrays. J. Neurochem. **78**(Suppl. 1): 110.
17. NGAI, J. 2001. Gene expression profiling in the nervous system. J. Neurochem. **78**(Suppl. 1): 110.
18. SHIMIZU, E. *et al.* 1997. Glutamate dehydrogenase mRNA is immediately induced after phencyclidine treatment in the rat brain. Schizophr. Res. **25:** 251–258.

A Single Dose of Methamphetamine Rescues the Blunted Dopamine D_1-Receptor Activity in the Neocortex of D_2- and D_3-Receptor Knockout Mice

CLAUDIA SCHMAUSS,[a,b] SARA B. GLICKSTEIN,[a] MELLA ADLERSBERG,[b] SHU-CHI HSIUNG,[b] AND HADASSAH TAMIR[a,b]

[a]Department of Psychiatry, Columbia University College of Physicians & Surgeons, New York, New York 10032, USA

[b]Department of Neuroscience, New York State Psychiatric Institute, New York, New York 10032, USA

ABSTRACT: Knockout mice deficient for dopamine D_2 and D_3 receptors exhibit blunted c-*fos* responses to D_1-agonist stimulation. A single dose of methamphetamine (METH), however, leads to a long-term reversal of these blunted c-*fos* responses in both mutants, and the same effect is obtained with a single administration of a full D_1-agonist. Consistent with the predominant c-*fos* expression in the neocortex induced by METH itself, METH pretreatment leads to the largest D_1-agonist-stimulated c-*fos* responses in the neocortex of these mutants. For example, a pronounced blunting of neocortical c-*fos* responses is detected in the prefrontal cortex, a region in which D_1 receptors play a critical role in working memory. METH pretreated mutants, however, exhibit robust c-*fos* responses in this region that are indistinguishable from wild type. Recent studies indicate that different mechanisms operate in brains of D_2 and D_3 mutants to lead to decreased D_1-receptor activity. For example, drug-naive D_2, but not D_3, mutants show significantly decreased G protein activation in response to D_1-agonist stimulation, and METH pretreatment also rescues this abnormal molecular phenotype. Moreover, although the protein phosphatases (PP) 1/2A and 2B play a critical role in modulating G protein activation in wild type, their effect is either diminished (PP1/2A) or abolished (2B) in D_2 mutants. Interestingly however, METH pretreatment does not rescue the activities of these phosphatases in the mutants, suggesting that the long-term effects of a single dose of METH are mediated via effector systems that act downstream of G protein activation.

KEYWORDS: dopamine receptors; knockout mice; D_1 agonists; methamphetamine; immediate early genes; prefrontal cortex; G proteins

Address for correspondence: Claudia Schmauss, Department of Psychiatry, Columbia University College of Physicians & Surgeons, New York, NY 10032. Voice: 212-543-6505; fax: 212-543-6017.

schmauss@neuron.cpmc.columbia.edu

Ann. N.Y. Acad. Sci. 965: 21–27 (2002). © 2002 New York Academy of Sciences.

INTRODUCTION

A variety of stimuli elicit the induction of expression of the immediate early gene c-*fos*, a gene with very low baseline expression in the brain.[1] For example, both dopamine D_1-receptor agonists and psychomotor stimulants, such as cocaine and amphetamine, elicit robust c-*fos* responses in distinct anatomic circuitries of the brain.[1] Interestingly, however, mutant mice deficient for dopamine D_1 receptors fail to exhibit psychostimulant-induced c-*fos* responses, indicating that the expression of D_1 receptors is essential for the induction of c-*fos* expression elicited by these drugs.[2] Moreover, several studies indicate that the magnitude of D_1-receptor-dependent induction of c-*fos* expression is modulated by dopamine D_2 and D_3 receptors. Moratalla *et al.*[2] found anatomically restricted alterations in c-*fos* expression in response to haloperidol, a neuroletic drug that blocks the D_2-class of dopamine receptors, and other studies on mice deficient for D_2 and D_3 receptors, revealed blunted c-*fos* responses to D_1 agonists in these mutants.[3,4]

Here we summarize the results of studies that demonstrate a decreased agonist-promoted dopamine D_1-receptor activity in mice deficient for D_2 and D_3 receptors that can be completely rescued in a long-term manner by both a single, low dose of METH or a full D_1 agonist.[3–5] Furthermore, we briefly discuss results of our most recent studies[6] that begin to identify mechanisms leading to the decreased D_1-receptor activity in these mutants and that test whether METH affects these mechanisms.

MATERIALS AND METHODS

Animals

The generation of our D_2- and D_3-receptor knockout mice is described in Ref. 7. For the present study, the fifth generation of congenic C57Bl/6 mutants and their wildtype littermates was used. Male mice at postnatal age P60 to P90 were selected for the study. These animals were housed in groups of four to five animals per cage, and they had unrestricted access to food and water. Animals that received a drug treatment were returned to their home cage immediately after drug injection and remained there until they were killed by decapitation. All experiments were carried out in accordance with the *National Institutes of Health Guide for the Care and Use of Laboratory Animals* and were approved by the Institutional Animal Care and Use Committees at Columbia University and the New York State Psychiatric Institute.

Drug Treatments

The D_1-agonists SKF82958 and SKF81297, the D_1 antagonist SCH23390 and S-(+)-methamphetamine hydrochloride were purchased from Research Biochemicals, Inc. (Natick, MA). All drugs were dissolved in saline and administered intraperitoneally.

In Situ *Hybridization, RNA Extraction, and Northern Blotting*

For *in situ* hybridization experiments, brains were collected one hour after SKF82958 (1 mg/kg) administration to drug-naive or METH (5 mg/kg) pretreated animals, frozen in Freon, and stored at $-80°C$. Brains were cryosectioned at 16 μm, thaw mounted onto gelatin-coated slides, dried for 2 min at 37°C, and then refrozen at $-80°C$. Sections were thawed, postfixed in 4% paraformaldehyde for 10 min, washed twice in 0.5x SSC, and subsequently prehybridized in a humidified chamber using a solution containing 20% dextran sulfate, 10 mM dithiothreitol, 0.75M NaCl, 1x Denhardt's solution, 2 mM EDTA, 50% formamide, 10 mM tris-HCL, and 0.05 mg/mL tRNA for one hour at 42°C. The buffer was then replaced with fresh buffer containing an ^{35}S-labeled, antisense riboprobe comprising 540 nucleotides of the mouse c-*fos* mRNA[8] (1×10^6 cpm/300 μL), and hybridization was continued overnight at 55°C. Slides were washed in 2x SSC, 50% formamide, and 0.1% β-mercaptoethanol at 50°C for 2 h, treated with tRNA (0.1%) at 37°C for 30 min, and washed in 2x SSC, 50% formimide, and 0.1% β-mercaptoethanol at 55°C for 1 h. A final wash in 0.1x SSC and 0.1% β-mercaptoethanol was done at 55°C for 1 h. Slides were air-dried and exposed to Kodak MR film for 14 h. Darkfield images of the films were digitized using MCID image analysis system (St. Catherines, Ontario, Canada).

For RNA extraction, brains were rapidly removed and the entire forebrain or the forebrain neocortex was dissected as described in Ref 4. RNA was extracted using the guanidine/cesium chloride method. Twenty μg of total RNA, extracted from tissues pooled from two to four animals per genotype, was loaded onto formaldehyde/agarose gels. For Northern blot analysis, a ^{32}P-random-primed cDNA encoding nucleotides 2160 to 2690 of the mouse c-*fos* gene[8] was used. Optical densities of c-*fos* signals were measured as described,[4] and multiple means of optical densities were compared with a one-way analysis of variance (ANOVA; threshold of significance $p < 0.05$) and the significance of differences were determined by Duncan's Studentized Range Test for comparison of multiple means.

RESULTS

As shown previously,[4] in wildtype mice, administration of a full D$_1$ agonist leads to forebrain c-*fos* mRNA expression levels that are substantially higher than corresponding levels expressed in response to indirect dopamine receptor stimulation by METH. In the forebrain of mice deficient for D$_2$ and D$_3$ receptors, however, D$_1$ agonist-stimulated c-*fos* mRNA expression levels are significantly lower when compared to wild type. However, a single dose of METH (5 mg/kg), leads to a long-term (as much as two weeks) reversal of the blunted c-*fos* responses to D$_1$ agonist stimulation in the mutants (see Fig. 1 in Ref. 4).

The analysis of the anatomic distribution of c-*fos* mRNA expressed 60 min following administration of the full D$_1$ agonist SKF82958 (1 mg/kg) by *in situ* hybridization revealed blunted c-*fos* mRNA expression in D$_2$ and D$_3$ mutants throughout the forebrain neocortex, hippocampus, striatum, hypothalamus, and thalamus. A representative example of such experiments is shown in FIGURE 1. In this experiment, reduced c-*fos* mRNA expression levels are most evident in the medial frontal cortex of drug-naive D$_2$ and D$_3$ mutants. However, in METH pretreated mutants that received a challenge dose of SKF 1 week after METH administration, c-*fos* mRNA expression levels are indistinguishable from wild type. Interestingly, in wildtype mice, METH pretreatment has no effect on c-*fos* mRNA levels expressed in response to an SKF challenge administered 1 week later (FIG. 1).

- METH   + METH

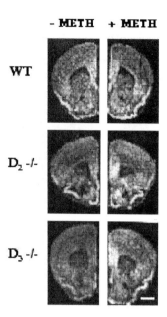

FIGURE 1. Darkfield autoradiographic image of an *in situ* hybridization experiment visualizing SKF-induced forebrain c-*fos* mRNA expressed in wild type and D_2-and D_3-receptor knockout mice. Representative sections of wild type (WT) and D_3 (−/−) and D_2 (−/−) mutants are taken at 5.5-mm rostral to the interaural line. In all genotypes, the application of SKF elicits an increase in c-*fos* mRNA relative to the basal expression evident in mice injected only with saline (not shown). Note reduced c-*fos* mRNA expression in both drug-naive D_2 and D_3 mutants, which is most apparent in the medial frontal cortex. Pretreatment with METH (5 mg/kg) administered one week prior to an SKF challenge, however, results in wild-type-like c-*fos* mRNA expression levels in both mutants.

FIGURE 2A shows mean optical densities (determined in at least four independent experiments) of c-*fos* mRNA signals detected on autoradiograms of Northern blots of total forebrain RNA of wild type, D_2, and D_3 mutants. Both mutants express less than 15% of the forebrain c-*fos* mRNA expressed in wild type. It should be noted that these significantly blunted c-*fos* mRNA responses of D_2 and D_3 mutants are not exclusively evident in response to the administration of the D_1 agonist SKF82958. In fact, c-*fos* responses to stimulation with another full D_1 agonist, SKF81297, are also blunted in both mutants, and these blunted responses can also be completely rescued by METH pretreatment.[5] Moreover, we found a complete absence of c-*fos* mRNA responses to both agonists in mice deficient for D_1 receptors, indicating that the induction of c-*fos* mRNA expression stimulated by SKF82958 and SKF81297 is strictly dependent on D_1 receptor activation.[5]

In contrast to full D_1 agonists, METH elicits forebrain c-*fos* mRNA responses that are most prominent in the neocortex (see Fig. 3 in Ref. 4). It is therefore of interest to note that METH pretreated D_2 and D_3 mutants show the largest increase in c-*fos* mRNA response to D_1-agonist stimulation in the forebrain neocortex. In fact,

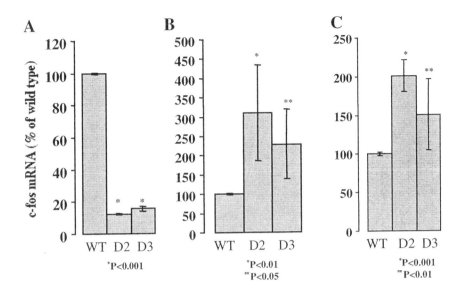

FIGURE 2. Comparison of optical densities (ODs) of c-*fos* mRNA signals of SKF82958-treated wild type and D$_2$ and D$_3$ mutant mice. c-*fos* mRNA expression levels were analyzed with Northern blots of total cytoplasmic RNA as described in the Materials and Methods section. c-*fos* expression levels were determined 60 min following a challenge dose of SKF82958 (1 mg/kg) (**A**) Mean (± S.E.M.) ODs of forebrain c-*fos* mRNA signals of drug-naive wild type and D$_2$ and D$_3$ mutants. (**B**) Mean (± S.E.M.) ODs of forebrain neocortical c-*fos* mRNA signals of METH-pretreated wild type and D$_2$ and D$_3$ mutants. (**C**) Mean (± S.E.M.) ODs of forebrain neocortical c-*fos* mRNA signals of SKF82958-pretreated wild type and D$_2$ and D$_3$ mutants.

as shown in FIGURE 2B, forebrain neocortical c-*fos* mRNA levels are 3- and 2-fold higher in D$_2$ and D$_3$ mutants, respectively, when compared to METH pretreated wild type.

Finally, to test whether the just-described long-term effects of a single dose of METH can also be mimicked by direct (one-time) stimulation of D$_1$ receptors with a full D$_1$ agonist, mice were pretreated with SKF82958 (1 mg/kg) instead of METH. Although SKF treatment of drug-naive mice induces similar levels of c-*fos* mRNA in forebrain neocortex and in structures of the extraneocortical (inner) forebrain mass (see Fig. 4 in Ref. 4), the same drug administered to SKF-pretreated animals elicits neocortical c-*fos* mRNA responses that, as summarized in FIGURE 2C, are still 2- and 1.5-fold higher in D$_2$ and D$_3$ mutants, respectively, when compared to SKF-pretreated wildtype.

In summary, the decreased agonist-promoted D$_1$-receptor activity of mice deficient for D$_2$ and D$_3$ receptors can be completely rescued in a long-term manner by a single dose of either METH or a full D$_1$ agonist. The effects of METH and, to a lesser extent, the D$_1$ agonist are most prominent in the forebrain neocortex.

DISCUSSION

The results summarized in the previous section illustrate that the constitutive inactivation of D_2 and D_3 receptors in knockout mice leads to a decrease in agonist-promoted D_1 receptor activity. However, an intermittent activation of D_1 receptors by either METH or a full D_1 agonist can rescue this abnormal phenotype in a long-term manner. Thus, the initiation of the long-term changes in the molecular responses to D_1 agonist stimulation induced by a single dose of METH are likely due to the (acute) one-time stimulation of D_1 receptors.

Interestingly, a single dose of METH leads to a long-term rescue of D_1-receptor-mediated c-*fos* responses only in brains with either low (preadolescent mice; see Ref. 4) or abnormally blunted c-*fos* mRNA expression levels (adult D_2 and D_3 mutants). We have recently begun to test for the physiological relevance of the findings described here. These studies have focused on the prefrontal cortex (PFC), where D_1 receptors play a critical role in the control of working memory.[9] Consistent with the results of our studies on the expression c-*fos* mRNA, more recent results of immunocytochemical studies revealed blunted c-*fos* protein in all three subregions (infralimbic, prelimbic, and cingulate) of the PFC.[5] METH pretreatment resulted in a significant increase in c-*fos* expressing neurons in D_2 mutants. In D_3 mutants, the rescue of prefrontal cortical c-*fos* responses, although evident, was less pronounced compared to D_2 mutants, and METH pretreatment had no effect on wild-type brains.[5] These data correlate well with the results of most recent studies that analyzed the performance of all three genotypes in a spatial working memory task. This study revealed that drug-naive D_2 and D_3 mutants exhibit a significant spatial working memory deficit. METH pretreatment of D_2 mutants completely rescues this deficit, but has only minimal effects on D_3 mutants (C.S., unpublished observation). Altogether, these data indicate that, in brains with compromised D_1-receptor function, a single dose of METH has long-term physiological consequences. It rescues the blunted D_1-receptor response to either exogenously administered agonists or endogenously released dopamine (released in response to a cognitive task).

A currently unresolved issue relates to the mechanisms that lead to the blunted D_1-receptor function in brains of D_2 and D_3 mutants and its rescue by a single dose of METH. We have recently reported results of [^{35}S]GTPγS binding experiments that revealed that the first step of D_1-receptor activation, namely G protein activation, is blunted in the forebrain neocortex of D_2 mutants and that METH pretreatment also rescues this blunted molecular phenotype.[6] Interestingly, however, the amount of [^{35}S]GTPγS bound to SKF-stimulated D_1 receptors expressed in brains of D_3 mutants is not significantly altered. Thus, the mechanisms leading to the decreased agonist-stimulated D_1-receptor activity obviously differ between both mutants.

We also found that distinct protein phosphatases (PP1/2A and PP2B) play a critical role in modulating the D_1-agonist-stimulated G protein activation (i.e., dephosphorylation of either receptor and/or G protein increase G protein activation in response to agonist stimulation). However, in contrast to wild type, in both D_2 and D_3 mutants, G protein activation in response to D_1 agonist stimulation with SKF82958 is only minimally affected by PP1/2A and PP2B inhibitors and METH pretreatment does not rescue the sensitivity to phosphatase inhibition.[6] This suggests that the long-term effects of a single dose of METH are mediated by effector systems that act downstream of G protein activation. Those could include the activity of adenylyl cyclase (and hence PKA) or the differential activation of principal transcriptional activators of FOS genes. Clearly, more research is needed to elucidate the mechanisms underlying the phenomena described here.

Finally, it remains to be tested whether, and if so when, a regimen of repeated intermittent stimulation of D$_1$ receptors with single applications of METH becomes ineffective in restoring a blunted D$_1$-receptor activity. This is particularly important in view of the fact that the subchronic administration of psychostimulants is associated with a progressive sensitization of neuronal systems.[10]

REFERENCES

1. HARLAN, R.E. & M.M. GARCIA. 1998. Drugs of abuse and immediate-early genes in the forebrain. Mol. Neurobiol. **16:** 221–267.
2. MORATALLA, R. *et al.* 1996. Cellular responses to psychomotor stimulant and neuroleptic drugs are abnormal in mice lacking the D1 dopamine receptor. Proc. Natl. Acad. Sci. USA **93:** 14928–14933.
3. JUNG, M.-Y. & C. SCHMAUSS. 1999. Decreased c-*fos* responses to dopamine D$_1$ receptor agonist stimulation in mice deficient for D$_3$ receptors. J. Biol. Chem. **274:** 29406–29412.
4. SCHMAUSS, C. 2000. A single dose of methamphetamine leads to a long term reversal of the blunted dopamine D1 receptor-mediated neocortical c-*fos* responses in mice deficient for D2 and D3 receptors. J. Biol. Chem. **275:** 38944–38948.
5. GLICKSTEIN, S.B. & C. SCHMAUSS. 2001. c-*fos* mRNA and protein responses to dopamine D1-agonist stimulation in the prefrontal cortex of mice deficient for D2 and D3 receptors. Society for Neuroscience Abstract 189.13. San Diego, CA.
6. HSIUNG, S.-C. *et al.* 2001. Decreased dopamine D1-receptor-activated binding of [35S]GTPγS in the neocortex of mice deficient for D2 receptors. Society for Neuroscience Abstract 379.9. San Diego, CA.
7. JUNG, M.-Y. *et al.* 1999. Potentiation of the D2-mutant motor phenotype in mice lacking dopamine D2 and D3 receptors. Neuroscience **91:** 911–924.
8. VAN BEVEREN, C. *et al.* 1983. Analysis of FBJ-MuSV provirus and c-fos (mouse) gene reveals that viral and cellular fos gene products have different carboxy termini. Cell **32:** 1241–1255.
9. WILLIAMS, G.V. & P.S. GOLDMAN-RAKIC. 1995. Modulation of memory fields by dopamine D1 receptors in prefrontal cortex. Nature **376:** 572–575.
10. CURRAN, E.J., H. AKIL & S.J. WATSON. 1996. Psychomotor stimulant- and opiate-induced c-*fos* mRNA expression patterns in the rat forebrain: comparisons between acute drug treatment and a drug challenge in sensitized animals. Neurochem. Res. **21:** 1425–1435.

Ibogaine Signals Addiction Genes and Methamphetamine Alteration of Long-Term Potentiation

EMMANUEL S. ONAIVI,[a,b] SYED F. ALI,[c] SANIKA S. CHIRWA,[d] JEAN ZWILLER,[e] NATHALIE THIRIET,[f] B. EMMANUEL AKINSHOLA,[g] AND HIROKI ISHIGURO[b]

[a]Department of Biology, William Paterson University, Wayne, New Jersey 07470, USA

[b]Molecular Neurobiology Branch, IRP, NIDA-NIH, Baltimore, Maryland 21224, USA

[c]Neurochemistry Laboratory, Division of Neurotoxicology Research, National Center for Toxicological Research/FDA, Jefferson, Arizona 72079, USA

[d]Department of Anatomy and Physiology, Meharry Medical College, Nashville, Tennessee 37308, USA

[e]INSERM U338, Center de Neurochemimie, Strasbourg, France

[f]Molecular Neuropsychiatry, NIDA-NIH, Baltimore, Maryland 21224, USA

[g]Department of Pharmacology, Howard University College of Medicine, Washington D.C. 20059, USA

ABSTRACT: The mapping of the human genetic code will enable us to identify potential gene products involved in human addictions and diseases that have hereditary components. Thus, large-scale, parallel gene-expression studies, made possible by advances in microarray technologies, have shown insights into the connection between specific genes, or sets of genes, and human diseases. The compulsive use of addictive substances despite adverse consequences continues to affect society, and the science underlying these addictions in general is intensively studied. Pharmacological treatment of drug and alcohol addiction has largely been disappointing, and new therapeutic targets and hypotheses are needed. As the usefulness of the pharmacotherapy of addiction has been limited, an emerging potential, yet controversial, therapeutic agent is the natural alkaloid ibogaine. We have continued to investigate programs of gene expression and the putative signaling molecules used by psychostimulants such as amphetamine in *in vivo* and *in vitro* models. Our work and that of others reveal that complex but defined signal transduction pathways are associated with psychostimulant administration and that there is broad-spectrum regulation of these signals by ibogaine. We report that the actions of methamphetamine were similar to those of cocaine, including the propensity to alter long-term potentiation (LTP) in the hippocampus of the rat brain. This action suggests that there may be a "threshold" beyond which the excessive brain stimulation that probably occurs with compulsive psychostimulant use results in the occlusion of LTP. The influence of ibogaine on immediate early genes

Address for correspondence: Emmanuel S. Onaivi, Department of Biology, William Paterson University, 300 Pompton Road, Wayne, NJ 07470. Voice: 973-720-3453; fax: 973-720-3730.
OnaiviE@WPUNJ.edu
Eonaivi@intra.nida.nih.gov

Ann. N.Y. Acad. Sci. 965: 28–46 (2002). © 2002 New York Academy of Sciences.

(IEGs) and other candidate genes possibly regulated by psychostimulants and other abused substances requires further evaluation in compulsive use, reward, relapse, tolerance, craving and withdrawal reactions. It is therefore tempting to suggest that ibogaine signals addiction gene products.

KEYWORDS: ibogaine; pharmacogenomics; pharmacotherapy: psychostimulant; gene chip; addiction; methamphetamine; haplotypes; SNPs; signal transduction; animal model

INTRODUCTION

The compulsive use of addictive substances despite adverse consequences continues to affect society, and the science underlying these addictions in general remains poorly understood. This is because the pharmacological treatment of drug and alcohol addiction has largely been disappointing. The good news is that the mapping of the human genetic code will enable us to identify potential gene products involved in human addictions and other diseases that have hereditary components. Indeed the compulsive use of addictive substances leading to neuroadaptation activates signal transduction pathways that regulate changes in gene expression.[1] Thus, genetic vulnerability and environmental factors are important determinants in transitions from casual drug use to compulsive use of addictive substances.[2] Addiction is therefore a polygenic disorder that affects the brain and peripheral tissues and does not follow simple Mendelian monogenic inheritance. While our knowledge of the pharmacogenomics and pharmacogenetics of addiction has yet to produce therapeutic targets to treat drug addicts, few findings of positive allelic association rarely withstand replication.[3] A genome-wide, parallel search to determine at-risk genes and programs of gene expression patterns using quantitative trait loci (QTLs) mapping of rodent strains and DNA microarray analysis reveals at best genetic heterogeneity and complexity of addictions.[3,4] Much effort recently has been focused on pharmacogenomics and addiction to opiates,[3] alcoholism and substance abuse,[5] genetic influences on smoking, and candidate genes.[6,7] Others have focused on the application of DNA microarrays to study human alcoholism,[8] or changes in non-human primate nucleus accumbens gene expression after chronic cocaine treatment,[9] and large-scale analysis of gene expression changes during acute and chronic exposure to Δ^9-THC in rats.[10]

Addiction is therefore a biological process[11] and a brain disease[12] that is not caused by one single gene, but rather involves multiple vulnerable genes,[3] with significant contribution from environmental factors, including the trigger by the availability of abused substance(s). Thus, as the usefulness of pharmacotherapy of addiction has been limited, an emerging potential, yet controversial therapeutic agen, is the natural alkaloid, ibogaine. We have continued to investigate programs of gene expression and the putative signaling molecules used by ibogaine and psychostimulants such as amphetamines in *in vivo* and *in vitro* models. Our work and that of others reveal that complex but defined signal transduction pathways are associated with the compulsive use of addictive substances and that the putative regulation of these signals by ibogaine may be linked to its broad spectrum of action on numerous biological systems.

MOLECULAR SIGNALS OF ADDICTION GENES

After over four decades of intensive research on the brain reward pathways in the development and the compulsive use of addictive substances, the dopamine circuits and hypothesis remain a difficult area and perhaps a major problem and hindrance to progress in unraveling the biology of addiction. For example, benzodiazepines, barbiturates, and inhalants do not increase dopamine levels, as do psychostimulants and opiates and most importantly other systems like gamma amino butyric acid (GABA), cholinergic, glutamatergic, adrenergic systems, cannabinomimetic and cAMP transduction pathways, which are involved in reward and relapse circuits in the brain. Additional evidence from knockout mice demonstrates that mutant mice without dopamine receptors and transporters continue to self-administer psycho-stimulants, whereas mutant mice without metabotrophic glutamate receptor (mGluR5) are completely unresponsive to cocaine even though their dopaminergic system remains intact. The link between learning and memory processes in addiction further indicates the complexity and polygenic nature of substance abuse vulnerability. Transition into compulsive drug use induces the expression of a number of genes from several biochemical pathways resulting in neuroadaptive changes in the brain.[1] Abused substances, as shown in FIGURE 1, are known to stimulate transcription of specific genes by activating the transcriptional regulators through appropriate transcriptional factors. Our working hypothesis is that ibogaine induces a synchronized state of programmed signal transduction and gene expression resulting in its broad-spectrum anti-addictive potential. As we reviewed recently,[13] a number of complex genetic markers and signaling molecules are stimulated or inhibited by transcriptional regulators and factors associated with specific programs of candidate genes. Indeed, a number of studies indicate that most drugs of abuse indirectly stimulate/inhibit transcription regulators and factors by a tangled, but precise web of signal transducers (FIG. 1).[1,13] Therefore, addictive substances are known to activate signal transduction pathways that regulate gene expression in the brain and peripheral organ systems in human and perhaps animal models. Addiction from drug abuse is now viewed as a brain disease, but we have to add that peripheral mechanisms, which are largely ignored, also contribute to the neurobiological disturbances and behavioral pathologies, such as compulsive drug use and craving.[1,14] Increasing evidence demonstrates that most drugs of abuse indirectly stimulate transcription of specific genes by increasing intracellular cAMP, which inevitably results in activation of multifunctional protein kinases and phosphorylation of several cellular proteins[1] (FIG. 1).

The current understanding of how transcription factors regulate gene expression is poor; however, the best characterized in the brain are the Fos/Jun family of immediate early gene (IEG) transcription factors and the CREB family of transcription factors as possible mediators of the effects of drug abuse on the regulation of gene expression.[1,15] Another example is the claim that ΔFosB might be a relatively sustained molecular "switch" that contributes to a state of addiction.[20] Some of the studies reported here indicate that acute ibogaine injection induces expression of the IEGs, *egr-1* and *c-fos*, in the mouse brain[16] (TABLE 1). This may be one way in which ibogaine is able to block the action of abused substances that cause addiction. The list of brain circuits involved in drug abuse continues to grow. Significant amounts of data implicate some role for dopaminergic pathways in drug addiction, but other

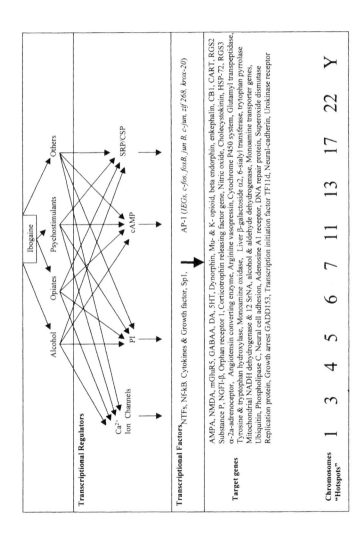

FIGURE 1. Hypothetical "putative" pharmacogenomic effects of ibogaine, showing putative regulation of ibogaine on the effects of substances with addiction potential on transcriptional regulators, factors, target genes and a listing of chromosomal "hot spots" of candidate genes involved with substance addiction. The hypothesis is that the broad-spectrum action of ibogaine forms a basis for its anti-addiction properties.

TABLE 1. Effect of ibogaine on c-fos and egr-1 gene expression

	egr-1		c-fos	
	Control	Ibogaine	Control	Ibogaine
NAc	5.78 ± 0.61	7.50 ± 0.37*	1.45 ± 0.13	1.95 ± 0.41
CPU	7.23 ± 0.26	12.4 ± 0.72**	1.15 ± 0.06	2.40 ± 0.50*
FCx	9.65 ± 0.75	17.4 ± 1.3**	1.23 ± 0.13	3.30 ± 0.14*
DG	3.87 ± 0.31	11.5 ± 0.81**	1.53 ± 0.29	6.65 ± 0.76*
CA1	6.50 ± 0.52	7.70 ± 0.52	1.60 ± 0.26	2.75 ± 0.26*
CA3	4.87 ± 0.40	9.10 ± 1.10*	1.78 ± 0.26	2.40 ± 0.67
Septum	3.90 ± 0.71	8.10 ± 0.83**	1.47 ± 0.07	5,27 ± 0.77

$*p < 0.01$; $** p < 0.001$, following Newmann-Keul's t-test after ANOVA.

circuits like opioid peptides and GABA are also involved (FIG.1). Furthermore, it has been demonstrated that the cannabinoid system may be involved in the neuronal processes underlying relapse to cocaine-seeking behavior in the rat model[17]. It is interesting that cannabinoid receptors, which are encoded by the CB1 gene, are one of the most abundant neuroreceptors in the mammalian brain. There is increasing evidence that cannabinoids inhibit neurotransmitter release via specific presynaptic CB1 receptors.[18] One of the recent advances in cannabinoid research is the identification of a series of endogenous modulators called endocannabinoids (e.g., anandamide, 2-arachidonyl glycerol and noladin ether).[19] It appears that this previously unknown cannabinoid physiological control system might be a key player in the neural mechanism of addiction. Cannabinoid receptor gene may be a piece of the genetic puzzle in addiction and perhaps may be part of the solution. The cannabinoid receptor antagonist (SR 141716) prevents acquisition of drinking behavior in alcohol-preferring rats, and SR 141716 has been found to block the acquisition, but not the expression, of cocaine- and morphine-induced conditioned place preference in rats.[21] These observations support the hypothesis that neurobiological events underlie the acquisition to a greater extent than those events mediating the expression of the positive-reinforcing properties of abusive drugs, including alcohol. Taken together, it appears that drugs of abuse alter intracellular messenger pathways into short- and long-term changes in target gene expression by the appropriate signal-regulated transcription factors (FIG. 1). Unfortunately, the relationship between these intracellular signaling and transcriptional regulations of the candidate genes involved with compulsive use of drugs is unclear at the moment.

The application of DNA microarrays as discussed here to study candidate genes that may be involved in human addiction has generated numerous genes whose role in addiction may not be readily obvious. There are problems with pharmacogenomics and large variability in microarray data, as discussed below. The important questions therefore are: (1) What is the significance of so many genes being transcribed after compulsive substance use? and (2) How can we pin down what are the important genes that induce the drug-dependent state or a relapse state after cessation from compulsive substance use? The preliminary preclinical and clinical data obtained with ibogaine demonstrate a broad spectrum of action on multiple systems that may account for its anti-addictive potential.

GENETIC APPROACHES FOR THE ANALYSIS OF ADDICTION

While significant advances have been made in demonstrating the role of specific gene products (or lack of) in animal models of addiction, Progress has been slow in identifying genes that affect risk of addiction in humans. In addition the identification of the genes involved in complex polygenic traits may be difficult because the principles learned about single-gene single-disease inheritance may not be relevant to polygenic and multifactorial inheritance as in polysubstance abuse and addictions.[24] It is even more difficult to pin down the cellular transcription cascades with the behavioral manifestation of compulsive drug-seeking and drug-taking despite horrendous consequences.[20] Several studies have also linked genetic and environmental factors combining to influence the process by which repeated exposure leads to addiction. For the genetic factors a large number of vulnerable candidate genes may be involved in addictions, with no single gene sufficient or necessary to cause addiction. For the environmental factors, the contribution of the environment is obvious in that genetic vulnerability can only lead to addiction when the substance of abuse is readily available.[3] Because drug addiction is a genetically complex and polygenic disease involving different stages, a number of genetic approaches for the analysis of addiction continue to evolve from pharmacogenetics to pharmacogenomic approaches in which the entire genome and its expression are evaluated to scan and map genetic variation across the entire human genome. Others have proposed that micro- and minisatellite polymorphisms play a role in the expression of many genes.[24] The human genome is highly polymorphic and mutations in the human genome lead to genetic polymorphisms in the population. The frequency of mutation in transgenes is now receiving considerable attention, since proteins synthesized in recombinant DNA biological systems are subject to genetic alteration through mutation and selection.[23] The complex polygenic trait in addiction may be multifactorial, since both genetic and environmental factors play a role in the cause.[23,24] As a result, these genes exists in the population with many functional alleleomorphic variants. Thus, there is a reasonable chance that an individual will inherit a threshold number of functional variants beyond which there is an appreciable effect on the phenotype.[24] Therefore, disease markers in the human sequences can be targeted with a complete genetic map of haplotypes and single nucleotide polymorphisms (SNPs). Haplotypes are sets of genetic markers that are close enough on a chromosome to be inherited together. Similarly, SNPs act as markers in genome-wide scanning for disease-causing genes to be traced through generations to identify genetic differences between people affected and unaffected by addiction. So, SNPs and haplotypes can be used to unravel the genetic differences that make some people more addiction-prone than others. It can therefore be deduced that a SNP and haplotypic genetic maps across the entire genome will be of great use in finding genes that are involved in addiction. However, using SNPs alone can be difficult and expensive, partly because it is currently hard to trace individual SNPs in the genome. But using haplotypes eases some of these difficulties, and makes it easier to identify variation in the genome because each haplotype contain a group of SNPs that tend to be inherited together. These haplotypes are found by analyzing genotype data to create a series of markers that have linkage disequilibrium in a gene.

Genotyping uses genomic DNA, PCR-RFLP, sequencing, and the like to examine the association between genes and addiction. For example, a genetic association for cigarette smoking behavior was reported between allele 9 of a dopamine transporter gene polymorphism (SLC6A3-9) and lack of smoking, late initiation of smoking, and length of quitting.[25,26] After extracting DNA from peripheral blood, SLC6A3 3', a variable number of tandem repeat (VNTR) genotypes were determined by PCR amplification and agarose gel electrophoresis by these investigators. In another study, alcohol and aldehyde dehydrogenase genotyping was undertaken to examine the allele frequencies at the ADH1, ADH2, and ADH3 loci among Alaska natives.[27] This is because alcohol and aldehyde dehydrogenase involved in alcohol metabolism are polymorhic and account for the ethnic differences in alcohol metabolism. The study's findings suggest that the Alaska natives are not protected from the risk of alcoholism in the way that Asians who possess the ALDH2*2 genotype are considered to have a negative risk factor. Nor do there appear to be any generalized differences between Alaska native alcoholics and members of the general population with respect to alcohol and aldehyde dehydrogenase.[27] The role of ibogaine (if any) in the genetics of alcohol and smoking addiction is provocative at best in the absence of microarray data before and after treatment of any these addictions with ibogaine.

The use of microarrays to study gene expression in alcoholism and drug addiction has yielded reams of data, but there is currently little information on the effect of ibogaine, if any, on "addiction genes." But cell and animal studies have consistently indicated that changes in gene expression in the brain appear to be responsible for tolerance, dependence, craving, and relapse to substance abuse.[28,29] Thus, DNA hybridization arrays for gene expression analysis[30] has been applied to addiction research to simultaneously examine changes in the expression of thousands of genes both in animal models of addiction and human addict samples. This is accomplished by microarray hybridization of immobilized gene-specific sequences on a solid-state matrix (e.g., nylon membranes, glass microscope slides, or silicon/ceramic chips) with labeled nucleic acids from human addicts and controls who are not addicts. The samples could also be from animal models of various stages of addiction and their respective controls. A number of studies have applied DNA microarrays to study human drug and alcohol addiction with a significant number of genes and gene products identified. The application of DNA microarray to study human alcoholism used postmortem human brain tissue from the frontal cortex that had been exposed to the chronic effects of alcohol[31] and nerve cells[32] that have been exposed to a few days of ethanol. The results demonstrated that 163 genes from the 4000 genes in the arrays differed by 40% or more from the frontal cortex tissue between alcoholics and nonalcoholics.[31] These investigators found that addiction to alcohol alters gene expression, which may change the programming and circuitry of the superior frontal cortex.[31] Chronic cocaine-mediated changes in non-human primate nucleus accumbens gene expression have been demonstrated by cDNA hybridization array analysis.[33] In another study, large-scale cDNA microarrays were employed to assess gene expression changes during acute and chronic exposure to Δ^9-THC in rats in comparison to vehicle-treated animals.[34] These studies and others further support and confirm that changes in gene expression, particularly in the brain and perhaps in the peripheral organ systems, contribute to drug and alcohol and addiction.

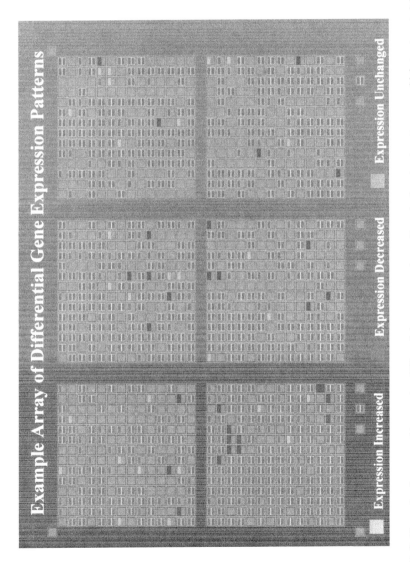

FIGURE 2. Example of array used to examine differential gene expression patterns in drug treatment versus vehicle treatment. A labeled RNA probe is applied to the array to provide expression profiling of changes in gene expression between experimental samples and controls.

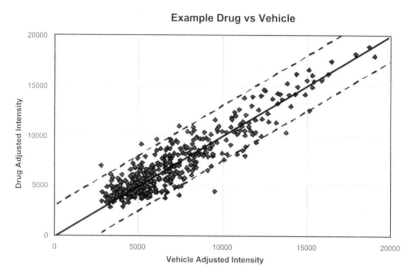

FIGURE 3. Scattergram of the example of the array results from FIGURE 2.

FIGURE 1 shows a number of the target genes whose expression is altered by abused substances. FIGURE 2 shows a prototypical example of a differential gene expression pattern using an array probed with RNA from different treatment, and the scattergram example of the arrays is shown in FIGURE 3. The important question is whether ibogaine has an effect in reversing the genetic effects of alcohol and drug abuse that contribute to addiction. Once a gene has been identified as playing some role in addiction, gene targeting by homologous recombination makes it possible to create knockout animals without specific gene(s) of interest. Gene-targeting strategies therefore provide an avenue for studying the function of a gene after its deletion. Thus, transgenic mice or knockout mice, with null mutation of specific genes obtained by homologous recombination have been used to study the relevance of some genes in different aspects of drug dependence and addiction.[35] A number of examples of genes inactivated using gene knockout techniques or mice transgenically overexpressing specific genes, antisense oligodeoxynucleotide (ODN); and other genetic manipulation strategies have been applied to study various aspects of addiction with a view to finding pharmacogenetic treatment for substance addiction. Mice lacking genes for the 5HT1B, PKCγ, GABA$_A$ receptor subunits, dopamine receptor subtypes, transporter and the vesicular monoamine transporter, tyrosine hydroxylase (*Th*), hypoxanthine-guanine phosphoribosyltransferase (HPRT), P-glucoprotein-*mdr1a*, p53, opioid receptor systems, pre-proenkephalin, isoforms of CREB, TGFα, IGF-I, *fyn*, neuronal acetylcholine receptor subunits (nAChR),[35] substance P, and cannabinoid CB1 receptor have all been studied for their potential influence on alcohol and drug response traits (FIG. 1).[22] Some problems have been identified with the use of transgenic animals, as discussed below; but the development of tissue-specific inducible knock-out mice and other conditionally regulated transgenics may become useful in validating the role(s) of these candidate genes in addictions.

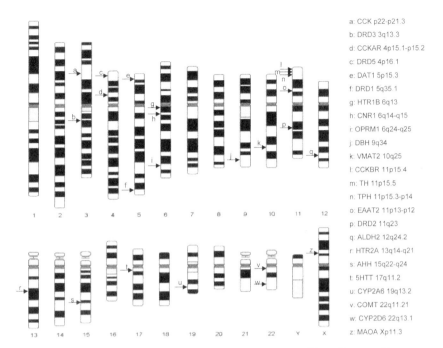

a: CCK p22-p21.3
b: DRD3 3q13.3
d: CCKAR 4p15.1-p15.2
c: DRD5 4p16.1
e: DAT1 5p15.3
f: DRD1 5q35.1
g: HTR1B 6q13
h: CNR1 6q14-q15
i: OPRM1 6q24-q25
j: DBH 9q34
k: VMAT2 10q25
l: CCKBR 11p15.4
m: TH 11p15.5
n: TPH 11p15.3-p14
o: EAAT2 11p13-p12
p: DRD2 11q23
q: ALDH2 12q24.2
r: HTR2A 13q14-q21
s: AHH 15q22-q24
t: 5HTT 17q11.2
u: CYP2A6 19q13.2
v: COMT 22q11.21
w: CYP2D6 22q13.1
z: MAOA Xp11.3

FIGURE 4. Addiction "hot spots" in human chromosomes. These "hot spots" are associations between genetic variants and substance abuse. ABBREVIATIONS: CCK, cholecystokinin; DRD1-5, dopamine receptor D1-5; CCKAR, cholecystokinin receptor type A; DAT1, dopamine transporter; HTR1B, serotonin receptor 1B; CNR1, cannabinoid receptor type 1; OPRM1, opioid receptor mu 1; DBH, dopamine beta-hydroxylase; VMAT2, vesicular monamine transporter 2; CCKBR, cholecystokinin receptor B; TH, tyrosine hydroxylase; TPH, trypophan hydroxylase; EAAT2, glutamate transporter; ALDH2, aldehyde dehydrogenase 2; HTR2A, serotonin receptor 2A; AHH, aryl hydrocarbon hydroxylase; 5HTT, serotonin transporter; CYP2A6, cytochrome P450 subfamily 2A6; COMT, catechol-*O*-methyltransferase; CYP2D6, cytochrome P450 subfamily 2D6; MAOA, monoamine oxidase A.

Mapping of quantitative trait loci (QTLs) is growing in importance in contributing to the identification of chromosomal "hot spots" that contain specific genes that influence all aspects of substance addiction. The specific regions of the chromosomes that contain specific genes that have been implicated in alcohol and drug addiction is shown in FIGURE 4. These chromosomal "hot spots" are by no means exhaustive because other abused substances influence genes on chromosome 1, 2, 7, and Y that have not been listed in FIGURE 4. These unbiased searches of the whole genome using various markers indicate the complexity of alcohol and drug addiction.

METHAMPHETAMINE ALTERS LONG-TERM POTENTIATION

Ibogaine in a number of studies has been shown to influence multiple central nervous system pathways, which has led us to postulate that the broad spectrum of action of ibogaine-like compounds may be important in their anti-addiction potential[13,36] The previous study in the mouse model of withdrawal indicated that ibogaine reversed the withdrawal aversions from chronic administration of psychostimulants like cocaine.[36] The follow-up studies described below examined the *in vivo* and *in vitro* action of another psychostimulant, methamphetamine. Methamphetamine is an indirect-acting catecholaminergic agent used in the treatment of hyperkinetic states in children or in the management of obesity.[37] It is a simple chemical derivative of ephedrine, an active ingredient of several cold remedies. Synthesis of methamphetamine is simple and straightforward, a factor that probably accounts for its widespread availability. This is of particular concern since methamphetamine produces prominent euphoric effects, a property that renders it subject to abuse[38]. Inappropriate doses or prolonged use of methamphetamine cause psychosis, disturbances in perception, and memory dysfunction.[39] The exact neural mechanisms that underlie these behavioral responses are not completely known. However, animal studies have shown that amphetamines induce phosphorylation of several proteins, including cAMP-responsive element binding protein (CREB). They also induce immediate early gene expressions, particularly those involving the CREB pathway.[40] One intriguing feature is that CREB phosphorylation and target gene activations require both DA1 dopaminergic and NMDA glutamatergic receptor activations.[41] Both NMDA receptors, and CREB pathways have been implicated in cellular processes involved in cognition. For example, memory consolidation is thought to require the stabilization of changes in synaptic efficacy through new synaptic growth. A cascade of biochemical events involving excitatory amino acid receptors, CREB-mediated gene expressions, and new protein synthesis triggers these structural changes.[42, 43]

Thirty Long-Evans hooded rats were used in the study and randomly divided into groups of 10 animals. Two groups were given methamphetamine (1 or 10 mg/kg i.p.) every day for 90 days, whereas the third group was treated with saline solution during the same period. All animals were subjected to behavioral assessments prior to and at weekly intervals during treatments. In brief: spontaneous locomotor activity and stereotype behavior were measured in computer-controlled-activity cages equipped with infrared emitters and detectors. After 90 days of treatment, animals were prepared for the removal of both hippocampal lobes. One set of hippocampal lobes was collected in vials according to treatment groups and stored in liquid nitrogen for the molecular analysis. The other hippocampuses were sliced to preserve a greater portion of the Schaffer collateral-commissural projections terminating in the same plane in CA1 regions and were randomly selected and transferred onto a recording slice chamber for the electrophysiological studies (a total of 8–10 slices were examined per animal group). Glass microelectrodes filled with saline solution were used to record population spikes (PS) in the CA1 region. Baseline responses were activated at 0.2 Hz, whereas 100 Hz for 1 sec was used for LTP. The population spikes were amplified via a 2-channel AC differential pre-amplifier (band pass: 100 Hz to 1 KHz). Rectangular pulses (60–100 µA, 0.1 msec) were delivered through photoelectric current isolation units regulated by a Grass stimulator. The amplified voltage potentials were viewed on an oscilloscope and taped for off-line analysis. The changes in DA1 and DA2A receptor gene expression in the hippocampus was performed by semi-quantitative competitive reverse transcriptase-polymerase chain

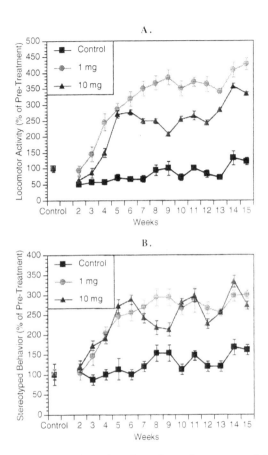

FIGURE 5. Effects of chronic methamphetamine on locomotor activity and stereotype behavior. Methamphetamine was administered 10 min prior to behavioral testing, and each trial was run for 20 min, respectively. Data represents the mean $\pm$ SEM ($n = 10$) in each case. Both locomotor (**A**) and stereotype (**B**) behaviors were found to be significantly different, from 2–3 weeks ($p < 0.05$, ANOVA with Dunnett's multiple comparisons tests).

reaction (RT-PCR), using constructed PCR mimics as normalized internal standards.[44]

FIGURE 5 shows the behavioral effects of methamphetamine during the chronic treatment. The spontaneous locomotor activity and sterotype behaviors were significantly increased, demonstrating the well-established pyschostimulant sensitization, probably attributable to increased release of dopamine. Overall, therefore, the chronic treatment with methamphetamine produced significant increases in DA1 and DA2A gene expression in rat hippocampus, as shown in FIGURE 6. In terms of bioelectrical recordings, the basic criterion for detection of LTP was that there be a post-tetanic response enhancement of at least 40% above baseline population spike, sus-

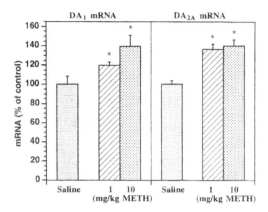

FIGURE 6. The amount of specific mRNA for DA1 and DA2A receptors. Data show that DA1 and DA2A gene expression increased in the hippocampal cells in rats chronically treated with methamphetamine, relative to control aimals given saline. *Asterisk* denotes significant differences (p <0.05, ANOVA with Dunnett's multiple comparison tests).

tained beyond 15 min. In this regard, high-frequency titanic stimulation readily produced LTP in 5 of 5 hippocampal slices obtained from the control animals (PS amplitude: pre-tetanus, 0.95 ± 0.02 mV; 30 min post-tetanus, 1.45 ± 0.04 mV; N = 5). In contrast, 2 of 6 hippocampal slices obtained from the low-dose group exhibited LTP (PS amplitude: pre-tetanus, 1.2 ± 0.2 mV; 30 min post-tetanus 1.42 ± 0.11 mV; N = 6), and none of the slices from the high-dose group developed LTP (PS amplitude: pre-tetanus, 0.8 ± 0.03 mV; 30 min post-tetanus, 0.68 0.04 mV, N = 4 slices). We report that similar to the actions of cocaine, methamphetamine increased both stereotypic and spontaneous locomotor activity and increased the expression of DA1 and DA2A receptor in the hippocampus of these animals. Furthermore, while synaptic transmission remained unaltered, the propensity to induce long-term potentiation (LTP) in the hippocampus was altered by methamphetamine. We deduced that if the effects of methamphetamine were mediated via increased release of dopamine, then the data would suggest that there might be a "threshold" beyond which excessive activation of the dopaminergic system, as probably occurs with chronic methamphetamine administration, results in antagonism of LTP expression. This is consistent with reports that methamphetamine is internalized into nerve terminals via the dopamine transporter and that the process results in a competitive blockade of dopamine re-uptake.[45] Within the terminal, methamphetamine presumably displaces dopamine in vesicles, and this contributes towards the enhanced release of dopamine into the synaptic cleft. Methamphetamine itself activates dopamine receptors indirectly, *albeit* with a lower efficacy. The foregoing actions invariably heighten behavioral responses mediated by dopamine receptor activations, including enhanced locomotion and stereotypy.

The significant increases in DA1 and DA2A transcripts is suggestive of an increased synthesis of DA1 and DA2A receptors transduced by coupling to guanine nucleotide–binding G-protein that regulate the activities of adenylate cyclase and phospholipase C.[45] Specifically, the stimulation of DA1 receptor increases cAMP and potentiates the activation of certain voltage-gated Ca^{2+} channels and multifunctional Ca^{2+}/calmodulin-dependent kinase II (CaMKII). In addition it is known that CREB is activated via phosphorylation by cAMP-dependent protein kinase A and CamKII, which in turn causes synergistic increases in CREB-mediated transcriptions and gene expression. While it was unexpected to discover a decrease in the propensity to induce LTP in slices obtained from methamphetamine-treated rats in the hippocampus, some reports suggest that dopaminergic systems partly mediate LTP. Indeed the expression of long-term potentiation in the striatum of methamphetamine-sensitized rats which was suppressed by NMDA receptor antagonist was reported by Nishioku *et al.*[47] and that tetanic stimulation induced long-term depression (LTD) of the field in the striatum of saline-treated rats. LTP in the hippocampus and LTD in the cerebellum are well-established models of synaptic plasticity that require the activation of certain classes of AMPA and NMDA glutamate receptors, which has recently been linked to the recall of the memories of addiction.[48] A single dose of cocaine exposure *in vivo* was shown to induce long-term potentiation in VTA dopamine neurons, which may be involved in the early stages of the development of drug addiction.[49] There are extrinsic dopaminergic inputs to the hippocampus, such as the mesolimbic dopaminergic pathway, that interact with DA1 and DA5 dopaminergic receptors, presumably on CA1 pyramidal cells.[50] Also, the use of retrograde fluorescent tracers showed that dopaminergic fibers projecting from the VTA and substantia nigra areas innervate the CA1 field. Thus the induction and maintenance of LTP seems to be dependent on *de novo* RNA transcription and protein synthesis.[51] The signal transduction mechanisms that initiate these processes may involve the dopamine/cAMP/CREB cascades.[46] Moreover, dopamine receptor antagonists abolish the maintenance of LTP across CA3/CA1 synapses.[52,53] In particular, blockade of either DA1 or DA2 receptor decreased the magnitude of the late-phase of LTP, two or more hours after induction.[52] In contrast, LTP-producing high-frequency stimulation of the CA1 Schaffer collateral synapses is facilitated by DA1/DA5 dopamine receptor activation.[52,53] How then do we explain the observed low LTP production in treated rats? Presuming that methamphetamine actions were mediated via dopamine/cAMP/CREB and gene expression in the hippocampus, it is feasible that some of these mechanisms are the same as those required for LTP.[54] If these mechanisms are already "maximally" activated by the drug, additional activation as a consequence of tetanic stimulations to produce LTP may not occur, resulting in occlusion of LTP development[53]. Interestingly, greater LTD was observed in cocaine-treated animals.[49] In summary, chronic methamphetamine administration produced behavioral sensitization in rats that may be associated with enhanced expression of DA1 and DA2A gene expression and a modification to the characteristics of synaptic transmission in the hippocampus. The data obtained add to the growing body of evidence indicating that modification of the hippocampus by drugs of abuse may play a role in altering nervous system plasticity, which may partly underlie dysfunctional mnemonic behaviors. It appears that the nature of recall of memories for the compulsive drug use and relapses that sustain addiction may be associated with the neural circuits involved with learning and memory. It is therefore tempting to speculate that the effects of ibogaine on psychostimulant abuse may involve action on the molecular processes associated with signals of addiction genes in learning and memory.

IBOGAINE PHARMACOGENOMICS

Because pharmacogenomics may be defined as the science of the development of drug therapies based on knowledge of the human genome, pharmacogenetic data are needed to determine a role (if any) of ibogaine pharmacogenomics. The pharmacogenetic approach that accesses genetic variation between individual's responses to drugs and in animal studies with both selected lines and inbred strains have provided clear evidence of genetic influence. Although, the genes identified by the pharmacogenetic approach indicate the presence or influence of genes in addiction, identifying the specific genes that make an animal sensitive or resistant to a given drug effect is difficult.[22] However, the advent of new powerful molecular techniques including genomewide scanning and microarray approaches that lead to the identification of specific genes or regions of the chromosomes will allow the function of candidate genes to be analyzed. The promise of pharmacogenomics in addiction research will pay off when therapies based on human genome using variation in DNA and gene expression are used to find new therapeutic targets. The determination of at-risk programs of gene expression patterns involved in addiction may ultimately lead to the identification of new drug targets from the analysis of the genome and expression data.

IBOGAINE INDUCES IMMEDIATE EARLY GENES

There are excellent reviews on the immediate early genes (IEGs)[54,55] and other inducible transcription factors (ITFs).[56] IEGs are a set of transcription factors that are expressed rapidly after stimulation of a variety of cell surface receptors. It has previously been reported that ibogaine injection induces expression of IEGs, *egr-1* and c-*fos*, in mouse brain.[16] Whether the IEGs could be a common biochemical mechanism(s) that underlie addiction is not established, but all drugs of abuse activate IEGs in the brain with differences in brain regions activated. Thus, different classes of abused substances activate IEGs in different brain regions and in some cases overlapping areas of IEG activation have been reported.[55] While common neuropharmacological mechanisms responsible for the activation of IEG expression in forebrain involve dopaminergic and glutamatergic systems, this may not be limited to addictive substances. There are no reports of addiction to ibogaine, which also activates IEGs, as shown in TABLE 1. Furthermore, not all addictive substances activate the release of dopamine in the brain, and therefore the expression of IEGs may be viewed as one of the markers for neuronal activation in the CNS that may not be the common biochemical mechanisms in addiction.

A number of studies have shown that different groups of addictive substances increases the expression of certain IEGs or ITFs in the brain, although each drug appears to induce a particular neuroanatomical pattern of expression, suggesting activation of distinct sets of neurons.[16,55] For example, patterns of c-*fos* expression have been studied after administration of alcohol and surprisingly, these patterns are significantly different from the ones produced by cocaine.[55] Since these genes encode transcription factors, their activation is likely to play a key role in the transduction of short-lived environmental signals into long-lasting changes in the cell function. Activation of c-*fos* in the brain can be induced by a diverse group of stimuli.[58] The inducibility of c-*fos* can now be regarded as a tool to study neuronal activation in different systems in the brain, while *egr-1* has been shown to be involved in neuronal plasticity of hippocampus, especially in LTP.[59] The ibogaine study reported here used adult C57 mice from the NCTR breeding colony. The mice were injected with saline or ibogaine, 50 mg/kg, i.p. ($n = 6$–8), and 30 minutes later animals were given an overdose of pentobarbital (50 mg/kg, i.p) and perfused transcardially with 0.9% saline (10 ml), followed by 1% paraformaldehyde in phosphate-buffered saline (pH 7.2, 50 ml). The brains were frozen in isopentane at $-40°C$, and stored at $-80°C$. Coronal tissue sections (10 μm thick) were thaw-mounted onto gelatin-coated glass slides and stored at $-80°C$. *In situ* hybridization with riboprobe for *egr-1* and c-*fos* was performed as previously described by Thiriet *et al.*[60] with [^{35}S]uridine triphosphate (UTP)-labeled RNA probes. In brief: sections were delipidated, acetylated, and prehybridized for 10 min at 60°C in 50% formamide, $1 \times$ SSC (150 mM NaCl and 15 mM sodium citrate, pH 7.0), dehydrated and air-dried. Thirty microliters of the labeled probe, diluted to 60,000 dpm/μL with hybridization buffer (50% formamide, $4 \times$ SSC, 10% dextran sulfate and 10 mM dithiothreitol), were placed on tissue sections and covered with cover slips. Hybridization was carried out overnight at 52°C. Hybridization medium was then washed off and the sections were washed twice in 50% formamide, $1 \times$ SSC at 55°C for 1 hr, followed by two washes in $2 \times$ SSC (5 min, room temperature). Sections were incubated in a 10-mM Tris-HCl buffer (pH 8.0) containing 100 mM NaCl, 1 mM EDTA, and 6.10^{-3} U/ml RNase for 30 min at 37°C. The slides were then rinsed, dehydrated, and exposed to X-ray film for 2–4 days. To obtain quantitative results, densitometry was determined with a Biocom 2000 image analyzer and the results were expressed in kilobecquerel per gram tissue, using [^{14}C]microscales for calibration as previously described.[60]

Acute injection of ibogaine produced the induction of IEGs, *erg-1* and c-*fos*, in selected regions of mouse brain (TABLE 1). *In situ* hybridization for *egr-1* showed a prominent high signal in caudate-putamen (Cpu), frontal cortex (FCx), septal area, as well as in the CA3 and dentate gyrus (DG) subfields of hippocampus. The *egr-1* mRNA was less induced in nucleus accumbens (NAc) and hippocampal CA1. Similar treatment of ibogaine increased c-*fos* mRNA in Cpu, FCx, and septum, as well as DG and CA1 region of hippocampus. No prominent induction of *egr-1* and c-*fos* was found in other regions of the brain. Quantitative analysis revealed that ibogaine induced statistically significant expression of *egr-1* and c-*fos* in those areas of the brain when compared to controls (TABLE 1). It is noteworthy that induction of both genes was highest in DG (197% and 334% increase for *egr-1* and c-*fos*, respectively). IEG expression was only induced by about 30% in the Nac, an increase that did not reach statistical significance in the case of c-*fos* induction. The data show that acute ibogaine injection induced IEGs, *egr-1* and c-*fos*, in different regions of the mouse brain. It has been reported that stimulants like cocaine or amphetamines induce IEGs, *egr-1* and c-*fos*, as well as the transcription factors, AP-1 and NFκB, in different brain regions.[16] Because of the complex pharmacology and broad spectrum of action of ibogaine, this activation of IEGs may be linked to increase in dopaminergic, serotonergic, and glutamatergic neurotransmission.[16] Evidence that glutamate may be more essential and central than dopamine in addiction was obtained from knockout mice.[57] This is because in dopamine receptor subtypes and transporter knockout mice, cocaine remains addictive, whereas in the knockout mice, without metabotrophic glutamate receptor (mGluR5), the mutant mice are completely unresponsive to cocaine, even though their dopaminergic system remains intact.[57]

CURRENT PROBLEMS IN PHARMACOGENOMICS

Some of the current problems in pharmacogenomics are summarized below.

- lack of complete genetic maps of SNPs, SSLPs, and haplotypes that can predict variation across the entire human genome and be capable of identifying disease genes (e.g., addiction genes);
- the requirement of accurate and cheap genotyping;
- problems associated with compensation in gene knockout animals;
- site-specific action in the brain;
- changes in levels or processing of proteins or peptides (these are thought to be more relevant to function than changes in gene expression, or the production of new mRNAs; it is known that changes in some mRNA levels do not always produce changes in proteins);
- lack of unifying biochemical mechanism for addiction;
- ethical considerations (e.g., the use individual versus pooled samples); and
- large variability in array data.

This list is by no means exhaustive as analysis of the human genome continues with the promise that specific therapies may be tailored to individual problems in the future, particular in the field of substance abuse.

REFERENCES

1. TORRES, G. & J.M. HOROWITZ. 1999. Drugs of abuse and brain gene expression. Psychosom. Med. **61:** 630–650.
2. TSUANG, M.T. *et al.* 1999. Genetic and environmental influences on transitions in drug use. Behav. Genet. **29:** 473–479.
3. LICHTERMANN, D. *et al.* 2000. Pharmacogenomics and addiction to opiates. Eur. J. Pharmacol. **410:** 269–279.
4. JIMENEZ-SANCHEZ, G. *et al.* 2001. Human disease genes. Nature **409:** 853–823.
5. ENOCH, M-A. & D. GOLDMAN. 1999. Genetics of alcoholism and substance abuse. Addict. Disord. **22:** 289–298.
6. ROSSING, M.A. 1998. Genetic influences on smoking: candidate genes. Environ. Hlth. Perspect. **106:** 231–238.
7. ARINAMI, T., H.H. ISHIGURO & E.S. ONAIVI. 2000. Polymorphisms in genes involved in neurotransmission in relation to smoking. Eur. J. Pharmacol. **410:** 215–226.
8. LEWOHL, J.M. *et al.* 2001. Application of DNA microarrays to study human alcoholism. J. Biomed. Sci. **8:** 28–36.
9. FREEMAN, W.M. *et al.* 2001. Chronic cocaine-mediated changes in non-human primate nucleus accumbens gene expression. J. Neurochem. **77:** 542–549.
10. KITTLER, J.T. *et al.* 2000. Large-scale analysis of gene expression changes during acute and chronic exposure to D9-THC in rats. Physio. Genomics **3:** 175–185.
11. NESTLER, E.J. & D. LANDSMAN. 2001. Learning about addiction from the genome. Nature **409:** 834–835.
12. WISE, R.A. 2000. Addiction becomes a brain disease. Neuron **26:** 27–33.
13. ONAIVI, E.S., B.E. AKINSHOLA & S.F. ALI. 2001. Changes in gene expression and signal transduction following ibogaine treatment. *In* The Alkaloid. K. Alper & S.D. Glick, Eds. **56:** 135–153. Academy Press. New York.
14. LESHNER, A. 1997. Addiction is a brain disease, and it matters. Science **278:** 45–47.

15. NESTLER, E.J. 1993. Cellular responses to chronic treatment with drugs of abuse. Crit. Rev. Neurobiol. **7**: 23–39.
16. ALI, S.F., N. THIRIET & J. ZWILLER. 1999. Acute ibogaine injection induces expression of the immediate early genes, *egr-1* and *c-fos*, in mouse brain. Mol. Brain Res. **74**: 237–241.
17. DE VRIES, T.J., Y. SHAHAM, J.R. HOMBEG, *et al.* 2001. A cannabinoid mechanism in relapse to cocaine seeking. Nat. Med., **7**: 1151–1154.
18. HANUS, L., S. ABU-LAFI, E. FRIDE, *et al.* 2001. 2-arachidonyl glyceryl ether, an endogenous agonist of the cannabinoid CB1 receptor. Proc. Natl. Acad. Sci. USA **98**: 3662–3665.
19. NESTLER, E.J. 2000. Genes and addiction. Nat. Genet. **26**: 277–281.
20. SERRA, S., M.A.M. CARAI, G. BRUNETTI, *et al.* 2001. The cannabinoid receptor antagonist SR 141716 prevents acquisition of drinking behavior in alcohol-preferring rats. Eur. J. Pharmacol. **430**: 369–371.
21. CRABBE, J.C. & T.J. PHILLIPS. 1998. Genetics of alcohol and other abused drugs: drug and alcohol dependence. **51**: 61–71.
22. CONNEALLY, P.M. 1994. Human genetic polymorphisms. Dev. Biol. Stand. **83**: 107–110.
23. COMINGS, D.E. 1998. Polygenic inheritance and micro/minisatellites. Mol. Psychiat. **3**: 21–31.
24. SABOL, S.Z, M.L. NELSON, C. FISHER, *et al.* 1999. A genetic association for cigarette smoking behavior. Hlth. Psychol. **18**: 7–13.
25. LERMAN, C., N.E. CAPORASO, J. AUDRAIN, *et al.* 1999. Evidence suggesting the role of specific genetic factors in cigarette smoking. Hlth. Psychol. **18**: 14–20.
26. SEGAL, B. 1999. ADH and ALDH polymorphisms among Alaska Natives entering treatment for alcoholism. Alaska Med. **41**: 9–12.
27. NESTLER, E. J. & D. LANDSMAN. 2001. Learning about addiction from the genome. Nature **409**: 834–835.
28. RAYL, A.J.S. 2001. Microarrays on the mind: technology shows alcohol abuse changes brain's molecular programming circuitry. The Scientist **15**: 1–6.
29. FREEMAN, W.M., D.J. ROBERTSON & K.E. VRANA. 2000. Fundamentals of DNA hybridization arrays for gene expression analysis. Biotechniques **29**: 1042–1055.
30. LEWOHL, J.M., L. WANG, M.F. MILES, *et al.* 2000. Gene expression in human alcoholism: Microarray analysis of frontal cortex. Alc. Clin. Exp. Res. **24**: 1873–1882.
31. MILES, M.F. 1995. Alcohol's effects on gene expression, Alc. Hlth. Res. World **19**: 237–243.
32. FREEMAN, W.M., M.A. NADER, S.H. NADER, *et al.* 2001. Chronic cocaine-mediated changes in non-human primate nucleus accumbens gene expression. J. Neurochem. **77**: 542–549.
33. KITLER, J.T., E.V. GRIGORENKO, C. CLAYTON, *et al.* 2000. Large-scale analysis of gene expression changes during acute and chronic exposure to D9-THC in rats. Physiol. Genom. **3**: 175–185.
34. PICH, E.M. & M.P. EPPING-JORDAN. 1998. Transgenic mice in drug dependence research. Ann. Med **30**: 390–396
35. ONAIVI, E.S., S.F. ALI & A. CHAKRABARTI. 1998. *In vivo* ibogaine blockade and *in vitro* PKC action of cocaine. Ann. N.Y. Acad. Sci. **844**: 227–244.
36. MITLER, M.A., R. HAJDUKOVIC & M.K. ERMAN. 1993. Treatment of narcolepsy with methamphetamine. Sleep **16**: 306–317.
37. MILLER, M.A. & N.J. KOZEL. 1991. Methamphetamine Abuse: Epidemiologic Issues and Implications. NIDA Res. Monographs No. 115.
38. KLEVEN, M.S. & L.S. SEIDEN. 1992. Methamphetamine-induced neurotoxicity: structure activity relationships. Ann. N.Y. Acad. Sciences **654**: 292–301.
39. KONRADI, C., R.L. COLE, S. HECKERS & S.E. HYMAN. 1994. Amphetamine and dopamine-induced immediate early gene expression in striatal neurons depends on postsynaptic NMDA receptors and calcium. J. Neurosci. **16**: 4231–4239.
40. SCHWARZSCHILD, M.A., R.L. COLE & S.E. HYMAN. 1997. Glutamate, but not dopamine, stimulates stress-activated protein kinase and AP-1-mediated transcription in striatal neurons. J. Neurosci. **17**: 3455–3466.
41. MARTIN, K.C. & B.E. DERRICK. 1996. Cell adhesion molecules, CREB, and the formation of new synaptic connections. Neuron **17**: 567–570.

42. MEBERG, P.J., E.G. VALCOURT & A. ROUTTENBERG. 1995. Protein F1/GAP-43 and PKC gene expression patterns in hippocampus are altered 1-2 h after LTP. Mol. Brain. Res. **34:** 343–346.

43. ONAIVI, E.S., C. BISHOP-ROBINSON, E.D. MOTLEY, *et al.* Neurobiological actions of cocaine in the hippocampus. Ann. New York Acad. Sci. **801:** 76–94.

44. SONDERS, M.S., S.-J. ZHU, N.R. ZAHNISER, *et al.* 1997. Multiple ionic conductances of the human dopamine transporter: the actions of dopamine and psychostimulants. J. Neurosci. **17:** 960–974.

45. GRANDY, D.K., Y.A. ZHANG, C. BOUVIER, *et al.* 1991. Multiple human D5 dopamine receptor genes: a functional receptor. Proc. Natl. Acad. Sci. USA **88:** 9175–9179.

46. NISHIOKU, T., T. SHIMAZOE, Y. YAMAMOTO, *et al.* 1999. Expression of long-term potentiation of the striatum in methamphetamine-sensitized rats. Neurosci. Lett. **268:** 81–84.

47. NESTLER, E.J. 2001. Total recall—the memory of addiction. Science **292:** 2266–2267.

48. UNGLESS, M.A., J.L. WHISTLER, R.C. MALENKA & A. BONCI. 2001. Single cocaine exposure in vivo induces long-term potentiation in dopamine neurons. Nature **411:** 583–587.

49. MONSMA, F.J., L.C. MAHAN, L.D. MCVITTIE, *et al.* 1990. Molecular cloning and expression of a D1 dopamine receptor linked to adenyl cyclase activation. Proc. Natl. Acad. Sci. USA. **87:** 6723–6727.

50. OTANI, S. & Y. ARI. 1993. Biochemical correlates of long-term potentiation in hippocampal synapses. Int. Rev. Neurobiol. **35:** 1–41.

51. FREY, U., H. SCHOEDER & H. MATTHIES. 1990. Dopaminergic antagonists prevent long-term maintenance of posttetanic LTP in the CA1 region of rat hippocampal slices. Brain Res. **522:** 69–75.

52. HUANG, Y-Y. & E.R. KANDEL. 1995. D1/D5 receptor agonists induce a protein synthesis-dependent late potentiation in the CA1 region of the hippocampus. Proc. Natl. Acad. Sci. USA **92:** 2446–2450.

53. SCHULZ, S., H. SIEMER, M. KRUG & V. HOLT. 1999. Direct evidence for biphasic cAMP responsive element-binding protein phosphorylation during long-term potentiation in the rat dentate gyrus in vivo. J. Neurosci. **19:** 5683–5692.

54. HOPE, B.T. 1998. Cocaine and the AP-1 transcription factor complex. Ann. N.Y. Acad. Sci. **844:** 1–6.

55. HARLAN, R.E. & M.M. GARCIA. 1998. Drugs of abuse and immediate-early genes in the forebrain. Mol. Neurobiol. **16:** 221–267.

56. RYABININ, A.E. 2000. ITF mapping after drugs of abuse: pharmacological versus perceptional effect. Acta Neurobiol. Exp. **60:** 547–555.

57. HOLLON, T. 2002. Phenotype offers new perception on cocaine. The Scientist **16:** 16–21.

58. HERRERA, D.G. & H.A. ROBERTSON. 1995. Activation of c-fos in the brain. Prog. Neurobiol. **50:** 83–107.

59. WORLEY, P.F., R.V. BHAT, J.M. BARABAN, *et al.* 1993. Threshold for synaptic activation of transcription factors in hippocampus: correlation with long-term enhancement. J. Neurosci. **13:** 4776–4786.

60. THIRIET, N., N. HUMBLOT, C. BURGUN, *et al.*. 1998. Cocaine and fluoxetine induce the expression of the hVH-5 gene encoding MAP kinase phosphatase. Mol. Brain Res. **62:** 150–157.

The Nitric Oxide Releasing Agent Sodium Nitroprusside Modulates Cocaine-Induced Immediate Early Gene Expression in Rat Brain

NATHALIE THIRIET, DOMINIQUE AUNIS, AND JEAN ZWILLER

INSERM U-338, Centre de Neurochimie, 67084 Strasbourg, France

ABSTRACT: The nitric oxide (NO)/cGMP pathway triggers key events in synaptic phenomena involved in learning and memory. Using *in situ* hybridization, the present report demonstrates that NO released by sodium nitroprusside regulates *egr-1*, *c-fos*, and *junB* immediate early gene expression in rat forebrain. These genes, which are rapidly and transiently induced in response to diverse extracellular stimulation, coordinate alterations in gene expression underlying neuronal plasticity. Intracerebroventricular injection of sodium nitroprusside induced immediate early gene expression, which was highest in the nucleus accumbens. On the other hand, sodium nitroprusside abolished the cocaine-induced early gene expression in the dopaminergic projection fields nucleus accumbens, caudate-putamen, and frontal cortex. Further studies are warranted to explore the potential of the NO/cGMP/cGMP-dependent protein kinase pathway to modify cocaine-related behavioral effects.

KEYWORDS: *c-fos*; *egr-1*; guanylyl cyclase; immediate early gene; *junB*; nitric oxide; sodium nitroprusside; rat forebrain

INTRODUCTION

Signaling pathways that increase cyclic GMP (cGMP) are implicated in various aspects of brain physiological functions, including neurotransmission and cell proliferation/differentiation.[1,2] They are also involved in many pathological events, such as neurodegenerative diseases. The most extensively cGMP signal transduction pathway studied is the one triggered by nitric oxide (NO). In neurons, NO is produced by neuronal or endothelial isoforms of NO synthase, and can easily diffuse from the producing to neighboring cells.[3] In the intracellular compartment, the major target of NO is represented by the heme group of soluble guanylyl cyclase (sGC) to which NO binds to promote the synthesis of the second messenger cGMP.[4] The NO/cGMP pathway is coupled to the glutamatergic neurotransmission, triggering key events in synaptic phenomena involved in learning and memory.[5] In addition to

Address for correspondence: Jean Zwiller, Unité INSERM U338, Centre de Neurochimie, 5, rue Blaise Pascal, 67084 Strasbourg Cedex, France. Voice: 33 3 88 45 67 27; fax: 33 3 88 60 08 06.

zwiller@neurochem.u-strasbg.fr

Ann. N.Y. Acad. Sci. 965: 47–54 (2002). © 2002 New York Academy of Sciences.

NO/sGC, the atrial, brain, and C-type natriuretic peptides, ANP, BNP, and CNP, also increase cGMP synthesis, but via the stimulation of membrane-bound guanylyl cyclases, GC-A and GC-B, with CNP preferentially stimulating the GC-B receptor.[6]

Several laboratories, including ours, have shown that acute administration of cocaine produces a rapid and transient induction of several immediate early genes (IEG) in rat brain structures, including *c-fos* and *egr-1*.[7–11] Cocaine-induced IEG expression results mainly from the stimulation of dopaminergic receptors,[12,13] although the serotonergic system may also participate in the gene induction in response to cocaine.[7,11,14] Because several IEGs encode transcription factors, their activation is likely to play a major role in the establishment of long-term neuroadaptations taking place in the brain in response to cocaine administration.

We have shown in a previous report that the natriuretic peptide CNP regulates the activity of dopaminergic neurons. In effect, i.c.v. injection of this peptide inhibits both cocaine-induced IEG expression and extracellular dopamine (DA) increase in the caudate-putamen (CPu).[15] Given that both CNP and NO are well characterized for signaling through the cGMP transduction pathway, in the present study we investigated whether the NO generator sodium nitroprusside (SNP) was also able to regulate cocaine-induced IEG expression.

MATERIALS AND METHODS

Male Wistar rats (250–300 g) were housed in individual cages with free access to food and water and maintained on a 12-h light–dark lighting schedule at 21°C. All experiments were carried out in accordance with the European Community Council Directive. For i.c.v. guide cannula implantation, rats were anesthetized with ketamine (100 mg/kg, i.p.) and placed in a stereotaxic frame. The i.c.v. guide cannula was slowly lowered into the brain at the following coordinates: anteroposterior, −0.5 mm to lambda; mediolateral, 0 mm; dorsoventral, −4.5 mm, according to Paxinos and Watson.[16] Experiments were performed four days after implantation. The correct placement of cannulae was verified on tissue sections. SNP (Sigma, USA) was administered i.c.v. using a Hamilton syringe, with a calibrated needle reaching the ventral coordinate −5.5 mm. Fifty μg SNP in a 10-μL solution were administered over a 1-min period. Fifteen min after SNP administration, animals were injected i.p. with saline (NaCl 0.9%) or cocaine (20 mg/kg; Sigma, USA).

Forty-five minutes after i.p. drug injection, animals were given an overdose of pentobarbital (100 mg/kg, i.p.) and were then perfused transcardially with saline (50 mL) followed by 1% paraformaldehyde in phosphate-buffered saline (pH 7.2, 250 mL). The brains were removed and kept overnight at 4°C in 15% sucrose, frozen in isopentane at −40°C, and then stored at −80°C. Coronal tissue sections (10 mm thick) were thaw-mounted onto gelatin-coated glass slides and stored at −80°C. *In situ* hybridization with [^{35}S] (UTP)-labeled riboprobes for *c-fos, egr-1,* and *junB* was performed as previously described.[14] The slides were exposed to X-ray film (Biomax-MR, Kodak, USA) for 3 to 7 days. For quantitative analysis, densitometry was performed with an image analyzer and the results expressed in kBq/g tissue, using [^{14}C] microscales (Amersham, UK) for calibration. ANOVA followed by Student–Newman–Keuls multiple comparisons test was used for statistical analysis.

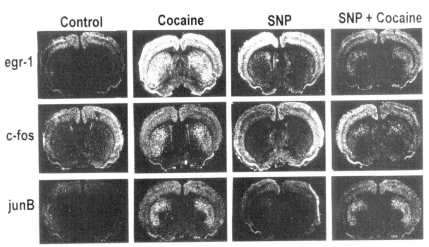

FIGURE 1. Immediate early gene expression in response to SNP and cocaine. Negative prints of *in situ* autoradiograms showing mRNA expression of *egr-1, c-fos,* and *junB* in rat-brain coronal sections (10 µm) taken at the level of striatum (approximately 0.3 mm anterior to bregma) and probed with [^{35}S] antisense riboprobes. Rats were injected i.c.v. with 50 µg SNP or vehicle and 15 min later they were injected i.p. with 20 mg/kg cocaine or 0.9% NaCl (Control). They were sacrificed 45 min after cocaine injection.

RESULTS

Effect of SNP on Cocaine-Induced IEG Expression

We investigated the effect of an i.c.v. injection of SNP, a NO-releasing agent, on cocaine-induced IEG expression in rat forebrain. FIGURE 1 illustrates the *egr-1, c-fos,* and *junB* mRNA expression observed in response to an i.p. injection of cocaine, in coronal sections taken at the level of striatum. After cocaine administration, the mRNA expression of the three genes was considerably enhanced in the CPu and in two cortical layers. When rats were given i.c.v. injections of SNP before cocaine was administered, the induction of the three genes was clearly reduced in the CPu. In addition, SNP alone was found to increase mRNA synthesis of *egr-1* to a certain extent. This effect was not the result of the injection procedure, since injection of the vehicle or of various pharmacological compounds did not produce any noticeable modification in IEG expression.

Quantitative Analysis of Immediate Early Gene Transcription

Quantitative densitometric analysis of IEG expression in well-delimited areas in response to the various treatments is shown in FIGURE 2. Acute cocaine administration caused an approximately 2.1-fold increase in *egr-1* expression in the shell part of the nucleus accumbens (NAc) and in the dorsal region of the CPu, and an 1.5-fold increase in the frontal cortex (FCx) (FIGURE 2a). I.c.v. administration of SNP induced a lesser but statistically significant increase of *egr-1* mRNA synthesis in the

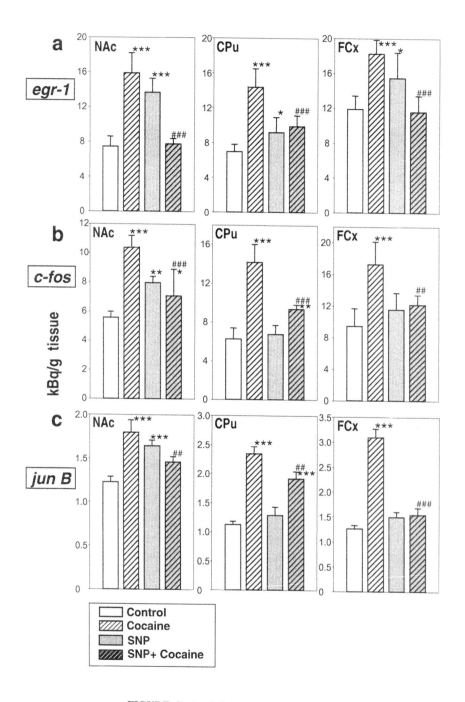

FIGURE 2. *See following page for legend.*

three structures examined. Pretreatment with SNP 15 min before i.p. cocaine injection abolished *egr-1* expression in the NAc and FCx, and strongly inhibited the expression in the CPu. It is noteworthy that, given the fact that SNP may act at sites very distant from the cannulation site and that NO released from SNP easily diffuses, only a small fraction of the injected SNP may actually be responsible for the observed effect. A 1.8-, 2.3-, and 1.8-fold increase in *c-fos* induction in response to cocaine was noted in the NAc shell, dorsal region of the CPu, and FCx, respectively (FIGURE 2b), and this expression was also significantly reduced in the three structures when SNP was administered before cocaine. Injection of SNP alone induced the *c-fos* gene only in the NAc. *JunB* expression was induced 1.5-, 2.1-, and 2.4-fold after cocaine treatment in the NAc, CPu, and FCx, respectively (FIGURE 2c). Pretreatment with SNP significantly reduced the cocaine-induced *junB* expression in the three structures considered, whereas SNP alone induced the *junB* gene expression only in the NAc, as seen for *c-fos*.

DISCUSSION

The present report demonstrates that NO, released by i.c.v. injection of sodium nitroprusside (SNP), abolished the cocaine-induced IEG expression in the striatum and in the frontal cortex. This result substantiates a previous observation that showed that cocaine-induced IEG expression was similarly inhibited by the neuropeptide CNP,[15] the natriuretic peptide preferentially expressed in the brain. Both NO and CNP are signaling through the second messenger cGMP signal transduction pathway, one class of target molecules for cGMP being cGMP-dependent protein kinases (PKGs).

In addition, we found that the i.c.v. administration of SNP alone caused a significant induction of the IEG *egr-1, c-fos,* and *junB* mRNAs in the NAc. This is in contrast to what was observed in the CPu and FCx, in which only the *egr-1* gene was induced, and this was barely statistically significant. Since the NAc is known to be mainly implicated in the processing of the emotional and motivational aspects of a drug or a behavior, our results suggest that NO may play some regulatory role in this function. It is difficult at present to explain why NO by itself produced significant transcription only in the NAc. It might come from a more effective expression of the sGC/cGMP/PKG system in this brain structure. We have previously shown that the stimulation of this pathway by NO increases mRNA expression of the IEGs *c-fos* and *junB*, as well as the DNA binding activity of the transcription factor AP-1 in PC12 cells.[17] Similar results were reported when the cGMP pathway was stimulated by NO in rat embryo fibroblasts and thyroid epithelial cells,[18] or by CNP in PC12

FIGURE 2. Densitometric analysis of *egr-1* (**a**), *c-fos* (**b**), and *junB* (**c**) mRNA expression from *in situ* autoradiograms. Comparable areas of the nucleus accumbens shell (NAc), the dorsal region of the caudate putamen (CPu), and frontal cortex (FCx) in sections from rats treated as described in legend to FIGURE 1, were quantified as kBq/g tissue. Results are expressed as mean ± SD ($n = 6$ to 8 sections from 4 animals). * $p < 0.05$; ** or ## $p < 0.01$; *** or ### $< p$ 0.001. *, significant when comparing treatment vs. saline control group and #, significant when comparing [SNP + cocaine] vs. cocaine group.

cells.[19] It was subsequently demonstrated that NO activates the *c-fos* promoter via the activation of PKG.[20] On the other hand, PKG overexpression was shown to greatly amplify the Egr-1 binding activity induced by the neurotransmitter serotonin or by growth factors.[21]

The current data show that SNP inhibited cocaine-induced *egr-1, c-fos,* and *junB* IEG expression in postsynaptic striatal and cortical neurons. In the striatum, this very likely occurs in medium-spiny GABAergic neurons that express the dopaminergic D1 receptor, since several arguments indicate that cocaine-induced IEG transcription takes place in neurons expressing the DA D1 receptor.[12,13,22] D1 receptor stimulation in medium-spiny neurons results in the elevation of intracellular cyclic AMP (cAMP) concentration, which may then be responsible for the cocaine-induced IEG transcription, via the activation of a transcription factor of the cAMP responsive element binding (CREB) family. It is tempting to speculate that SNP actually inhibited gene expression in the presynaptic neuron by the stimulation of sGC and the increase in intracellular cGMP concentration, which in turn resulted in a reduced dopamine release and thus in a lesser D1 receptor stimulation. The hypothesis of SNP controlling DA release is supported by a former report in which NO was found to alter the release of several neurotransmitters, including DA and 5-HT in the striatum, the effect being mediated by cGMP formation.[23] Cyclic GMP activates two mammalian isotypes of PKGs, the type II being an ubiquitous brain protein kinase.[24,25] The NO/sGC/PKG pathway was shown to modulate presynaptic activity in various situations, including catecholamine secretion from chromaffin cells,[26] or establishment of long-term potentiation.[27] In ciliary ganglion neurons, it was demonstrated that the activation of PKGL inhibits acetylcholine release at some point after calcium entry.[28] Alternatively, neurotransmitter release may be inhibited by the direct phosphorylation by PKG and subsequent inhibition of L-type[29] or N-type Ca^{2+} channels.[30]

In conclusion, the data presented herein confirm that activating the cGMP signal transduction pathway reduces the cocaine-induced immediate early gene transcription. Since these genes are known to play a key role in phenotypic long-term adaptations, it would be of interest to investigate whether NO also modulates the behavioral adaptations known to occur after repeated cocaine administration.

ACKNOWLEDGMENTS

The authors thank Mrs. Marie-Odile Revel for valuable technical support.

REFERENCES

1. SCHMIDT, H.H. & U. WALTER. 1994. NO at work. Cell **78:** 919–925.
2. HOFMANN, F., A. AMMENDOLA & J. SCHLOSSMANN. 2000. Rising behind NO: cGMP-dependent protein kinases. J. Cell Sci. **113:** 1671–1676.
3. BREDT, D.S. & S.H. SNYDER. 1990. Isolation of nitric oxide synthetase, a calmodulin-requiring enzyme. Proc. Natl. Acad. Sci. USA **87:** 682–685.
4. MIKI, N., Y. KAWABE & K. KURIYAMA. 1977. Activation of cerebral guanylate cyclase by nitric oxide. Biochem. Biophys. Res. Commun. **75:** 851–856.

5. FEDELE, E. & M. RAITERI. 1999. In vivo studies of the cerebral glutamate receptor/NO/ cGMP pathway. Prog. Neurobiol. **58:** 89–120.
6. KOLLER, K.J. *et al.* 1991. Selective activation of the B natriuretic peptide receptor by C-type natriuretic peptide (CNP). Science **252:** 120–123.
7. BHAT, R.V. & J.M. BARABAN. 1993. Activation of transcription factor genes in striatum by cocaine: role of both serotonin and dopamine systems. J. Pharmacol. Exp. Ther. **267:** 496–505.
8. TORRES, G. & C. RIVIER. 1994. Induction of c-fos in rat brain by acute cocaine and fenfluramine exposure: a comparison study. Brain Res. **647:** 1–9.
9. MORATALLA, R., H.A. ROBERTSON & A.M. GRAYBIEL. 1992. Dynamic regulation of NGFI-A (zif268, egr1) gene expression in the striatum. J. Neurosci. **12:** 2609–2622.
10. HOPE, B. *et al.* 1992. Regulation of immediate early gene expression and AP-1 binding in the rat nucleus accumbens by chronic cocaine. Proc. Natl. Acad. Sci. USA **89:** 5764–5768.
11. HUMBLOT, N. *et al.* 1998. The serotonergic system modulates the cocaine-induced expression of the immediate early genes egr-1 and c-fos in rat brain. Ann. N.Y. Acad. Sci. **844:** 7–20.
12. DRAGO, J. *et al.* 1996. D1 dopamine receptor-deficient mouse: cocaine-induced regulation of immediate early gene and substance P expression in the striatum. Neuroscience **74:** 813–823.
13. MAILLEUX, P., F. ZHANG & J.J. VANDERHAEGHEN. 1992. The dopamine D1 receptor antagonist SCH-23390 decreases the mRNA levels of the transcription factor zif268 (krox-24) in adult rat intact striatum—an in situ hybridization study. Neurosci. Lett. **147:** 182–184.
14. THIRIET, N. *et al.* 1998. Cocaine and fluoxetine induce the expression of the hVH-5 gene encoding a MAP kinase phosphatase. Mol. Brain Res. **62:** 150–157.
15. THIRIET, N. *et al.* 2001. C-type natriuretic peptide (CNP) regulates cocaine-induced dopamine increase and immediate early gene expression in rat brain. Eur. J. Neurosci. **14:** 1702–1708.
16. PAXINOS, G. & C. WATSON. 1997. The rat brain in stereotaxic coordinates, 3rd ed. Academic Press. Orlando, FL.
17. HABY, C. *et al.* 1994. Stimulation of the cyclic GMP pathway by NO induces expression of the immediate early genes c-fos and junB in PC12 cells. J. Neurochem. **62:** 496–501.
18. PILZ, R.B. *et al.* 1995. Nitric oxide and cGMP analogs activate transcription from AP-1-responsive promoters in mammalian cells. FASEB J. **9:** 552–558.
19. THIRIET, N. *et al.* 1997. Immediate early gene induction by natriuretic peptides in PC12 phaeochromocytoma and C6 glioma cells. Neuroreport **8:** 399–402.
20. IDRISS, S.D. *et al.* 1999. Nitric oxide regulation of gene transcription via soluble guanylate cyclase and type I cGMP-dependent protein kinase. J. Biol. Chem. **274:** 9489–9493.
21. ESTEVE, L. *et al.* 2001. Cyclic GMP-dependent protein kinase potentiates serotonin-induced Egr-1 binding activity in PC12 cells. Cell. Signalling **13:** 425–432.
22. DAUNAIS, J.B. & J.F. MCGINTY. 1996. The effects of D1 or D2 dopamine receptor blockade on zif/268 and preprodynorphin gene expression in rat forebrain following a short-term cocaine binge. Mol. Brain Res. **35:** 237–248.
23. GUEVARA-GUZMAN, R., P.C. EMSON & K.M. KENDRICK. 1994. Modulation of in vivo striatal transmitter release by nitric oxide and cyclic GMP. J. Neurochem. **62:** 807–810.
24. VAANDRAGER, A.B. & H.R. DE JONGE. 1996. Signalling by cGMP-dependent protein kinases. Mol. Cell. Biochem. **157:** 23–30.
25. DE VENTE, J. *et al.* 2001. Localization of cGMP-dependent protein kinase type II in rat brain. Neuroscience **108:** 27–49.
26. SCHWARZ, P.M. *et al.* 1998. Functional coupling of nitric oxide synthase and soluble guanylyl cyclase in controlling catecholamine secretion from bovine chromaffin cells. Neuroscience **82:** 255–265.
27. ZHUO, M. *et al.* 1994. Role of guanylyl cyclase and cGMP-dependent protein kinase in long-term potentiation. Nature **368:** 635–639.

28. GRAY, D.B. *et al.* 1999. A nitric oxide/cyclic GMP-dependent protein kinase pathway alters transmitter release and inhibition by somatostatin at a site downstream of calcium entry. J. Neurochem. **72:** 1981–1990.
29. HELL, J.W. *et al.* 1993. Differential phosphorylation of two size forms of the neuronal class C L-type calcium channel alpha 1 subunit. J. Biol. Chem. **268:** 19451–19457.
30. HELL, J.W. *et al.* 1994. Differential phosphorylation of two size forms of the N-type calcium channel alpha 1 subunit which have different COOH termini. J. Biol. Chem. **269:** 7390–7396.

Gene Expression Related to Synaptogenesis, Neuritogenesis, and MAP Kinase in Behavioral Sensitization to Psychostimulants

HIROSHI UJIKE, MANABU TAKAKI , MASAFUMI KODAMA, AND SHIGETOSHI KURODA

Department of Neuropsychiatry, Okayama University Medical School and Okayama University Graduate School of Medicine and Dentistry, Okayama, Japan

ABSTRACT: The most important characteristic of behavioral sensitization to psychostimulants, such as amphetamine and cocaine, is the very long-lasting hypersensitivity to the drug after cessation of exposure. Rearrangement and structural modification of neural networks in CNS must be involved in behavioral sensitization. Previous microscopic studies have shown that the length of dendrites and density of dendritic spines increased in the nucleus accumbens and frontal cortex after repeated exposure to amphetamine and cocaine, but the molecular mechanisms responsible are not well understood. We investigated a set of genes related to synaptogenesis, neuritogenesis, and mitogen-activated protein (MAP) kinase after exposure to methamphetamine. *Synaptophysin* mRNA, but not *VAMP2* (*synaptobrevin 2*) mRNA, which are considered as synaptogenesis markers, increased in the accumbens, striatum, hippocampus, and several cortices, including the medial frontal cortex, after a single dose of 4 mg/kg methamphetamine. *Stathmin* mRNA, but not *neuritin* or *narp* mRNA, which are markers for neuritic sprouting, increased in the striatum, hippocampus, and cortices after a single dose of methamphetamine. The mRNA of *arc*, an activity-regulated protein associated with cytoskeleton, but not of *alpha-tubulin*, as markers for neuritic elongation, showed robust increases in the striatum, hippocampus, and cortices after a single dose of methamphetamine. The mRNAs of *MAP kinase phosphatase-1 (MKP-1)* , *MKP-3*, and *rheb*, a ras homologue abundant in brain, were investigated to assess the MAP kinase cascades. *MKP-1* and *MKP-3* mRNAs, but not *rheb* mRNA, increased in the striatum, thalamus, and cortices, and in the striatum, hippocampus, and cortices, respectively, after a single methamphetamine. S*ynaptophysin* and *stathmin* mRNAs did not increase again after chronic methamphetamine administration, whereas the increases in *arc*, *MKP-1*, and *MKP-3* mRNAs persisted in the brain regions after chronic methamphetamine administration. These findings indicate that the earlier induction process in behavioral sensitization may require various plastic modifications, such as synaptogenesis, neuritic sprouting, neuritic elongation, and activation of MAP kinase cascades, throughout almost the entire brain. In contrast, later maintenance process of sensitization may require only limited plastic modification in restricted regions.

Address for correspondence: H. Ujike, M.D., Ph.D., Department of Neuropsychiatry, Okayama University Graduate School of Medicine and Dentistry, 2-5-1 Shikata-cho, Okayama 700-8558, Japan. Voice: +81-86-223-7151; fax:+81-86-235-7246.
hujike@cc.okayama-u.ac.jp

Ann. N.Y. Acad. Sci. 965: 55–67 (2002). © 2002 New York Academy of Sciences.

KEYWORDS: behavioral sensitization; methamphetamine; cocaine; plasticity; synaptogenesis; neuritogenesis; MAP kinase

1. INTRODUCTION

Behavioral sensitization or reverse tolerance induced in experimental animals by administration of psychostimulants, including methamphetamine, amphetamine, and cocaine, has been recognized and used in animal models of human methamphetamine psychoses and schizophrenia.[1,2] The rationale for so doing is based on the striking analogy between them, especially in the chronological quantitative and qualitative alterations in the response to psychostimulants. For example, repeated administration of a fixed dose of psychostimulants to rodents induces progressive augmentation in induced abnormal behaviors, such as increased hyperlocomotion and characteristic stereotypes. Such enhanced responses to drugs must be due to the development of altered function and supersensitivity in the host brain. Similar quantitative augmentation and qualitative alterations in response to psychostimulants is commonly observed in human methamphetamine psychoses.[3,4] Abuse of methamphetamine induces euphoria and hyperarousal in the user, but further repeated use induces gradual development of psychotic states, mainly characterized by acoustic hallucinations and delusions. The psychotic symptoms induced by methamphetamine recover relatively rapidly when use is discontinued, but they relapse readily after resumption of the drug, or sometimes in response to alcohol consumption or psychological stress (cross-sensitization). The susceptibility to relapse into psychostimulant-induced psychoses persists even after long-term abstinence; these psychoses are suspected of being the same as in the mechanisms underlying susceptibility to relapse seen in chronic schizophrenics. The most important characteristic of the sensitization phenomenon is the very long persistence of hyperresponsiveness to the drugs. Rats previously sensitized to methamphetamine remain hypersensitive to the psychomotor activating and rewarding effects of a subsequent dose after at least 6 months of abstinence.[5] When the life span of rats is considered, sensitization to the drug seems to be almost perpetual.

Various neurochemical adaptations have been found in the sensitization phenomenon, including up- or down-regulation of D1 dopamine,[6] sigma,[7–9] and neuropeptide receptors,[10–12] altered dopamine transporters mRNA,[13] changes in the alpha and beta subunits of trimeric G proteins[14–16] and enzymes for dopamine synthesis and metabolism,[2] increased adenylyl cyclase activity, cyclic AMP and protein kinase A,[17] increased calmodulin and activated CamK II,[18–20] and increased c-fos and AP-1 binding protein.[21,22] However, since these subcellular neurochemical adaptations are all transient or reversible, they must be converted to more lasting plastic brain changes during sensitization. Previous studies have shown that the protein synthesis inhibitors, anisomycin and cycloheximide, block the development of sensitization,[23,24] and that pups younger than 3 weeks old, which are too immature to develop neural networks, do not become sensitized to psychostimulants.[25,26] This evidence suggests that rearrangement of neural networks and circuitry must develop for the long-lasting plasticity required for sensitization to occur.

Lines of evidence from previous behavioral pharmacological studies have suggested that rearrangement of the neural networks shown in FIGURE 1[27] must develop

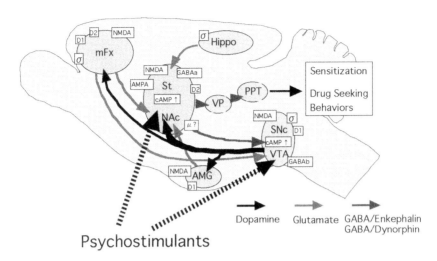

FIGURE 1. Rearrangement of neural network during development of behavioral sensitization to psychostimulants. KEY: mFX: medial frontal cortex; Hippo: hippocampus; St: striatum; NAc: accumbens; VP: ventral pallidum; PPT: pedunclopontine tegmentum nucleus; AMG: amygdala; SNc: substantia nigra pars compacta; VTA: ventral tegmentum area.

during the establishment of behavioral sensitization. The A10 dopaminergic pathway from the ventral tegmentum area (VTA) to mesolimbic areas, such as the nucleus accumbens and medial prefrontal cortex, plays an indispensable role in the development of psychostimulant-induced sensitization; it is also called the "rewarding system." Psychostimulants enhance dopamine release from the synaptic terminals of A10 dopamine neurons in the accumbens, and the "pleasant" or "high feeling" signals are transmitted to the PPT via the ventral pallidum, which ultimately results in drug-seeking behavior and abnormal stereotypy. The output signals from the accumbens may be highly regulated by the glutaminergic afferents from prefrontal cortex, amygdala, and hippocampus. Increased glutamate release in the accumbens also enhanced abnormal stereotyped behaviors. Thus, the VTA–accumbens–frontal cortex–accumbens–VTA circuitry may be constructed and strengthened during the development of sensitization and persist for a very long period. Moreover, microscopic studies with Golgi-staining have demonstrated anatomical changes as a result of exposure to psychostimulants corresponding to such enhanced synaptic connectivity or transduction efficacy in the circuitry.[28,29] Chronic exposure to AMP or cocaine produces an increase in the length of dendrites, the density of dendritic spines, and the number of branched spines on the major output cells of the accumbens and prefrontal cortex, but the precise molecular basis for such morphological changes in response to exposure to psychostimulants is not well understood. To further clarify it, in this study we used *in situ* hybridization and Western blots to assess a set of genes for synaptogenesis, neuritogenesis, and mitogen-activating protein (MAP) kinases, which are involved in very diverse plasticity.

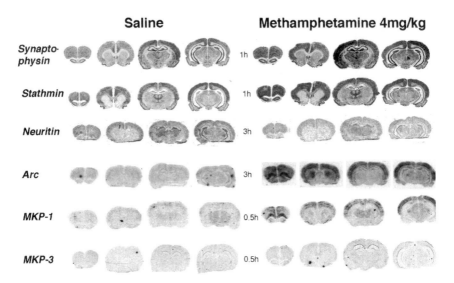

FIGURE 2. Changes in gene expression related to synaptogenesis, neuritogenesis, and MAP kinase phosphatase after a single exposure to methamphetamine. (**a**) *In situ* hybridization images; (**b**) temporal profiles of changes in gene expression. KEY: PFX: prefrontal cortex; CA1: CA1 region of the hippocampus; Cx: cortex. * $p < 0.05$, ** $p < 0.01$, *** $p < 0.001$.

2. GENES RELATED TO SYNAPTOGENESIS FOR THE SENSITIZATION PHENOMENON

The genes *synaptophysin*[30] and *VAMP-2* (also called as *synaptobrevin 2*)[31] were examined as markers for presynaptic plasticity and synaptogenesis. The molecules encoded by these genes are major integral membrane proteins of small presynaptic vesicles that participate in neurotransmitter exocytosis, and they are molecular indicators for synaptic densities. In naive rat brain, *synaptophysin* mRNA is most densely distributed in the hippocampus, whereas its density is moderate in parts of the cortex, such as the temporal cortex, parietal cortex, and occipital cortex, and minimal in the prefrontal cortex, striatum, accumbens, and amygdala (FIG. 2). One 4-mg/kg dose of methamphetamine significantly increased *synaptophysin* mRNA in the prefrontal cortex by about 50% 1 h later, in the temporal cortex 30 min later, in the striatum 1 h later, and in the occipital cortex, the CA1 and CA3 regions of the hippocampus, and the accumbens 3 h later[32] (FIG. 3). The increase in mRNA *synaptophysin* in all regions subsided within 6–24 h after methamphetamine administration. By contrast, *VAMP-2* mRNA was unchanged after an acute dose of methamphetamine. After chronic exposure to methamphetamine for 10 days, *synaptophysin* mRNA was no longer increased in any of the brain regions where increases had been observed after acute methamphetamine administration. These findings indicated that the role of *synaptophysin* in methamphetamine-induced sensitization differs in its early and late phases, in other words, in the induction phase and expression/establishment phase of sensitization. The finding that *synaptophysin* mRNA in-

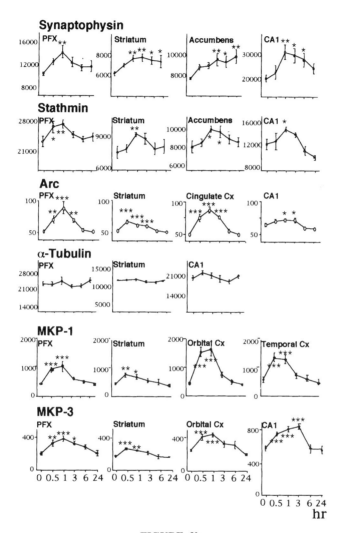

FIGURE 2b.

creased during the process of induction of sensitization not only in the accumbens and striatum, but also in unexpectedly broad areas of several regions of the cortex, including the prefrontal cortex and the hippocampus, was significant, because it implied that widespread synaptogenesis throughout the brain occurs in the early phase of the sensitization process. Previous studies have also revealed alteration of synapse-related molecules after psychostimulant exposure, including an increase in *synaptotagmin IV* mRNA,[33] a synaptic vesicle protein participating in Ca^{2+}-dependent and Ca^{2+}-independent interaction during membrane trafficking, in the striatum after

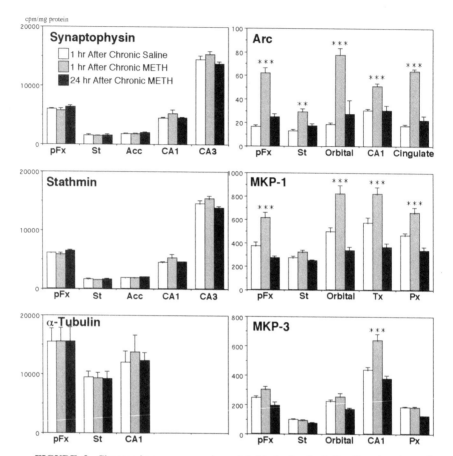

FIGURE 3. Changes in gene expression related to brain plasticity after chronic methamphetamine administration. KEY: METH: methamphetamine; PFX: prefrontal cortex; St: striatum; Acc: accumbens; CA1 and CA3: CA1 and CA3 regions of the hippocampus; Tx: temporal cortex; Px: parietal cortex. $**p < 0.01$, $***p < 0.001$.

cocaine administration. These findings indicate that increases in presynapse markers are not specific to the action of methamphetamine, but a common event after psychostimulant exposure. Increased synapse synthesis may reinforce synaptic connections and enhance neural transduction. Since the extent of synaptic vesicle protein correlates with the extent of neurotransmitter exocytosis, it may also contribute to molecular mechanisms underlying the enhanced dopamine release in the accumbens, striatum, and frontal cortex occurring after the sensitization phenomenon. Another study showed that phosphorylation of synapsin I, another synaptic vesicles docking protein, increased after repeated amphetamine adminsistration.[20,34] Phosphorylated synapsin I, an activated form, renders the dopamine pool in vesicles prone to release. Although methamphetamine-induced dopamine release is mainly caused by its action on the dopamine transporter, it has been suggested that Ca^{2+}-dependent and impulse-dependent exocytosis is also involved.[35] Thus, presynaptic modification by the three molecules mentioned previously must develop after psychostimulant administration, and it may contribute, at least partially, to enhanced dopamine release from the presynaptic terminals of the mesocorticolimbic and nigrostriatal projection after the sensitization phenomenon.

3. GENES RELATED TO NEURITE SPROUTING IN THE SENSITIZATION PHENOMENON

Presynaptic modifications are insufficient for the rearrangement of the neural networks, and corresponding postsynaptic modifications are needed. Three molecules, *stathmin, narp,* and *neuritin,* were examined as markers of neurite sprouting, the first step in neuritogenesis. *Stathmin* is a growth-associated cytosolic phosphoprotein present in the growth cones of neurite ends and is involved in neural plasticity.[36,37] *Narp* belongs to the pentraxin protein family and is expressed in neurites after neural activity.[38] *Narp* is thought to be involved in clustering receptors, such as AMPA glutaminergic receptors (receptor clustering enhances exponentially synaptic conduction).[39] Neuritin is a membrane protein and induces neurite branching.[40]

The distribution of *stathmin* mRNA in naive rat brain was found to be highest in the dentate gyrus of the hippocampus and almost the entire cortex, of a moderate density in the CA1 and CA3 areas of the hippocampus, and of minimal density in the striatum, accumbens, and amygdala (FIG. 2.). Acute methamphetamine administration increased mRNA *stathmin* by about 30% in the prefrontal cortex, striatum, accumbens, temporal cortex, and hippocampus CA1 0.5–1 h after the injection, and it returned to the basal level within 3 h[32] (FIG. 3). Neither *narp* nor *neuritin* mRNA changed after a single methamphetamine dose.

Stathmin is a cytoplasmic phosphoprotein that acts as a growth-associated protein (GAP), and it is involved in plastic adaptation, including regulation of cell proliferation and differentiation.[36,41] The stathmin family is composed of *stathmin, SCG 10,*[41,42] and two recently discovered molecules, *RB3*[43] and *SCLIP,*[44] all of which have been shown to be involved in plasticity. *Stathmin* binds to microtubules and inhibits their assembly, resulting in neuritogenesis through the regulation of dynamic microtubule instability.[45] The increase in *stathmin* mRNA in widespread brain areas after acute methamphetamine almost coincided with the increase in *synaptophysin* mRNA described earlier. These findings may indicate that robust neurite sprouting at postsynaptic sites during the early phase of sensitization occurs in concert with synaptogenesis at presynaptic sites, resulting in a robust and new generation of synaptic connections.

After chronic methamphetamine exposure, *stathmin* mRNA showed a slight decrease in the striatum and accumbens, but not in other brain regions. Another study, however, showed that the phosphorylated form of the GAP molecule, *neuromodulin* (GAP-43), which is its active form, increased in the striatum after chronic amphetamine administration.[34,46] Thus, *neuromodulin*, not *stathmin*, seems to be involved in neurite plasticity in the late phase of stimulant-induced sensitization.

4. GENES RELATED TO NEURITIC ELONGATION IN THE SENSITIZATION PHENOMENON

The development of new neural networks requires the outgrowth and elongation of axons and dendrites, and this must be accompanied by increased synthesis of neuritic components. Since *alpha-tubulin* is a cytoskeletal protein and component of microtubles,[47] and *arc* is an activity-regulated cytoskeleton-associated protein that is localized in the perikarya and dendritic processes and cosedimentates with actin,[48] their mRNAs were examined as markers for neuritic elongation.

After a single dose of methamphetamine adminsitration, arc increased sharply by 70–150% in the frontal cortex, orbital cortex, and cingulate cortex, and by 20–50% in the striatum and hippocampus[51] (FIG. 2). These increases peaked around 1 h after the methamphetamine injection, and the values returned to their basal levels after 6 h. The increases in arc mRNA in every brain region after methamphetamine injection were reversed by coadministration of SCH 23390, a D1 dopamine antagonist, or MK-801, a NMDA antagonist, and both compounds, SCH 23390 and MK-801, have been shown to prevent the development of sensitization to psychostimulants.[49,50] Microscopic autoradiography revealed that increased *arc* mRNAs after methamphetamine exposure in the parietal cortex was abundant in layers IV and VI, and those in the striatum existed mainly in the medium-sized neurons.[51] The D1 receptors in the cortex are mostly distributed in layer VI, which receives mesocortical dopaminergic projections. Accordingly, the enhanced dopamine release induced by methamphetamine may activate *arc* transcription via D1 dopamine receptors, at least in the cortical layer VI. After chronic methamphetamine exposure, the *arc* mRNA response to a methamphetamine challenge was similar to that seen after acute methamphetamine administration and occurred in similar brain regions. These results suggested that every methamphetamine dose, regardless of whether acute or chronic, widely stimulates *arc* synthesis in the brain, including in the hippocampus, corticostriatal, and striatocortical projections, and this may indicate neurite outgrowth and elongation in those areas.

Contrary to our expectations based on the arc findings, the alpha-tubulin mRNA level was constant after methamphetamine exposure,[32] which may mean that the amount of microtubulin was constant. Since disengagement and polymerization of *alpha-tubulin* plays a role in axonal and dendritic outgrowth, polymerization of *alpha-tubulin*, rather than increased synthesis, may be important for neuritogenesis in the sensitization phenomenon. Alternatively, other components of microtubules, for example, microtubule-associated proteins, may be more important for the neural plasticity during sensitization.

5. GENES RELATED TO REGULATION OF MAP KINASE IN THE SENSITIZATION PHENOMENON

The MAP kinase cascades have been shown to play a crucial role in various types of plasticity and adaptation, but its role in behavioral sensitization is still unknown. The MAP kinase family consists of two major subgroups, the extracellular signal-regulated kinase (ERK), which induces cell growth and proliferation (classic MAPK cascade), and the stress-activated protein kinase/c-Jun N-terminal kinase (SAPK/

JNK) and p38, which induce apoptosis, the stress reaction, and gene transcription (novel MAPK cascade). MAP kinases are activated and phosphorylated by MAPKK and MAPKKK and selectively inactivated and dephosphoryrated by mitogen-activated protein phosphatases (MKPs). Many kinds of MKPs are known, but *MKP-1* and *MKP-3* were examined because of their abundant distribution in the brain.[52,53] *Rheb*, a ras homologue, which is abundant in the brain and activates MAPK cascade,[54] was also examined.

MKP-1 mRNA is abundantly distributed in the cerebral cortex and thalamus of the naive rat, whereas *MKP-3* mRNA is restricted to the hippocampus[55] (FIG. 2). *MKP-1* mRNA significantly increased by about 60–300% in the several areas of the cortex, striatum, and thalamus, 0.5–1 h in response to acute and chronic methamphetamine administration (FIGS. 2b and 3). *MKP-3* mRNA had increased by about 50% in the cortex, striatum, and hippocampus 1 h after acute methamphetamine administration, but only in the hippocampus CA1 after chronic methamphetamine administration. Pretreatment with the D1 dopamine antagonist SCH 23390 completely abolished the increase in *MKP-1* and *MKP-3* mRNA levels induced by acute methamphetamine administration, but it was only partially abolished by the NMDA antagonist *MK-801*. The *MKP-1* protein level also increased in the cortex 3 h after acute and chronic methamphetamine administration. *Rheb* mRNA was unchanged after acute and chronic methamphetamine adminsitration. MKPs are inactivators of MAPK,[56,57] but they are directly activated by activation of MAPK. *MKP-1* is selectively activated by SAPK/JNK and p38, and *MKP-3* by ERK.[58,59] Therefore, the increase in *MKP-1* and *MKP-3* mRNAs observed after methamphetamine administration must indicate activation of SAPK/JNK and p38, and ERK, respectively. Taken together, these findings indicate that acute methamphetamine administration may activate both the classic and novel MAPK cascades in several areas of the cortex and striatum, the novel MAPK cascade in the thalamus, and the classic MAPK cascade in the hippocapmus. By contrast, chronic methamphetamine may activate selected MAPKs in restricted regions, that is, the novel MAPK cascade in the frontal cortex and the classic MAPK cascade in the hippocampus.

6. CONCLUSION

The differences in regulation of several genes related to morphological plasticity after acute and subchronic methamphetamine are quite significant, and they are summarized in TABLE 1. The behavioral sensitization phenomenon in response to psychostimulants is considered to consist of two distinct major processes: an early induction process and a later maintenance or expression process. Induction of sensitization has been shown to occur after administration of several doses of psychostimulants. The neurochemical changes in increased dopamine efflux and morphological changes in dendrites and spines in the accumbens and frontal cortex were demonstrated after chronic amphetamine administration. However, recent studies have shown that even a single exposure to amphetamine also induced long-term behavioral and neurochemical sensitization.[60] The neural adaptation during persistent sensitization, such as synaptogenesis and neuritogenesis, must begin with the first psychostimulant exposure, and thus the changes in gene expression seen after a sin-

TABLE 1. Transcriptional changes of neural plasticity-related genes in two phases of behavioral sensitization

	Behavioral Sensitization	
	Induction	Maintenance & Expression
Synaptogenesis		
Synaptophysin	↑ Cx, Acc, St, CA1, CA3	⇄
VAMP2	⇄	n.e.
Neuritic Sprouting		
Stathmin	↑ Cx, Acc, St, CA1	⇄/↓
Neuritin	⇄	n.e.
Narp	⇄	n.e.
Neuritic elongation		
Arc	↑↑↑ Cx, ST, CA1, CA3	↑↑↑ Cx, ST, CA1, CA3
alpha-Tubulin	⇄	⇄
MAP Kinase Cascade		
MKP-1	↑↑↑ CX, ST, Thal	↑ FX, ST
MKP-3	↑ CX, St, CA1, CA3	↑ CA1
Rheb	⇄	n.e.

gle dose of methamphetamine and during chronic administration should correspond to the molecular mechanisms of the induction and maintenance processes of sensitization, respectively. During the induction process of sensitization, various processes involved in the neural adaptation, synaptogenesis, sprouting, and elongation processes, and activation of MAPK cascades begin abruptly throughout almost the entire brain, including the striatum, accumbens, frontal and several areas of cortex, and hippocampus. In contrast, no additional synaptogenesis or sprouting seemed to be required during the maintenance process, because *synaptophysin* and *stathmin* transcription returned to their basal levels. Neurite elongation, indicated by the increased *arc* mRNA, may persist in those brain regions in response to every methamphetamine exposure, and this sustained neurite elongation during repeated methamphetamine administration may contribute to rearrangement of the neural networks for behavioral sensitization. Activation of the novel MAPK kinase cascade in the frontal cortex and classic MAPK cascade in the hippocampus as indicated by the increase in *MKP-1* and *MKP-3* mRNAs, respectively, also persisted during the maintenance process of sensitization. This may imply occurrence of apoptosis in the frontal cortex and neurogenesis in the hippocampus, which has not been demonstrated in the sensitization phenomenon. The actions and roles of many other plasticity-related genes should be investigated to further clarify the molecular mechanisms in very long-lasting neural adaptation during sensitization.

ACKNOWLEDGMENTS

This work was supported in part by a grant from the Zikei Institute of Psychiatry (Okayama, Japan).

REFERENCES

1. AKIYAMA, K., A. KANZAKI, K. TSUCHIDA & H. UJIKE. 1994. Methamphetamine-induced behavioral sensitization and its implications for relapse of schizophrenia. Schizophr. Res. **12:** 251–257.
2. ROBINSON, T.E. & J.B. BECKER. 1986. Enduring changes in brain and behavior produced by chronic amphetamine administration: a review and evaluation of animal models of amphetamine psychosis. Brain Res. Rev. **11:** 157–198.
3. SATO, M., C.C. CHEN, K. AKIYAMA & S. OTSUKI. 1983. Acute exacerbation of paranoid psychotic state after long-term abstinence in patients with previous methamphetamine psychosis. Biol. Psychiatry **18:** 429–440.
4. TATETSU, S. 1963. Methamphetamine psychosis. Folia Pstchiatr. Neurol. Jpn. Suppl. **7:** 377–380.
5. PAULSON, P.E., D.M. CAMP & T.E. ROBINSON. 1991. Time course of transient behavioral depression and persistent behavioral sensitization in relation to regional brain monoamine concentrations during amphetamine withdrawal in rats. Psychopharmacology (Berl.) **103:** 480–492.
6. UJIKE, H. *et al.* 1991. Lasting increase in D1 dopamine receptors in the lateral part of the substantia nigra pars reticulata after subchronic methamphetamine administration. Brain Res. **540:** 159–163.
7. ITZHAK, Y. 1994. Modulation of the PCP/NMDA receptor complex and sigma binding sites by psychostimulants. Neurotoxicol. Teratol. **16:** 363–368.
8. UJIKE, H. *et al.* 1992. Persistent supersensitivity of sigma receptors develops during repeated methamphetamine treatment. Eur. J. Pharmacol. **211:** 323–328.
9. UJIKE, H., K. TSUCHIDA, K. AKIYAMA & S. OTSUKI. 1992. Supersensitivity of sigma receptors after repeated administration of cocaine. Life Sci. **51:** PL31–PL36.
10. UJIKE, H., N. OGAWA & S. OTSUKI. 1988. Effects of acute and long-term treatment with methamphetamine on substance P concentration and receptor numbers in the rat brain. Brain Res. **453:** 136–142.
11. NAKASHIMA, M., S. KAJITA & S. OTSUKI. 1989. Reduction of rat striatal thyrotropin-releasing hormone receptors produced by repeated methamphetamine administration. Biol. Psychiatry **25:** 191–199.
12. WANG, J.Q. & J.F. MCGINTY. 1995. Alterations in striatal zif/268, preprodynorphin and preproenkephalin mRNA expression induced by repeated amphetamine administration in rats. Brain Res. **673:** 262–274.
13. SHILLING, P.D., J.R. KELSOE & D.S. SEGAL. 1997. Dopamine transporter mRNA is upregulated in the substantia nigra and the ventral tegmental area of amphetamine-sensitized rats. Neurosci. Lett. **236:** 131–134.
14. UJIKE, H., K. AKIYAMA & S. KURODA. 1996. Increased Gi alpha and Go alpha mRNAs in hippocampus after repeated methamphetamine administration. Neuroreport **7:** 2036–2040.
15. WANG, X.B. *et al.* 1997. rGbeta1: a psychostimulant-regulated gene essential for establishing cocaine sensitization. J. Neurosci. **17:** 5993–6000.
16. NESTLER, E.J. *et al.* 1990. Chronic cocaine treatment decreases levels of the G protein subunits Giα and Goα in discrete regions of rat brain. J. Neurochem. **55:** 1079–1082.
17. TERWILLIGER, R.Z. *et al.* 1991. A general role for adaptations in G-proteins and the cyclic AMP system in mediating the chronic actions of morphine and cocaine on neuronal function. Brain Res. **548:** 100–110.
18. GNEGY, M.E., G.H. HEWLETT, S.L. YEE & M.J. WELSH. 1991. Alterations in calmodulin content and localization in areas of rat brain after repeated intermittent amphetamine. Brain Res. **562:** 6–12.
19. SHIMIZU, Y. *et al.* 1997. Alterations of calmodulin and its mRNA in rat brain after acute and chronic administration of methamphetamine. Brain Res. **765:** 247–258.
20. IWATA, S.I. *et al.* 1997. Enhanced dopamine release and phosphorylation of synapsin I and neuromodulin in striatal synaptosomes after repeated amphetamine. J. Pharmacol. Exp. Ther. **283:** 1445–1452.
21. GRAYBIEL, A.M., R. MORATALLA & H.A. ROBERTSON. 1990. Amphetamine and cocaine induce drug-specific activation of the c-fos gene in striosome-matrix compartments and limbic subdivisions of the striatum. Proc. Natl. Acad. Sci. USA **87:** 6912–6916.

22. ISHIHARA, T. *et al.* 1996. Activator protein-1 binding activities in discrete regions of rat brain after acute and chronic administration of methamphetamine. J. Neurochem. **67:** 708–716.
23. KARLER, R., K.T. FINNEGAN & L.D. CALDER. 1993. Blockade of behavioral sensitization to cocaine and amphetamine by inhibitors of protein synthesis. Brain Res. **603:** 19–24.
24. SHIMOSATO, K. & T. SAITO. 1993. Suppressive effect of cycloheximide on behavioral sensitization to methamphetamine in mice. Eur. J. Pharmacol. **234:** 67–75.
25. FUJIWARA, Y. *et al.* 1987. Behavioral sensitization to methamphetamine in the rat: an ontogenic study. Psychopharmacology (Berl.) **91:** 316–319.
26. UJIKE, H. *et al.* 1995. Ontogeny of behavioral sensitization to cocaine. Pharmacol. Biochem. Behav. **50:** 613–617.
27. UJIKE, H., M. TAKAKI & S. KURODA. 2002. Neural plasticity-related genes and the behavioral sensitization phenomenon. Psychiatry Clin. Neurosci. In press.
28. ROBINSON, T.E. & B. KOLB. 1997. Persistent structural modifications in nucleus accumbens and prefrontal cortex neurons produced by previous experience with amphetamine. J. Neurosci. **17:** 8491–8497.
29. ROBINSON, T.E. & B. KOLB. 1999. Alterations in the morphology of dendrites and dendritic spines in the nucleus accumbens and prefrontal cortex following repeated treatment with amphetamine or cocaine. Eur. J. Neurosci. **11:** 1598–1604.
30. MARQUEZE-POUEY, B., W. WISDEN, M.L. MALOSIO & H. BETZ. 1991. Differential expression of synaptophysin and synaptoporin mRNAs in the postnatal rat central nervous system. J. Neurosci. **11:** 3388–3397.
31. ARCHER, B.T., III *et al.* 1990. Structures and chromosomal localizations of two human genes encoding synaptobrevins 1 and 2. J. Biol. Chem. **265:** 17267–17273.
32. TAKAKI, M. *et al.* 2001. Increased expression of synaptophysin and staathmin mRNAs after methamphetamine administration in rat brain. Neuroreport **12:** 1055–1060.
33. DENOVAN-WRIGHT, E.M. *et al.* 1998. Acute administration of cocaine, but not amphetamine, increases the level of synaptotagmin IV mRNA in the dorsal striatum of rat. Mol. Brain Res. **55:** 350–354.
34. IWATA, S. *et al.* 1996. Increased in vivo phosphorylation state of neuromodulin and synapsin I in striatum from rats treated with repeated amphetamine. J. Pharmacol. Exp. Ther. **278:** 1428–1434.
35. CASTANEDA, E., J.B. BECKER & T.E. ROBINSON. 1988. The long-term effects of repeated amphetamine treatment in vivo on amphetamine, KCl and electrical stimulation evoked striatal dopamine release in vitro. Life Sci. **42:** 2447–2456.
36. HIMI, T. *et al.* 1994. Differential localization of SCG10 and p19/stathmin messenger RNAs in adult rat brain indicates distinct roles for these growth-associated proteins. Neuroscience **60:** 907–926.
37. SOBEL, A. 1991. Stathmin: a relay phosphoprotein for multiple signal transduction? Trends Biochem. Sci. **16:** 301–305.
38. TSUI, C.C. *et al.* 1996. Narp, a novel member of the pentraxin family, promotes neurite outgrowth and is dynamically regulated by neuronal activity. J. Neurosci. **16:** 2463–2478.
39. O'BRIEN, R.J. *et al.* 1999. Synaptic clustering of AMPA receptors by the extracellular immediate-early gene product Narp. Neuron **23:** 309–323.
40. NAEVE, G.S. *et al.* 1997. Neuritin: a gene induced by neural activity and neurotrophins that promotes neuritogenesis. Proc. Natl. Acad. Sci. USA **94:** 2648–2653.
41. SUGIURA, Y. & N. MORI. 1995. SCG10 expresses growth-associated manner in developing rat brain, but shows a different pattern to p19/stathmin or GAP-43. Brain Res. Dev. Brain Res. **90:** 73–91.
42. MCNEILL, T.H., N. MORI & H.W. CHENG. 1999. Differential regulation of the growth-associated proteins, GAP-43 and SCG-10, in response to unilateral cortical ablation in adult rats. Neuroscience **90:** 1349–1360.
43. BEILHARZ, E.J. *et al.* 1998. Neuronal activity induction of the stathmin-like gene RB3 in the rat hippocampus: possible role in neuronal plasticity. J. Neurosci. **18:** 9780–9789.
44. OZON, S., T. BYK & A. SOBEL. 1998. SCLIP: a novel SCG10-like protein of the stathmin family expressed in the nervous system. J. Neurochem. **70:** 2386–2396.

45. BELMONT, L.D. & T.J. MITCHISON. 1996. Identification of a protein that interacts with tubulin dimers and increases the catastrophe rate of microtubules. Cell **84:** 623–631.
46. GNEGY, M.E., P. HONG & S.T. FERRELL. 1993. Phosphorylation of neuromodulin in rat striatum after acute and repeated, intermittent amphetamine. Brain Res. Mol. Brain Res. **20:** 289–298.
47. MILLER, F.D. *et al.* 1987. Isotypes of alpha-tubulin are differentially regulated during neuronal maturation. J. Cell Biol. **105:** 3065–3073.
48. LYFORD, G.L. *et al.* 1995. Arc, a growth factor and activity-regulated gene, encodes a novel cytoskelton-associated protein that is enriched in neuronal dendrites. Neuron **14:** 43–445.
49. KARLER, R., L.D. CALDER, I.A. CHAUDHRY & S.A. TURKANIS. 1989. Blockade of "reverse tolerance" to cocaine and amphetamine by MK-801. Life Sci. **45:** 599–606.
50. UJIKE, H. *et al.* 1989. Effects of selective D-1 and D-2 dopamine antagonists on development of methamphetamine-induced behavioral sensitization. Psychopharmacology (Berl.) **98:** 89–92.
51. KODAMA, M. *et al.* 1998. A robust increase in expression of arc gene, an effector immediate early gene, in the rat brain after acute and chronic methamphetamine administration. Brain Res. **796:** 273–283.
52. GASS, P. *et al.* 1996. Transient expression of the mitogen-activated protein kinase phosphatase MKP-1 (3CH134/ERP1) in the rat brain after limbic epilepsy. Brain Res. Mol. Brain Res. **41:** 74–80.
53. MUDA, M. *et al.* 1996. MKP-3, a novel cytosolic protein-tyrosine phosphatase that exemplifies a new class of mitogen-activated protein kinase phosphatase. J. Biol. Chem. **271:** 4319–4326.
54. YAMAGATA, K. *et al.* 1994. rheb, A growth factor- and synaptic activity-regulated gene, encodes a novel Ras-related protein. J. Biol. Chem. **269:** 16333–16339.
55. TAKAKI, M. *et al.* 2001. Two kinds of mitogen-activated protein kinase phosphatases, MKP-1 and MKP-3, are differently activated by acute and chronic methamphetamine treatment in the rat brain. J. Neurochem. **79:** 679–688.
56. FRANKLIN, C.C. & A.S. KRAFT. 1997. Conditional expression of the mitogen-activated protein kinase (MAPK) phosphatase MKP-1 preferentially inhibits p38 MAPK and stress-activated protein kinase in U937 cells. J. Biol. Chem. **272:** 16917–16923.
57. MUDA, M. *et al.* 1996. The dual specificity phosphatases M3/6 and MKP-3 are highly selective for inactivation of distinct mitogen-activated protein kinases. J. Biol. Chem. **271:** 27205–27208.
58. BOKEMEYER, D. *et al.* 1996. Induction of mitogen-activated protein kinase phosphatase 1 by the stress-activated protein kinase signaling pathway but not by extracellular signal-regulated kinase in fibroblasts. J. Biol. Chem. **271:** 639–642.
59. CAMPS, M. *et al.* 1998. Catalytic activation of the phosphatase MKP-3 by ERK2 mitogen-activated protein kinase. Science **280:** 1262–1265.
60. VANDERSCHUREN, L.J. *et al.* 1999. A single exposure to amphetamine is sufficient to induce long-term behavioral, neuroendocrine, and neurochemical sensitization in rats. J. Neurosci. **19:** 9579–9586.

Prenatal Exposure to Methamphetamine in the Rat

Ontogeny of Tyrosine Hydroxylase mRNA Expression in Mesencephalic Dopaminergic Neurons

JOANA GOMES-DA-SILVA,[a,b,c] ALBERTO PÉREZ-ROSADO,[d]
ROSARIO DE MIGUEL,[d] JAVIER FERNÁNDEZ-RUIZ,[d]
M. CAROLINA SILVA,[b,c] AND M. AMÉLIA TAVARES[a,c]

[a]Institute of Anatomy, Medical School of Porto, University of Porto, Portugal

[b]Institute for Biomedical Sciences Abel Salazar (ICBAS), University of Porto, Portugal

[c]Institute of Molecular and Cell Biology (IBMC), University of Porto, Portugal

[d]Department of Biochemistry, Faculty of Medicine, Complutense University, Madrid, Spain

ABSTRACT: Methamphetamine (Meth) is an illicit substance known to interfere with catecholaminergic systems and a popular recreational drug among young adult women, that is, in gestational age. Tyrosine hydroxylase (TH), the rate-limiting enzyme of the synthetic pathway of catecholamines, is a good marker to assess potential effects of Meth in catecholaminergic (particularly in dopaminergic) systems. In the rat, prolonged neonatal Meth exposure altered several dopaminergic markers (TH activity and gene expression) in substantia nigra pars compacta (SN) and in caudate-putamen (TH activity) when animals matured. However, it was never verified whether gestational exposure to Meth might compromise TH enzyme in the pups during the neonatal immature periods. The present study was designed to address this issue by analyzing TH gene expression, measured by in situ hybridization in SN and ventral tegmental area (VTA), dopaminergic areas that are well characterized as target areas for Meth, and in rats prenatally exposed to this psychostimulant. To this end, dated pregnant Wistar rat dams received 5 mg Meth hydrochloride/kg body weight/day. It was administered subcutaneously from gestational day 8 until 22. The control group was pair-fed and saline injected, using the same experimental protocol as for Meth-treated dams. On the day of birth (postnatal day 0, PND 0), litters were culled to 8 pups, sex-balanced whenever possible, and were followed until the day of sacrifice (PND 7, 14, or 30). Meth treatment differentially affected TH mRNA levels in VTA and SN, in an age- and gender-dependent manner. Thus, TH mRNA levels were decreased in the VTA of PND 7 and PND 14 females gestationally exposed to Meth; this effect was not evident in males or on PND 30. TH mRNA levels also tend to decrease in SN of PND 14 females gestationally exposed to Meth. Collectively, the present results indicated that gestational Meth exposure affects TH gene expression in the postnatal life, a

Address for correspondence: Joana Gomes-da-Silva, Neurobehaviour Unit, Institute of Molecular and Cell Biology (IBMC), R. Campo Alegre, 823, 4150-180 Porto, Portugal. Voice: 351-22-6074900; fax: 351-22-6099157.

josilva@ibmc.up.pt

Ann. N.Y. Acad. Sci. 965: 68–77 (2002). © 2002 New York Academy of Sciences.

phenomenon that appears to be transient, since it is no longer evident by the end of the first month of life in the rat.

KEYWORDS: methamphetamine; tyrosine hydroxylase; prenatal; postnatal; rat; Wistar rat; substantia nigra; ventral tegmental area; gene expression

INTRODUCTION

Methamphetamine (Meth) is a methylated analog of amphetamine that is known to interfere with several neurotransmitter systems, especially the dopaminergic systems (reviewed in Refs. 1 and 2). Chronic exposure to Meth is described as resulting in long-term alterations of the normal brain function in rodents (reviewed in Ref. 2), nonhuman primates,[3] and humans.[4–7] Experimental exposure to other psychostimulants (cocaine, amphetamine) during gestation alters the patterns of development of the offspring, interfering with the normal development of brain circuitries, as evidenced by morphological and functional alterations in the postnatal period, which can be either transient or permanent (reviewed in Refs. 8–10). These effects include derangement of the dopaminergic systems after prenatal exposure to cocaine, which is evident in the prenatal[11] and postnatal periods.[12,13] Although the studies that characterize the effects of developmental exposure to Meth are relatively scarce, a recent review advanced that the development of neural circuitries might be affected, mainly due to the action of Meth upon the developing dopaminergic and serotonergic systems.[14] In fact, in the rat, prenatal Meth exposure altered monoaminergic markers in caudate-putamen in the postnatal period.[15] Since tyrosine hydroxylase (TH, tyrosine 3-monooxygenase) catalyses the conversion of L-tyrosine to L-3,4-dihydroxyphenylalanine (L-DOPA),[16] it is a good marker to assess potential effects of Meth in developing catecholaminergic (particularly, dopaminergic) systems (reviewed in Ref. 17). The TH enzyme acts early in the development of the central nervous system (CNS), and is connected to the differentiation of neuronal groups.[18,19] It is supposed that TH interferes with the neurochemical processes that control axonal guidance, neuronal recognition, and synaptogenesis (reviewed in Ref. 20). TH is transiently expressed in neuronal groups that, existing only in the fetal period, play an important role on the development of not only catecholaminergic neurons but also of other neuronal groups (reviewed in Ref. 20). Because TH appears to be permanently affected following chronic exposure to Meth,[21] it is possible that the early action of these psychostimulants upon TH gene expression might affect critical processes in dopaminergic development, altering the pattern of maturation of TH containing neurons. This would result in disruption of the DA system itself and of its target areas, potentially leading to long-term changes.[22] The present study aimed to verify whether gestational Meth exposure in the rat could alter TH gene expression in SN and in VTA of developing male and female rats, in an ontogenic manner. To this aim, TH mRNA expression was measured in both mesencephalic areas at three different ages of the first month of life — postnatal days (PND) 7, 14, and 30, which correspond to key ages of development in this species.

MATERIAL AND METHODS

Animals, Treatments, and Sampling

Nulliparous Wistar female rats (60 days old) purchased from the colony of the Gulbenkian Institute for Science, Oeiras, Portugal, were bred in the Institute of Anatomy, Medical School of Porto. Institutional guidelines were followed for animal care. The animals were kept in a room with controlled photoperiod (7:00 A.M.–7:00 P.M.) and temperature ($22 \pm 1°C$). At the onset of breeding, adult females (over 8 weeks old) were placed with males from 8:00 P.M. to 8 A.M. A vaginal smear was then performed; the detection of spermatozoa or vaginal plug was considered a positive mark for pregnancy, and this day was considered GD 1.

Prenatal Exposure to Meth

Females with dated pregnancies were placed in individual cages, and assigned to the experimental groups. From GD 8 until GD 22, females received a dose of 5 mg/kg body weight/day of (±)Meth hydrochloride (SIGMA Chemical Company, St. Louis, MO), prepared in a 0.9% saline vehicle. Meth or saline were injected twice a day, subcutaneously (s.c.). Each dose was split equally, the first injected between 8:30 and 9:00 A.M., and the second between 5:00 and 6:30 P.M., during the daylight phase. Daily food consumption (weight difference to a known value) was registered during the Meth exposure period (GD 8–GD 22). The control groups were pair-fed and saline injected. From GD 8 to GD 22, each female was injected with 0.9% saline, s.c., in a dosage isovolumetric to the Meth dose injected in females of the same weight. Also, each pair-fed female received the average amount of food daily that the Meth-injected females in the same group ate the same gestational day. This procedure allowed the number of dams involved in this study to be kept to the minimum, due to the occurrence of miscarriages and mortality in Meth-treated dams, as well as differences in weight evolution in the control and Meth-treated females.

After the first meal on the day of birth (PND 0), litters were reduced whenever possible to eight animals, sex-balanced—four females and four males. Pups were weaned on PND 21. Rats were sacrificed by decapitation on PND 7, 14, and 30. The whole brain was quickly removed, frozen by immersion in 2-methylbutane over dry ice, and kept at −80°C until assayed.

In situ Hybridization of TH mRNA

Coronal brain sections (20 mm) corresponding to the SN/VTA area (referenced to the atlas of Paxinos and Watson[23]) were cut in a cryostat at −20°C, collected in RNAse-free gelatinized slides, and kept at −80°C until assayed. The analysis of TH mRNA levels was carried out according to Garcia-Gil et al.,[24] with minor modifications previously described.[25] Briefly, slides were allowed to dry at room temperature for 10 min. Then they were fixed in 4% paraformaldehyde prepared in PBS, dehydrated and delipidated in an ethanol-chloroform series, and rehydrated. After washing in 1% sodium citrate buffer and in distilled water, sections were hybridized overnight in hybridization buffer. The probe used for the hybridization was complementary to bases 1223–1252 (DuPont, ITISA, Madrid, Spain) of the TH cDNA. The oligonucleotide probe was 3′-end labeled with [^{35}S]-dATP (2.5×10^5 dpm per section; Amersham Pharmacia Biotech., Madrid, Spain), using terminal deoxynucleoti-dyl-transferase (Boehinger Mannheim, Barcelona, Spain). Slides were then washed, exposed to X-ray films (Hyperfilm βmax, Amersham Iberica, Madrid, Spain) for 5 days, and developed for 6 min at 20°C (D-19, Kodak). The intensity of the hybrid-ization signal was assessed by measuring the gray levels in the autoradiographic films, using a computer-assisted videodensitometer (ImageQuant 3,3, Molecular Di-namics). Values were expressed as arbitrary units of optical density (referred to a ref-erence scale of gray levels) and represent means + standard error of the mean (SEM) of three to six animals per group, proceeding from three or four distinct litters per treatment.

Statistics

For data analysis, the normality of distribution was tested and three-way analysis of variance (ANOVA; age × gender × treatment) was applied to the results in both brain areas, as required, followed by an appropriate *post hoc* test (Student–Newman–Keuls).

RESULTS

The levels of TH mRNA in the SN of PND 7, 14, and 30 male and female rats, gestationally exposed to Meth (GD 8 until GD 22) or vehicle and pair-fed, are shown in FIGURE 1. In SN, TH gene expression varies with age [$F(2, 48) = 34.43$, $p < 0.0001$] and decreases throughout the first month of postnatal life, from PND 7 to PND 14, and from this age to PND 30. The effect of gestational Meth exposure is only apparent as a trend in the three-way interaction age × treatment × gender [F(2,

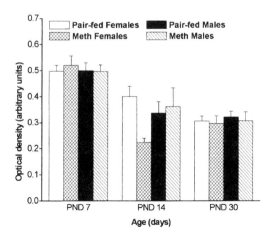

FIGURE 1. TH mRNA levels in the substantia nigra of male and female PND 7, 14, and 30 rats, prenatally exposed to Meth or saline and pair-fed. Values shown are mean + SEM of 3 to 8 determinations per group, expressed in arbitrary units of optical density.

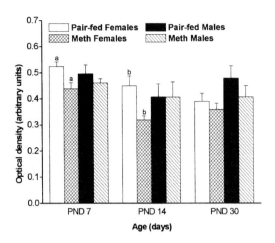

FIGURE 2. TH mRNA levels in the VTA of male and female PND 7, 14, and 30 rats, prenatally exposed to Meth or saline and pair-fed. Values shown are mean + SEM of 2 to 6 determinations per group, expressed in arbitrary units of optical density. Columns with the same letter (a or b) are statistically different ($p < 0.05$).

48) = 2.76, $p = 0.0732$], reflecting the tendency of PND 14 Meth-exposed females to have lower TH gene expression in SN than their controls. However, these results only represent a nonsignificant tendency, as mentioned earlier. In SN, TH gene expression does not vary with the other variables (gender and treatment) or interaction of variables.

FIGURE 2 represents the levels of TH gene expression in the VTA of PND 7, 14, and 30 male and female rats, gestationally exposed to Meth (GD 8 until GD 22) or vehicle and pair-fed. In VTA, TH mRNA expression is significantly affected by Meth treatment [$F(1, 42) = 7.45$, $p < 0.01$] and also varied with age [$F(2, 42) = 5.26$, $p < 0.01$]. In PND 7 and 14, Meth-exposed females have lower TH mRNA expression than the respective pair-fed controls ($p < 0.05$, at both ages). In PND 30, this effect is only tendential. Overall, in VTA, TH gene expression in PND 7 is higher than in PND 14 and 30 rats, regardless of treatment (gestational Meth exposure and respective pair-fed controls). TH gene expression is not affected by gender or by the interaction of variables.

Representative autoradiograms of slide-mounted brain sections of PND 7, 14, and 30 female rats, prenatally exposed to Meth or saline and pair-fed, that were used for the analysis of TH mRNA levels in SN and in VTA, are shown in FIGURE 3.

DISCUSSION

In the present work, the hypothesis tested was whether Meth exposure during the prenatal period of development of the rat might alter TH gene expression in mesencephalic dopaminergic areas during postnatal development. To achieve this objective, pregnant Wistar rats were administered Meth throughout the period of prenatal

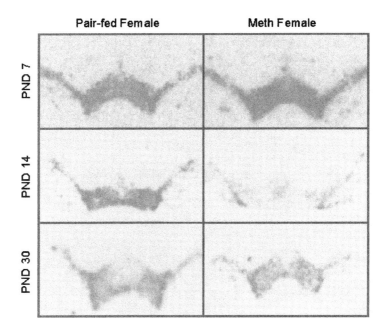

FIGURE 3. Representative autoradiograms for the analysis of TH mRNA levels in slide-mounted brain sections of PND 7, 14, and 30 female rats, prenatally exposed to Meth or saline and pair-fed.

development of dopaminergic systems, and pups were analyzed at key ages (PND 7, 14, and 30) of the first month of postnatal life. Male and female pups were assessed, since gender is a relevant factor concerning the action of Meth.[25,26]

The dopaminergic areas analyzed in the present study (SN and VTA) underlie the control of important behaviors (locomotion, motivation) and emotions (affection), and are deeply involved in phenomena associated with brain reward and addiction to drugs of abuse (reviewed in Refs. 27 and 28). SN and VTA are brain areas that start to differentiate early in the prenatal period,[18] and by GD 18 and 21 the morphology and distribution of TH-containing neurons resemble those of the adult rat brain.[19] In the fetal rat, TH gene expression is detected first at GD 13 in the ventral caudal mesencephalon, using *in situ* hybridization of TH mRNA.[29] By GD 18, it is possible to differentiate the developing VTA (midline) and SN (winglike lateral extensions), and by the time of birth the cells that express TH correspond to those in the adult.[29] In the present study, Meth exposure occurs from GD 8 until GD 22, thus covering the whole period of prenatal ontogeny of TH gene expression in the ventral mesencephalon in the rat.

The results presented here show that PND 7 and 14 female rats gestationally exposed to Meth have lower TH gene expression in the VTA. The hypothesis that TH gene expression might be altered by prenatal exposure to other drugs of abuse was analyzed in a few studies, with distinct outcomes. Prenatal exposure to cocaine

(40 mg/kg/day, s.c., from GD 8 to GD 20) did not alter several dopaminergic markers in preweanling (PND 21) male and female Sprague-Dawley rats, namely, mRNA levels of TH and dopamine transporter (DAT) in SN and VTA, D1 and D2 receptors in dorsolateral or medial caudate-putamen, nucleus accumbens core, and shell.[30] It was suggested that either the experimental paradigm employed has no effect, or by PND 21 the effects may be resolved.[30] Our findings that prenatal Meth exposure altered TH gene expression in VTA on PND 7 and 14, but not on PND 30, confirm the relevance of age in the analysis of the effects of exposure to psychostimulants. Prenatal ethanol exposure throughout pregnancy also alters dopaminergic gene expression in adult male Sprague-Dawley rat offspring,[31] decreasing DAT mRNA in SN and VTA and TH mRNA in VTA, but has no significant effect on either TH or norepinephrine transporter mRNA expression in the locus coeruleus. Accordingly, the present results show that prenatal Meth decreases TH gene expression in VTA and, as was reported for prenatal ethanol,[31] SN appears to be less susceptible. However, the effects observed in VTA occur only in females and are resolved by PND 30. It was previously reported by us that prolonged neonatal Meth exposure altered TH gene expression in the SN of PND 30 rats[25] in a gender-dependent manner; only males evidenced such alterations. The combined observations indicate substantial differences in the effects of developmental Meth exposure, depending on such factors as gender and timing of drug exposure. The molecular mechanisms that lead to the alteration in TH gene expression after Meth exposure are still unclear. TH gene expression is modulated by a complex group of mechanisms, including transcriptional processes, which alter *de novo* protein synthesis (reviewed in Refs. 32 and 33). Mitogen-activated (MAP) kinases, cyclic-adenosine-monophosphate-dependent (c-AMP) and Ca^{2+}/calmodulin-dependent protein kinases are second messengers involved in the induction of immediate early genes that induce TH gene (this topic was previously reviewed by some of us[34]). The major response elements in the proximal promoter region of TH gene are activating protein-1 (AP-1) and cAMP responsive element (CRE),[35,36] and these elements are induced following Meth exposure,[37–40] depending on the type of exposure (acute or chronic) and the time of evaluation.[41] The involvement of such biochemical indicators in modulating *in vivo* TH gene expression after Meth exposure is complex, and factors such as duration of Meth exposure and the developmental stage of the subjects will probably determine the response.

The present report is the first that demonstrates that gestational Meth exposure affects TH mRNA levels in VTA in an age and gender-dependent manner. TH gene expression in the VTA of PND 7 and PND 14 females that have been gestationally exposed to Meth was significantly lower than in respective controls; this effect is not evident in males and is no longer evident on PND 30. The involvement of VTA in phenomena related to brain reward and addiction to drugs of abuse[27,28] raises the concern of whether the differences found in female offspring might translate into functional alterations of the CNS. In SN, TH gene expression at PND 7, 14, or 30 is not affected by gestational exposure to Meth, although PND 14 Meth-exposed female rats tend to have lower TH gene expression than the respective pair-fed controls. Collectively, the present results indicate that Meth exposure during gestation can affect TH gene expression in postnatal life, a phenomenon that appears to be transient, since it is no longer evident by the end of the rats' first month of life.

CONCLUSIONS

Prenatal exposure to Meth alters TH gene expression in the VTA of female rat offspring. Male rats do not exhibit changes in TH mRNA expression in SN or VTA. The decrement of TH gene expression in the VTA at PND 7 and 14 female rats that were prenatally exposed to Meth is no longer observed in the end of the first month of life.

ACKNOWLEDGMENTS

This work was supported by Project PECS/C/SAU/87/95 (JNICT/FCT) and Programa de Financiamento Plurianual (IBMC) and J. Gomes da Silva was supported by PRAXIS BD 9279/96 Sub-Programa Ciência e Tecnologia do 2° Quadro Comunitário de Apoio. We thank M. Manuela Pacheco for assistance with animal handling and technical support throughout the development of this project.

REFERENCES

1. SEIDEN, L.S. & G.A. RICAURTE. 1987. Neurotoxicity of methamphetamine and related drugs. *In* Psychopharmacology: The Third Generation of Progress, H. Y. Meltzer, Ed.: 356–366. Raven Press. New York.
2. GIBB, J.W. *et al.* 1997. Neurotoxicity of amphetamines and their metabolites. NIDA Res. Monogr. **173:** 128–145.
3. VILLEMAGNE, V. *et al.* 1998. Brain dopamine neurotoxicity in baboons treated with doses of methamphetamine comparable to those recreationally abused by humans: evidence from [11C]WIN-35,428 positron emission tomography studies and direct in vitro determinations. J. Neurosci. **18:** 419–427.
4. MCCANN, U.D. *et al.* 1998. Reduced striatal dopamine transporter density in abstinent methamphetamine and methcathinone users: evidence from positron emission tomography studies with [11C]WIN-35,428. J. Neurosci. **18:** 8417–8422.
5. ERNST, T., L. CHANG, M. LEONIDO-YEE & O. SPECK. 2000. Evidence for long-term neurotoxicity associated with methamphetamine abuse: A 1H MRS study. Neurology **54:** 1344–1349.
6. VOLKOW, N.D. *et al.* 2001. Higher cortical and lower subcortical metabolism in detoxified methamphetamine abusers. Am. J. Psychiatry **158:** 383–389.
7. VOLKOW, N.D. *et al.* 2001. Association of dopamine transporter reduction with psychomotor impairment in methamphetamine abusers. Am. J. Psychiatry **158:** 377–382.
8. MIDDAUGH, L.D. 1989. Prenatal amphetamine effects on behavior: possible mediation by brain monoamines. Ann. N.Y. Acad. Sci. **562:** 308–318.
9. DOW-EDWARDS, D., L. MAYES, L. SPEAR & Y. HURD. 1999. Cocaine and development: clinical, behavioral, and neurobiological perspectives—A symposium report. Neurotoxicol. Teratol. **21:** 481–490.
10. MAYES, L.C. 1999. Developing brain and in utero cocaine exposure: effects on neural ontogeny. Dev. Psychopathol. **11:** 685–714.
11. MEYER, J.S. & S.A. DUPONT. 1993. Prenatal cocaine administration stimulates fetal brain tyrosine hydroxylase activity. Brain Res. **608:** 129–137.
12. MILLER, M.W., R. WAZIRI, S. BARUAH & D.M. GILLIAM. 1995. Long-term consequences of prenatal cocaine exposure on biogenic amines in the brains of mice: the role of sex. Brain Res. Dev. Brain Res. **87:** 22–28.
13. CHOI, S.J., E. MAZZIO, M.G. KOLTA & K.F. SOLIMAN. 1998. Prenatal cocaine exposure affects postnatal dopaminergic systems in various regions of the rat brain. Ann. N.Y. Acad. Sci. **844:** 293–302.

14. FROST, D.O. & J. CADET. 2000. Effects of methamphetamine-induced neurotoxicity on the development of neural circuitry: a hypothesis. Brain Res. Brain Res. Rev. **34:** 103–118.
15. ACUFF-SMITH, K.D., M.A. SCHILLING, J.E. FISHER & C.V. VORHEES. 1996. Stage-specific effects of prenatal d-methamphetamine exposure on behavioral and eye development in rats. Neurotoxicol. Teratol. **18:** 199–215.
16. NAGATSU, T., M. LEVITT & S. UDENFRIEND. 1964. Tyrosine hydroxylase. The initial step in norepinephrine biosynthesis. J. Biol. Chem. **239:** 2910–2917.
17. VORHEES, C.V. & C. PU. 1995. Ontogeny of methamphetamine-induced neurotoxicity in the rat model. NIDA Res. Monogr. **158:** 149–171.
18. SPECHT, L.A., V.M. PICKEL, T.H. JOH &. D.J. REIS. 1981. Light microscopic immunocytochemical localisation of tyrosine hydroxylase in prenatal rat brain. I. Early ontogeny. J. Comp. Neurol. **199:** 233–245.
19. SPECHT, L.A., V.M. PICKEL, T.H. JOH & D.J. REIS. 1981. Light-microscopic immunocytochemical localization of tyrosine hydroxylase in prenatal rat brain. II. Late ontogeny. J. Comp. Neurol. **199:** 255–276.
20. FERNÁNDEZ-RUIZ, J.J., F. RODRIGUEZ, M. NAVARRO & J.A. RAMOS.1992. Maternal cannabinoid exposure and brain development: changes in the ontogeny of dopaminergic neurons. In Marihuana/Cannabinoids: Neurobiology and Neurophysiology, I.I. Murphy and A. Bartke, Eds.: 119–164. CRC Press. Boca Raton, FL.
21. TRULSON, M.E., M.S. CANNON, T.S. FAEGG & J.D. RAESE. 1985. Effects of chronic methamphetamine on the nigral-striatal dopamine system in rat brain: tyrosine hydroxylase immunochemistry and quantitative light microscopic studies. Brain Res. Bull. **15:** 569–577.
22. BONNIN, A. et al. 1994. Changes in tyrosine hydroxylase gene expression in mesencephalic catecholaminergic neurons of immature and adult male rats perinatally exposed to cannabinoids. Brain Res. Dev. Brain Res. **81:** 147–150.
23. PAXINOS, G. & C. WATSON. 1986. The Rat Brain in Stereotaxic Coordinates. Academic Press. New York.
24. GARCÍA-GIL, L. et al. 1998. Perinatal Δ^9-tetrahydrocannabinol exposure did not alter dopamine transporter and tyrosine hydroxylase mRNA levels in midbrain dopaminergic neurons of the adult male and female rats. Neurotoxicol. Teratol. **20:** 549–553.
25. GOMES-DA-SILVA, J. et al. 2000. Neonatal methamphetamine in the rat: evidences for gender-specific differences upon tyrosine hydroxylase in the nigrostriatal dopaminergic system. Ann. N.Y. Acad. Sci. **914:** 431–438.
26. WAGNER, G.C., T.L. TEKIRIAN & C.T. CHEO. 1993. Sexual differences in sensitivity to methamphetamine toxicity. J. Neural Transm. Gen. Sect. **93:** 67–70.
27. KOOB, G.F. 1992. Drugs of abuse: anatomy, pharmacology and function of reward pathways. Trends Pharmacol. Sci. **13:** 177–184.
28. KOOB, G.F. 1998. Circuits, drugs, and drug addiction. Adv. Pharmacol. **42:** 978–982.
29. BURGUNDER, J.M. & W.S. YOUNG III. 1990. Ontogeny of tyrosine hydroxylase and cholecystokinin gene expression in the rat mesencephalon. Brain Res. Dev. Brain Res. **52:** 85–93.
30. DE BARTOLOMEIS, A. et al. 1994. Dopaminergic and peptidergic mRNA levels in juvenile rat brain after prenatal cocaine treatment. Brain Res. Mol. Brain Res. **21:** 321–332.
31. SZOT, P., S.S. WHITE, R.C. VEITH & D.D. RASMUSSEN. 1999. Reduced gene expression for dopamine biosynthesis and transport in midbrain neurons of adult male rats exposed prenatally to ethanol. Alcohol Clin. Exp. Res. **23:** 1643–1649.
32. KUMER, S.C. & K.E. VRANA. 1996. Intricate regulation of tyrosine hydroxylase activity and gene expression. J. Neurochem. **67:** 443–462.
33. DU, X. & L. IACOVITTI. 1997. Multiple signaling pathways direct the initiation of tyrosine hydroxylase gene expression in cultured brain neurons. Brain Res. Mol. Brain Res. **50:** 1–8.
34. HERNANDEZ, M. et al. 2000. Cannabinoid CB(1) receptors colocalize with tyrosine hydroxylase in cultured fetal mesencephalic neurons and their activation increases the levels of this enzyme. Brain Res. **857:** 56–65.
35. TANK, A.W. et al. 1998. Regulation of tyrosine hydroxylase gene expression by trans-synaptic mechanisms and cell-cell contact. Adv. Pharmacol. **42:** 25–29.

36. JOH, T.H. *et al.* 1998. Unique and cell-type-specific tyrosine hydroxylase gene expression. Adv. Pharmacol. **42:** 33–36.
37. SHENG, P. *et al.* 1996. Methamphetamine-induced neurotoxicity is associated with increased striatal AP-1 DNA-binding activity in mice. Brain Res. Mol. Brain Res. **42:** 171–174.
38. SHENG, P. *et al.* 1996. AP-1 DNA-binding activation by methamphetamine involves oxidative stress. Synapse **24:** 213–217.
39. ASANUMA, M., H. HIRATA & J.L. CADET. 1998. Attenuation of 6-hydroxydopamine-induced dopaminergic nigrostriatal lesions in superoxide dismutase transgenic mice. Neuroscience **85:** 907–917.
40. ASANUMA, M. *et al.* 2000. Direct interactions of methamphetamine with the nucleus. Brain Res. Mol. Brain Res. **80:** 237–243.
41. AKIYAMA, K., T. ISHIHARA & K. KASHIHARA. 1996. Effect of acute and chronic administration of methamphetamine on activator protein-1 binding activities in the rat brain regions. Ann. N.Y. Acad. Sci. **801:** 13–28.

Neuroadaptive Changes in NMDAR1 Gene Expression after Extinction of Cocaine Self-Administration

JOSÉ A. CRESPO,[a] JOSÉ M. OLIVA,[a] M. BEHNAM GHASEMZADEH,[b] PETER W. KALIVAS,[b] AND E. AMBROSIO[a]

[a]Departamento de Psicobiología, Universidad Nacional de Educación a Distancia (UNED), Ciudad Universitaria, 28040 Madrid, Spain

[b]Department of Physiology and Neuroscience, Medical University of South Carolina, Charleston, South Carolina 29425, USA

ABSTRACT: The aim of the present work was to study the time course effects in levels of mRNA encoding N-methyl-D-aspartate receptor subunit 1 (NMDAR1) after long-term cocaine self-administration (1 mg/kg/ injection) and its extinction using a yoked-box procedure. NMDAR1 content was measured by quantitative *in situ* hybridization histochemistry in prefrontal cortex, caudate-putamen, nucleus accumbens, olfactory tubercle, and piriform cortex immediately after cessation of the last session of cocaine self-administration (Day 0) and 1, 5, and 10 days after the extinction period. The results show that long-term cocaine self-administration and its extinction alter NMDAR1 gene expression in these forebrain regions, and that the changes depend upon the brain region examined and the type of cocaine administration (contingent, noncontingent, and saline). Compared to saline and noncontingent cocaine administration, contingent cocaine produced an up-regulation in NMDAR1 gene expression on Day 0 in all the brain regions analyzed. NMDAR1 levels of contingent animals decreased progressively in the absence of cocaine, and the decrement persisted 10 days after the extinction of cocaine self-administration behavior in all the forebrain areas, with the exception of olfactory tubercle. In contrast, noncontingent cocaine administration did not produce any change in NMDAR1 gene expression on Day 0, and extinction resulted in an increase of NMDAR1 mRNA content on Days 1 and 5 and returned to control (saline) values on Day 10. These results suggest that an interaction between environmental stimuli and the pharmacological action of cocaine during drug self-administration and its extinction may represent an important factor in the regulation of cocaine effects on NMDAR1 gene expression.

KEYWORDS: extinction; cocaine self-administration; glutamate; NMDAR1; gene expression; withdrawal

Address for correspondence: Emilio Ambrosio, Departamento de Psicobiología, Universidad Nacional de Educación a Distancia (UNED), Ciudad Universitaria, 28040 Madrid, Spain. Voice: 34-91-398 7974; fax: 34-91-398 6287.
eambrosio@psi.uned.es

Ann. N.Y. Acad. Sci. 965: 78–91 (2002). © 2002 New York Academy of Sciences.

INTRODUCTION

Addiction to cocaine continues to be a serious public health problem throughout the world. Acquiring detailed understanding of the effects of cocaine in the central nervous system is a critical factor in resolving this problem. Substantial evidence has accumulated over the last several years that the mesolimbic and mesocortical dopamine systems, which project from the ventral tegmental area to the nucleus accumbens and prefrontal cortex, respectively, are involved in cocaine reward function.[1] However, cocaine exhibits a complex pharmacology that includes significant interactions with several neurotransmitter systems in addition to dopamine. Thus, a number of studies have suggested a role for glutamate transmission in the expression of locomotor-stimulating, stereotypy-stimulating, and reinforcing effects of cocaine.[2–9]

Chronic cocaine administration produces an abundance of long-lasting neuroadaptations.[10–12] Most of the studies investigating neural plasticity associated with cocaine addiction have focused on changes in dopamine transmission. However, several studies have shown the involvement of excitatory amino acid neurotransmission in the nucleus accumbens and ventral tegmental area in the long-term neuroadaptations produced by repeated cocaine. These studies have demonstrated that repeated cocaine administration results in an increased elevation of extracellular glutamate levels in both the nucleus accumbens and ventral tegmental area that in part parallels the time course of behavioral sensitization.[7,13,14] In addition, repeated cocaine administration augments the behavioral activation elicited by an α-amino-3-hydroxy-5-mmethylisoxazole-4-propionic acid (AMPA) or N-methyl-D-aspartate (NMDA) agonist microinjected into the nucleus accumbens[6] as well as increases the level of immunoreactive GluR1 subunit of AMPA glutamate receptors in the nucleus accumbens[15] Moreover, inhibition of NMDA or AMPA receptors prevents the induction of cocaine sensitization.[16,17] Recently, it has been reported that stimulation of glutamate receptors in the nucleus accumbens augments the reinforcing effect of cocaine, although glutamate transmission in not required to maintain cocaine self-administration.[9] Little is known, however, about the neuroadaptation of regulatory elements of glutamatergic neurotransmission in cocaine withdrawal.

The majority of studies investigating cocaine-induced neuroadaptation use repeated noncontingent administration of the drug, while fewer studies employ cocaine self-administration. However, previous studies have shown that contingent administration of reinforcing events results in significant differences in neurobiological measures compared with the noncontingent delivery of the same reinforcing event.[18–24]

The aim of the present work was to study the time-course effects in levels of mRNA encoding N-methyl-D-aspartate receptor subunit 1 (NMDAR1)[25] after long-term cocaine self-administration and its extinction using a yoked-box procedure. This procedure allows testing of the relative differences related to contingent versus noncontingent cocaine administration.[26] The gene expression of NMDAR1 glutamate receptor subunit was measured by quantitative *in situ* hybridization histochemistry in forebrain regions—prefrontal cortex, caudate-putamen, nucleus accumbens, olfactory tubercle and piriform cortex—involved in cocaine-reinforcing effects.[27]

MATERIALS AND METHODS

Animals

Adult male Lewis rats (CRIFFA, France) weighing approximately 300–350 g at the beginning of their training were used. All animals were experimentally naive, housed individually in a temperature-controlled room (23°C) with a 12-h light–dark cycle (08:00–20:00 lights on) and given free access to Purina laboratory chow and tap water prior to initiation of the experiments. Animals used in this study were maintained in facilities according to European Union Laboratory Animal Care Rules.

Surgery

Experimentally naive subjects were surgically prepared with an i.v. catheter placed in the jugular vein. Polyvinylchloride tubing (0.064 i.d.) was implanted in the right jugular vein approximately at the level of the atrium under ketamine and diazepam anesthesia. The catheter was passed s.c. and exited in the midscapular region. The catheter then passed through a spring tether system (Alice King Chatham, USA) that was mounted to the skull of the rat with dental cement. All subjects were housed individually following surgery and given at least 7 days to recover.

Apparatus

Twelve operant chambers (Coulburn Instruments, USA) were used for cocaine self-administration studies. Two levers designed to register a response when 3.0 g of force was applied were placed 14 cm apart on the front wall of the chamber. A microliter injection pump (Harvard 22) was used to deliver i.v saline or drug injections to the rat. Drug delivery and operant data acquisition and storage were accomplished on IBM computers (Med Associates, USA).

Experimental Procedure

Cocaine-reinforced behavior was studied according to a procedure described previously.[28] Briefly stated, before surgical implantation of the i.v. catheter, animals were trained to lever-press for food reinforcement under a fixed ratio-five (FR5) schedule of reinforcement. Initially, a single lever press on the left-hand lever resulted in delivery of a food pellet (45 mg, Noyes Pellets, USA) and turned on a stimulus light above the lever. After responding was initiated, the response requirement to food delivery was raised in increments to 5 and a programmed 30-s time-out (TO) period, in which responses had no programmed consequences, followed each food pellet delivery (FR5:TO 30 s). When behavior was maintained under the FR5 schedule of food-reinforced behavior, the catheter was surgically implanted as described.

After the postoperative period, 72 littermate male Lewis rats were randomly assigned in triads to one of three conditions: (a) contingent i.v self-administration of 1 mg/kg/injection of cocaine (Cont) or (b) noncontingent i.v injections of either 1 mg/kg of cocaine (NonCont) or (c) saline (Saline) yoked to the intake of the self-administering subject. Initially, substitution of food delivery by cocaine began under a FR1 schedule of reinforcement and was subsequently raised to FR5. In this case, a programmed 30-s time-out, in which responses had no programmed consequences, followed each cocaine injection (FR5:TO 30 s). Animals were allowed to self-administer cocaine in daily 2-h sessions between 9:00 and 14:00 h, 7 days a week for a minimum of 3 weeks. After stable behavior was established (less than 10% of variability in the number of injections for 5 sequential days), saline was substituted for 4 days in the operant chambers. After this first extinction period, cocaine self-administration behavior was reinstated and maintained for 2 weeks. Saline substitution was carried out again for 1, 5, and 10 days in the operant chambers. Immediately after the last day of cocaine self-administration in which the animals reached the stability criterion (Day 0) and after 1-day (Day 1), 5-day (Day 5) and 10-day (Day 10) period of extinction, animal brains of each triad were removed to be processed for quantitative *in situ* hybridization histochemistry. The number of subjects in each group of triads was 18 (Cont = 6; NonCont = 6: Saline = 6) and the total number of brains removed was 72 [4 groups of triads (Day 0, Day 1, Day 5 and Day 10) × 18].

Quantitative In Situ *Hybridization Histochemistry*

Brain sections (six slides/level; two sections/slide) were serially cut at 20 μm from 3.4 mm anterior to bregma to 2.2 mm posterior to bregma to include the medial prefrontal cortex (MPFC), caudate-putamen (CPU), nucleus accumbens (NAc), olfactory tubercle (TU), and piriform cortex (PIR), according to the Paxinos and Watson atlas.[29] These brain sections were adjacent to those of a previous study.[24] The sections were mounted onto gelatin-coated slides and stored at −80°C until the day of the assay. Quantitative *in situ* hybridization histochemistry for NMDAR1 glutamate receptor subunit was accomplished according to previously described procedures.[30,31] Briefly, oligodeoxyribonucleotide probes specific for NMDAR1 mRNA were made according to published cDNA sequences[25] and 3′-end-tailed with terminal deoxynucleotidyltransferase using ^{35}S-dATP nucleotide (DU Pont-NEN, USA). For prehybridization, cryostat sections were rinsed in 4% paraformaldehyde in 0.1 M phosphate buffer, pH 7.4 (10 min); 3 X phosphate-buffered saline (5 min); 0.1 M triethanolamine (pH 8.0) with 0.25% acetic acid anhydride (10 min); phosphate-buffered saline (5 min); and graded ethanol solutions (2 min each). Hybridization was performed in a buffer of 50% formamide, 0.3 M NaCl, 10 mM Tris (pH 8.0), 1 mM EDTA (pH 8.0), 10% dextran sulfate, 1 X Denhardt's solution, 100 mM dithiothreitol, and ≅ 30,000 dpm/μl labeled probe at 37°C overnight. Cold competition controls were hybridized with a 25-fold excess of unlabeled probe added to the hybridization buffer. Posthybridization washes were performed to a maximal stringency of 0.5 X standard saline citrate (SSC) at 60°C for 40 min. The sections were exposed to β-Max Hyperfilm (Amersham) for 3 weeks. All sections from all the extinction groups were processed for *in situ* hybridization in a single batch to ensure identical experimental conditions and treatment. Films were developed and optical densities of the autoradiograms analyzed with reference to coexposed standard ^{14}C-microscales (Amersham). Two slides per level (two slices/slide; two measurement/slice) in each animal were analyzed with a PC computer using the public-domain NIH Image program. Measurement were pooled from brain sections and the values averaged. Additional brain sections were cohybridized with a 100-fold excess of cold probes or with RNAse to assert the specificity of the signal. As expected, no hybridization signal was detected in these sections (data not shown).

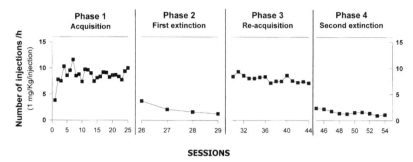

SESSIONS

FIGURE 1. Behavioral responses during cocaine self-administration behavior and its extinction in contingent, noncontingent, and saline groups. These behavioral data correspond to the response of cocaine (1 mg/kg/ infusion) contingent self-administering animals because noncontingent and saline subjects passively received cocaine (1 mg/kg/ infusion) or saline while the contingent animals self-administer. Cocaine self-administration behavior and its extinction are presented divided into four consecutive phases: acquisition and maintenance (phase 1); first-extinction (phase 2); reacquisition (phase 3); and second-extinction (phase 4). In both acquisition phases the number of cocaine injections/hour was clearly higher than the number of saline injections/hour during both extinction phases. In the days 0 (last day of cocaine i.v. self-administration), 1, 5, and 10 of the second-extinction phase brain of animals in the triads ($N = 18$ in each triad: contingent, $n = 6$; noncontingent, $n = 6$; saline, $n = 6$) were removed to be processed for quantitative *in situ* histochemical study. See details in the text. *Ordinate*: Number of cocaine or saline injections per hour in 2-h sessions of i.v. cocaine or saline self-administration. *Abscissa*: Sessions of i.v cocaine or saline self-administration .

Statistical Analyses

A one-way analysis of variance (ANOVA) was performed for each brain region and day of extinction (0, 1, 5, and 10) with the type of cocaine administration (Cont, NonCont, or Saline) serving as independent variable. Subsequently, other one-way ANOVAs were performed for each brain region and type of cocaine administration to analyze the time-course effects of type of cocaine administration with the day of extinction serving as independent variable. If a significant interaction F score was measured, post hoc comparisons between type of cocaine administration or day of extinction were conducted using a Student Newman Keul's test. Differences were considered significant if the probability of error was less than 5%.

RESULTS

FIGURE 1 shows the behavioral data corresponding to contingent group since the noncontingent and saline groups did not have the possibility of responding: In both groups the subjects received cocaine (1 mg/kg/injection) or saline passively when the contingent animals self-administer the drug. In FIGURE 1, contingent cocaine administration and its extinction is presented in four consecutive phases: Acquisition and maintenance (phase 1); First Extinction (phase 2); Reacquisition (phase 3); and

Second Extinction (phase 4). The behavioral responding pattern that emerges from FIGURE 1 suggests that cocaine was serving as a positive reinforcer. Thus, cocaine maintained robust responding compared to responding under saline in first and second extinction phases. In addition, in both phases of acquisition and maintenance (last 15 days of phase 1 and 15 days of phase 3), the number of cocaine injections/ hour was clearly higher than the number of saline injections/hour. Moreover, both extinction phases were very similar, suggesting that extinction occurred in all the subjects in a very consistent manner.

The one-way ANOVAs performed for each brain region revealed that NMDAR1 mRNA levels were different across all the days of extinction. On Day 0 there was a statistically significant effect of the type of cocaine administration on NMDAR1 gene expression in all the brain regions analyzed (MPFC: $F_{2,12} = 16.04$, $p < 0.001$; CPU: $F_{2,12} = 18.89$, $p > 0.001$; NAc: $F_{2,12} = 13.17$, $p < 0.01$; TU: $F_{2,12} = 7.42$, $p < 0.01$; PIR: $F_{2,12} = 10.15$, $p < 0.01$). Levels of mRNA encoding NMDAR1 glutamate receptor subunit in the Cont group were significantly higher than NonCont and Saline groups. No statistical differences were found between NonCont and Saline groups. On Day 1 NMDAR1 mRNA content of both cocaine groups was higher than Saline in all the brain areas ($p < 0.05$), with the exception of NAc. No statistical differences were found between both cocaine groups. On Day 5, there was a statistically significant effect of the type of cocaine administration in all the forebrain regions of our study (MPFC: $F_{2,10} = 20.86$, $p < 0.001$; CPU: $F_{2,10} = 24.49$, $p < 0.001$; NAc: $F_{2,10} = 13.20$, $p < 0.01$; TU: $F_{2,10} = 48.55$, $p < 0.001$; PIR: $F_{2,12} = 26.65$, $p < 0.001$). mRNA levels encoding NMDAR1 glutamate receptor subunit were significantly decreased in the Cont group compared to the NonCont group in all brain areas ($p < 0.05$). No statistical differences were found between the Cont and Saline groups, with the exception of CPU ($p < 0.05$). However, NMDAR1 content in the NonCont group was higher than the Saline group in all brain regions ($p < 0.05$). On Day 10, the statistical analysis revealed a significant effect of the type of cocaine administration on NMDAR1 gene expression in all the forebrain regions (MPFC: $F_{2,11} = 22.94$, $p < 0.001$; CPU: $F_{2,11} = 7.79$, $p < 0.05$; NAc: $F_{2,11} = 18.68$, $p < 0.001$; PIR: $F_{2,11} = 21.98$, $p < 0.001$), with the exception of TU. NMDAR1 mRNA levels in the Cont group were significantly decreased compared to the NonCont and Saline groups in all the brain regions analyzed ($p < 0.05$), with the exception of TU.

The overall one-way ANOVA performed to analyze the time-course effects of Cont administration on NMDAR1 gene expression across the extinction period also revealed statistical differences in all the brain regions (MPFC: $F_{3,16} = 23.94$, $p < 0.001$; CPU: $F_{3,16} = 12.61$, $p < 0.001$; NAc: $F_{3,16} = 24.04$, $p < 0.01$; TU: $F_{3,16} = 5.55$, $p < 0.05$; PIR: $F_{3,16} = 8.39$, $p < 0.01$). NMDAR1 mRNA levels on Day 0 in Cont animals were significantly higher than Day 5 ($p < 0.05$) and Day 10 ($p < 0.05$). No statistical differences in Cont groups were found between Day 0 and Day 1 in any forebrain region. However, on Day 1 NMDAR1 mRNA levels were higher than in Day 5 ($p < 0.05$) and Day 10 ($p < 0.05$) in all the brain areas studied, with the exception of TU. Cont NMDAR1 mRNA content on Day 5 was only higher than Day 10 in the MPFC and not in the rest of the regions.

In the case of NonCont animals, the one-way ANOVA that analyzed the time-course effects of noncontingent cocaine administration on NMDAR1 gene expression also showed statistical significant differences (MPFC: $F_{3,13} = 23.90$, $p < 0.001$; CPU: $F_{3,13} = 19.21$, $p < 0.001$; NAc: $F_{3,13} = 3.48$, $p < 0.05$; TU: $F_{3,13} = 14.13$, $p <$

TABLE 1. Content of mRNA encoding NMDAR1 glutamate receptor subunit in rat forebrain regions during the extinction of i.v. cocaine self-administration behavior

	MPFC	CPU	NAc	TU	PIR
Cont					
0	428 ± 47	353 ± 55	431 ± 41	563 ± 115	598 ± 110
1	327 ± 34	264 ± 33	351 ± 58	421 ± 79	502 ± 87
5	186 ± 13	108 ± 5	136 ± 21	203 ± 14	196 ± 26
10	63 ± 8	72 ± 11	35 ± 5	182 ± 23	135 ± 22
NonCont					
0	194 ± 7	133 ± 8	147 ± 67	208 ± 17	201 ± 12
1	332 ± 12	248 ± 29	281 ± 65	409 ± 21	412 ± 22
5	322 ± 15	274 ± 12	293 ± 20	397 ± 16	401 ± 20
10	215 ± 20	142 ± 8	136 ± 8	287 ± 42	331 ± 17
Saline					
0	178 ± 31	131 ± 26	148 ± 23	196 ± 14	174 ± 32
1	193 ± 28	144 ± 28	161 ± 31	182 ± 16	186 ± 29
5	188 ± 24	193 ± 21	173 ± 29	205 ± 19	191 ± 27
10	179 ± 19	140 ± 20	167 ± 26	189 ± 14	204 ± 24

NOTE: the values are the mean $\pm$ SEM express as d.p.m. ($\times 10$).

0.001; PIR: $F_{3,13} = 26.66$, $p < 0.01$). NonCont NMDAR1 gene expression was significantly lower on Day 0 compared to Day 1 ($p < 0.05$) and Day 5 ($p < 0.05$) in all the brain areas, with the exception of the expression on Day 1 in the NAc that did not reach statistical significance. Compared to Day 10, NonCont NMDAR1 mRNA content on Day 0 was also significantly lower in PIR and TU ($p < 0.05$), and no statistical differences were found between Day 0 and Day 10 in the rest of brain areas analyzed. Similarly, there was no statistical significance between NMDAR1 mRNA levels on Day 1 and Day 5 in any of the brain areas analyzed. However, NMDAR1 mRNA levels on Day 1 and Day 5 were significantly higher than Day 10 in MPFC, CPU and PIR ($p<0.05$). In addition, NMDA mRNA gene expression on Day 1 was higher than Day 10 in TU ($p< 0.05$).

In Saline animals, the overall one-way ANOVA performed to analyze the time-course effects of saline administration on NMDAR1 gene expression during the extinction showed no statistical differences between any day and brain area.

FIGURES 2–6 show an overall view of the time-course effects of extinction of cocaine self-administration on NMDAR1 mRNA content in all the brain regions of the present study. The data are represented considering mean Saline values of TABLE 1 as 100%. It is clear from FIGURES 2–6 that in all forebrain regions Cont cocaine administration produced an increase in NMDAR1 gene expression on Day 0 (last session of cocaine self-administration) that was progressively decreasing across the rest of the extinction days. On the contrary, compared to Day 0, NonCont cocaine administration produced an increase in NMDAR1 gene expression on Day 1 and Day 5. This increment in NMDAR1 mRNA levels of NonCont animals returned to Saline values on Day 10.

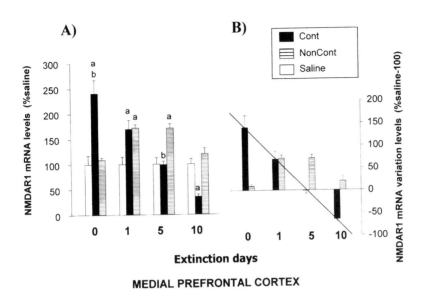

FIGURE 2. Time-course effects of extinction of cocaine self-administration on NMDAR1 mRNA levels in rat medial prefrontal cortex of contingent (Cont), noncontingent (NonCont), and saline (Saline) groups. The values are represented considering mean Saline values of each triad in TABLE 1 as 100%. (**A**) Percentage of NMDAR1 gene expression change in Cont and NonCont groups with respect to Saline group of each triad. (**B**) An overall view of the variations in NMDAR1 gene expression across the extinction period of both cocaine Cont and NonCont groups. Experimental design has been described in the MATERIALS AND METHODS section. (**a**) Values that are significantly different ($p < 0.05$) from Saline group; (**b**) values that are significantly different ($p < 0.05$) from the NonCont group.

DISCUSSION

The results of the present work show that long-term cocaine self-administration and its extinction alter NMDAR1 gene expression in forebrain regions involved in cocaine-reinforcing effects. A similar pattern of change in NMDAR1 mRNA content was found in all the brain areas of our study, but the magnitude and significance of the changes depend upon the brain region examined and the type of cocaine administration (contingent, noncontingent, and saline). Compared to saline and noncontingent cocaine administration, contingent cocaine produced an upregulation in NMDAR1 gene expression on the last day of drug intake in all the brain regions analyzed. Levels of mRNA encoding NMDAR1 receptor subunit of contingent animals decreased progressively in the absence of cocaine, and this decrement persisted 10 days after the extinction of cocaine self-administration behavior in all the forebrain areas, with exception of TU. In contrast, noncontingent cocaine administration did not produce any change in NMDAR1 gene expression on the last session of cocaine intake, and withdrawal of the drug resulted in an increase of NMDAR1 mRNA content on Days 1 and 5 of extinction. This increase returned to control (saline) values

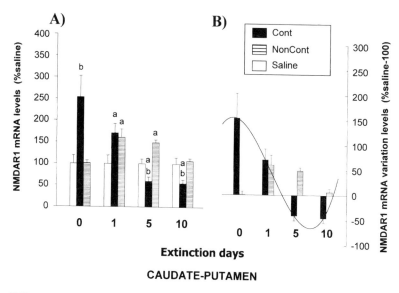

FIGURE 3. Time-course effects of extinction of cocaine self-administration on NMDAR1 mRNA levels in rat caudate-putamen of contingent (Cont), noncontingent (Non-Cont), and saline (Saline) groups. The values are represented considering mean Saline values of each triad in TABLE 1 as 100%. (**A**) Percentage of NMDAR1 gene expression change in Cont and NonCont groups with respect to Saline group of each triad. (**B**) Overall view of the variations in NMDAR1 gene expression across the extinction period of both cocaine Cont and NonCont groups. Experimental design has been described in the MATERIAL AND METHODS section. (**a**) Values that are significantly different ($p < 0.05$) from Saline group; (**b**) values that are significantly different ($p < 0.05$) from the NonCont group.

10 days later of the last noncontingent administration session. These results suggest that an interaction between environmental stimuli and the pharmacological action of cocaine during drug self-administration and its extinction may represent an important factor in the regulation of cocaine effects on NMDAR1 gene expression. In addition, the maintained decrement of levels of mRNA encoding NMDAR1 receptor subunit 10 days after contingent cocaine extinction does not suggest a response to short-term compensatory adaptation in brain function of that forebrain region.

The progressive decrease in NMDAR1 mRNA content across the extinction period of contingent animals may constitute a downregulation response to elevated levels of extracellular glutamate. Likewise, the upregulation in NMDAR1 gene expression found on Day 0 may be a consequence of reduced extracellular glutamate levels produced by contingent cocaine self-administration. We and others have shown that repeated noncontingent cocaine administration reduces basal extracellular glutamate levels in the nucleus accumbens,[7,13] but alterations in NMDAR1 gene expression were not found after repeated cocaine noncontingent administration (15 and 30 mg/kg) in the nucleus accumbens, striatum ventral, tegmental area, and prefrontal cortex.[31] In the present work we also did not find any changes in NMDAR1 mRNA content in noncontingent animals on Day 0. Thus, given that doses and route

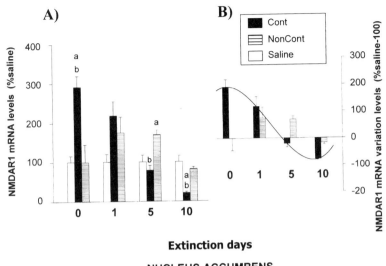

Extinction days

NUCLEUS ACCUMBENS

FIGURE 4. Time-course effects of extinction of cocaine self-administration on NMDAR1 mRNA levels in rat nucleus accumbens of contingent (Cont), noncontingent (NonCont), and saline (Saline) groups. The values are represented considering mean Saline values of each triad in TABLE 1 as 100%. (**A**) The percentage of NMDAR1 gene expression change in Cont and NonCont groups with respect to Saline group of each triad. (**B**) Overall view of the variations in NMDAR1 gene expression across the extinction period of both cocaine Cont and NonCont groups. Experimental design has been described in the MATERIAL AND METHODS section. (**a**) Values that are significantly different ($p < 0.05$) from Saline group; (**b**) values that are significantly different ($p < 0.05$) from the NonCont group.

of contingent and noncontingent cocaine administration in the present study are similar, the upregulation of NMDAR1 gene expression found on Day 0 may be related to other factors, such as environmental stimuli associated with operant-cocaine-reinforced behavior. In this respect, it has recently been suggested that interaction of NMDA glutamatergic and D_1 dopaminergic receptors in the nucleus accumbens may modulate gene regulation and intracellular events involved in acquisition of appetitive instrumental learning.[32]

The brain regions analyzed in this study are part of the proposed rewarding circuitry of mesocorticolimbic dopaminergic system.[1,27] Glutamatergic and dopaminergic convergence in some areas of this circuitry may participate in the modulation of cocaine-reinforcing properties. For example, in the nucleus accumbens dopaminergic projections converge arising from dopamine neurons in the ventral tegmental area[33] and glutamatergic afferents from prefrontal cortex, hippocampus, basolateral amygdala, and periventricular thalamic nucleus.[34–38] In addition, dopamine axon terminals and glutamate afferents converge on the same medium spiny nucleus accumbens neurons and are also in direct axo-axonal apposition to each other.[39,40] This morphological disposition may facilitate glutamatergic and dopaminergic interaction to modulate cocaine-reinforcing effects. In a parallel study carried out with

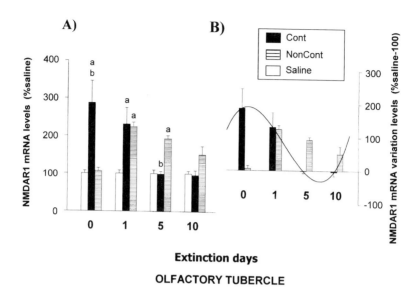

FIGURE 5. Time-course effects of extinction of cocaine self-administration on NMDAR1 mRNA levels in rat olfactory tubercle of contingent (Cont), noncontingent (Non-Cont), and saline (Saline) groups. The values are represented considering mean Saline values of each triad in TABLE 1 as 100%. (**A**) Percentage of NMDAR1 gene expression change in Cont and NonCont groups with respect to Saline group of each triad. (**B**) Overall view of the variations in NMDAR1 gene expression across the extinction period of both cocaine Cont and NonCont groups. Experimental design has been described in the MATERIAL AND METHODS section. (**a**) Values that are significantly different ($p < 0.05$) from Saline group; (**b**) values that are significantly different ($p < 0.05$) from the NonCont group.

brain slices adjacent to those of the present study, we have found a significant decrease in the binding to D_2-like dopaminergic receptor family (D_2, D_3, D_4) in the nucleus accumbens of cocaine contingent and noncontingent animals, compared to saline subject.[41] This finding is compatible with a high dopamine release in both cocaine groups during cocaine self-administration. Considering together the results of that study and those of the present work, it is tempting to speculate that, in the particular conditions of our experiments, the interaction between environmental stimuli and pharmacological cocaine properties might produce an increase in dopamine release and a decrease in glutamate release which, in turn, would result in a downregulation of NMDAR1 gene expression in the nucleus accumbens of contingent animals. This hypothesis must be viewed with caution because much work is needed to establish a structural and functional relationship between dopaminergic and glutamatergic neurotransmission in cocaine self-administration. Although the relevance of the reported changes in NMDAR1 gene expression of the present study clearly will require further analysis, this work provides data on enduring changes in the levels of mRNA encoding the ionotropic NMDAR1 glutamate receptor subunit after long-term cocaine administration and its extinction in brain regions associated with the behavioral effects of cocaine. These findings are in accordance with other

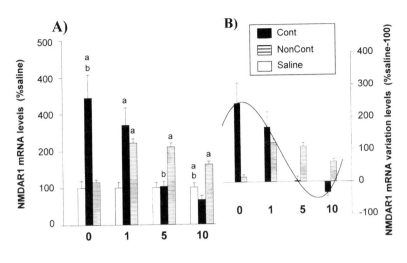

Extinction days

PIRIFORM CORTEX

FIGURE 6. Time-course effects of extinction of cocaine self-administration on NMDAR1 mRNA levels in rat piriform cortex of contingent (Cont), noncontingent (Non-Cont), and saline (Saline) groups. The values are represented considering mean Saline values of each triad in TABLE 1 as 100%. (**A**) Percentage of NMDAR1 gene expression change in Cont and NonCont groups with respect to Saline group of each triad. (**B**) Overall view of the variations in NMDAR1 gene expression across the extinction period of both cocaine Cont and NonCont groups. Experimental design has been described in the MATERIAL AND METHODS section. (**a**) Values that are significantly different ($p < 0.05$) from Saline group; (**b**) values that are significantly different ($p < 0.05$) from the NonCont group.

studies reporting a role for glutamate neurotransmission in cocaine-seeking behavior[9,31] and suggest that alterations in the expression of glutamate receptor subunit mRNAs may participate in cocaine dependence.

ACKNOWLEDGEMENTS

We are grateful to R. Ferrado for technical assistance. Cocaine chlorhydrate was kindly provided by Dirección General de Estupefacientes (Spain). This work was supported by Grants DGESIC PM97-0027 and Plan Nacional sobre Drogas 2000-2003.

REFERENCES

1. KOOB, G.F & F.E. BLOOM. 1988. Cellular and molecular mechanisms of drug dependence. Science **242:** 715–722
2. PULVIRENTI, L., R. MALDONADO-LÓPEZ & G.F. KOOB. 1992. NMDA receptors in the nucleus accumbens modulate intravenous cocaine but not heroine self-administration in the rat. Brain Res. **594:** 327–330.

3. KALIVAS, P.W. & J.E. ALESDATTER. 1993. Involvement of N-methyl-D-aspartate receptor stimulation in the ventral tegmental area and amygdala in behavioral sensitization to cocaine. J. Pharmacol. Exp. Ther. **267**: 86–495.
4. SCHENK, S. *et al.* 1993. Development and expression of sensitization to cocaine reinforcing's reinforcing properties: role of NMDA receptors. Psychopharmacology **111**: 332–338
5. FITZGERALD L.W. *et al.* 1996. Drug of abuse and stress increase the expression of GluR1 and NMDAR1 glutamate receptor subunits in the ventral tegmental area: common adaptations among cross sensitization agents. J. Neurosci. **16**: 274–282.
6. BELL, K. & P.W. KALIVAS. 1996. Context-specific cross sensitization between systemic cocaine and intra-accumbens AMPA infusion in rats. Psychopharmacology **127**: 377–383.
7. PIERCE, R.C. *et al.* 1996. Repeated cocaine augments excitatory amino acid transmission in the nucleus accumbens only in rats having developed behavioral sensitization. J. Neurosci. **16**: 1550–1560.
8. PIERCE, R.C. & P.W. KALIVAS. 1997. The NMDA antagonist, dizocilpine (MK-801), attenuates cocaine self-administration without affecting meso-accumbens dopamine transmission. Psychopharmacology **133**: 188–195.
9. CORNISH, J.L., P. DUFFY & P.W. KALIVAS. 1999. A role for nucleus accumbens glutamate transmission in the relapse to cocaine-seeking behavior. Neuroscience **93**: 1359–1367.
10. NESTLER, E.J. 1993. Cellular responses to chronic treatment with drugs of abuse. Crit. Rev. Neurobiol. **7**: 23–39.
11. HYMAN, S.E. 1996. Addiction to cocaine and amphetamine. Neuron **16**: 901–904.
12. PIERCE, R.C. & P.W. KALIVAS. 1997. A circuitry model of the expression of behavioral sensitization to amphetamine-like psychostimulants. Brain Res. Rev. **25**: 192–216.
13. REID, M.S. & S.P. BERGER. 1996. Evidence for sensitization of cocaine-induced nucleus accumbens glutamate release. NeuroReport **7**: 1325–1329.
14. KALIVAS, P.W. & P. DUFFY. 1998. Repeated cocaine administration alters extracellular glutamate in the ventral tegmental area. J. Neurochem. **70**: 1497–1502.
15. CHURCHILL, L., M.B. GHASEMZADEH & P.W. KALIVAS. 1997. Glutamate receptor subunits (GluR1 and NMDAR1) increase in the nucleus accumbens of rats 3 weeks after repeated cocaine exposure. Soc. Neurosci. Abstr. **23**: 260.
16. KARLER, R., L.D. CALDER & J.B. BEDINGFIELD. 1994. Cocaine behavioral sensitization and the excitatory amino acids. Psychopharmacology **115**: 305–310.
17. WOLF, M.E. 1998. The role of excitatory amino acids in behavioral sensitization to psychomotor stimulants. Prog. Neurobiol. **54**: 1–42.
18. DWORKIN, S.I., L.J. PORRINO & J.E. SMITH. 1992. Importance of behavioral controls in the analysis of ongoing events. *In* Neurobiological Approaches to Brain-Behavior Interaction. J. Frascella and R.M. Brown, Eds.: 173–188. National Institute on Drug Abuse Research Monograph 124. U.S. Government Printing Office. Washington, D.C.
19. DWORKIN, S.I., C. CO & J.E. SMITH. 1995. Rat brain neurotransmitter turnover rates altered during withdrawal from chronic cocaine administration. Brain Res. **682**: 116–126.
20. DWORKIN, S.I., S. MIRKIS & J.E. SMITH. 1995. Response-dependent versus response-independent presentation of cocaine: differences in the letal effects of the drug. Psychopharmacology **117**: 262–266.
21. WILSON, J.M. *et al.* 1994. Amygdala dopamine levels are markedly elevated after self- but not passive-administration of cocaine. Brain Res. **668**: 39–45.
22. HEMBY, S.E. *et al.* 1997. Differences in extracellular dopamine concentration in the nucleus accumbens during response-independent cocaine administration in the rats. Psychopharmacology **133**: 7–16.
23. GALICI, R. *et al.* 2000. Comparison of noncontingent versus contingent cocaine administration on plasma corticosterone levels in rats. Eur. J. Pharmacol. **387**: 59–62.
24. CRESPO, J.A. *et al.* 2001. Extinction of cocaine self-administration produces a differential time-related regulation of proenkephalin gene expression in rat brain. Neuropsychopharmacology **25**: 185–194.

25. STANDAERT, D.G. *et al.* 1994. Organization of N-methyl-D-aspartate glutamate receptor gene expression in the basal ganglia of the rat. J. Comp. Neurol. **343:** 1–16.
26. SMITH, J.E. & S.I. DWORKING. 1986. Neurobiological substrates of drug self-administration. *In* Opiate Receptor Subtypes and Brain Function. R.M. Brown, D. H. Clouet and D.P. Friedman, Eds.: 127–145. National Institute on Drug Abuse Research Monograph 71. U.S. Government Printing Office. Washington, D.C.
27. KOOB, G.F. 1992. Drugs of abuse: anatomy, pharmacology and function of reward pathways. Trends Pharmacol. Sci. **13:** 177–184.
28. AMBROSIO, E. *et al.* 1996. Cardiovascular effects of cocaine during operant cocaine self-administration. Eur. J. Pharmacol. **315:** 43–51.
29. PAXINOS, G. & C. WATSON. 1998. The Rat Brain in Stereotaxic Coordinates. Academic Press. San Diego, CA.
30. TESTA, C.M. *et al.* 1995. Differential expression of mGluR5 metabotropic glutamate receptor mRNA by rat striatal neurons. J. Comp. Neurol. **354:** 241–252.
31. GHASEMZADEH, M.B. *et al.* 1999. Neuroadaptations in ionotropic and metabotropic glutamate receptor mRNA produced by cocaine treatment. J. Neurochem. **72:** 157–165.
32. SMITH-ROE, S.L. & A.E. KELLEY. 2000. Coincident activation of NMDA and dopamine D_1 receptors within the nucleus accumbens core is required for appetitive instrumental learning. J. Neurosci. **20:** 7737–7742.
33. FALLON, J.H. & R.Y. MOORE. 1978. Catecholamine innervation of basal forebrain .IV.Topography of the dopamine projection to the basal forebrain and striatum. J. Comp. Neurol. **180:** 545–580.
34. BERENDSE, H.W. *et al.* 1992. Topographical organization and relationship with ventral striatal compartments of prfrontal corticostriatal projections in the rat. J. Comp. Neurol. **316:** 314–367.
35. BERENDSE, H.W. & H.J. GROENEWEGEN. 1990. Organization of the thalamostriatal projections in the rat, with special emphasis on the ventral striatum. J. Comp. Neurol. **299:** 187–228.
36. BROG, J.S. *et al.* 1993. The patterns of afferent innervation of the core and shell in "accumbens" part of the ventral striatum: immunohistochemical detection of retrogradely transported Fluoro-Gold. J. Comp. Neurol. **338:** 255–278.
37. PHILLIPSON, O.T. & A.C. GRIFFITHS. 1985. The topographic order of inputs to the nucleus accumbens in the rat. Neuroscience **16:** 275–296.
38. WRIGHT, C.I., V.J. BEIJER & H.J. GROENEWEGEN. 1996. Basal amygdaloid complex afferents to the rat nucleus accumbens are compartmentally organized. J. Neurosci. **16:** 1877–1893.
39. MEREDITH, G.E., C.M.A. PENNARTZ & H.J. GROENEWEGEN. 1993. The cellular framework for chemical signalling in the nucleus accumbens. Prog. Brain Res. **99:** 3–24.
40. SESACK, S.R. & V.M. PICKEL. 1990. In the medial nucleus accumbens, hippocampal and catecholaminergic terminals converge on spiny neurons and are in apposition to each other. Brain Res. **527:** 266–272.
41. AMBROSIO, E. & J.A. CRESPO. 2000. Neuroadaptive changes in dopaminergic and glutamatergic systems during cocaine withdrawal. *In* Recent Advances in the Neurobiology of Drug Addiction. Proceedings of 6th Internet World Conference for Biomedical Sciences–Internet Association for Biomedical Sciences (INABIS)–2000. M. García-Rojo, Ed. Presentation 25.

Preclinical Evaluation of GBR12909 Decanoate as a Long-Acting Medication for Methamphetamine Dependence

MICHAEL H. BAUMANN,[a] JENNIFER M. PHILLIPS,[a]
MARIO A. AYESTAS,[a] SYED F. ALI,[b] KENNER C. RICE,[c]
AND RICHARD B. ROTHMAN[a]

[a]Clinical Psychopharmacology Section, Intramural Research
Program (IRP), National Institute on Drug Abuse (NIDA),
National Institutes of Health (NIH), Baltimore, Maryland USA

[b]Neurochemistry Laboratory, Division of Neurotoxicology,
National Center for Toxicological Research (NCTR), Food and
Drug Administration (FDA), Jefferson, Arkansas USA

[c]Laboratory of Medicinal Chemistry, National Institute of Diabetes
and Digestive and Kidney Diseases (NIDDK), National Institutes of Health,
Bethesda, Maryland USA

ABSTRACT: Methamphetamine (METH) abuse is a growing health problem, and no treatments for METH dependence have been identified. The powerful addictive properties of METH are mediated by release of dopamine (DA) from nerve terminals in mesolimbic reward pathways. METH stimulates DA release by acting as a substrate for DA transporter (DAT) proteins, thereby triggering efflux of DA from cells into the synapse. We have shown that blocking DAT activity with high-affinity DA uptake inhibitors, like GBR12909, can substantially reduce METH-evoked DA release in vitro, suggesting GBR12909 may have potential as a pharmacotherapy for METH dependence. The purpose of the present study was to examine the neurobiological effects of a long-acting oil-soluble preparation of GBR12909 (1-[2-[bis(4-fluorophenyl)methoxy]ethyl]-4-(3-hydroxy-3-phenylpropyl) piperazinyl decanoate, or GBR-decanoate). Male rats received GBR-decanoate (480 mg/kg, i.m.) or its oil vehicle, and were tested using a variety of methods one and two weeks later. Ex vivo autoradiography showed that GBR-decanoate decreases DAT binding in DA-rich brain regions. In vivo microdialysis in the nucleus accumbens revealed that GBR-decanoate elevates baseline levels of extracellular DA and antagonizes the ability of METH to evoke DA release. The dopaminergic effects of GBR-decanoate were sustained, lasting for at least two weeks. Rats pretreated with GBR-decanoate displayed enhanced locomotor responses to novelty at one week, but not two weeks, postinjection. Administration of the D_2/D_3 receptor agonist quinpirole (10 and 100 μg/kg, s.c.) decreased locomotor activity and suppressed plasma prolactin levels; quinpirole-induced responses were not altered by GBR-

Address for correspondence: Michael H. Baumann, Ph.D., Clinical Psychopharmacology Section, IRP, NIDA, NIH, 5500 Nathan Shock Drive, Baltimore, MD 21224. Voice: 410-550-1754; fax: 410-550-2997

mbaumann@intra.nida.nih.gov

Ann. N.Y. Acad. Sci. 965: 92–108 (2002). © 2002 New York Academy of Sciences.

decanoate. Thus, GBR-decanoate is able to elevate basal synaptic DA levels and block METH-evoked DA release in a persistent manner, without significant perturbation of DA receptor function. The findings suggest that GBR-decanoate, or similar long-acting agents, should be evaluated further as potential treatment adjuncts in the management of METH addiction in humans.

KEYWORDS: methamphetamine; cocaine; pharmacotherapies; drug addiction; DA transporter; GBR-decanoate; GBR12909; psychomotor stimulants

INTRODUCTION

Methamphetamine (METH) abuse and its associated medical complications are growing health concerns in the United States.[1,2] The most serious abuse of METH has been confined to western states such as California and Arizona, but recent findings indicate that this problem is spreading nationwide.[3,4] Moreover, dramatic increases in the trafficking and misuse of METH are occurring throughout the world in places like Japan, the Philippines, Thailand, North Korea, and Australia.[5,6] Despite the extent of the METH problem, few treatment options are available and no pharmacotherapies specifically targeted for METH dependence have been reported. It is worth noting that medication development efforts aimed at treating addiction to cocaine (another widely abused stimulant) have been largely unsuccessful[7,8] Consequently, the discovery and development of effective pharmacotherapies for stimulant dependence represents a formidable challenge for biomedical research.

A first step in the search for medications to treat METH dependence involves determining neurobiological effects of the drug in animal models. Preclinical evidence shows that habit-forming properties of METH, and other illicit stimulants, are mediated by activation of DA neurotransmission in mesolimbic reward circuits.[9] In particular, METH causes nonexocytotic release of DA from nerve terminals by acting as a substrate for DA transporter (DAT) proteins, thereby facilitating the reverse transport of DA out of cells into the extracellular space.[10–12] Thus, METH-induced DA release is a DAT-dependent process. The crucial role of DAT in mediating the addictive effects of psychomotor stimulants has prompted us to examine DAT ligands, like the DA uptake blocker GBR12909 (1-[2-[bis(4-fluorophenyl)methoxy]ethyl]-4-(3-phenylpropyl) piperazine), as potential therapeutic agents and as tools to test the DA hypothesis of addiction.[13–15]

GBR12909 displays a number of unique properties that are consistent with its use as a pharmacotherapy for stimulant dependence. At the molecular level, GBR12909 binds with high affinity and selectivity to DAT proteins, thereby blocking DA uptake in nervous tissue.[16–18] Once bound to DAT, GBR12909 exhibits "pseudoirreversible" binding that is characterized by slow dissociation of the drug from its binding site.[19] The precise nature of the interaction between GBR12909 and DAT is not fully understood, but it has been shown that GBR analogs bind to DAT polypeptides in a region that is distinct from the region where cocaine analogs bind.[20,21] At the organismic level, GBR12909 penetrates into the brain very slowly upon systemic administration in rats.[22] *In vivo* microdialysis studies demonstrate that GBR12909 produces dose-dependent elevations in extracellular DA in rat brain; the drug-induced rise in dialysate DA is slow in onset, modest in magnitude, and sustained in duration.[14,19] Because GBR12909 binds to DAT sites, pretreatment with the drug

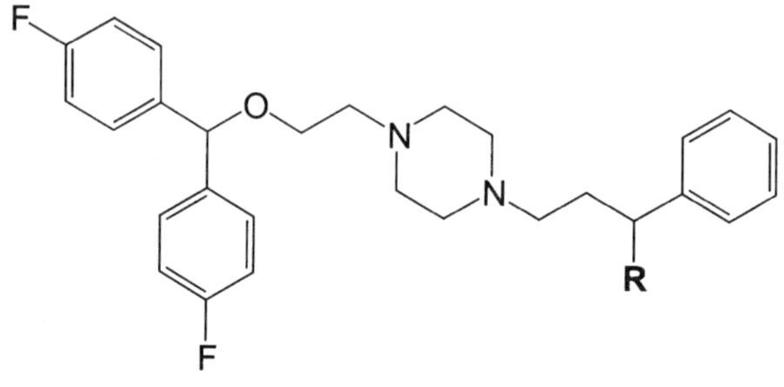

GBR-12909, **R** = H

GBR-hydroxy, **R** = OH

GBR-decanoate, **R** = $OCOC_9H_{19}$

FIGURE 1. Chemical structures of GBR12909, GBR-hydroxy, and GBR-decanoate.

antagonizes amphetamine-induced release of DA *in vivo.*[14,23] Perhaps more importantly, GBR12909 suppresses cocaine self-administration in animals[24,25] and appears to be less reinforcing than abused stimulants.[26,27] Taken together, the preclinical data suggest that GBR12909 might be a useful pharmacological adjunct in the management of stimulant addictions. Clinical safety trials with this medication are currently underway.[28]

There are numerous impediments to successful treatment of stimulant-dependent patients, including high dropout rates and lack of compliance with medication regimens.[29] In order to circumvent issues related to patient noncompliance, we have developed a long-acting depot formulation of GBR12909 (1-[2-[bis(4-fluorophenyl)methoxy]ethyl]-4-(3-hydroxy-3-phenylpropyl) piperazyl decanoate, or GBR-decanoate) that can be administered as a single i.m. injection.[30,31] FIGURE 1 illustrates the chemical structure of GBR12909, along with its hydroxy and decanoate analogs. In a preliminary report, Glowa *et al.*[30] showed that one dose of GBR-decanoate suppresses cocaine self-administration behavior in rhesus monkeys for up to one month. The suppressive effect of GBR-decanoate is selective for cocaine self-administration, since the drug had little effect on food-reinforced behavior. Like other depot preparations,[32,33] GBR-decanoate is an oil-soluble prodrug that slowly releases an active hydroxylated derivative (1-[2-[bis(4-fluorophenyl)methoxy]ethyl]-4-(3-hydroxy-3-phenylpropyl) piperazine, or GBR-hydroxy) into the circulation. GBR-hydroxy is a potent and selective inhibitor of DAT binding, similar to GBR12909 itself; in binding assays using [^{125}I]3β-(4-iodophenyl)tropan-2β-carboxylic acid methyl ester ([^{125}I]RTI-55) to label DAT and 5-HT transporters (SERT), GBR-hydroxy displays high affinity for DAT ($Ki = 2.2 \pm 0.1$ nM) and low affinity for SERT ($Ki = 117 \pm 7$ nM). Not surprisingly, GBR-hydroxy blocks [^{3}H]DA uptake with greater potency than [^{3}H]5-HT uptake.[31] In agreement with the *in vitro* findings, FIGURE 2 shows that i.v. administration of GBR-hydroxy to rats produces slow-onset elevations in extracellular DA, but not 5-HT, in the nucleus accumbens.

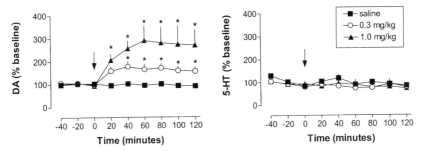

FIGURE 2. Effects of acute administration of GBR-hydroxy on extracellular DA (*left panel*) and 5-HT (*right panel*) in the nucleus accumbens of conscious rats. Data are mean ± SEM for $n = 5$ rats per group, expressed as % of baseline. Baseline levels of dialysate DA and 5-HT were 2.50 ± 0.31 and 0.47 ± 0.07 nM, respectively. * = $p < 0.05$ with respect to vehicle controls at a given time point.

With regard to the above-mentioned findings, we were interested in evaluating the potential utility of GBR-decanoate as a long-acting medication for METH dependence. To achieve this aim, the neurobiological consequences of GBR-decanoate treatment in rats were examined using a variety of methods. All rats received single i.m. injections of GBR-decanoate (1 mL/kg of a 48% solution, or 480 mg/kg) or its sesame oil vehicle, and groups of rats were tested one or two weeks later. First, the ability of GBR-decanoate to affect DAT and SERT binding was examined using *ex vivo* autoradiography, with [^{125}I]RTI-55 as the radiolabeled ligand. Next, the effect of GBR-decanoate on METH-induced release of DA and 5-HT was evaluated by *in vivo* microdialysis in the nucleus accumbens. Finally, the impact of GBR-decanoate on DA receptor function was evaluated by assessing responsiveness to the D_2/D_3 agonist quinpirole. Quinpirole-evoked inhibition of locomotor activity and suppression of prolactin secretion were used as indices of presynaptic and postsynaptic D_2/D_3 receptor sensitivity, respectively.

MATERIALS AND METHODS

Animals

Male Sprague-Dawley rats (Charles River, Wilmington, MA) weighing 300–350 g were housed two per cage in standard vivarium conditions (lights on from 0700–1900 h) with food and water freely available. Animals were maintained in facilities fully accredited by the American Association of the Accreditation of Laboratory Animal Care (AAALAC), and experiments were performed in accordance with the Institutional Care and Use Committee of the National Institute on Drug Abuse (NIDA), Intramural Research Program (IRP).

Chemicals

GBR-decanoate was prepared by esterification of the hydroxyl analog of GBR12909 (1-[2-]bis(4-fluorophenyl)methoxy[ethyl]-4-(3-hydroxy-3-phenylpropyl)piperazine), which we abbreviate GBR-hydroxy.[30,31] [^{125}I]RTI-55 (SA = 2200 Ci/mmol), also known as [^{125}I]CFT, was prepared as described.[34] Sodium pentobarbital was purchased from Sigma (St. Louis, MO), whereas methoxyflurane (Metofane) was purchased from Pittman-Moore (Phillipsburg, NJ). (+)-Methamphetamine HCl was generously provided by NIDA Drug Supply (Rockville, MD) and (−)-quinpirole was a gift from Dr. Srihari Tella. All other reagents were purchased from Sigma.

Transporter Autoradiography

Autoradiographic methods were used to assess the effects of GBR-decanoate on transporter binding in brain tissue. Rats were housed two per cage and received single i.m. injections of GBR-decanoate (1 mL/kg of a 48% solution, or 480 mg/kg) or sesame oil vehicle in their home cages. Separate groups of rats were sacrificed 6–7 days later (one week) and 13–14 days later (two weeks). On the day of sacrifice, rats were brought into a testing room and allowed 1 h to acclimate to the surroundings. Subsequently, rats were decapitated. Brains were removed, frozen in isopentane, and stored at −80°C. DAT and SERT sites were visualized in 30 μM sections of brain tissue using minor modifications of published methods.[35] Briefly, slide-mounted sections were placed in Lipshaw racks and preincubated in binding buffer (55 mM sodium phosphate with 0.1% bovine serum albumin, pH = 7.4) for 30 min at 4°C. The preincubation step was performed to wash away any residual unbound GBR-hydroxy in tissue. Slides were subsequently rinsed, transferred to cytomailers, and incubated with 0.01 nM [^{125}I]RTI-55 diluted in binding buffer. Incubations were carried out for 60 min at 4°C in the presence of 100 nM paroxetine for DAT binding or 5 μM benztropine for SERT binding. Nonspecific binding was determined in the presence of 10 μM indatraline. Incubations were terminated by two washes of ice-cold binding buffer. Slides were dried, dessicated overnight, and apposed to radiosensitive film (Hyperfilm, Amersham, Arlington Heights, IL) for 4–8 days. A MacIntosh Apple Power G3 computer and a scanner were used to digitize the sections from film. The NIH Image 1.62 program, available on the Internet at http://rsb.info.nih.gov/nih-image, was used to construct standard curves and quantify relative optical densities in discrete brain regions.

In Vivo Microdialysis Experiments

In vivo microdialysis methods were used to characterize the neurochemical effects of GBR-decanoate treatment. The rats used in the microdialysis experiments received sodium pentobarbital (60 mg/kg, i.p.) for surgical anesthesia. An indwelling jugular catheter made of Silastic Medical Grade tubing (Dow Corning, Midland, MI) was implanted. Each rat was then placed in a stereotaxic apparatus, and a plastic intracerebral guide cannula (CMA 12, CMA/Microdialysis, Acton, MA) was implanted 2 mm above the nucleus accumbens (ML ± 1.4 mm and AP + 1.6 mm from bregma, DV + 6.2 mm from dura) according to published methods.[36] The guide cannulae were positioned so that microdialysis probes would reside within the core region of the nucleus accumbens, close to the lateral border of the medial shell region. The guide cannula was fixed to the skull using stainless-steel screws and dental acrylic. Animals were singly housed postoperatively. After 7–10 days of recovery, rats received single i.m. injections of GBR-decanoate (1 mL/kg of a 48% solution, or 480 mg/kg) or sesame oil in their home cages. Rats were tested in the microdialysis paradigm 6–7 days later (one week) and 13–14 days later (two weeks). Separate groups of rats were used for the one-week and two-week experiments.

On the evening before an experiment, rats were moved to the testing room and lightly anesthetized with Metofane. A microdialysis probe with a 2- × 0.5-mm exchange surface (CMA/12, CMA/Microdialysis) was lowered into the guide cannula, and an extension tube (PE-50) was attached to the jugular catheter. Each rat was placed into its own plastic container and connected to a tethering system that allowed motor activity within the container. Ringers' solution containing 147.0 mM NaCl, 4.0 mM KCl, 1.8 mM $CaCl_2$ was pumped through the probe overnight at 0.5 μL/min. On the next morning, 10 μL dialysate samples were collected at 20-min intervals. Samples were immediately assayed for DA and 5-HT by high-pressure liquid chromatography coupled to electrochemical detection (HPLC-EC).[36] When three stable baseline samples were obtained, each rat received an i.v. challenge injection of METH (0.3 mg/kg) or saline, followed by a second i.v. injection of METH (1.0 mg/kg) or saline one hour later. Microdialysate samples were collected throughout the experiment until one hour after the second METH injection.

Aliquots of the dialysate (5 μL) were injected onto a microbore HPLC column (3 μm, C18, 100 × 1 mm, Bioanalytical Systems Inc., West Lafayette, IN) that was coupled to an amperometric detector (Model LC-4C, BAS, Inc.). A glassy carbon electrode was set at a potential of +650 mV relative to Ag/AgCl reference. A mobile phase consisting of 150 mM monochloroacetic acid, 150 mM NaOH, 2.5 mM sodium octanesulfonic acid, 250 μM disodium EDTA, with1 mL triethylamine, 6% MeOH, 6% CH_3CN per liter of water (final pH = 5) was pumped (Model 260D, ISCO, Lincoln, NE) at a rate of 60 μL/min. Chromatographic data were acquired online and exported to a MAXIMA 820 software system (Waters Associates, Milford, MA) for peak amplification, integration, and analysis. Standards of DA and 5-HT were run daily before dialysate samples, and standard curves were linear over a wide range of concentrations (1–1000 pg). A monoamine standard mix containing DA, 5-HT, and their respective acid metabolites was injected before and after the experiment to ensure the validity of the constituent retention times. Peak heights of unknowns were compared to peak heights of standards and the lower limit of detection (3 × baseline noise) was100 fg/ 5 μL sample.

Quinpirole Challenge Experiments

The DA D_2/D_3 receptor agonist, quinpirole,[37,38] was used as a probe to examine DA receptor responsiveness in rats pretreated with GBR-decanoate or vehicle. Rats were housed two per cage and received single i.m. injections of GBR-decanoate (1 mL/kg of a 48% solution, or 480 mg/kg) or sesame oil in their home cages. Separate groups of rats were tested 6–7 days later (one week) and 13–14 days later (two weeks). On the morning of an experiment, each rat received a s.c. challenge injection of quinpirole (10 or 100 μg/kg) or saline vehicle. Rats were immediately placed into plexiglass arenas that were equipped with photocell sensors for determining horizontal locomotor activity (Omnitech, Columbus, OH). Rats were not acclimated to the chambers before testing, since we were interested in determining the locomotor response to a novel environment. Exploratory locomotor activity, defined as distance traveled in cm, was determined on the basis of photocell beam breaks in the horizontal plane as the rat moved about the arena. Activity was measured over 5-min intervals, and each rat received a summed score that consisted of the total activity during the first 30 min postinjection. The data were recorded via a digital multiplexer and transferred to a computerized spreadsheet for analysis.

After the 30-min locomotor test, rats were quickly transported to a separate room and decapitated. Trunk blood was collected into heparinized tubes (100 µL of 1000 IU/mL heparin) and centrifuged at 2500 rpm for 10 min. Plasma was decanted and stored at –80°C. Prolactin was assayed by double-antibody radioimmunoassay using materials provided by the National Hormone and Pituitary Program (A.F. Parlow, UCLA Medical Center, Torrance, CA, USA) and the NIDDK (Rockville, MD, USA), as previously described[39] Antiserum directed against rat prolactin (rPRL-S-9) was diluted 1:437,500 and rPRL-RP-3 was the reference standard. [^{125}I]Prolactin was obtained from Covance Laboratories (Vienna, VA, USA). Plasma samples (50 µL) were analyzed in duplicate within a single assay, and the intraassay coefficient of variability was 8.5%.

Data Analysis

For the autoradiography experiments, DAT and SERT binding densities in specific brain regions were compared using one-factor (pretreatment) analysis of variance. In the microdialysis experiments, the first three samples collected before any treatment were considered baseline, and all subsequent monoamine measures were expressed as a percent of this baseline. Dialysate transmitter data were evaluated by one-factor (acute drug treatment) and two-factor (pretreatment × acute treatment) analysis of variance. For the quinpirole challenge experiments, locomotor activity data and plasma prolactin levels were analyzed by two-factor (pretreatment × acute treatment) analysis of variance. When significant F values were obtained, Duncan's Multiple Range test was performed to compare group means. $p < 0.05$ was chosen as the minimum criterion for statistical significance.

RESULTS

Transporter Autoradiography

The data in FIGURE 3 demonstrate that a single injection of GBR-decanoate significantly reduces the density of [^{125}I]RTI-55-labeled DAT binding sites in DA-rich regions of the brain. One week after GBR-decanoate injection, DAT binding was decreased by 33% in caudate nucleus ($F[1,6] = 20.67, p < 0.001$) , 34% in nucleus accumbens core ($F[1,6] = 6.77, p < 0.01$), and 39% in nucleus accumbens shell ($F[1,6] = 9.65, p < 0.01$). The reductions in DAT binding were sustained, lasting for at least two weeks. No changes in SERT binding were noted between rats pretreated with GBR-decanoate or oil at either time point (data not shown). Previous experience with GBR12909 suggests that such decreases in DAT binding are probably due to persistent occupation of DAT by GBR-hydroxy rather than drug-induced downregulation DAT.[13,15,26]

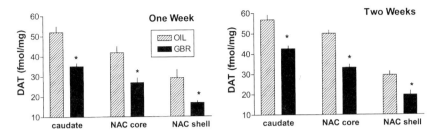

FIGURE 3. Effects of GBR-decanoate (GBR) pretreatment on [^{125}I]RTI-55-labeled DAT binding in rat forebrain. Rats were treated with single i.m. injections of GBR (1 mL/ kg of a 48% solution, or 480 mg/kg) or sesame oil vehicle. One week (*left panel*) and two weeks (*right panel*) later, groups of rats were decapitated and brains were removed. Slide-mounted sections of brain tissue were incubated with 0.01 nM [^{125}I]RTI-55 under DAT-specific conditions (i.e., in the presence of 100 nM paroxetine to prevent binding of radiolabeled ligand to 5-HT transporters). Each value is fmol/mg protein, expressed as mean ± SEM for $n = 4$ rats per group. Control levels of DAT binding in caudate nucleus, nucleus accumbens core, and nucleus accumbens shell were 52.1 ± 2.8, 41.9 ± 4.0, and 29.2 ± 3.1 fmol/mg protein, respectively. * = $p < 0.05$ with respect to vehicle controls in a specified brain region.

TABLE 1. Effects of GBR-decanoate or its sesame oil vehicle on baseline levels of dialysate DA and 5-HT in rat nucleus accumbens

Treatment, test day[a]	Dialysate DA (nM)[b]	Dialysate 5-HT (nM)
OIL, one week	1.93 ± 0.30	0.41 ± 0.05
GBR, one week	4.80 ± 1.15*	0.44 ± 0.09
OIL, two weeks	1.69 ± 0.37	0.36 ± 0.05
GBR, two weeks	3.95 ± 0.64*	0.41 ± 0.09

[a]Male rats received i.m. injections of GBR-decanoate (1 mL/kg of a 48% solution, or 480 mg/ kg) or its sesame oil vehicle. Rats were subjected to microdialysis sampling in the nucleus accumbens at one week and two weeks after i.m. injections, as described in Materials and Methods. Separate groups of rats were used for the one-week and two-week tests.
[b]Dialysate samples were assayed for DA and 5-HT by HPLC-EC.[36] Data are nM concentrations, expressed as mean ± SEM for $n = 6$–7 rats per group. * $p < 0.05$ (Duncan's) when compared to vehicle pretreated group at a given time point.

In Vivo *Microdialysis Data*

TABLE 1 shows the baseline levels of extracellular DA and 5-HT in dialysate samples obtained from the nucleus accumbens of rats treated with GBR-decanoate or sesame oil vehicle. One week after GBR-decanoate injection, rats pretreated with drug displayed significant 2.5-fold elevations in baseline extracellular DA (4.80 ± 1.15 nM) compared to controls (1.93 ± 0.30 nM). The data in FIGURE 4 illustrate that GBR-decanoate antagonizes the DA-releasing capability of METH. At the one-week test session, i.v. METH produced dose-related increases in dialysate DA levels, and prior treatment with GBR-decanoate significantly reduced METH-induced stimula-

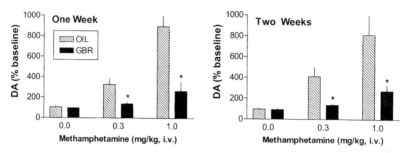

FIGURE 4. Effects of GBR-decanoate (GBR) pretreatment on METH-induced DA release in the nucleus accumbens of conscious rats. Rats received single i.m. injections of GBR (1 mL/kg of a 48% solution, or 480 mg/kg) or sesame oil vehicle. One week (*left panel*) and two weeks (*right panel*) later, rats undergoing *in vivo* microdialysis received i.v. challenge injections of METH (0.3 and 1.0 mg/kg) or saline vehicle, as described in Materials and Methods. Dialysate samples were assayed for DA by HPLC-EC. [36] Data are peak DA responses measured 20 min after METH, expressed as % baseline (mean ± SEM) for $n = 6–7$ rats per group. Baseline levels of dialysate DA are shown in TABLE 1. * = $p < 0.05$ with respect to vehicle-pretreated group that received METH.

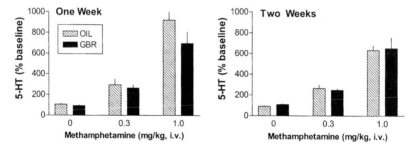

FIGURE 5. Effects of GBR-decanoate (GBR) pretreatment on METH-induced 5-HT release in the nucleus accumbens of conscious rats. Rats received single i.m. injections of GBR (1 mL/kg of a 48% solution, or 480 mg/kg) or sesame oil vehicle. One week (*left panel*) and two weeks (*right panel*) later, rats undergoing *in vivo* microdialysis received i.v. challenge injections of METH (0.3 and 1.0 mg/kg) or saline vehicle, as described in Materials and Methods. Dialysate samples were assayed for 5-HT by HPLC-EC. [36] Data are peak 5-HT responses measured 20 min after METH, expressed as % baseline (mean ± SEM) for $n = 6–7$ rats per group. Baseline levels of dialysate 5-HT are shown in TABLE 1.

tion of DA release at 0.3 mg/kg ($F[1,23] = 6.14$, $p < 0.02$) and 1.0 mg/kg ($F[1,23] = 7.70$, $p < 0.01$) challenge doses. At the two-week time point, rats pretreated with GBR-decanoate still had significant elevations in baseline extracellular DA (3.95 ± 0.64 nM) compared to controls (1.69 ± 0.37 nM). Additionally, rats receiving GBR-decanoate exhibited blunted METH-induced DA release at 0.3 mg/kg ($F[1,23] = 11.43$, $p < 0.002$) and 1.0 mg/kg ($F[1,23] < 10.29$, $p < 0.004$) doses.

The data in FIGURE 5 demonstrate that GBR-decanoate does not alter 5-HT release produced by METH. One week after GBR-decanoate injection, baseline extra-

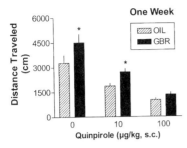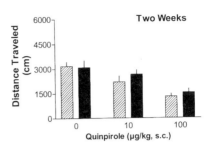

FIGURE 6. Effects of GBR-decanoate (GBR) pretreatment on quinpirole-induced inhibition of exploratory locomotor activity in rats. Rats received single i.m. injections of GBR (1 mL/kg of a 48% solution, or 480 mg/kg) or sesame oil vehicle. One week (*left panel*) and two weeks (*right panel*) later, rats received s.c. challenge injections of quinpirole (10 and 100 mg/kg) or saline vehicle. Each rat was placed into a plexiglass arena, and horizontal locomotor activity was determined by photocell beam breaks as the rat moved about the arena. Values are distance traveled in cm during 30 min postinjection, expressed as mean ± SEM for $n = 6$–7 rats per group. * = $p < 0.05$ with respect to vehicle-pretreated group that received the same dose of quinpirole.

cellular 5-HT levels were similar in drug-treated (0.44 ± 0.09 nM) and oil-treated (0.41 ± 0.05 nM) groups. FIGURE 5 shows that i.v. METH increased dialysate 5-HT levels at 0.3 mg/kg ($F[1,18] = 42.17$, $p < 0.001$) and 1.0 mg/kg ($F[1,18] = 70.96$, $p < 0.0001$), and exposure to GBR-decanoate did not alter METH-evoked 5-HT responses. When tested at two weeks, extracellular 5-HT levels were similar in drug- (0.41 ± 0.09 nM) and oil-pretreated (0.36 ± 0.05 nM) rats. As observed at one week, GBR-decanoate had no effect on METH-induced 5-HT release.

Quinpirole Challenge Data

FIGURE 6 shows the effects of GBR-decanoate injection on inhibition of locomotor activity produced by quinpirole. One week after GBR-decanoate injection, rats pretreated with drug displayed a significantly enhanced baseline locomotor response to novelty (4505 ± 510 cm) when compared to controls (3278 ± 462 cm). Quinpirole produced a dose-related decrease in locomotor activity all rats ($F[2,36] = 39.40$, $p < 0.0001$), and GBR-decanoate affected this response ($F[1,36] = 10.07$, $p < 0.01$). Specifically, *post hoc* tests revealed that rats receiving GBR-decanoate had higher levels of activity at the 0-µg/kg (i.e., control; $F[1,12] = 5.18$, $p < 0.05$) and 10-µg/kg ($F[1,12] = 11.45$, $p < 0.01$) quinpirole challenge doses. The apparent difference in sensitivity to quinpirole between groups was due to elevated baseline activity in GBR-decanoate rats. At the two-week time point, baseline locomotor responses to novelty were comparable between drug- (3082 ± 422 cm) and oil-pretreated (3172 ± 255 cm) groups. Quinpirole-induced suppression of locomotor activity was similar, regardless of pretreatment condition.

The data in FIGURE 7 illustrate the influence of prior exposure to GBR-decanoate on quinpirole-induced suppression on prolactin secretion. One week after GBR-decanoate, quinpirole decreased prolactin secretion ($F[2,36] = 10.46$, $p < 0.001$), and this effect was similar in both pretreatment groups. At the two-week time point,

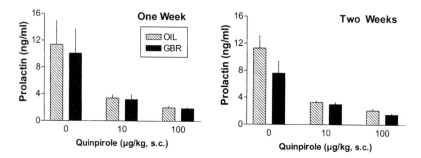

FIGURE 7. Effects of GBR-decanoate (GBR) pretreatment on quinpirole-induced suppression of prolactin secretion in rats. Rats received single i.m. injections of GBR (1 mL/kg of a 48% solution, or 480 mg/kg) or sesame oil vehicle. One week (*left panel*) and two weeks (*right panel*) later, rats received s.c. challenge injections of quinpirole (10 and 100 mg/kg) or saline vehicle. Rats were decapitated 30 min later and trunk blood was collected. Plasma prolactin was determined by double-antibody radioimmunoassay methods. [39] Values are ng/mL, expressed as mean ± SEM for $n = 6$–7 rats per group. * = $p < 0.05$ with respect to vehicle-pretreated group that received the same dose of quinpirole.

quinpirole decreased plasma prolactin levels to a similar extent in drug- and oil-pretreated rats.

DISCUSSION

The main purpose of the present experiments was to evaluate the neurobiological effects of a depot formulation of GBR12909, GBR-decanoate. With respect to the use of GBR-decanoate as a medication, we were particularly interested in the ability of this drug to influence METH-induced neurotransmitter release. GBR12909 is a high-affinity DA uptake inhibitor that is being tested in humans as a treatment for stimulant dependence,[28] and the decanoate derivative has been synthesized in an attempt to generate long-lasting pharmacological activity *in vivo*.[31] Our findings demonstrate several important consequences of GBR-decanoate treatment in rats, namely, (1) reductions in [^{125}I]RTI-55-labeled DAT binding, (2) elevations in baseline extracellular DA, and (3) inhibition of METH-evoked DA release. The dopaminergic effects produced by GBR-decanoate were persistent, lasting for at least two weeks after a single injection. Moreover, the actions of the drug appear to be DA-specific, since no changes in 5-HT neurotransmission were detected. It is noteworthy that rats pretreated with GBR-decanoate displayed enhanced locomotor responses to novelty, but this hyperactivity was transient, subsiding by two weeks postinjection. Finally, GBR-decanoate had little influence on responsiveness to the DA D_2/D_3 receptor agonist quinpirole, suggesting that GBR-decanoate does not dramatically alter DA receptor function.

A fundamental assumption governing the interpretation of our findings is that the effects of GBR-decanoate are mediated by a slow release of GBR-hydroxy into the bloodstream, with subsequent pseudoirreversible binding of GBR-hydroxy to DAT sites in the brain.[30,31] While we have no direct pharmacokinetic evidence to validate this notion, the present autoradiographic data show that GBR-decanoate produces significant decreases in *ex vivo* DAT binding (FIG. 3). The reductions in [^{125}I]RTI-55 binding are DAT-specific, since GBR-decanoate does not alter SERT binding. Moreover, the decreases in [^{125}I]RTI-55-labeled DAT binding parallel the neurochemical effects of GBR-decanoate suggesting a correlative relationship between these variables. Kunko *et al.*[40] observed that subchronic infusion of GBR12909 to rats (30 mg/kg/day for 7 days), which mimics the administration GBR-decanoate employed here, dramatically reduces the β_{max} for DAT binding in the striatum and nucleus accumbens. The decrease in DAT binding density is persistent, lasting for days after cessation of GBR12909 infusion. We believe that subchronic infusion of GBR12909, or by analogy administration of GBR-decanoate, causes long-term reductions in DAT binding via persistent occupation of transporter sites by the treatment drugs. Alternatively, it is possible that GBR analogs might diminish DAT binding by triggering internalization and proteolysis of DAT proteins.[41,42] Further experiments will be required to determine the precise molecular mechanism whereby GBR analogs decrease DAT binding.

Reductions in DAT binding produced by GBR-decanoate appear to have a number of functional consequences. For instance, the modest and sustained elevation of baseline extracellular DA produced by GBR-decanoate (see TABLE 1) is consistent with the ability of GBR-hydroxy to bind pseudoirreversibly to DAT sites, thereby causing prolonged inhibition of DA reuptake.[19,31] As depicted in FIGURE 2, acute i.v. injection of GBR-hydroxy causes a slow and steady rise in extracellular DA that reaches a plateau; this effect is reminiscent of the increase in dialysate DA evoked by i.v. GBR12909.[14] A persistent increase in baseline extracellular DA could be therapeutically relevant with regard to treating stimulant dependence. Preclinical evidence indicates that chronic administration of stimulants like cocaine and METH causes central DA dysfunction.[43,44] Indeed, high doses of METH induce neurotoxic depletions of DA in the brains of nonhuman primates and people.[45,46] Symptoms of stimulant withdrawal in humans include anhedonia, depression, and suicidal ideation, which might reflect deficits in brain DA.[47,48] GBR-decanoate, by increasing basal synaptic DA in the brain, might ease the dysphoria of stimulant withdrawal and correct a hypodopaminergic state.

Perhaps the most striking feature of GBR-decanoate treatment is the ability of the drug to nearly eliminate METH-induced DA release in a persistent manner (FIG. 4). It is noteworthy that this effect was DA-specific, since METH-induced 5-HT release is unaffected. From a molecular perspective, METH stimulates the release of monoamine transmitters (i.e., DA, 5-HT, and NE) by a nonexocytotic diffusion-exchange mechanism involving transporter proteins in nerve cell membranes.[49,50] The *in vivo* microdialysis data presented in FIGURES 4 and 5 show that acute METH administration evokes marked dose-related elevations in both DA and 5-HT in rat nucleus accumbens, and this observation agrees with the work of others.[51,52] Transporter proteins, such as DAT and SERT, play a pivotal role in mediating the neurochemical effects of METH, because these proteins serve as gateways for the passage of drug molecules into cells in exchange for transmitter molecules that flow out. We have shown previously that blocking DAT sites with GBR12909 can prevent the DA-releasing action of METH *in vitro*.[53] The present data demonstrate that GBR-decanoate can selectively antagonize METH-induced DA release *in vivo*.

Because DA release in the nucleus accumbens is implicated in the addictive properties of METH and other stimulants,[9] it seems possible that GBR-decanoate might reduce the positive reinforcing properties of illicit stimulants. Consistent with this notion, GBR12909 and GBR-decanoate are known to reduce cocaine self-administration in rats and monkeys.[24,25,30] More recent findings from Glowa et al.,[54] show that GBR12909 also attenuates METH self-administration in monkeys. Stimulant dependence, like other substance use disorders, is a chronic relapsing disease. Methamphetamine addicts in treatment are often poorly compliant and have high dropout rates.[29,55] Similar problems with schizophrenic patients have been addressed in part by the development of long-acting depot preparations of antipsychotic medications, such as haloperidol decanoate.[56] Based on the data from the present study, it seems plausible that METH addicts who take GBR-decanoate as a medication may not experience the reinforcing effects of METH in the event of relapse. Under such circumstances, METH abuse would be predicted to cease.

Our neurochemical data may shed light on the specific mechanisms whereby GBR12909 and GBR-decanoate suppress ongoing stimulant self-administration. We hypothesize that GBR-decanoate might reduce cocaine and METH self-administration by a process involving both DA and 5-HT systems. First, by blocking stimulant-evoked elevations in synaptic DA, GBR-type compounds can reduce the habit-forming properties of illicit stimulants, as described above. Second, because GBR-decanoate and GBR-hydroxy do not alter 5-HT transmission, the serotonergic effects produced by stimulant drugs remain unimpeded (see FIG. 5). It is well accepted that pharmacological treatments leading to increased synaptic 5-HT are not reinforcing. For example, increased serotonergic transmission decreases brain stimulation reward,[57] produces conditioned place aversions,[58] and reduces the positive reward value of stimulants both in animals and humans.[59,60] Thus, in the presence of GBR-type compounds, illicit stimulants like METH may become very effective 5-HT releasing agents that lack positive reinforcing qualities. On the other hand, several studies in rats demonstrate that pretreatment with monoamine reuptake inhibitors can enhance the discriminative stimulus properties of cocaine,[61,62] suggesting the possibility that GBR-decanoate might actually amplify the effects of illicit stimulants. Such uncertainties indicate that any clinical studies testing the safety and efficacy of GBR compounds should proceed with caution.

An important question with regard to the use of GBR-decanoate as a medication is whether the drug causes adverse effects. For instance, it might be predicted that prolonged blockade of DA uptake, and the ensuing elevations in synaptic DA, might alter downstream DA receptor function. Indeed, there is substantial evidence showing that repeated exposure to amphetamine or cocaine produces desensitization of DA D_2 autoreceptors in mesolimbic pathways.[63,64] In our study, the D_2/D_3 receptor agonist quinpirole was used as a probe to assess DA receptor sensitivity in rats pretreated with GBR-decanoate or vehicle. Low doses of quinpirole are known to inhibit exploratory activity in rodents, and most investigators agree that quinpirole-induced locomotor suppression is mediated via activation of DA D_2 autoreceptors[37,65] (although see Ref. 66). Rats receiving GBR-decanoate display enhanced locomotor responses to novelty when tested at the one-week time point, but this heightened activity disappears by two weeks postinjection (FIG. 6). The observed hyperactivity could be secondary to elevations in baseline extracellular DA produced by GBR-decanoate. Importantly, the ability of quinpirole to suppress loco-motor activity was similar in rats pretreated with GBR-decanoate or oil vehicle at both time points. Thus, based on the present locomotor activity data, we found little evidence for changes in D_2 autoreceptor function after GBR-decanoate treatment.

Prolactin is a protein hormone whose secretion from the anterior pituitary is ton-ically inhibited by hypothalamic DA release.[67] The prolactin-inhibiting action of DA is mediated by the direct binding of DA to D_2 receptors expressed on pituitary lactotrophs. In the present study, we used quinpirole-induced inhibition of prolactin secretion as an index of postsynaptic DA receptor sensitivity.[67,68] Baseline circulat-ing prolactin levels are similar in rats receiving GBR-decanoate or vehicle. Further-more, quinpirole produces marked decreases in circulating prolactin regardless of pretreatment condition (FIG. 7). These results indicate that GBR-decanoate does not alter DA receptor function in the anterior pituitary or in hypothalamic circuits cou-pled to neuroendocrine secretion.

In summary, the data presented herein show that GBR-decanoate produces long-lasting decreases in DAT binding, elevations in baseline extracellular DA, and profound reductions in METH-evoked DA release. These effects are most likely due to persistent occupation of DAT sites by GBR-hydroxy. Interestingly, we observed no significant changes in DA receptor function in rats receiving GBR-decanoate, de-spite profound changes in presynaptic DA function. A key question to be answered is what degree of DAT occupancy by GBR-hydroxy is necessary to attenuate METH-induced DA release. Studies using positron emission tomography in baboons indicate that doses of GBR12909 producing DAT occupancy levels of 30–40% can substantially reduce amphetamine-induced DA release.[23] In humans, a 100-mg dose of GBR12909 occupies 30–40% of DAT sites in the caudate nucleus,[69] and this dose of drug does not elicit stimulant-like subjective effects in normal volunteers.[70] Sim-ilar levels of DAT occupancy were obtained here in rats pretreated with GBR-decanoate. Thus, it seems feasible that daily oral administration of GBR12909, or periodic injections of GBR-decanoate, could significantly antagonize dopaminergic effects of METH and facilitate abstinence in METH-dependent individuals. Careful-ly controlled clinical trials with these medications should be conducted to determine the efficacy of such intervention.

ACKNOWLEDGMENT

This work was generously supported by the NIDA, IRP.

REFERENCES

1. ANONYMOUS. 1995. Increasing morbidity and mortality associated with abuse of meth-amphetamine—United States, 1991–1994. MMWR Morb. Mort. Wkly. Rep. **44:** 882–886.
2. ALBERSON, T.E., R.W. DERLET & B.E. VAN DOOZEN. 1999. Methamphetamine and the expanding complications of amphetamines. West. J. Med. **170:** 214–219.
3. http://www.usdoj.gov/ndic/pubs/647/meth.htm
4. RAWSON, R.A., M.D. ANGLIN & W. LING. 2002. Will the methamphetamine problem go away? J. Addict. Dis. **21:** 5–19.

5. http://www.un.org/ga/20special/featur/amphet.htm
6. NATIONAL INSTITUTE ON DRUG ABUSE. 1999. Epidemiological Trends in Drug Abuse. Vol. II: Proceedings of the International Epidemiology Work Group on Drug Abuse. NIH Publication No. 00-4530.
7. McCANCE, E.F. 1997. Overview of potential treatment medications for cocaine dependence. NIDA Res. Monogr. **175**: 36–72.
8. CARROLL, F.I., L.L HOWELL & M.J. KUHAR. 1999. Pharmacotherapies for treatment of cocaine abuse: preclinical aspects. J. Med. Chem. **42**: 2721–2736.
9. WISE, R.A. 1996. Neurobiology of addiction. Curr. Opin. Neurobiol. **6**: 243–251.
10. KUCZENSKI, R. & D.S. SEGAL. 1994. Neurochemistry of amphetamine. In Amphetamine and Its Analogs—Psychopharmacology, Toxicology, and Abuse. A.K. Cho and D.S. Segal, Eds.: 81–113. Academic Press. San Diego.
11. RUDNICK, G. 1997. Mechanisms of biogenic amine neurotransmitter transporters. In Neurotransmitter Transporters— Structure, Function, and Regulation. M.E.A. Reith, Ed.: 73–100. Humana Press. Totowa, NJ.
12. ROTHMAN, R.B. et al. 2000. Neurochemical neutralization of methamphetamine with high-affinity nonselective inhibitors of biogenic amine transporters: a pharmacological strategy for treating stimulant abuse. Synapse **35**: 222–227.
13. ROTHMAN, R.B. 1990. High affinity dopamine uptake inhibitors as potential cocaine antagonists. Life. Sci. **46**: PL21–PL221.
14. BAUMANN, M.H. et al. 1994. GBR12909 attenuates cocaine-induced activation of mesolimbic dopamine neurons in the rat. J. Pharmacol. Exp. Ther. **271**: 1216–1222.
15. ROTHMAN, R.B. & J.R. GLOWA. 1995. A review of the effects of dopaminergic agents on humans, animals, and drug seeking behavior, and its implications for medication development: focus on GBR12909. Mol. Neurobiol. **11**: 1–19.
16. ANDERSEN, P.H. 1989. The dopamine inhibitor GBR12909: selectivity and molecular mechanism of action. Eur. J. Pharmacol. **166**: 493–504.
17. ROTHMAN, R.B. et al. 1993. Identification of a GBR12935 homolog, LR111, which is over 4000-fold selective for the dopamine transporter, relative to serotonin and norepinephrine transporters. Synapse **14**: 34–39.
18. ROTHMAN, R.B. et al. 1994. Studies of the biogenic amine transporters. IV. Demonstration of a multiplicity of binding sites in rat caudate membranes for the cocaine analog [^{125}I]RTI-55. J. Pharmacol. Exp. Ther. **270**: 296–309.
19. ROTHMAN, R.B. et al. 1991. GBR12909 antagonizes the ability of cocaine to elevate extracellular levels of dopamine. Pharmacol. Biochem. Behav. **40**: 387–397.
20. VAUGHAN, R.A. 1995. Photoaffinity-labeled ligand binding domains on dopamine transporters identified by peptide mapping. Mol. Pharmacol. **47**: 956–964.
21. VAUGHAN, R.A. & M.J. KUHAR. 1996. Dopamine transporter ligand binding domains. J. Biol. Chem. **271**: 21672–21680.
22. POGUN, S., U. SCHEFFEL & M.J. KUHAR. 1991. Cocaine displaces [^{3}H]WIN35428 binding to dopamine uptake sites in vivo more rapidly than mazindol and GBR12909. Eur. J. Pharmacol. **198**: 203–205.
23. VILLEMAGNE, V.L. et al. 1999. GBR12909 attenuates amphetamine-induced striatal dopamine release as measured by [^{11}C]raclopride continuous infusion PET scans. Synapse **33**: 268–273.
24. TELLA, S.R. 1995. Effects of monoamine reuptake inhibitors on cocaine self-administration in rats. Pharmacol. Biochem. Behav. **51**: 687–692.
25. GLOWA, J.R. et al. 1995. Effects of dopamine reuptake inhibitors on food and cocaine maintained responding. II: comparisons with other drugs and repeated administrations. Exp. Clin. Psychopharmacol. **3**.
26. TELLA, S.R. et al. 1996. Differential reinforcing effects of cocaine and GBR-12909: biochemical evidence for divergent neuroadaptive changes in the mesolimbic dopaminergic system. J. Neurosci. **16**: 7416–7427.
27. WOJNICKI, F.H. & J.R. GLOWA. 1996. Effects of drug history on the acquisition of responding maintained by GBR12909 in rhesus monkeys. Psychopharmacology **123**: 34–41.
28. PRETI, A. 2000. Vanoxerine, National Institute on Drug Abuse. Curr. Opin. Investig. Drugs **2**: 241–251.

29. BATTJES, R.J., L.S. ONKEN & P.J. DELANY. 1999. Drug abuse treatment entry and engagement: report of a meeting on treatment readiness. J. Clin. Psychol. **55:** 643–657.
30. GLOWA, J.R. *et al.* 1996. Sustained decrease in cocaine-maintained responding in rhesus monkeys with 1-[2-[bis(4-fluorophenyl)methoxy]ethyl]-4-(3-hydroxy-3-phenylpropyl) piperazinyl decanoate, a long-acting ester derivative of GBR 12909. J. Med. Chem. **39:** 4689–4691.
31. LEWIS, D.B. *et al.* 1999. Oxygenated analogs of 1-[2-(diphenylmethoxy)ethyl]- and 1-[2-[bis-(4-fluorophenyl)methoxy]ethyl] 4-(3-phenylpropyl)piperazines (GBR12935 and GBR12909) as potential extended-action cocaine-abuse therapeutic agents. J. Med. Chem. **42:** 5029–5042.
32. DREYFUSS, J. *et al.* 1976. Release and elimination of ^{14}C-fluphenazine enanthate and decanoate esters administered in sesame oil to dogs. J. Pharm. Sci. **65:** 502–507.
33. FLORENCE, A.T. & W.R. VEZIN. 1981. Prolongation of the action of intramuscular formulations of phenothiazines. *In* Optimization of Drug Delivery. H. Bundgaard, A. Bagger Hansen, and H. Kofod, Eds.: 93–111. Munkgaard Publishing. Copenhagen.
34. ROTHMAN, R.B. *et al.* 1998. Studies of the biogenic amine transporters. VII. Characterization of a novel cocaine binding site identified with [^{125}I]RTI-55 in membranes prepared from human, monkey and guinea pig caudate. Synapse **28:** 322–338.
35. STALEY, J.K. *et al.* 1994. Visualizing dopamine and serotonin transporters in the human brain with the potent cocaine analog [^{125}I]RTI-55: in vitro binding and autoradiographic characterization. J. Neurochem. **62:** 549–556.
36. BAUMANN, M.H. *et al.* 2000. Effects of phentermine and fenfluramine on extracellular dopamine and serotonin in rat nucleus accumbens: therapeutic implications. Synapse **36:** 102–113.
37. SVENSSON, K. *et al.* 1994. Behavioral and neurochemical data suggest functional differences between dopamine D2 and D3 receptors. Eur. J. Pharmacol. **263:** 235–243.
38. HEIDBREDER C.A. & M.H. BAUMANN. 2001. Autoregulation of dopamine synthesis in subregions of the rat nucleus accumbens. Eur. J. Pharmacol. **411:** 107–113.
39. BAUMANN, M.H. *et al.* 2000. Differential neuroendocrine responsiveness to morphine in Lewis, Fischer 344, and ACI inbred rats. Brain Res. **858:** 320–326.
40. KUNKO, P.M., R.J. LOELOFF & S. IZENWASSER. 1997. Chronic administration of the selective dopamine uptake inhibitor, GBR12909, but not cocaine, produces marked decreases in dopamine transporter density. Naunyn-Schmiedebergs Arch. Pharmacol. **356:** 562–569.
41. DANIELS, G.M. & S.G. AMARA. 1999. Regulated trafficking of the human dopamine transporter. J. Biol. Chem. **274:** 35794–35801.
42. MELIKIAN, H.E. & K.M. BUCKLEY. 1999. Membrane trafficking regulates the activity of the human dopamine transporter. J. Neurosci. **19:** 7699–7710.
43. SEIDEN, L.S., K.E. SABOL & G.A. RICAURTE. 1993. Amphetamine: effects on catecholamine systems and behavior. Annu. Rev. Pharmacol. Toxicol. **33:** 639–677.
44. KUHAR, M.J. & N.S. PILOTTE. 1996. Neurochemical changes in cocaine withdrawal. Trends Pharmacol. Sci. **17:** 260–264.
45. WILSON, J.M. *et al.* 1996. Striatal dopamine nerve terminal markers in human chronic methamphetamine users. Nat. Med. **2:** 699–703.
46. VILLEMAGNE, V.L. *et al.* 1998. Brain dopamine neurotoxicity in baboons treated with doses of methamphetamine comparable to those recreationally abused by humans: evidence from [^{11}C]WIN-35,428 positron emission tomograpgy studies and direct in vitro determinations. J. Neurosci. **18:** 419–427.
47. GAWIN, F. 1991. Cocaine addiction: psychology and neurophysiology. Science **253:** 1580–1586.
48. KALECHSTEIN, A.D. *et al.* 2000. Psychiatric comorbidity of methamphetamine dependence in a forensic sample. J. Neuropsychiatry Clin. Neurosci. **12:** 480–484.
49. RUDNICK, G. & J. CLARK. 1993. From synapse to vesicle: the reuptake and storage of biogenic amine neurotransmitters. Biochimica et Biophysica Acta **1144:** 249–263.
50. WALL, S.C., H. GU & G. RUDNICK. 1995. Biogenic amine flux mediated by cloned transporters stably expressed in cultured cell lines: amphetamine specificity for inhibition and efflux. Mol. Pharmacol. **47:** 544–550.

51. KUCZENSK, R. *et al.* 1995. Hippocampus norepinephrine, caudate dopamine and serotonin, and behavioral responses to stereoisomers of amphetamine and methamphetamine. J. Neurosci. **15:** 1308–1317.
52. MELEGA, W.P. *et al.* 1995. Pharmacokinetic and pharmacodynamic analysis of the action of amphetamine and D-methamphetamine on dopamine terminals. J. Pharmacol. Exp. Ther. **274:** 90–96.
53. ROTHMAN, R.B. *et al.* 2000. Methamphetamine dependence: medication development efforts based on a dual deficit model of stimulant addiction. Ann. N.Y. Acad. Sci. **914:** 71–81.
54. GLOWA, J.R. *et al.* 2001. Effects of GBR12909 on responding maintained under a progressive-ratio schedule of methamphetamine delivery in rhesus monkeys. Drug Alcohol Depend. **63:** S55–S56.
55. MAGLIONE, M., B. CHAO & M.D. ANGLIN. 2000. Correlates of outpaient drug-treatment drop-out among methamphetamine users. J. Psychoact. Drugs **32:** 221–228.
56. DAVIS, J.M. *et al.* 1993. Dose response of prophylactic antipsychotics. J. Clin. Psychiatry **54**(Suppl.): 24–30.
57. HARRISON, A.A. & A. MARKOU. 2001. Serotonergic manipulations both potentiate and reduce brain stimulation reward in rats: involvement of serotonin1A receptors. J. Pharmacol. Exp. Ther. **297:** 31–325.
58. MARONA-LEWICKA, D. *et al.* 1996. Reinforcing effects of certain serotonin-releasing amphetamine derivatives. Pharmacol. Biochem. Behav. **53:** 99–105.
59. BRAUER, L.H. *et al.* 1996. Evaluation of phentermine and fenfluramine, alone and in combination, in normal, healthy volunteers. Neuropsychopharmacology **14:** 233–241.
60. REA, W.P., R.B. ROTHMAN & T.S. SHIPPENBERG. 1998. Evaluation of the conditioned reinforcing effects of phentermine and fenfluramine in the rat: concordance with clinical studies. Synapse **30:** 107–111.
61. CUNNINGHAM, K.A. & P.M. CALLAHAN. 1991. Monoamine reuptake inhibitors enhance the discriminative state induced by cocaine in the rat. Psychopharmacology **104:** 177–180.
62. KLEVEN, M.S. & W. KOEK. 1998. Discriminative stimulus properties of cocaine: enhancement by monoamine reuptake inhibitors. J. Pharmacol. Exp. Ther. **284:** 1015–1025.
63. WHITE, F.J. & R.Y. WANG. 1984. Electrophysiological evidence for A10 dopamine autoreceptor subsensitivity following chronic D-amphetamine treatment. Brain Res. **309:** 283–292.
64. HENRY, D.J., M.A. GREENE & F.J. WHITE. 1989. Electrophysiological effects of cocaine in the mesoaccumbens dopamine system: repeated administration. J. Pharmacol. Exp. Ther. **251:** 833–839.
65. DEPOORTERE, R., G. PERRAULT & D.J. SANGER. 1996. Behavioural effects in the rat of the putative dopamine D3 receptor agonist 7-OH-DPAT: comparison with quinpirole and apomorphine. Psychopharmacology **124:** 231–240.
66. STAHLE, L. 1992. Do autoreceptors mediate dopamine agonist-induced yawning and suppression of exploration? A critical review. Psychopharmacology **106:** 1–14.
67. BEN JONATHAN, N. & R. HNASKO. 2001. Dopamine as a prolactin (PRL) inhibitor. Endocr. Rev. **22:** 724–763.
68. KURASHIMA, M. *et al.* 1996. Inhibitory effects of putative dopamine D3 receptor agonists, 7-OH-DPAT and quinpirole, on prolactin secretion in rats. Pharmacol. Biochem. Behav. **53:** 379–383.
69. WONG, D.F. *et al.* 1999. In vivo human dopamine transporter occupancy of a potential cocaine treatment agent. Soc. Neurosci. Abstr. **29:** 242.
70. SÖGAARD U. *et al.* 1990. A tolerance study of single and multiple dosing of the selective dopamine uptake inhibitor GBR 12909 in healthy subjects. Int. Clin. Psychopharmacol. **5:** 237–251.

Appetite Suppressants as Agonist Substitution Therapies for Stimulant Dependence

RICHARD B. ROTHMAN,[a] BRUCE E. BLOUGH,[b] AND MICHAEL H. BAUMANN[a]

[a]Clinical Psychopharmacology Section, NIDA, NIH, Baltimore, Maryland 21224, USA

[b]Chemistry and Life Sciences, Research Triangle Institute, Research Triangle Park, North Carolina 27709, USA

ABSTRACT: Several lines of evidence support a dual-deficit model of stimulant withdrawal in which decreases in synaptic dopamine (DA) and serotonin (5-HT) contribute to withdrawal symptoms, drug craving, and relapse. According to the dual-deficit model, DA dysfunction during withdrawal underlies anhedonia and psychomotor disturbances, whereas 5-HT dysfunction gives rise to depressed mood, obsessive thoughts, and lack of impulse control. The model suggests that medications capable of normalizing stimulant-induced DA and 5-HT deficits should be effective treatment adjuncts. Furthermore, the model may explain why medications targeting only one neurotransmitter system (i.e., DA) have failed to treat cocaine dependence. Amphetamine-type appetite suppressants are logical choices for neurochemical normalization therapy of stimulant dependence, yet few clinical studies have tested anorectics in this regard. The chief purpose of the present work is to profile the activity of various anorectic agents at DA, 5-HT, and NE transporters, in order to identify possible medications for stimulant dependence. Compounds were tested *in vitro* for their ability to stimulate release and inhibit uptake of [³H]DA, [³H]NE, and [³H]5-HT. Selected compounds were tested *in vivo* for their ability to elevate extracellular levels of DA and 5-HT in rat nucleus accumbens. The results show that clinically available appetite suppressants display a wide range of activities at monoamine transporters. However, no single medication possesses equal potency at DA and 5-HT transporters, suggesting that none of the anorectics is ideally suited for treatment of stimulant addictions. Future efforts should focus on developing new medications that possess the desired therapeutic activity but lack the adverse effects associated with older amphetamine-type anorectics.

KEYWORDS: methamphetamine; appetite suppressant; agonist substitution therapy; dual-deficit model; stimulant withdrawal

INTRODUCTION

Cocaine and methamphetamine are major drugs of abuse in the United States. These stimulants are generally acknowledged to be among the most addictive substances known,[1–3] and long-term stimulant abuse is associated with considerable

Address for correspondence: Richard B. Rothman M.D., Ph.D., Clinical Psychopharmacology Section, IRP, NIDA, NIH, 5600 Nathan Shock Drive, Baltimore, MD 21224. Voice: 410-550-1487; fax: 410-550-2997.

rrothman@intra.nida.nih.gov

Ann. N.Y. Acad. Sci. 965: 109–126 (2002). © 2002 New York Academy of Sciences.

morbidity and mortality.[3,4] The comorbidity of drug abuse with psychiatric disorders, as well as the clinical presentation of primary stimulant dependence, [5–7] indicates that efforts to develop new and effective treatments for stimulant addictions is
an important goal of biomedical research. The association of intravenous drug use
with the spread of HIV [8,9] heightens the importance of this effort to society.

Despite intensive investigation, effective pharmacotherapy for stimulant addiction remains a research goal rather than a clinical reality. Formidable barriers exist
to the development of any medication, as it often takes many years and millions of
dollars to bring a drug from its initial discovery to final approval by the Food and
Drug Administration.[10] As reviewed elsewhere, additional barriers hinder the development of medications specifically targeted for substance-abuse disorders.[11] These
hurdles are sufficiently prohibitive that major pharmaceutical firms do not place a
high priority on identifying medications for treating stimulant addiction. Therefore,
the development of such pharmacotherapies is a task left to the public sector. In this
regard, a logical place to look for potential treatment agents is among the medications already approved for human use. In this paper, we will describe our efforts to
characterize clinically approved amphetamine-type appetite suppressants as potential treatment agents for cocaine and methamphetamine dependence.

The use of stimulant-like medications to treat stimulant addictions is an approach
described as "agonist substitution" therapy. This strategy involves administering
medications that are less potent and less addictive than cocaine or methamphetamine, but that nevertheless decrease stimulant abuse because of shared neurochemical properties with the illicit drugs.[12] Viewed from this perspective, agonist
substitution therapy could be described as neurochemical "normalization" therapy:
by substituting for the abused drug, the treatment drug "normalizes" dysregulated
neurochemistry. Neurochemical normalization therapy has generated effective treatments for nicotine dependence[13] and opioid dependence,[14,15] and this approach has
recently been explored for the treatment of cocaine dependence.[16–20]

An important first step in the development of successful normalization therapy
for stimulant addictions is determining the neurobiological consequences of long-
term stimulant abuse. A major hypothesis driving medication discovery efforts for
cocaine addiction is the so-called "dopamine (DA) hypothesis," which proposes that
chronic cocaine exposure leads to a functional DA deficit.[21,22] This hypothesis has
been tested extensively by double-blind placebo-controlled clinical trials of medications known to increase central DA transmission. Unfortunately, none of the medications assessed thus far has demonstrated efficacy for treating cocaine dependence
(for review, see Ref. 23). While a variety of factors can account for the lack of efficacy seen in these trials,[24] it seems possible that the DA hypothesis may be insufficient to explain the complex underpinnings of cocaine addiction. Indeed, converging
lines of evidence indicate that cocaine withdrawal is accompanied by deficits in serotonin (5-HT) function, as well as DA function, in the brain.[25–31] For example, *in
vivo* microdialysis studies in rats have shown that withdrawal from repeated cocaine
injections is accompanied by decreases in basal extracellular levels of both DA and
5-HT in the brain.[28,32–34]

Based on the findings just-mentioned, we have proposed a dual-deficit model of
stimulant withdrawal in which drug-induced DA and 5-HT dysfunction contributes
to withdrawal symptomatology, drug craving, and relapse.[30,35–37] According to the

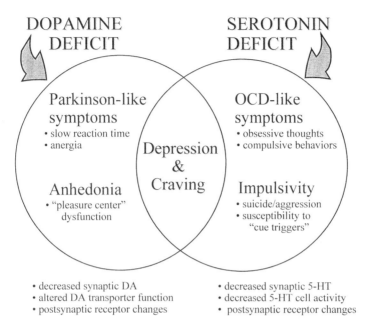

FIGURE 1. The dual-deficit model of psychostimulant withdrawal. According to the model, withdrawal from chronic stimulant use leads to decreased synaptic availability of DA and 5-HT, which contributes to withdrawal symptoms, drug craving, and relapse. DA dysfunction underlies anhedonia and psychomotor disturbances, whereas 5-HT dysfunction causes depressed mood, obsessive thoughts, and lack of impulse control. Protracted withdrawal phenomena are postulated to contribute significantly to relapse.

dual-deficit model (FIG. 1), decreased synaptic DA during stimulant withdrawal underlies anhedonia and psychomotor retardation, whereas decreased synaptic 5-HT gives rise to depressed mood, obsessive thoughts, and lack of impulse control. Consistent with this model, rats receiving repeated injections of abused stimulants exhibit neurobiological changes similar to those observed in human patients with major depression.[31,36,38,39] The dual-deficit model predicts that pharmacotherapies capable of normalizing the proposed abnormalities in DA and 5-HT function should be effective in treating stimulant dependence. Indeed, drugs that release DA (phentermine, amphetamine) and 5-HT (fenfluramine) display properties that are consistent with effective treatment of substance use disorders.[35,40–43]

Clinically available appetite suppressants, such as phentermine, diethylpropion, and phendimetrazine, are logical candidates for neurochemical normalization therapy of stimulant dependence. As depicted in FIGURE 2, these medications and the other anorectic agents considered in this paper are structurally related to amphetamine (i.e., phenylethylamines). Furthermore, most of these drugs share behavioral properties with abused stimulants, but are less potent and less addictive.[44–47] Interestingly, the neurochemical mechanism underlying the behavioral actions of many

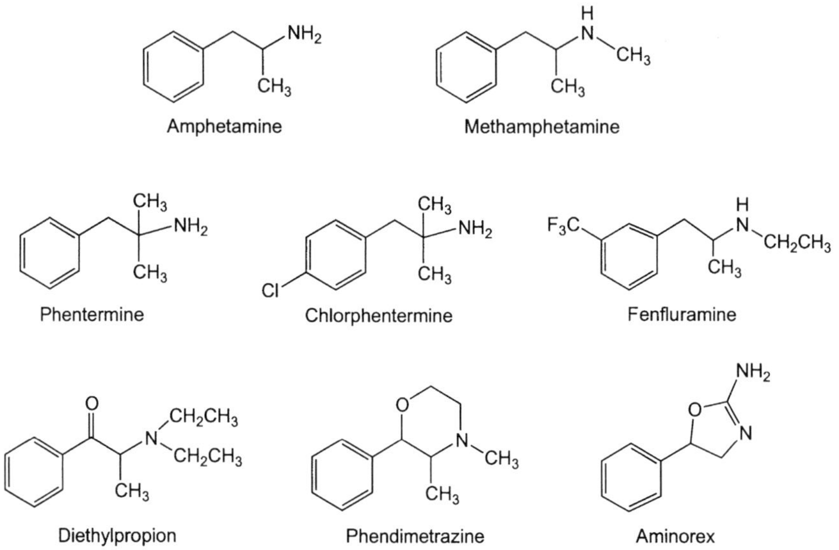

FIGURE 2. Chemical structures of selected amphetamine-type appetite suppressants.

anorectic drugs is not well studied. Depending on the drug tested, these agents can increase extracellular levels of DA, 5-HT, or both transmitters, in the brain.[37,48–50] According to the dual-deficit hypothesis, the ideal normalization pharmacotherapy should elevate extracellular levels of DA and 5-HT to a similar extent, and the balance between stimulation of DA and 5-HT transmission has important therapeutic implications. For example, anorectic agents like phentermine that stimulate DA transmission, possess the undesirable qualities of locomotor activation and abuse liability. Drug treatments that stimulate 5-HT transmission, on the other hand, can antagonize phentermine-induced motor activation,[37] phentermine-related reward,[35] and phentermine-associated subjective effects.[51] Thus, elevations in synaptic 5-HT appear to counteract undesirable effects mediated by elevations in synaptic DA. Consistent with this hypothesis, the phentermine/fenfluramine combination is not self-administered by rats.[52]

An additional rationale for considering appetite suppressants as potential pharmacotherapies for stimulant dependence is the substantial overlap between neural circuits controlling feeding behavior and those involved in self-administration of abused drugs.[53–55] Food deprivation enhances the acquisition of stimulant self-administration behavior, suggesting there are similarities between hunger for food and "hunger" for abused drugs. Thus, both food consumption and drug self-administration are homeostatic deficit-driven processes. When stimulant addiction is viewed as dysregulated appetitive behavior, it seems reasonable to theorize that medications used to combat obesity (i.e., excessive food consumption) could also treat drug addiction (i.e., excessive drug intake).[37,56] Thus, we speculated that amphetamine-type appetite suppressants might be effective in the treatment of substance-abuse disorders. Consistent with this hypothesis, a variety of appetite suppressants decrease cocaine and methamphetamine self-administration in animal species.[52,57–60]

It is well accepted that illicit stimulants like cocaine and methamphetamine interact with DA transporters (DAT), norepinephrine transporters (NET), and 5-HT transporters (SERT) in nervous tissue.[61,62] More specifically, cocaine binds to monoamine transporters, thereby blocking transmitter reuptake. Methamphetamine acts as a substrate for monoamine transporters, thereby stimulating nonexocytotic transmitter release. In both cases, the immediate consequence of drug/transporter interactions is elevation of the synaptic levels of DA, NE, and 5-HT throughout the neuraxis.[63–66] Perhaps by analogy, it is often assumed that amphetamine-type appetite suppressants act at monoamine transporters to release DA, NE, and 5-HT, but this hypothesis has not been rigorously tested for many anorectics. Because of the critical role of DAT, NET, and SERT proteins in mediating the actions of abused stimulants and anorectic medications, we have developed uptake and release assays as tools to examine the effects of drugs on monoamine transporter function. The chief purpose of the work described herein is to examine the profile of activity of various amphetamine-type appetite suppressants at DAT, NET, and SERT, in order to identify possible candidate medications for normalization therapy of stimulant dependence.

MATERIALS AND METHODS

Animals

Male Sprague-Dawley rats (300–450 g) were obtained from Charles River Laboratories (Wilmington, MA). The animal housing facilities were fully accredited by the American Association of the Accreditation of Laboratory Animal Care (AAA-LAC), and all experiments were performed within the guidelines delineated in the Institutional Care and Use Committee of the National Institute on Drug Abuse (NIDA), Intramural Research Program (IRP).

Transporter Assays

The assays used to characterize reuptake and release of [^{3}H]DA, [^{3}H]NE, and [^{3}H]5HT were performed according to published methods.[67] Briefly, a crude synaptosomal tissue preparation from rat caudate (for DA reuptake and release assays) or from whole brain minus caudate (for NE and 5HT reuptake and release assays) was obtained by homogenizing freshly excised tissue in ice-cold 10% sucrose using 12 strokes of a Potter-Elvehjem homogenizer. The homogenate was centrifuged at 1000 g for 10 min. Supernatants were retained on ice and used immediately in reuptake and release assays.

All assays were performed in Krebs-phosphate buffer (pH 7.4) containing 154.4 mM NaCl, 2.9 mM KCl, 1.1 mM CaCl$_2$, 0.83 mM MgCl$_2$, 5 mM glucose, 1 mg/mL ascorbic acid, and 50 μM pargyline. For [^{3}H]DA, [^{3}H]NE, and [^{3}H]5HT release assays, 1 μM reserpine was added to the sucrose solution and assay buffer. [^{3}H]NE reuptake and release assays were performed in the presence of 5 nM RTI-229 to prevent reuptake of [^{3}H]NE into dopaminergic nerves. [^{3}H]5HT reuptake and release assays were performed in the presence of 100 nM nomifensine and 100 nM GBR12909 to prevent reuptake of [^{3}H]5HT into noradrenergic and dopaminergic nerves. For the reuptake assays, incubation times were 15, 10, and 30 min for [^{3}H]DA, [^{3}H]NE, and [^{3}H]5HT, respectively.

For release assays, synaptosomal preparations were incubated to steady state with 5 nM [^{3}H]DA (30 min), 7 nM [^{3}H]NE (60 min), or 5 nM [^{3}H]5HT (60 min). Synaptosomes preloaded with [^{3}H]neurotransmitter were added to test tubes containing test drugs and incubated for 5 min ([^{3}H]DA and [^{3}H]5HT) or 30 min ([^{3}H]NE). At the designated time, the assay was filtered using a Packard Filtermate Harvester. Nondisplaceable tritium was measured by incubations in the presence of 100 μM tyramine for [^{3}H]5-HT release and 10 μM tyramine for [^{3}H]DA and [^{3}H]NE release. The filters were dried for an hour at 60°C and counted using the Packard Topcount-NXT™ Microplate Scintillation and Luminescence Counter. Retained tritium was counted by a Taurus liquid scintillation counter at 40% efficiency after an overnight extraction in 3 mL Cytoscint (ICN).

In Vivo *Microdialysis*

Surgical implantation of indwelling jugular catheters and intra-accumbens guide cannulae was carried out as previously described.[63] Guide cannulae were aimed at the nucleus accumbens according to the coordinates of Paxinos and Watson.[68] Rats were singly housed after surgery and allowed to recover for at least one week. On the evening prior to testing, extension tubes were connected to catheters and microdialysis probes (2-mm × 0.5-mm exchange surface, CMA/12, CMA/Microdialysis) were inserted into the nucleus accumbens via the previously implanted guide cannulae. Each rat was placed into its own plexiglass arena and then connected to a tethering system that allowed movement within the container. Probes were perfused *in situ* with artificial cerebrospinal fluid (aCSF) containing 150 mM NaCl, 3.0 mM KCl, 1.4 mM CaCl$_2$, 0.8 mM MgCl$_2$, overnight at 0.5 μL/min. The next morning, dialysate samples were collected at 20-min intervals. Samples were immediately assayed for DA and 5-HT by microbore high-pressure liquid chromatography with electrochemical detection (HPLC-EC), as described elsewhere.[37] Three baseline samples were collected before any treatments, and all subsequent DA and 5-HT measures were expressed as a percent of this baseline. Probe recoveries of DA and 5-HT ranged from 18% to 20%. Drug solutions were prepared immediately before use, and doses are expressed as the salt.

Data Analysis

For the *in vitro* data, IC_{50} values (for inhibition of reuptake) and EC_{50} values (for stimulation of release) were determined using the nonlinear least-square curve-fitting program MLABPC (Civilized Software, Bethesda, MD). In the reuptake assays, apparent K_i values were calculated from IC_{50} values using well-described methods.[69] In the release assays, "specific" displaceable tritium was calculated as the difference between total retained tritium and nondisplaceable tritium. As described earlier,[67] in release experiments the apparent K_i of reuptake blockers was determined by measuring the EC_{50} value of a releasing agent in the absence (EC_{50-1})

and presence (EC_{50-2}) of the blocking agent. The K_i was calculated according to the following equation: $K_i = [\text{Test Drug}]/(EC_{50-2}/EC_{50-1} - 1]$. For the microdialysis experiments, the first three samples collected before any treatment were considered baseline, and all subsequent monoamine measures were expressed as a percent of this baseline. Data were evaluated by one-way (acute drug treatment) ANOVA with repeated measures. Sources of reagents and chemicals are published.[70]

RESULTS AND DISCUSSION

Traditionally, it has been difficult to use simple *in vitro* test assays to discriminate between drugs that are monoamine uptake blockers and those that are substrate-type releasers. This problem arises because both types of drugs interact with the same transporter proteins to elevate extracellular levels of neurotransmitter.[61,62] Thus, a releasing agent might be incorrectly identified as an uptake blocker because releasers display potent activity in assays measuring [³H]neurotransmitter uptake. To circumvent this problem, neurotransmitter release is often determined *in vitro* using superfusion assay systems.[71,72,73] In this approach, tissue slices or synaptosomes are preloaded with [³H]neurotransmitter and then placed in superfusion chambers. Physiological medium is perfused through the chambers and the medium is assayed for released neurotransmitter. This method essentially generates a time course of neurotransmitter release for each drug concentration tested. Not surprisingly, using this method to generate dose-response curves or screen large numbers of compounds is a time-consuming process.

Our laboratory has recently developed a rapid high-throughput method for measuring release of [³H]DA, [³H]NE, and [³H]5-HT from nervous tissue *in vitro*.[67] The basic strategy employed in the release assay is to first incubate synaptosomes with [³H]neurotransmitter for sufficient time to achieve steady state. At steady state, test drugs are added to synaptosomes, and after 5 min the reaction is terminated by rapid filtration. Transmitter "release" is quantified by measuring the amount of tritium retained on the filter: decreases in retained tritium reflect increases in [³H]neurotransmitter released. A key requirement of our release assay is the inclusion of reserpine in the assay buffer; reserpine prevents accumulation of neurotransmitters in synaptic vesicles, thereby maximizing the amount of preloaded [³H]neurotransmitter available for substrate-induced release. The addition of reserpine greatly amplifies the signal-to-noise ratio of the assay.

The activity of transporter blockers can be readily distinguished from that of transporter substrates using our *in vitro* release assay. For instance, FIGURE 3 compares the effects of indatraline (a transporter blocker) and methamphetamine (a transporter substrate) on [³H]neurotransmitter release. Indatraline is a nonselective uptake inhibitor that has high affinity for DAT, NET, and SERT, yet this drug displays very weak activity in release assays. By contrast, the transporter substrate, methamphetamine causes dose-dependent release of [³H]DA, [³H]NE, and [³H]5-HT. Methamphetamine is much more potent at releasing DA and NE when compared to its effects on 5-HT, consistent with the known pharmacology of this drug.[67,70] The data in FIGURE 4 demonstrate that low concentrations of indatraline antagonize methamphetamine-induced release of [³H]DA, shifting the methamphetamine re-

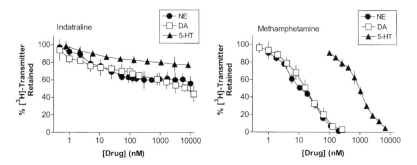

FIGURE 3. Effects of the reuptake blocker indatraline (*left panel*) and the transporter substrate methamphetamine (*right panel*) on the release of [³H]DA, [³H]NE, and [³H]5-HT in synaptosomes. Release assays were carried out as described in Materials and Methods. Each point is the mean ± SD (*n* = 3). (Data are from Rothman *et al.*[67])

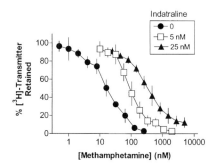

FIGURE 4. Effects of indatraline (5 nM and 25 nM) on methamphetamine-evoked release of [³H]DA. Release assays were carried out as described in Materials and Methods. Each point is the mean ± SD (*n* = 3). (Data are from Rothman *et al.*[67])

lease curve to the right. Thus, indatraline blocks the DA-releasing activity of meth-amphetamine by binding to DAT sites in the tissue. The apparent K_i value for indatraline (~2 nM) calculated from the shift of the methamphetamine release curve is similar to its K_i value for inhibition of [³H]DA uptake (1.9 nM). These findings show that our assay systems can discriminate releasers from uptake blockers. More-over, the assays can be used to evaluate the pharmacological profile of test drugs at all three monoamine transporters under similar experimental conditions.

Using *in vitro* uptake and release assays, we characterized the interaction of var-ious transporter substrates and uptake blockers at DAT, NET, and SERT proteins. With specific reference to the dual-deficit model discussed in the Introduction (FIG. 1), we hoped to identify compounds that cause substrate-type release of DA and 5-HT with similar potency. The *in vitro* data are summarized in TABLE 1. Of the clinically available appetite suppressants, no compound releases both DA and 5-HT with equal potency. For example, phentermine and (+)-amphetamine are 13-fold and 71-fold more potent at DA release than 5-HT release. It is important to note that

TABLE 1. Pharmacological profile of selected agents in the DA, NE, and 5-HT release and uptake inhibition assays

Drug	NE Release EC_{50} (nM ± SD)	NE Uptake K_i (nM ± SD)	5-HT Release EC_{50} (nM ± SD)	5-HT Uptake K_i (nM ± SD)	DA Release EC_{50} (nM ± SD)	DA Uptake K_i (nM ± SD)
Appetite suppressants and their metabolites						
Phentermine	39.4±6.6	244±15	3511±253	>10,000	262±21	1580±80
(+)-Amphetamine	7.07±0.95	38.9±1.8	1765±94	3830±170	24.8±3.5	34.0±6.0
(−)-Ephedrine	72.4±10.2	225±36	>10,000	>10,000	1350±124	4398±213
Diethylpropion	>10,000	>10,000	>10,000	>10,000	>10,000	>10,000
2-Ethylamino- propiophenone	360±29	99.6±6.6	3840±240	2118±98	1014±80	>10,000
N,N-Diethyl- pseudoephedrine	>10,000	>10,000	>10,000	>10,000	>10,000	>10,000
Phendimetrazine	8300±445	>10,000	>10,000	>10,000	>10,000	>10,000
Appetite suppressants removed from clinical use						
(+)-Fenfluramine	302±20	1290±152	51.7±6.1	150±5	>10,000	>10,000
(±)-Fenfluramine	739±57	1987±205	79.3±11.5	269±7	>10,000	>10,000
Aminorex	26.4±2.8	54.5±4.8	193±23	1244±106	49.4±7.5	21±67
Chlorphentermine	>10,000	451±66	30.9±5.4	338±6	2650±273	3940±110
Abused Stimulants						
(−)-Methamphetamine	28.5±2.5	234±14	4640±243	14000±644	416±20	4840±178
(+)-Methamphetamine	12.3±0.7	48.0±5.1	736±45	2137±98	24.5±2.1	114±11
(±)-MDMA	77.4±3.4	462±18	56.6±2.1	238±13	376±16	1572±59

NOTE: From Rothman et al.[70] Each value is the mean ± SD of three experiments.

TABLE 1. *Continued*

Drug	NE Release EC_{50} (nM ± SD)	NE Uptake K_i (nM ± SD)	5-HT Release EC_{50} (nM ± SD)	5-HT Uptake K_i (nM ± SD)	DA Release EC_{50} (nM ± SD)	DA Uptake K_i (nM ± SD)
Endogenous Substrates						
Tyramine	40.6±3.5	72.5±5.0	2775±234	1556±95	119±11	106±6
Norepinephrine	>10,000	63.9±1.6	>10,000	>10,000	869±51	357±27
Dopamine	66.2±5.0	40.3±4.4	>10,000	6489±200	86.9±9.7	38.3±1.6
5HT	>10,000	3013±266	44.4±5.3	16.7±0.9	>10,000	2703±79
Transporter Inhibitors						
GBR12935	>10,000	277±23	>10,000	289±29	>10,000	4.9±0.31
GBR12909	>10,000	79.2±4.9	>10,000	73.2±1.5	>10,000	4.3±0.30
Cocaine	>10,000	779±30	>10,000	304±10	>10,000	478±25
Mazindol	>10,000	2.88±0.17	>10,000	272±11	>10,000	25.9±0.6
Desipramine	>10,000	8.32±1.19	>10,000	350±13	>10,000	5946±193
Fluoxetine	>10,000	688±39	>10,000	9.58±0.88	>10,000	>10,000
Citalopram	>10,000	4332±295	>10,000	2.40±0.09	>10,000	>10,000
RTI-55	>10,000	5.89±0.53	>10,000	1.00±0.03	>10,000	0.83±0.09
RTI-229	>10,000	19.5±0.6	>10,000	362±13	>10,000	2.15±0.24
Indatraline	>10,000	12.6±0.5	>10,000	3.10±0.09	2810±777	1.90±0.05

phentermine and (+)-amphetamine display their highest potency at stimulation of NE release rather than DA release. As described elsewhere,[74] diethylpropion is totally inactive at monoamine transporters. The *in vivo* activity of this compound is most likely attributable to the *N*-deethylated metabolite, 2-ethylaminopropiophenone,[75] which blocks DA uptake and releases 5-HT with about the same potency. Phendimetrazine, similar to diethylpropion, is inactive in the transporter assays used here. It seems possible that the activity of phendimetrazine is mediated by one or more bioactive metabolites.[76] For example, it has been reported that phendimetrazine is extensively metabolized to form the *N*-demethylated metabolite, phenmetrazine. The hypothesis that phenmetrazine mediates the activity of phendimetrazine awaits confirmation.

Appetite suppressants that were once clinically available (i.e., they are now removed from the market), or were once considered for clinical use, have interesting pharmacological profiles. (+)-Fenfluramine and (±)-fenfluramine are prototypical 5-HT releasing agents that were widely prescribed appetite suppressants, until their removal from the market due to the occurrence of cardiac valve abnormalities in some patients.[77,78] Our data show that (+)-fenfluramine potently releases 5-HT, but this agent also releases NE. The narrow margin of separation between the effects of (+)-fenfluramine on SERT and NET (~5-fold) suggests that this agent probably releases both 5-HT and NE *in vivo*. Both (±)- and (+)-fenfluramine display very low potency in assays measuring DAT activity. Aminorex, an anorectic medication that caused an epidemic of pulmonary hypertension during the 1960s,[79] releases DA and 5-HT with similar potency. Like phentermine and (+)-amphetamine, aminorex displays its highest potency as an NE releaser. The *para*-chloro analog of phentermine, chlorphentermine, is a rather selective 5-HT releaser that blocks NE uptake and DA uptake at much higher doses.

Regarding stimulants of abuse, (+)-methamphetamine is a powerful releaser of DA and NE, as described earlier. (±)-MDMA displays significant releasing activity at all three monoamine transporters, but its most potent actions are on 5-HT and NE release. A wide range of reuptake inhibitors was tested in our assay systems: these drugs included therapeutic agents such as fluoxetine and abused stimulants like cocaine. As predicted, reuptake blockers had minimal activity in release assays, but were quite potent in uptake inhibition assays.

The microdialysis data in FIGURES 5–7 depict the effects of selected appetite suppressants on extracellular DA and 5-HT in the rat nucleus accumbens. FIGURE 5 shows that (+)-methamphetamine and aminorex produce dose-related elevations in dialysate levels of DA and 5-HT. The fact that (+)-methamphetamine causes parallel increases in both DA and 5-HT is surprising based on the *in vitro* release data showing this drug is 30-fold selective for DAT versus SERT. While we are unable to explain such discrepancies in the data, the microdialysis findings clearly demonstrate that the profile of drug-induced extracellular transmitter release *in vivo* may not match the profile of transporter activity determined *in vitro*. Therefore, substrate-type releasers that appear selective *in vitro* may not be selective when administered in the intact organism. The data in FIGURE 6 illustrate that addition of a *para*-chloro group on the phenyl ring of phentermine dramatically affects transporter activity (see FIGURE 2 for structures). While phentermine is predominately a DA releaser, chlorphentermine is predominately a 5-HT releaser. Thus, halogen substitution on

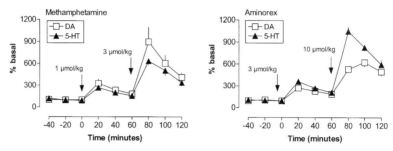

FIGURE 5. Effects of (+)-methamphetamine (*left panel*) and aminorex (*right panel*) on extracellular DA and 5-HT in rat nucleus accumbens. Rats received i.v. doses of drug at time zero and 60 min later. Dialysate samples were collected at 20-min intervals and immediately assayed for DA and 5-HT by HPLC-EC. Data are mean ± SEM expressed as % baseline (*n* = 5–6 rats/group).

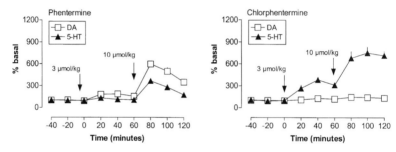

FIGURE 6. Effects of phentermine (*left panel*) and chlorphentermine (*right panel*) on extracellular DA and 5-HT in rat nucleus accumbens. Rats received i.v. doses of drug at time zero and 60 min later. Dialysate samples were collected at 20-min intervals and immediately assayed for DA and 5-HT by HPLC-EC. Data are mean ± SEM expressed as % baseline (*n* = 5–6 rats/group).

the phenyl ring confers specificity for SERT substrate activity. FIGURE 7 depicts the effects of (±)-fenfluramine and (+)-fenfluramine on extracellular DA and 5-HT. Consistent with the known pharmacology of these agents, both drugs produce dose-related elevations in dialysate 5-HT without significant effects on DA. The microdialysis data with fenfluramine agree with the *in vitro* profile shown in TABLE 1.

A number of general conclusions emerge from the *in vitro* data presented here. First, all of the substrate-type releasing agents possess significant pharmacological activity in assays measuring [³H]neurotransmitter uptake. Therefore, it is essential that candidate medications be tested in release assays and uptake assays to determine the precise nature of drug-transporter interaction. A second important finding is that all stimulants capable of releasing DA also release NE with equal or greater potency. Indeed, the potency of amphetamine-type drugs to produce stimulant-like subjective effects in humans correlates with their potency at releasing NE, rather than DA.[70] These findings support the notion that NE release mediates at least some of the sub-

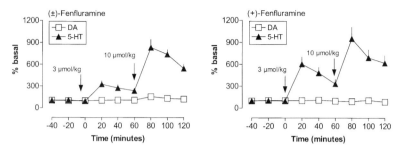

FIGURE 7. Effects of (±)-fenfluramine (*left panel*) and (+)-fenfluramine (*right panel*) on extracellular DA and 5-HT in rat nucleus accumbens. Rats received i.v. doses of drug at time zero and 60 min later. Dialysate samples were collected at 20-min intervals and immediately assayed for DA and 5-HT by HPLC-EC. Data are mean ± SEM expressed as % baseline (*n* = 5–6 rats/group).

jective effects produced by stimulant drugs in people. Finally, the present data demonstrate that subtle changes in the molecular structure of amphetamine-type compounds can dramatically affect biological activity. The most obvious example of this effect is seen with phentermine and chlorphentermine; phentermine is a preferential NE and DA releaser, whereas chlorphentermine is a rather selective 5-HT releaser.

Based on the *in vivo* data presented here, the only agents that would likely release neuronal DA and 5-HT at therapeutic doses are (+)-methamphetamine and aminorex. Obviously, the clinical utility of these agents is limited by serious side effects. The high abuse potential of (+)-methamphetamine is widely accepted,[59] though slow-release formulations of this drug might be well tolerated and have lowered abuse potential. In fact, the preliminary findings of Grabowski *et al.* [Grabowski, personal communication] suggest that (+)-methamphetamine exhibits efficacy as a treatment for cocaine dependence. As mentioned previously, aminorex was removed from clinical use due to its association with primary pulmonary hypertension. We have recently shown that aminorex, and other amphetamine-type drugs known to increase the risk for developing primary pulmonary hypertension (fenfluramines, chlorphentermine) share the common feature of being SERT substrates.[50] On the other hand, not all SERT substrates are associated with primary pulmonary hypertension, and we have argued that it will be possible to develop 5-HT releasing agents devoid of significant pulmonary toxicity.[56] Taken together, the *in vitro* and *in vivo* findings show that amphetamine-type appetite suppressants have a wide range of activities at monoamine transporters, with each drug exhibiting its own unique profile of actions.

In previous studies, we have explored the possibility that coadministration of phentermine (a DA releaser) and fenfluramine (a 5-HT releaser) might be an effective strategy for treating stimulant dependence.[35] With regard to the dual-deficit model, combined administration of phentermine and fenfluramine (phentermine/fenfluramine) would be predicted to elevate extracellular levels of DA and 5-HT in the brain, thereby normalizing monoamine dysfunction in abstinent stimulant addicts.[35,37,48] In agreement with this notion, phentermine/(±)-fenfluramine [or phentermine/(+)-fenfluramine] reduces cocaine self-administration behavior in rats and monkeys.[52,58] There is one report demonstrating that the phentermine/fenfluramine mixture suppresses methamphetamine self-administration in rats.[59] Perhaps more importantly, preliminary studies suggest that phentermine/fenfluramine alleviates withdrawal symptoms in abstinent human cocaine addicts, indicating that this medication could be a useful pharmacological adjunct in treatment.[18,42,43] Unfortunately, as mentioned earlier, (±)-fenfluramine and (+)-fenfluramine were removed from the market due to the occurrence of cardiac valve abnormalities in some patients taking these drugs. There are currently no 5-HT releasing agents available for clinical use, so the therapeutic potential of this class of drugs can no longer be evaluated in people.

Our findings with diethylpropion and phendimetrazine are particularly intriguing. Both of these anorectic medications are considered weak psychomotor stimulants due to their shared properties with illicit drugs like cocaine. For example, diethylpropion and phendimetrazine are self-administered by animals,[44,80] and both drugs exhibit discriminative stimulus properties that generalize to cocaine.[46,47] While it might be assumed that diethylpropion and phendimetrazine interact with monoamine transporters, our *in vitro* data clearly show these agents are inactive at DAT, NET, and SERT. One hypothesis consistent with the available data is that diethylpropion and phendimetrazine are "prodrugs" that are converted to bioactive metabolites upon systemic administration. In the case of diethylpropion, the *N*-deethylated metabolite, 2-ethylaminopropiophenone, appears to be the active metabolite, since this compound has considerable activity at DAT and SERT. Regrettably, this metabolite exhibits much higher potency at NET relative to DAT and SERT, suggesting diethylpropion may have sympathomimetic side effects that limit its usefulness as a medication for stimulant dependence [see Ref. 20]. Nevertheless, the idea of using prodrugs as pharmacotherapies for substance-use disorders deserves further study. Prodrugs might prove useful in the treatment of stimulant addictions, because such agents necessarily limit the amount of active medication entering the brain. This feature of "slow kinetics" would be predicted to reduce the abuse potential of medications, especially those with strong DA-releasing activity.

In summary, a variety of clinical and preclinical evidence suggests that drugs capable of releasing both DA and 5-HT will be effective medications for neurochemical normalization therapy of stimulant addictions. Using simple high-throughput *in vitro* methods to screen the activity of compounds at monoamine transporters, we have found that none of the clinically available amphetamine-type appetite suppressants are equipotent substrates for DAT and SERT proteins. Furthermore, most of the existing anorectic medications are associated with serious side effects: DA-releasing agents display high abuse potential, whereas 5-HT-releasing agents are associated with pulmonary hypertension and cardiac valve disease. Despite these problems, there is sufficient evidence to support the use of amphetamine-type agents in treating stimulant dependence. The work of Grabowski and coworkers is especially noteworthy in this regard.[17] These investigators carried out a double-blind placebo-controlled clinical trial to evaluate the efficacy of a sustained-release formulation of (±)-amphetamine in treating cocaine dependence. Their findings demonstrate that patients receiving medication had increased retention in treatment and decreased cocaine-positive urines, when compared to unmedicated patients. Thus, more clinical testing of anorectic agents as treatments for stimulant addictions is warranted. Future medication discovery efforts should focus on identifying new compounds that possess the desired substrate activity at DAT and SERT, but that lack the adverse effects of stimulants developed decades ago.

REFERENCES

1. GONZALEZ CASTRO, F. *et al.* 2000. Cocaine and methamphetamine: differential addiction rates. Psychol. Addict. Behav. **14:** 390–396.
2. MUSTO, D.F. 1992. Cocaine's history, especially the American experience. Ciba Found. Symp. **166:** 7–14.
3. DAS, G. 1993. Cocaine abuse in North America: a milestone in history. J. Clin. Pharmacol. **33:** 296–310.
4. ANONYMOUS. 1995. Increasing morbidity and mortality associated with abuse of methamphetamine—United States, 1991–1994. Morb. Mortal. Wkly. Rep. **44:** 882–886.
5. KALECHSTEIN, A.D. *et al.* 2000. Psychiatric comorbidity of methamphetamine dependence in a forensic sample. J. Neuropsychiatry Clin. Neurosci. **12:** 480–484.
6. REGIER, D.A. *et al.* 1990. Comorbidity of mental disorders with alcohol and other drug abuse. J. Am. Med. Assoc. **264:** 2511–2518.
7. MILLER, N.S. 1994. Prevalence and treatment models for addiction in psychiatric populations. Psychiatric Ann. **24:** 399–406.
8. HALKITIS, P.N., J.T. PARSONS & M.J. STIRRATT. 2001. A double epidemic: crystal methamphetamine drug use in relation to HIV transmission among gay men. J. Homosex. **41:** 17–35.
9. BATKI, S.L. 1990. Drug abuse, psychiatric disorders, and AIDS. Dual and triple diagnosis. West. J. Med. **152:** 547–552.
10. DIMASI, J.A. *et al.* 1995. Research and development costs for new drugs by therapeutic category. A study of the US pharmaceutical industry. Pharmacoeconomics **7:** 152–169.
11. VOCCI, F. *et al.* 1995. Overview: medications development for the treatment of drug abuse. NIDA Res. Monogr. **149:** 4–15.
12. GORELICK, D.A. 1998. The rate hypothesis and agonist substitution approaches to cocaine abuse treatment. Adv. Pharmacol. **42:** 995–997.
13. HENNINGFIELD, J.E. 1995. Nicotine medications for smoking cessation. N. Engl. J. Med. **333:** 1196–1203.
14. KREEK, M.J. 1996. Opiates, opioids and addiction. Mol. Psychiatry **1:** 232–254.
15. LING, W., R.A. RAWSON & M.A. COMPTON. 1994. Substitution pharmacotherapies for opioid addiction: from methadone to LAAM and buprenorphine. J. Psychoact. Drugs **26:** 119–128.
16. GRABOWSKI, J. *et al.* 1997. Replacement medication for cocaine dependence: methylphenidate. J. Clin. Psychopharmacol. **17:** 485–488.
17. GRABOWSKI, J. *et al.* 2001. Dextroamphetamine for cocaine-dependence treatment: a double-blind randomized clinical trial. J. Clin. Psychopharmacol. **21:** 522–526.
18. KAMPMAN, K.M. *et al.* 2000. The combination of phentermine and fenfluramine reduced cocaine withdrawal symptoms in an open trial. J. Subst. Abuse Treat. **19:** 77–79.
19. WALSH, S.L., K.A. HABERNY & G.E. BIGELOW. 2000. Modulation of intravenous cocaine effects by chronic oral cocaine in humans. Psychopharmacology **150:** 361–373.
20. ALIM, T.N. *et al.* 1995. Diethylpropion pharmacotherapeutic adjuvant therapy for inpatient treatment of cocaine dependence: a test of the cocaine-agonist hypothesis. Clin. Neuropharmacol. **18:** 183–195.
21. DACKIS, C.A. & M.S. GOLD. 1985. Pharmacological approaches to cocaine addiction. J. Subst. Abuse Treat. **2:** 139–145.
22. DACKIS, C.A., M.S. GOLD & A.L. POTTASH. 1986. Central stimulant abuse: neurochemistry and pharmacotherapy. Adv. Alcohol Subst. Abuse **6:** 7–21.

23. GORELICK, D.A. 1997. Pharmacologic therapies for cocaine and other stimulant addiction. *In* Principles of Addiction Medicine. A.W. Graham & T.K. Schultz, Eds. American Society of Addiction Medicine. Chevy Chase, MD.
24. CARROLL, K.M., C. NICH & B.J. ROUNSAVILLE. 1997. Variability in treatment-seeking cocaine abusers: implications for clincal pharmacotherapy trials. NIDA Res. Monogr. **175:** 137–157.
25. KUHAR, M.J. & N.S. PILOTTE. 1996. Neurochemical changes in cocaine withdrawal. Trends Pharmacol. Sci. **17:** 260–264.
26. WEISS, F. *et al.* 1992. Neurochemical correlates of cocaine and ethanol self-administration. Ann. N.Y. Acad. Sci. **654:** 220–241.
27. CUNNINGHAM, K.A., J.M. PARIS & N.E. GOEDERS. 1992. Chronic cocaine enhances serotonin autoregulation and serotonin uptake binding. Synapse **11:** 112–123.
28. PARSONS, L.H., G.F. KOOB & F. WEISS. 1995. Serotonin dysfunction in the nucleus accumbens of rats during withdrawal after unlimited access to intravenous cocaine. J. Pharmacol. Exp. Ther. **274:** 1182–1191.
29. BAUMANN, M.H., K.M. BECKETTS & R.B. ROTHMAN. 1995. Evidence for alterations in presynaptic serotonergic function during withdrawal from chronic cocaine in rats. Eur. J. Pharmacol. **282:** 87–93.
30. BAUMANN, M.H. & R.B. ROTHMAN. 1998. Serotonergic dysfunction during cocaine withdrawal: implications for cocaine-induced depression. *In* Drug Abuse Handbook. S.B. Karch, Ed.: 463–484. CRC Press. Boca Raton.
31. LEVY, A.D., M.H. BAUMANN & L.D. VAN DE KAR. 1994. Monoaminergic regulation of neuroendocrine function and its modification by cocaine. Front. Neuroendocrinol. **15:** 85–156.
32. PARSONS, L.H., A.D. SMITH & J.B. JUSTICE, JR. 1991. The effect of chronic cocaine on basal extracellular dopamine in the nucleus accumbens. Synapse **9:** 60–65.
33. ROBERTSON, M.W., C.A. LESLIE & J. BENNETT, JR. 1991. Apparent synaptic dopamine deficiency induced by withdrawal from chronic cocaine treatment. Brain Res. **538:** 337–339.
34. ROSETTI, Z.L., J. HMAIDAN & G.L. GESSA. 1992. Marked inhibition of mesolimbic dopamine release: a common feature of ethanol, morphine, cocaine and amphetamine abstinence in rats. Eur. J. Pharmacol. **221:** 227–234.
35. ROTHMAN, R.B. *et al.* 1998. Phentermine and fenfluramine: preclinical studies in animal models of cocaine addiction. Ann. N.Y. Acad. Sci. **844:** 59–74.
36. BAUMANN, M.H. & R.B. ROTHMAN. 1998. Alterations in serotonergic responsiveness during cocaine withdrawal in rats: similarities to major depression in humans. Biol. Psychiatry **44:** 578–591.
37. BAUMANN, M.H. *et al.* 2000. Effects of phentermine and fenfluramine on extracellular dopamine and serotonin in rat nucleus accumbens: therapeutic implications. Synapse **36:** 102–113.
38. LIN, D., G.F. KOOB & A. MARKOU. 1999. Differential effects of withdrawal from chronic amphetamine or fluoxetine administration on brain stimulation reward in the rat—interactions between the two drugs. Psychopharmacology **145:** 283–294.
39. MARKOU, A. & G.F. KOOB. 1991. Postcocaine anhedonia. An animal model of cocaine withdrawal. Neuropsychopharmacology **4:** 17–26.
40. YU, Y.L. *et al.* 1997. Amphetamine and fenfluramine suppress ethanol intake in ethanol-dependent rats. Alcohol **14:** 45–48.
41. HALLADAY, A.K. *et al.* 1999. Differential effects of monoaminergic agonists on alcohol intake in rats fed a tryptophan-enhanced diet. Alcohol **18:** 55–64.
42. HITZIG, P. 1993. Combined dopamine and serotonin agonists: a synergistic approach to alcoholism and other addictive behaviors. Maryland Med. J. Feb. 153–157.
43. ROTHMAN, R.B., T.M. GENDRON & P. HITZIG. 1994. Combined use of fenfluramine and phentermine in the treatment of cocaine addiction: a pilot case series. J. Subst. Abuse Treat. **11:** 273–275.
44. GRIFFITHS, R.R. *et al.* 1976. Comparison of behavior maintained by infusions of eight phenylethylamines in baboons. Psychopharmacology **50:** 251–258.
45. CORWIN, R.L. *et al.* 1987. Anorectics: effects on food intake and self-administration in rhesus monkeys. Alcohol Drug Res. **7:** 351–361.

46. EVANS, S.M. & C.E. JOHANSON. 1987. Amphetamine-like effects of anorectics and related compounds in pigeons. J. Pharmacol. Exp. Ther. **241:** 817–825.
47. WOOD, D.M. & M.W. EMMETT OGLESBY. 1988. Substitution and cross-tolerance profiles of anorectic drugs in rats trained to detect the discriminative stimulus properties of cocaine. Psychopharmacology **95:** 364–368.
48. SHOAIB, M. *et al.* 1997. Behavioural and neurochemical characteristics of phentermine and fenfluramine administered separately and as a mixture in rats. Psychopharmacology **131:** 296–306.
49. BALCIOGLU, A. & R.J. WURTMAN. 1998. Effects of fenfluramine and phentermine (fenphen) on dopamine and serotonin release in rat striatum: in vivo microdialysis study in conscious animals. Brain Res. **813:** 67–72.
50. ROTHMAN, R.B. *et al.* 1999. Aminorex, fenfluramine, and chlorphentermine are serotonin transporter substrates: implications for primary pulmonary hypertension Circulation **100:** 869–875.
51. BRAUER, L.H. *et al.* 1996. Evaluation of phentermine and fenfluramine, alone and in combination, in normal, healthy volunteers. Neuropsychopharmacology **14:** 233–241.
52. GLATZ, A.C. *et al.* 2002. Inhibition of cocaine self-administration by fluoxetine or D-fenfluramine combined with phentermine. Pharmacol. Biochem. Behav. **71:** 197–204.
53. WISE, R.A. 1997. Drug self-administration viewed as ingestive behaviour. Appetite **28:** 1–5.
54. POTHOS, E.N., L. HERNANDEZ & B.G. HOEBEL. 1995. Chronic food deprivation decreases extracellular dopamine in the nucleus accumbens: implications for a possible neurochemical link between weight loss and drug abuse. Obes. Res. 3(Suppl 4): 525S–529S.
55. CARR, K.D. 1996. Feeding, drug abuse, and the sensitization of reward by metabolic need. Neurochem. Res. **21:** 1455–1467.
56. ROTHMAN, R.B. & M.H. BAUMANN. 2000. Neurochemical mechanisms of phentermine and fenfluramine: therapeutic and adverse effects. Drug Dev. Res. **51:** 52–65.
57. WOJNICKI, F.H.E. *et al.* 1999. Effects of phentermine on responding maintained under multiple fixed-ratio schedules of food-presentation and cocaine-delivery in the rhesus monkey. J. Pharmacol. Exp. Ther. **288:** 550–560.
58. GLOWA, J.R. *et al.* 1997. Phentermine/fenfluramine decreases cocaine self-administration in rhesus monkeys. Neuroreport **8:** 1347–1351.
59. MUNZAR, P. *et al.* 1999. Effects of dopamine and serotonin-releasing agents on methamphetamine discrimination and self-administration in rats. Psychopharmacology **141:** 287–296.
60. STAFFORD, D. *et al.* 2001. A comparison of cocaine, GBR 12909, and phentermine self-administration by rhesus monkeys on a progressive-ratio schedule. Drug Alcohol Depend. **62:** 41–47.
61. RUDNICK, G. & J. CLARK. 1993. From synapse to vesicle: the reuptake and storage of biogenic amine neurotransmitters. Biochim. Biophys. Acta **1144:** 249–263.
62. AMARA, S.G. & M.S. SONDERS. 1998. Neurotransmitter transporters as molecular targets for addictive drugs. Drug Alcohol Depend. **51:** 87–96.
63. BAUMANN, M.H. *et al.* 1994. GBR12909 attenuates cocaine-induced activation of mesolimbic dopamine neurons in the rat. J. Pharmacol. Exp. Ther. **271:** 1216–1222.
64. KUCZENSKI, R. *et al.* 1995. Hippocampus norepinephrine, caudate dopamine and serotonin, and behavioral responses to the stereoisomers of amphetamine and methamphetamine. J. Neurosci. **15:** 1308–1317.
65. MELEGA, W.P. *et al.* 1995. Pharmacokinetic and pharmacodynamic analysis of the actions of D-amphetamine and D-methamphetamine on the dopamine terminal. J. Pharmacol. Exp. Ther. **274:** 90–96.
66. PEPPER, J. *et al.* 2001. Inhibition of MAO-A fails to alter cocaine-induced increases in extracellular dopamine and norepinephrine in rat nucleus accumbens. Brain Res. Mol. Brain Res. **87:** 184–189.
67. ROTHMAN, R.B. *et al.* 2000. Neurochemical neutralization of methamphetamine with high affinity non-selective inhibitors of biogenic amine transporters: a pharmacological strategy for treating stimulant abuse. Synapse **35:** 222–227.

68. PAXINOS, G. & C. WATSON. 1982. The Rat Brain in Stereotaxic Coordinates. Academic Press. New York.
69. ROTHMAN, R.B. *et al.* 1998. Studies of the biogenic amine transporters. VII. Characterization of a novel cocaine binding site identified with [^{125}I]RTI-55 in membranes prepared from human, monkey and guinea pig caudate. Synapse **28**: 322–338.
70. ROTHMAN, R.B. *et al.* 2001. Amphetamine-type central nervous system stimulants release norepinephrine more potently than they release dopamine and serotonin. Synapse **39**: 32–41.
71. RAITERI, M., F. ANGELINI & G. LEVI. 1974. A simple apparatus for studying the release of neurotransmitters from synaptosomes. Eur. J. Pharmacol. **25**: 411–414.
72. CRESPI, D. *et al.* 1997. Carrier-dependent and Ca(2+)-dependent 5-HT and dopamine release induced by (+)-amphetamine, 3,4-methylendioxymethamphetamine, p-chloroamphetamine and (+)-fenfluramine. Br. J. Pharmacol. **121**: 1735–143.
73. GOBBI, M., A. PARAZZOLI & T. MENNINI. 1998. In vitro studies on the mechanism by which (+)-norfenfluramine induces serotonin and dopamine release from the vesicular storage pool. Naunyn Schmiedebergs Arch. Pharmacol. **358**: 323–327.
74. YU, H. *et al.* 2000. Uptake and release effects of diethylpropion and its metabolites with biogenic amine transporters. Bioorg. Med. Chem. **8**: 2689–2692.
75. DANGOR, C.M., A.H. BECKETT & A.M. VELTMAN. 1986. Simultaneous determination of amfepramon and its two major metabolites in biological fluids by gas liquid chromatography. Arzneimittelforschung **36**: 1307–1310.
76. BECKETT, A.H. & A. RAISI. 1976. Bioavailability in man of phendimetrazine from various dosage forms. J. Pharm. Pharmacol. **28**(Suppl.): 40P.
77. CONNOLLY, H.M. *et al.* 1997. Valvular heart disease associated with fenfluramine-phentermine. N. Engl. J. Med. **337**: 581–588.
78. CONNOLLY, H.M. & M.D. MCGOON. 1999. Obesity drugs and the heart. Curr. Probl. Cardiol. **24**: 745–792.
79. GURTNER, H.P. 1990. Aminorex pulmonary hypertension. *In* The Pulmonary Circulation: Normal and Abnormal. A.P. Fishman, Ed.: 397–411. Univ. of Pennsylvania Press. Philadelphia.
80. GOTESTAM, K.G. & B.E. ANDERSSON. 1975. Assessment of reinforcing properties of amphetamine analogues in self-administering rats. Postgrad. Med. J. **51**(Suppl. 1): 80–83.

Behavioral Consequences of Methamphetamine-Induced Neurotoxicity in Mice: Relevance to the Psychopathology of Methamphetamine Addiction

YOSSEF ITZHAK[a] AND SYED F. ALI[b]

[a]*Department of Psychiatry and Behavioral Science, University of Miami School of Medicine, Miami, Florida, USA*

[b]*Neurochemistry Laboratory, Division of Neurotoxicology, National Center for Toxicological Research/FDA, Jefferson, Arkansas, USA*

ABSTRACT: Methamphetamine (METH) is a major drug of abuse in the United States. A high dose of METH given to mice and rats causes long-lasting depletion of tyrosine hydroxylase activity, dopamine (DA), and DA-transporter (DAT) binding sites in the striatum. In human METH-abusers, a marked decrease of the DAT in the caudate putamen was observed. Despite intensive investigations of the mechanism associated with METH-induced neurotoxicity, the behavioral consequences of this phenomenon are not clear. We used the mouse model of METH-induced neurotoxicity to investigate the response of the animals to the psychomotor-stimulating effect of METH and the rewarding effect of the drug. Mice pre-exposed to a neurotoxic dose of METH developed a marked sensitization to the psychomotor-stimulating effect of METH, which lasted for more than two months. The rewarding effect of METH was determined by the conditioned place preference (CPP) paradigm. Mice pre-exposed to the neurotoxic dose of METH showed reduced sensitivity to the rewarding effect of METH compared with control animals. While CPP was maintained for three months in the control group, the conditioned response in the METH pre-exposed animals lasted only a few days. These findings indicate that METH neurotoxicity is associated with opposing and long-lasting behavioral outcomes: (a) sensitization to the psychomotor-stimulating effect of the drug and (b) desensitization to the rewarding properties of the drug. These consequences may be relevant to the psychopathology of METH abuse. Sensitization is pertinent to compulsive drug-seeking behavior that is accompanied by desensitization to the rewarding effect of METH.

KEYWORDS: neurotoxicity; reward; sensitization; psychostimulants; methamphetamine

Address for correspondence: Yossef Itzhak, Ph.D., Department of Psychiatry & Behavioral Sciences, 1011 NW 15th Street, Gautier Building, Room 503, University of Miami School of Medicine, Miami, Florida 33136, USA. Voice: 305-243-4635; fax: 305-243-2771.

yitzhak@med.miami.edu

Ann. N.Y. Acad. Sci. 965: 127–135 (2002). © 2002 New York Academy of Sciences.

INTRODUCTION

Methamphetamine (METH) is a psychostimulant and a major drug of abuse in many parts of the United States. Amphetamines inhibit the re-uptake of dopamine (DA), leading to reverse transport of DA from the cytoplasm to the extracellular space.[14] In addition, amphetamines are substrates for the vesicular monoamine transporter, causing a rise in the extravesicular cytosolic DA level, which in turn contributes to the reverse transport of DA into the extracellular space.[23]

A high dose of METH results in neurotoxicity associated with a marked decrease in tyrosine hydroxylase activity, DA, and DA-transporter (DAT) binding sites in the striatum.[6,7,13] A similar depletion in striatal DA nerve terminal markers in post-mortem, chronic METH users had been reported.[26] Recent studies suggest that METH-induced dopaminergic neurotoxicity may arise from the formation of oxygen-based free radicals such as superoxide and peroxynitrite.[1] Although many studies had focused on the mechanism underlying the development of METH-induced neurotoxicity, little attention was given to the behavioral consequences of exposure to a neurotoxic dose regimen of METH.

Mice exposed to a neurotoxic dose of METH became sensitized to the locomotor-stimulating effect of a low dose of METH given three days after the high dose.[10,11] This finding suggested that depletion of striatal dopaminergic markers did not blunt the development of behavioral sensitization to subsequent METH injection.[10,11] Rats treated with a neurotoxic dose of METH were sensitized to the stereotypic effects caused by subsequent METH administration.[24,25] In addition, rats exposed to a neurotoxic dose of METH developed signs of cognitive impairment in various tasks of learning and memory paradigms.[3,5]

METH-induced psychosis has been the focus of many investigations,[4] and some evidence suggests a correlation between the diminished level of the DAT in the caudate/putamen, prefrontal cortex, and nucleus accumbens and the severity of psychiatric symptoms in METH abusers.[21] However, the relationship between METH-induced neurotoxicity and abnormal behavior remains largely unclear. Here we describe our recent findings on the short- and long-term consequences of METH-induced dopaminergic neurotoxicity on the psychomotor-stimulating effect as well as the rewarding properties of METH in Swiss Webster mice. The psychomotor-stimulating effect of METH, and the acquisition and maintenance of METH-induced conditioned place preference (CPP) were investigated during a period of 3 days to 3 months after exposure to a neurotoxic dose of METH. The CPP paradigm is utilized to determine the rewarding effects of abused substances. We postulated that the results of these studies may be relevant to the psychopathology of humans abusing high doses of METH.

EFFECT OF A NEUROTOXIC DOSE OF METH ON THE STRIATAL DOPAMINERGIC MARKERS

Male Swiss Webster mice were administrated METH ($5\ mg/kg \times 3$) and sacrificed 3, 14, or 95 days later. Three days after METH administration the level of striatal DA, 3,4-dihydoxyphenylacetic acid (DOPAC), homovanillic acid (HVA), and DAT were $38 \pm 2\%$, $46 \pm 4\%$, $44 \pm 4\%$ and $36 \pm 3\%$ of control, respectively (TABLE 1).

TABLE 1. The concentrations of dopamine (DA) and its metabolites 3,4-dihydoxyphenylacetic acid (DOPAC) and homovanillic acid (HVA) and DA transporter (DAT) binding sites in the striatum of control and METH-treated mice

	DA	DOPAC	HVA	DAT
Control	675 ± 12	112 ± 5	98 ± 6	1823 ± 35
METH				
Day 3	256 ± 10 (38%)*	46 ± 4 (41%)*	44 ± 3 (44%)*	656 ± 24 (36%)*
Day 14	283 ± 17 (42%)*	58 ± 6 (52%)*	62 ± 4 (63%)*	802 ± 41 (44%)*
Day 95	405 ± 11 (60%)*	71 ± 6 (63%)*	73 ± 5 (74%)*	1130 ± 57 (62%)*

NOTE: The level of the dopaminergic markers were measured 3, 14, and 95 days after the administration of METH (5 mg/kg × 3). The concentration of DA, DOPAC, and HVA are expressed in ng/100 mg tissue, and the concentration of the DAT in fmol/mg protein. Values in parentheses are % of control. The level of the dopaminergic markers remained significantly (*$p < 0.05$) below control values ($n = 18$) on day 3 ($n = 6$), day 14 ($n = 6$), and day 95 ($n = 10$).

The level of the dopaminergic markers remained low compared to control values 14 days and 95 days after METH administration, but a time-dependent recovery was observed (TABLE 1). The level of the dopaminergic markers was determined 3, 14, and 95 after METH administration because these time points coincided with the CPP experiment. On day 4 the acquisition of METH-induced CPP began; on day 14 the first test for place preference was conducted, and on day 94 the last test for place preference was performed.

EFFECT OF A NEUROTOXIC DOSE OF METH ON MICE LOCOMOTOR ACTIVITY

Control and METH-treated (5 mg/kg × 3) mice were challenged with a low dose of METH (1 mg/kg) three days after the administration of the high dose of METH, and locomotor activity was recorded by infrared beam interrupt (Opto-Varimex Mini; Columbus Instruments, Columbus, OH). Results in TABLE 2 indicate that the pre-exposure to the high dose of METH resulted in significant ($p < 0.05$) sensitization to the locomotor-stimulating effect of METH. This finding confirms our previous observations.[10,11]

To determine whether the sensitized response to METH persists 74 days after the exposure to the high dose of METH, the two groups of the CPP experiment (control and METH-pretreated mice) were challenged with 1 mg/kg METH, and locomotor activity was recorded. Results in TABLE 2 indicate that mice pre-exposed to the high dose of METH were sensitized to the locomotor-stimulating effect of METH compared to the control group, suggesting that sensitization to the locomotor-stimulating effect of METH is long-lasting.

The animals' response to the psychomotor-stimulating effect of METH was tested on day 74 because it corresponded to day 61 after the CPP testing began (TABLE 3). On day 60 of the CPP testing, a priming injection of 0.5 mg/kg METH produced a marked preference of the control group for the drug-paired compartment, but the preference of the METH group for the drug-paired compartment was significantly

TABLE 2. Comparison between METH-induced hyperlocomotion in control and METH pre-exposed mice

	Activity counts (60 min)	
	Day 3	Day 74
Control	7,324 ± 687	7,5844 ± 901
METH	12,664 ± 932*	12,0344 ± 1123*

NOTE: In the first experiment, two groups of mice, control ($n = 6$) and METH (5 mg/kg × 3; $n = 6$) pretreated mice received a single injection of METH (1 mg/kg) 3 days after the administration of the high dose. METH induced significantly higher locomotor activity in the METH pre-exposed group compared with the control group (*p <0.05); suggesting the development of sensitization. In a second experiment, control ($n = 10$) and METH (5 mg/kg × 3; $n = 10$) pretreated mice that were trained on the CPP paradigm were challenged with 1 mg/kg METH 74 days after the neurotoxic dose of METH was administered. Day 74 corresponds to day 61 post-CPP testing (see also TABLE 3). The METH group was significantly more sensitive to METH-induced hyperactivity compared to the control group (*p <0.05). However, the same METH group was less sensitive to the rewarding effect of METH than was the control group (see TABLE 3, day 60).

TABLE 3. Comparison between the acquisition, maintenance, and reinstatement of conditioned place preference (CPP) in the control and METH pre-exposed mice

	Difference in time between drug- and saline-paired compartments (sec ± SEM) post-CPP (day)							
	1	8	15	22	29	58	60	81
Control	325 ± 41	405 ± 33	354 ± 51[#]	332 ± 28[#]	318 ± 24[#]	155 ± 18[#]	425 ± 39	311 ± 41[#]
METH	108 ± 27*	119 ± 22*	41 ± 21	36 ± 12	22 ± 18	27 ± 10	112 ± 18*	46 ± 21

NOTE: The acquisition of CPP was performed with 0.5 mg/kg METH and saline in alternate days for a total of 8 days. On day 1 and 8 following the acquisition of CPP (post-CPP) the METH group showed significantly lower preference for the drug-paired compartment compared with the control group (*p <0.01). On day 15, 22, and 29 the control group, but not the METH group, maintained the conditioned response ([#]p <0.005 compared with the pre-CPP time). On day 58, the conditioned response of the control group diminished, but was still significant compared to the pre-CPP time ([#]p <0.05). On day 60 the two groups received a priming injection of METH (0.5 mg/kg), and the preference of the mice for the two compartments was measured under the influence of the drug. The priming injection of METH fully reinstated the place preference of the control group; the response of the METH group was significantly lower than control (*p <0.01). After 3 weeks on day 81, the animals were re-tested with saline injection. Only the control group maintained highly significant place preference ([#]p <0.005).

lower than control (TABLE 3). Thus, this experimental design allowed us to establish that the *same group* of mice which was desensitized to the rewarding effect of METH was sensitized to the psychomotor-stimulating effect of the drug. In addition, the *same group* of mice (control) that was sensitive to the rewarding effect of METH was significantly less sensitive to the psychomotor-stimulating effect of the drug compared with the METH group (TABLES 2 and 3).

EFFECT OF A NEUROTOXIC DOSE OF METH ON THE ACQUISITION AND MAINTENANCE OF CONDITIONED PLACE PREFERENCE (CPP)

Experiments were carried out essentially as we described previously.[9,15] The acquisition of CPP with 0.5 mg/kg METH resulted in marked preference of the control group for the drug-paired compartment (325 ± 41 s) while the preference of the METH group for the drug-paired compartment was significantly lower (108 ± 27 s; $p <0.01$) (TABLE 3; post-CPP day 1). Further testing of the animals, once a week, with a priming injection of saline revealed that the conditioned response of the control group remained highly significant for 4 weeks and was attenuated after 8 weeks (TABLE 3; day 58 post-CPP). However, the conditioned response of the METH group remained lower on day 8 (TABLE 3), and after that it became statistically insignificant until day 58 (TABLE 3). On day 60, animals were given a priming injection of METH (0.5 mg/kg), and their preference for the two compartments of the cage was tested under the influence of the drug. Results in TABLE 3 indicate that the priming injection of METH robustly reinstated the preference of the control group for the drug-paired compartment, while the reinstatement of place preference in the METH group remained significantly lower. To determine whether a single priming injection of METH caused long-lasting conditioned response, animals were tested with saline injection three weeks later (TABLE 3; day 81). Results indicate that only the control group remained highly conditioned in preference for the drug-paired compartment while the METH group lost the conditioned response.

SUMMARY AND DISCUSSION

The major finding of the present study is that METH-induced neurotoxicity is associated with long-lasting sensitization to the psychomotor-stimulating effect of METH and a marked desensitization to the rewarding effect of the drug. Most studies have focused on the development of sensitization to the motor-stimulating effects of psychostimulants. One of the prevalent theories concerning the relevance of sensitization to the development of addiction is the "incentive-sensitization" view. According to this hypothesis, the brain regions that are sensitized to the drug are not the ones that mediate the euphoric effects of the drug (termed "drug liking"), but rather are the ones that mediate the incentive significance of the drug (termed "drug wanting").[16–18] The results of the present study demonstrate the concurrent development of *sensitization* and *desensitization* to the effects of METH. Accordingly, sensitization may be related to compulsive drug-seeking behavior (drug wanting), while desensitization may correspond to tolerance or reduced sensitivity to the rewarding effect of the drug (the drug-liking component), which may lead to a "binge" consumption of METH.

Three days after exposure to a neurotoxic dose of METH the mice became sensitized to the locomotor-stimulating effect of the drug (TABLE 2). Although this finding may imply that sensitization is a result of neurotoxicity, we have previously reported that repeated administration of a low dose of METH (1 mg/kg) for five days, a schedule that did not produce dopaminergic neurotoxicity, also caused sensitization to the locomotor-stimulating effect of METH.[8] These findings suggest that sensitization is not a result of neurotoxicity, but rather the consequence of the previous exposure to the drug. Although it is unclear whether a low, intermittent administration of METH produced long-lasting sensitization, results of the present study show that the neurotoxic dose of METH produced long-lasting sensitization, that is, 74 days after the initial exposure to METH (TABLE 2). The enduring, sensitized response of the METH group to a challenge injection of METH on day 74 cannot be attributed to the exposure of the animals to the low dose of METH (0.5 mg/kg) during the CPP training period because the control group (TABLE 2) was also trained on the CPP with the same dose of METH. Thus, the only difference between the two groups that were tested on day 74 (TABLE 2) is the pre-exposure of one group to the neurotoxic dose of METH. The results indicate that pre-exposure to the neurotoxic dose of METH results in long-lasting sensitized response.

Of interest is the finding that sensitization to METH developed despite the significant depletion of striatal dopaminergic markers. This finding is in agreement with our previous studies showing that induction of sensitization to METH is not affected by the depletion of dopaminergic markers.[10,11] Also, pre-exposure to a neurotoxic dose of METH did not affect spontaneous locomotor activity in Swiss Webster mice.[11] Depletion of dopaminergic markers in the striatum, as well as in the nucleus accumbens (NAC), of C57BL/6 mice by the neurotoxin 1-methyl-4-phenyl-1,2,3,6-tetrahydropyridine (MPTP) did not affect the induction of sensitization to cocaine, but it exacerbated the expression of the sensitized response.[12] Taken together, it appears that intact dopaminergic transmission in the striatum and NAC is not a prerequisite for the development of behavioral sensitization to psychostimulants. However, intact dopaminergic transmission in the striatum may be necessary for the full appreciation of the rewarding effect of METH.

The acquisition of CPP in the METH group was significantly lower than in the control group (TABLE 3). The differences between the two groups persisted throughout the experiment—that is, three months after the initial exposure to METH. The acquisition of CPP began on day 4 after METH administration, a time point when levels of striatal dopaminergic markers were significantly lower than control values (TABLE 1). The first test day in the CPP paradigm corresponded to day 14 after the initial exposure to METH. Results indicate that on day 14 striatal dopaminergic markers were still below control values (TABLE 1). The last test day in the CPP paradigm corresponded to day 94 after the exposure to the neurotoxic dose of METH, and on day 95 striatal dopaminergic markers were still below control values. The lack of maintaining a conditioned response in the CPP paradigm may correlate with the sustained reduced levels of the dopaminergic markers or may just correspond to the lower acquisition of CPP in the METH group.

The results of the present study also showed a difference between the control and the METH groups in the reinstatement of CPP. While the priming injection of METH resulted in robust place preference in the control group, the response of the METH group to the priming injection of METH was significantly lower (TABLE 3). It appears that the variation between the two groups in the acquisition of CPP resulted in further differences in the maintenance and the reinstatement of the conditioned response. Notably, the conditioned response of the control group was long-lasting after the initial acquisition of CPP (until day 58), as well as after the reinstatement of CPP by the priming injection of METH; the conditioned response was maintained for three additional weeks (TABLE 3). Together, these findings suggest that METH-associated cues produced long-lasting conditioned response in the control group.

Previous studies suggested that the rat striatum is more sensitive than the NAC to METH-induced neurotoxicity.[2,19] If we predict that in the present study METH produced greater striatal than NAC neurotoxicity in the mouse, this assumption cannot explain the marked desensitization of the METH group to the rewarding effect of METH. The NAC is the major limbic structure involved in the rewarding effects of many abused substances. Because, in the present study, the levels of dopaminergic markers were determined in the entire striatum of the mouse, we may only conclude that there is an association between striatal dopaminergic neurotoxicity and desensitization to the rewarding effect of METH. Moreover, results indicate that desensitization to the rewarding effect of METH was accompanied by sensitization to the psychomotor-stimulating effect of the drug.

The mechanism underlying the desensitization to the rewarding effect of METH needs further investigation. From the studies that show that DAT knockout mice acquired cocaine-induced CPP[22] and cocaine self-administration[20] as wild-type mice, it is unclear whether METH-induced depletion of the DAT impaired the acquisition of CPP or whether the initial exposure to the drug was sufficient to cause tolerance to the rewarding effect of METH. If tolerance is one of the consequences of METH-induced neurotoxicity, then a higher dose of MET—for example, 1 mg/kg instead of 0.5 mg/kg—may be required to induce more significant CPP in the METH group. However, since our previous studies showed that the acquisition of CPP with 1 mg/kg METH produced an equal or less conditioned response compared to those with 0.5 mg/kg (unpublished results), we did attempt to induce CPP with a higher dose of METH.

The acquisition of CPP requires the application of learning and memory. We reported that the co-administration of scopolamine, a muscarinic cholinergic antagonist known to impair learning and memory, with cocaine blocked cocaine-induced conditioned responses such as CPP and place-dependent hyperlocomotion in mice.[9] Thus, the reduced CPP response in the METH group may be due to cognitive deficits associated with the dopaminergic neurotoxicity. Rats exposed to a neurotoxic dose of METH showed signs of cognitive impairment in various tasks of learning and memory.[3,5]

However, an impediment of learning and memory is probably not the only mechanism that attenuates the acquisition of CPP. Specific manipulation of the reward process may also diminish the development of the conditioned response. We reported that the neuronal nitric oxide synthase (nNOS) inhibitor, 7-nitroindazole, blocked nicotine-induced CPP, but not LiCl-induced conditioned place aversion (CPA) in mice.[15] The finding that the nNOS inhibitor had a differential effect on CPP and CPA suggests the following: (a) The nNOS inhibitor did not impair learning and memory. (b) The acquisition of reward-induced place preference involves not only learning and memory but also a specific discrimination process of the reward stimuli that can be selectively diminished by the nNOS inhibitor, and not only by a drug that impairs learning and memory (e.g., scopolamine). Accordingly, METH neurotoxicity may influence multiple neural processes that are necessary for the establishment of CPP.

In summary, the present study suggests that pre-exposure to a neurotoxic dose of METH produced different responses to the psychomotor stimulation and the rewarding effects of the drug. The development of sensitization to the psychomotor stimulation and desensitization to the rewarding effects of METH may be relevant to the psychopathology of METH abuse.

ACKNOWLEDGMENTS

This work was supported by Awards RO1DA08584 and DA12867 from the National Institute on Drug Abuse.

REFERENCES

1. CADET, J.L. & C. BRANNOCK. 1998. Free radicals and pathobiology of brain dopamine systems. Neurochem. Int. **32:** 117–131.
2. CASS, W.A. 1997. Decrease in evoked overflow of dopamine in rat striatum after neurotoxic dose of methamphetamine. J. Pharmacol. Exp. Ther. **280:** 105–113.
3. CHAPMAN, D.E., G.R. HANSON, R.P. KESNER & K.A. KEEFE. 2001. Long-term changes in basal ganglia function after a neurotoxic regimen of methamphetamine. J. Pharmacol. Exp. Ther. **296:** 520–527.
4. ELLISON, G. 1994. Stimulant-induced psychosis, the dopamine theory of schizophrenia, and the habenula. Brain Res. Brain Res. Rev. **19:** 223–139.
5. FRIEDMAN, S.D., E. CASTANEDA & G.K. HODGE. 1998. Long-term monoamine depletion, differential recovery, and subtle behavioral impairment following methamphetamine-induced neurotoxicity. Pharmacol. Biochem. Behav. **61:** 35–44.
6. GIBB, J.W., M. JOHNSON & G.R. HANSON. 1990. Neurochemical basis of neurotoxicity. Neurotoxicology **11:** 317–321.
7. GIBB, J.W. & F.J. KOGAN. 1979. Influence of dopamine synthesis on methamphetamine-induced changes in striatal and adrenal tyrosine hydroxylase activity. Naunyn Schmiedeberg's Arch. Pharmacol. **310:** 185–187.
8. ITZHAK, Y. 1997. Modulation of cocaine- and methamphetamine-induced behavioral sensitization by inhibition of brain nitric oxide synthase. J. Pharmacol. Exp. Ther. **282:** 521–527.
9. ITZHAK, Y. & J.L. MARTIN. 2000. Scopolamine inhibits cocaine-conditioned but not unconditioned stimulant effects in mice. Psychopharmacology **152:** 216–223.
10. ITZHAK, Y., C. GANDIA, P.L. HUANG & S.F. ALI. 1998. Resistance of neuronal nitric oxide synthase-deficient mice to methamphetamine-induced dopaminergic neurotoxicity. J. Pharmacol. Exp. Ther. **284:** 1040–1047.
11. ITZHAK, Y., J.L. MARTIN, S.F. ALI & M.D. NORENBERG. 1997. Depletion of striatal dopamine transporter does not affect psychostimulant-induced locomotor activity. Neuroreport **8:** 3245–3249.
12. ITZHAK, Y., J.L. MARTIN, M.D. BLACK & S.F. ALI. 1999. Effect of the dopaminergic neurotoxin MPTP on cocaine-induced locomotor sensitization. Pharmacol. Biochem. Behav. **63:** 101–107.
13. KOGAN, F.J., W.K. NICHOLS & J.W. GIBB. 1976. Influence of methamphetamine on nigra and striatal tyrosine hydroxylase activity and on striatal dopamine levels. Eur. J. Pharmacol. **36:** 363–371.
14. KUCZENSKI, R. 1983. Biochemical action of amphetamine and stimulants. *In* Stimulants: Neurochemical, Behavioral and Clinical Perspectives. I. Cress, Ed.: 21–61. Raven Press. New York.
15. MARTIN, J.L. & Y. ITZHAK. 2000. 7-Nitroindazole blocks nicotine-induced conditioned place preference but not LiCl-induced conditioned place aversion. Neuroreport **115:** 39–47.
16. ROBINSON, T.E. & K.C. BERRIDGE. 1993. The neural basis of drug craving: an incentive-sensitization theory of addiction. Brain Res. Rev. **18:** 247–291.
17. ROBINSON, T.E. & K.C. BERRIDGE. 2000. The psychology and neurobiology of addiction: an incentive-sensitization view. Addiction **2:** S91–117.
18. ROBINSON, T.E. & K.C. BERRIDGE. 2001. Incentive-sensitization and addiction. Addiction **96:** 103–114.
19. ROBINSON, T.E., J. YEW, P.E. PAULSON & D.M. CAMP. 1990. The long-term effects of neurotoxic doses of methamphetamine on the extracellular concentration of dopamine measured with microdialysis in striatum. Neurosci. Lett. **110:** 193–198.

20. ROCHA, B.A., F. FUMAGALLI, R.R. GIANETDINOV, *et al.* 1998. Cocaine self-administration in dopamine transporter knockout mice. Nature Neurosci. **1:** 132–137.
21. SEKINE, Y., M. IYO, Y. OUCHI, *et al.* 2001. Methamphetamine-related psychiatric symptoms and reduced brain dopamine transporter studies with PET. Am. J. Psychiatry **158:** 1206–1214.
22. SORA, I., C. WICHEMS, N. TAKAHSHI, *et al.* 1998. Cocaine reward models: conditioned place preference can be established in dopamine and serotonin-transporter knockout mice. Proc. Natl. Acad. Sci. USA **95:** 7699–7704.
23. SULZER, D., T-K. CHEN, Y.Y. LAU, *et al.* 1995. Amphetamine redistributes dopamine from synaptic vesicles to the cytosol and promotes reverse transport. J. Neurosci. **15:** 4102–4108.
24. WALLACE, T.L., G.A. GUDELSKY & C.V. VORHEES. 1999. Methamphetamine-induced neurotoxicity alters locomotor activity, stereotypic behavior, and stimulated dopamine release in the rat. J. Neurosci. **19:** 9141–9148.
25. WALLACE, T.L., G.A. GUDELSKY & C.V. VORHEES. 2001. Neurotoxic regimen of methamphetamine produces evidence of behavioral sensitization in rats. Synapse **39:** 1–7.
26. WILSON, J.M., K.S. KALASINKY, A.I. LEVEY, *et al.* 1996. Striatal dopamine nerve terminal markers in human, chronic methamphetamine users. Nature Med. **2:** 699–703.

Estrogen, Anti-Estrogen, and Gender Differences in Methamphetamine Neurotoxicity

DEAN E. DLUZEN AND JANET L. McDERMOTT

Department of Anatomy, Northeastern Ohio Universities College of Medicine (NEOUCOM), Rootstown, Ohio 44272, USA

ABSTRACT: In Part 1 of this report, we review data on the effects of estrogen (E), the anti-E tamoxifen (TMX), and testosterone (T) on methamphetamine (METH)-induced neurotoxicity in female and male CD-1 mice. Treatment of gonadectomized females with a physiological regimen of E significantly diminished the amount of striatal dopamine (DA) depletion to METH compared with non-E-treated mice. If these E-treated mice received coadministered TMX, the neuroprotective effects of E were abolished. However, TMX administration to either intact female or male mice appeared to exhibit a neuroprotective effect. Whereas E administration one week before METH treatment serves as a neuroprotectant, reversing the treatment order (METH→one week→E) failed to indicate any neurorestorative effects for E. This striatal DA-preserving effect of E was gender specific, because males receiving an identical treatment of E followed by METH failed to show any evidence of neuroprotection, nor did the predominantly male gonadal steroid hormone T afford any neuroprotection in gonadectomized male or female mice. In the second part of the report, we direct our attention toward examining some of the means by which E can exert this neuroprotective effect. The findings that gonadectomized female, but not intact male, mice treated with E show a significant reduction in body temperature can contribute to the gender-specific METH neuroprotection. E also diminishes the initial amounts of DA evoked by METH, as observed when E is coinfused with METH into superfused striatal tissue fragments of gonadectomized female and male mice. By contrast, T tends to increase METH-evoked DA responses. Finally, differences in mRNA levels were obtained between male and female mice treated with METH. Intact female mice tend to show greater levels of striatal glial fibrillary acidic protein and decreased levels of plasminogen activator inhibitor-1 compared with males. Each of these factors, combined with our previous findings that E can inhibit DA transporter function, represent significant events contributing to E/gender-dependent effects on METH neurotoxicity.

KEYWORDS: tamoxifen; testosterone; dopamine; nigrostriatal; sex differences; Parkinson's disease; thermoregulation; GFAP; PAI-1

Address for correspondence: Dean Dluzen, Department of Anatomy, NEOUCOM, 4209 State Route 44, P.O. Box 95, Rootstown, OH 44272-0095. Voice: 330-325-6300; fax: 330-325-5913.
ded@neoucom.edu

Ann. N.Y. Acad. Sci. 965: 136–156 (2002). © 2002 New York Academy of Sciences.

INTRODUCTION

Since the initial reports of gender differences in neurodegeneration to neurotoxins that target the nigrostriatal dopaminergic (NSDA) system with males showing more severe deterioration,[1–8] a great deal of interest and speculation has been generated in order to understand this difference. The significance of this observation is not simply of academic interest, because gender differences have been shown to exist for methamphetamine (METH) toxicity[9] and for the putative NSDA neurodegenerative disorder Parkinson's disease.[10–15] It appears that the gonadal steroid hormone, estrogen (E) may represent a significant component involved in these gender differences. Overall, E levels can range between two- and tenfold greater in women. In addition, E, when administered to ovariectomized female rodents, has been shown to decrease the amount of striatal dopamine (DA) depletions to neurotoxins that target the NSDA system, including MPTP,[5,16,17] 6-OHDA,[18] and METH.[7,19] Reductions in MPTP-induced DA depletion by E have also been observed within male mice.[17,20] This basic finding that E can function as a neuroprotectant of the NSDA system (reviewed in Refs. 5, 12, and 21–24) raises two fundamental questions: (1) What are the characteristics of this phenomenon? and (2) What are the bases for this effect? In this brief review we attempt to accomplish two goals with regard to these effects of gender and role of E on METH-induced neurotoxicity. In Part 1, some of the critical variables associated with gender/hormonal modulation of METH-induced neurotoxicity of the NSDA system are summarized. In Part 2, some of the approaches we have applied to understand the bases for these gender/hormonal modulatory effects are presented.

PART 1: CHARACTERIZATION OF GENDER/HORMONAL MODULATION OF METH-INDUCED NEUROTOXICITY

Effects in the Male and Testosterone

The robust nature of E's function as a neuroprotectant within ovariectomized females is summarized in FIGURE 1. The data contained in FIGURE 1 illustrate that E administration (0.1-mg, 21-day release estradiol pellet, s.c.; Innovative Research of America) in gonadectomized female mice followed by METH (20 mg/kg i.p. × 4 at 2-h intervals) treatment one week after E preserves both corpus striatal (CS) dopamine (DA) concentrations (FIG. 1A) and potassium-stimulated DA release (FIG. 1B) compared with non-E-treated mice.[19] This E treatment does not *prevent* CS DA neurotoxicity, because the DA concentration levels obtained are significantly reduced compared with vehicle controls (10,808 vs. 16,563 pg/mg) but *preserves* CS DA function because levels are significantly increased over those obtained with non-E-treated mice receiving METH (4423 pg/mg). Such findings call into question the potential for E to exert this effect in the male. Accordingly, gonadectomized male mice were treated with E followed by METH in a manner identical to that performed in the female. CS DA concentrations from these males were then determined at one week post-METH and are displayed in FIGURE 2A. For this, as well as for the remaining experiments in Part 1, we present only data from CS DA concentrations because the DA release data showed a similar pattern of responsiveness to that shown

A.

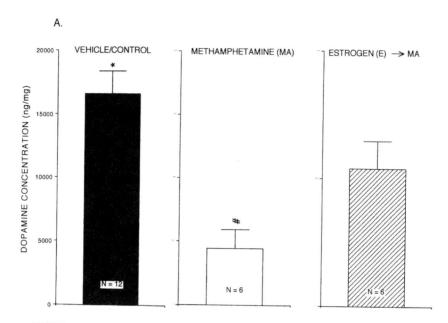

FIGURE 1. (A) Summary of corpus striatal (CS) dopamine concentrations (mean+SEM in pg/mg) from gonadectomized CD-1 female mice: (1) treated or not with estrogen (E: 0.1 mg estradiol, 21-day release pellet, s.c.; Innovative Research of America) pooled into a vehicle/control group, (2) gonadectomized female mice administered methamphetamine (METH: 20 mg/kg × 4 i.p. injections at 2-h intervals), and (3) gonadectomized+E–treated female mice administered METH (E→METH). CS dopamine concentrations of E-treated mice were significantly increased compared to those of mice not receiving E, but were significantly decreased compared to those of the vehicle/controls (as indicated by differing superscript and pattern notations). **(B)** Summary of potassium stimulated (30 mM K^+) dopamine release *in vitro* (pg/mg/min) of superfused tissue fragments derived from the contralateral CS of the treatment groups described for A. These K^+-stimulated dopamine release rates showed a pattern very similar to those of the dopamine concentrations in A, with maximal responses obtained in the vehicle/control, intermediate responses in the E-treated mice and lowest responses within the METH group. These data suggest that treatment with E diminishes, but does not prevent, the degree of neurotoxicity resulting from METH, as indicated by the changes observed in CS dopamine concentrations **(A)** and K^+-stimulated release **(B)**. (Data adapted from Gao and Gluzen.[19])

in FIGURES 1A and B. The data contained in FIGURE 2A provide no indication that E can function as a neuroprotectant within gonadectomized male mice, inasmuch as DA concentrations of these males did not differ significantly from that of gonadectomized females receiving METH. Rather, they were significantly lower than those of gonadectomized, E-treated females receiving METH. It should be noted that these males were treated with a regimen of E identical to that used with females. Because an identical E treatment within gonadectomized female and male rodents may not produce equivalent serum estradiol levels,[25] it remains possible that higher doses of E in the male may act as a neuroprotectant in the male. What these data do tell us is that females are clearly more sensitive to the neuroprotectant capacity of E.

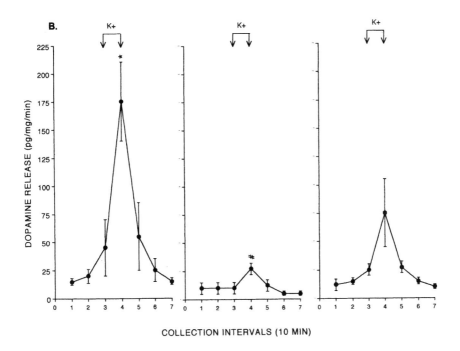

COLLECTION INTERVALS (10 MIN)

FIGURE 1. *Continued.*

The next issue addressed was that of the predominantly male gonadal steroid hormone testosterone (T). We tested the effects of T treatment in both gonadectomized females and males. Analogous to those of tests for E, a T pellet (5-mg, 21-day release) was implanted s.c. and followed one week later by METH. For neither gender was there any suggestion that T could function as a neuroprotectant.[26] CS DA concentrations for both gonadectomized+T–treated females and males receiving METH were statistically equivalent to each other as well as to gonadectomized, non-E-treated females; and concentrations were significantly decreased compared with gonadectomized+E females receiving METH (FIG. 2B). These results, demonstrating an absence of a neuroprotectant effect by T, are similar to those reported for NSDA neurotoxicity induced by MPTP.[27,28] A lack of neuroprotection by T was also reported in cell cultures of SK-N-SH cells subjected to serum deprivation,[29] but T-dependent neuroprotection was observed within similarly perturbed human fetal brain tissue cells.[30]

Effects of E as a Neurorestorant

When administered before treatment with a NSDA neurotoxin, E can function as a neuroprotectant. That is, E can effectively decrease the amount of CS DA depletions within gonadectomized female rodents. In the following experiment, we examined the potential for E to restore CS DA levels in mice previously treated with a

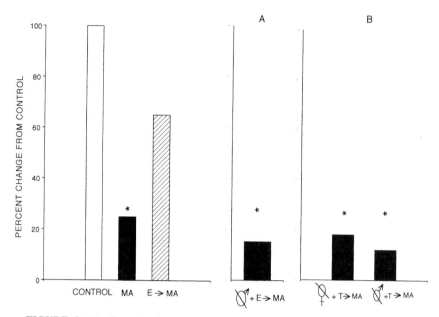

FIGURE 2. The first three bars contain the dopamine concentration data of FIGURE 1 expressed in percent depletion from vehicle/controls (100%) to provide a means for comparison with subsequent treatments in this report. (**A**) The effects of E treatment in gonadectomized male CD-1 mice on METH-induced depletion of CS dopamine concentrations. The amount of METH-induced depletion from gonadectomized, E-treated males was statistically equivalent to that of gonadectomized females not receiving E and significantly reduced compared with that of gonadectomized, E-treated females receiving METH. (**B**) The effects of testosterone treatment (T: 5-mg, 21-day release pellet) in gonadectomized female and male CD-1 mice on METH-induced depletion of CS dopamine concentration. The amount of METH-induced depletion of CS dopamine concentrations from these T-treated mice were statistically equivalent to that of METH-treated gonadectomized females administered METH and significantly decreased compared with that of gonadectomized, E-treated females administered METH. These data suggest that, unlike that in the female (FIG. 1), E cannot function as a neuroprotectant against METH-induced neurotoxicity in gonadectomized male mice (**A**). In addition, treatment with T does not afford any apparent neuroprotection against METH-induced neurotoxicity in either gonadectomized female or male mice (**B**). Bars with * indicate groups that were statistically equivalent, and bars with different pattern notations indicate groups that differ statistically. (Data adapted from Gao and Dluzen.[26])

neurotoxin regimen of METH. In effect, we reversed the order of the treatments, now applying a protocol of METH→(1 week)→E as opposed to that of E→(1 week)→METH, as used for the data of FIGURES 1 and 2. With this approach we found no indication for any restorative effects of E when administered one week post-METH.[19] The percent depletion of striatal DA concentrations from METH→E mice was 30%, which was similar to that of METH alone (33%) and significantly lower than that of E→METH mice (65%), as presented in FIGURE 1A. Future work in this area will be required to determine whether the administration of E at more immediate time intervals post-METH can serve to decrease the amount of METH-induced NSDA neurotoxicity. It has been reported that E's capacity to protect against insults of the central nervous system (e.g., ischemia) can occur after the application of this caustic treatment.[31] Accordingly, it will be critical to test whether E can exert any neuroprotectant actions when applied soon after METH treatment (minutes→hours) like those observed with ischemia.

Effects of the Anti-E, Tamoxifen

Since E, either through endogenous sources[7] or by supplemental administration (FIG. 1A), can serve as an effective neuroprotectant of the NSDA system, an important issue to consider involves the effects of conditions under which E is diminished or rendered inactive. The salient results achieved by diminishing E, as achieved with gonadectomy, are shown in FIGURE 1. Other means of decreasing E effectiveness can involve treatment with an anti-E, like tamoxifen (TMX). Testing the effects of TMX on METH-induced NSDA neurotoxicity is significant for the following reasons: (1) It permits an assessment of the effects of this anti-E on the central nervous system; (2) it allows us to consider actions on E α or β receptors, because TMX is not believed to interact with the E β receptor;[32] and (3) TMX has been proposed to be used as a prophylactic in women at risk for breast cancer;[33,34] therefore its use, particularly its use with premenopausal women, may become more widespread in the near future. Initial attempts to test this effect of TMX involved treating gonadectomized female mice with a coadministration of E and TMX (5-mg, 21-day release pellet). In this way, we could determine whether the addition of TMX to E-treated mice would alter the degree of neuroprotection normally afforded by E alone (FIG. 1). When the effects of METH in these E/TMX-treated mice were compared with E-treated mice, the CS DA concentrations of the former were significantly decreased, but were not significantly different from those of gonadectomized, non-E-treated females.[19] These data demonstrate that TMX can abolish the neuroprotectve capacity of E as tested in gonadectomized females (FIG. 3A). A similar abolition of E neuroprotection with TMX was observed with the neurotoxin MPTP.[35] When tested with TMX alone, there was no evidence that this anti-E served as a neuroprotectant in gonadectomized female mice (FIG. 3B).

Effects in Intact Mice

We were particularly interested in testing the effects of TMX in intact female mice. Intact females show greater NSDA neuroprotection than males,[1–8] and there exist estrous cycle variations in NSDA neuroprotection.[7] Therefore, this experiment would enable us to determine whether TMX treatment would inhibit the capacity for endogenous E to function as a neuroprotectant. Intact females were implanted with a pellet containing TMX followed by METH treatment at one week post-TMX. For controls, intact females receiving either no hormone treatment or intact females treated with an E pellet were used. In addition, to assess potential gender/hormonal interactions, intact males treated with TMX or E were included in this experiment. As in the previous experiments, CS DA concentration determinations were performed at one week post-METH. We anticipated that TMX treatment of intact females would decrease the display of neuroprotection and these females would show significantly decreased CS DA compared with intact, untreated female mice. Our

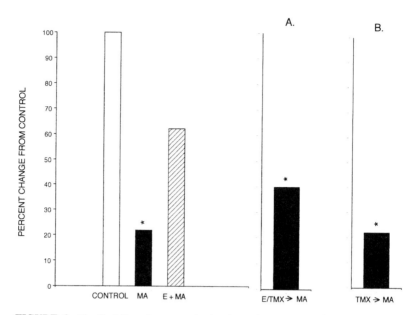

FIGURE 3. The first three bars contain the dopamine concentration data of FIGURE 1 expressed in percent depletion from vehicle/controls (100%) to provide a means for comparison with subsequent treatments in this report. **(A)** Gonadectomized female mice receiving coadministration of E and the anti-E, tamoxifen (TMX: 5-mg, 21-day release pellet) showed a depletion of CS dopamine concentration that was statistically equivalent to that of gonadectomized females not receiving E and significantly decreased compared to that of gonadectomized, E-treated females. **(B)** Treatment of gonadectomized females with TMX resulted in CS dopamine concentrations that were statistically equivalent to those of gonadectomized females not receiving E and significantly decreased compared with that of gonadectomized, E-treated females. These data suggest that TMX treatment of gonadectomized, E-treated female mice antagonizes the capacity for E to function as a neuroprotectant (FIG. 3A) and, by itself, TMX does not act as a neuroprotectant against METH-induced neurotoxicity within gonadectomized female mice (FIG. 3B). Bars with * indicate groups that were statistically equivalent, and bars with different pattern notations indicate groups that differ statistically. (These data are adapted from Gao and Dluzen.[19])

data showed quite the opposite effect. Intact female mice treated with TMX had CS DA concentrations that were significantly greater than intact females not receiving any exogenous hormonal treatment following METH (FIG. 4A).[36] This result implies that TMX can exert a neuroprotective effect on METH-induced NSDA neurodegeneration within intact female mice. The apparent discrepancy in the capacity for TMX to function as a neuroprotectant in intact female mice but abolish the neuroprotective effect of E in gonadectomized female mice (FIG. 3A) may be related to the mixed agonist–antagonist actions exerted by TMX.[37] A similar neuroprotective effect was observed with a supplemental E treatment in intact females (FIG. 4A). Intriguingly, this neuroprotectant effect of TMX was also observed in intact males; however, E treatment provided no evidence of neuroprotection in these mice (FIG. 4B). In this regard, neither intact nor gonadectomized males (FIG. 2A) show any neu-

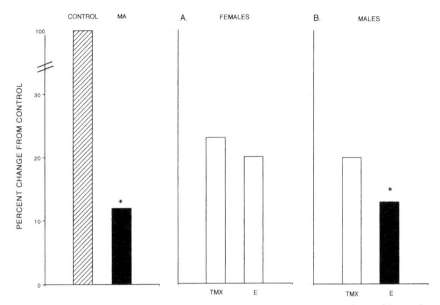

FIGURE 4. The first two bars contain the CS dopamine concentrations of intact females treated with the vehicle for METH (control = 100%), and the percent depletion from this control value as obtained from intact females treated with METH. **(A)** Intact females treated with either TMX or E followed by METH showed CS dopamine concentrations that were significantly increased compared to those of intact females treated with METH. **(B)** Intact males treated with TMX, but not E, showed CS dopamine concentrations that were significantly increased compared to those of intact females treated with METH. These data suggest that TMX treatment of intact female and male mice and E treatment of intact females can produce a neuroprotectant effect against METH-induced neurotoxicity. Bars with * indicate groups that were statistically equivalent, and bars with different pattern notations indicate groups which differ statistically. (Data adapted from Dluzen et al.[36])

roprotection when treated with a regimen of E that was capable of producing neuroprotection in intact or gonadectomized females. A final observation of significance in this experiment was the finding that treatment of intact males with E produced a salient acute toxicity to METH. FIGURE 5 presents the mortality rates from the treatment groups of this experiment. Although the overall mortality rates obtained from these treatments, as defined by mortality within 24 hours post-METH, were generally low (<23%), mortality levels rose to 59% in intact males treated with E. This acute toxicity was even more striking than that illustrated in FIGURE 5, because several of these E-treated, intact males died before receiving the full regimen of METH treatment, with males dying in some cases after the second or third METH administration. At present we have no explanation for this acute METH-induced toxicity, which is confined to intact+E–treated male mice, but its magnitude highlights its significance. The rapidity of this effect suggests a cardiovascular involvement. In collaboration with Charles Pilate of the Department of Physiology at NEOUCOM, we have measured heart rates in intact male mice treated or not with E and found no

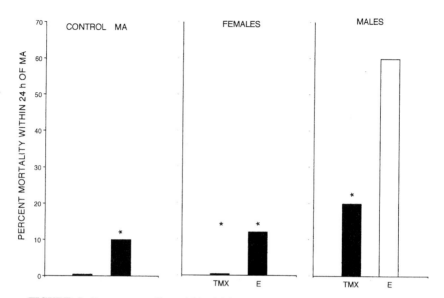

FIGURE 5. Percent mortality within 24 hours post-METH treatment for treatment groups in FIGURE 4. With the exception of the E-treated males, mortality rates were relatively low and not statistically different among the treatment groups (controls = 0%, METH = 10%, females + TMX = 0%, females + E = 11%, males + TMX = 22%). The mortality percent of the intact males treated with E (59%) was significantly greater than all other treatment groups. These data suggest that treatment of intact male mice with E greatly enhances the acute toxicity resulting from METH treatment. Bars with * indicate groups that were statistically equivalent, and bars with different pattern notations indicate groups that differ statistically. (Data adapted from Dluzen et al.[36])

statistically significant difference between these groups from these preliminary findings. On the contrary, heart rates tended to be decreased in E-treated mice (mean+SEM bpm = $727+7$, $n = 4$) compared to non-E-treated ($770+20$ bpm, $n = 3$) intact mice. In addition to determination of heart rates, we have also measured heart (left ventricle) catecholamine concentrations between intact male mice treated or not with E. The data from these determinations reveal a tendency for norepinephrine concentrations within the left ventricle of E-treated mice to be increased (mean+SEM pg/mg = $846+36$, $n = 4$), compared with the non-E-treated males ($681+75$ pg/mg, $n = 3$).

PART 1 SUMMARY

TABLE 1 contains a summary of the characterization for some of the hormonal/ gender influences upon METH-induced neurotoxicity of the nigrostriatal dopaminergic (NSDA) system. Our data reveal that E, but not T, can exert a neuroprotective effect on METH-induced NSDA neurotoxicity. These neuroprotective effects of E on METH-induced NSDA neurotoxicity appear to be gender specific, since no evidence for neuroprotection was obtained in either gonadectomized or intact male

TABLE 1. Summary of estrogen gender modulatory effects of methamphetamine (MA)-induced NSDA neurotoxicity

	EVIDENCE FOR PROTECTION AGAINST MA	NO EVIDENCE OR INDICATION FOR PROTECTION AGAINST MA
SPECIFICITY	17β-E	TESTOSTERONE
GENDER	♀ + E & ♀(gonadectomized) + E	♂ + E & ♂(gonadectomized) + E
ANTI-E	♀ + TMX & ♂ + TMX	♀(gonadectomized) + E/TMX
E-RESTORANT		♀(gonadectomized) → MA → E (1 week)

mice receiving E. The anti-E TMX can abolish the neuroprotective effects of E when coadministered with E in gonadectomized female mice. When intact mice are treated with TMX, however, there is an indication that this anti-E can function as a neuroprotectant in female, as well as in male, mice. Finally, we observed that intact male mice treated with E show enhanced sensitivity to the acute toxicity of METH. For reasons that remain obscure, these E-treated intact males show excessive mortality rates when exposed to METH.

PART 2: BASES FOR GENDER/ESTROGEN NEUROPROTECTION OF THE NSDA SYSTEM

E as a Central Nervous System Neuroprotectant

Understanding the means by which E can function as a central nervous system neuroprotectant is not a simple endeavor. FIGURE 6 illustrates the plethora of E actions through which this gonadal steroid hormone may function as a modulatory neuroprotectant of the central nervous system. In the upper portion of this figure, putative actions on the NSDA system are indicated that will enable E to function as a neuroprotectant at this site. It has been reported that E can affect DA release,[38–40] uptake,[41–47] synthesis,[48,49] receptors,[50,51] and interactions with other hormones.[52] In addition to this relatively specific action on the NSDA system, E can produce a

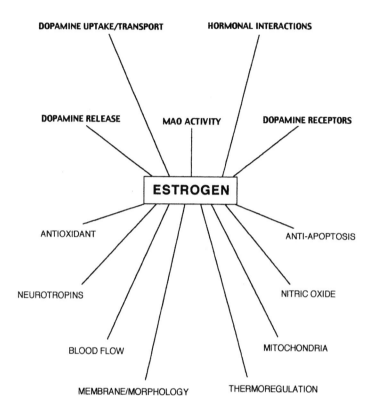

FIGURE 6. Illustration indicating the multifarious means by which the gonadal steroid hormone estrogen (E) can function as a neuroprotectant within the central nervous system. In the upper portion of this illustration putative modulatory effects of E on the nigrostriatal dopaminergic system[38–52] are shown that can serve as a neuroprotectant against METH-induced neurotoxicity. The lower portion of this illustration shows more generalized effects of E on the central nervous system through which E can function as a neuroprotectant. (Information adapted from Dluzen *et al.*[12])

variety of more generalized effects within the central nervous system that allow it to exert neuroprotection. These effects have been summarized in detail previously,[12] and can include actions on neurotrophins, blood flow, membrane morphology, mitochondria, nitric oxide, apoptosis, anti-oxidation, and thermoregulation. From this summary, it is clear that the capacity for E to act as a NSDA neuroprotectant can be quite complex and may involve one or several events and/or interactions among events to result in its final action as a neuroprotectant. In Part 2, we relate approaches we have been using to assess some of the mechanisms by which E can function as a neuroprotectant of the NSDA system to METH.

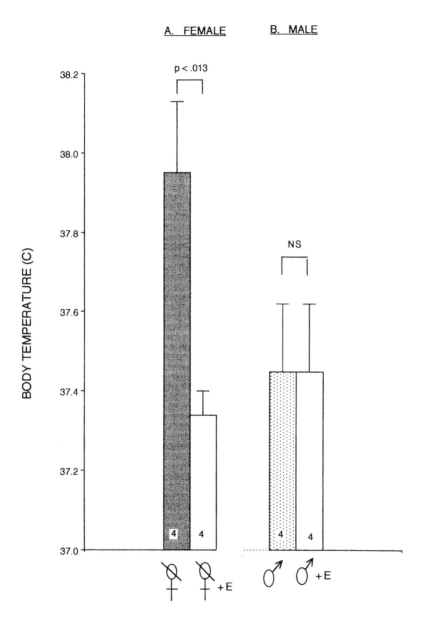

FIGURE 7. Summary of body temperatures (mean+SEM in °C) from gonadectomized female **(A)** and intact male **(B)** mice treated or not with E. Body temperatures of gonadectomized females treated with E are significantly decreased, whereas no statistically significant changes in body temperatures were obtained in intact males treated with E. These data suggest that an additional means by which E can contribute to neuroprotection against METH-induced neurotoxicity in females is through reducing their body temperature, which can decrease METH's ability to effectively produce neurotoxicity in the NSDA system. (Data adapted from Gao and Dluzen.[19])

Effects of E on Body Temperature

An important component of METH-induced neurotoxicity is temperature. Increases in body temperature as achieved by increasing core or ambient temperature have been shown to increase the degree of neurotoxicity, whereas reductions in body temperature diminish the neurotoxicity.[53–55] Moreover, METH itself increases body temperature.[56] Therefore, in this experiment we assessed the effects of E on body temperature. Gonadectomized female mice treated with E show a significant reduction in body temperature (FIG. 7A). By contrast, intact male mice receiving an identical E treatment protocol failed to show any statistically significant change in body temperature (FIG. 7B). In this way, the presence of higher E levels in the female has the capacity to diminish body temperature, which can decrease METH's effectiveness in producing neurotoxicity within the NSDA system. While exact interpretations of the body temperature effects associated with NSDA neurotoxicity require additional work,[57] this function remains an important contributing factor associated with the attenuated METH-induced neurotoxicity obtained in females.

Direct and Immediate Effects of E and T on METH-Induced CS DA Responses

Upon initial exposure to METH, a marked increase in DA output is observed. This METH-induced DA response represents the initial effects produced by this neurotoxin and may indicate an important component of the resultant NSDA neurodegeneration that occurs to METH. This follows because it has been demonstrated that an excess efflux of extracellular DA can damage the NSDA system.[58,59] Accordingly, events that have the ability to decrease this initial DA response may exert a favorable influence on diminishing NSDA neurotoxicity. We examined whether E could produce such an effect in this experiment. CS tissue fragments of gonadectomized female mice were superfused in vitro under conditions in which METH was infused directly into these tissue fragments either in the presence or absence of E (300 nM) in the medium. The amount of DA evoked by METH (10 μM) when E was contained within the medium was markedly reduced compared to that of preparations with no E in the medium (FIG. 8A).[60] A similar reduction to MPP^+-evoked DA output was observed in the presence of E in gonadectomized female rats as tested under both in vitro[61] and in vivo[25,62] paradigms. This result prompted us to examine whether this response would be present in males. Because we found no evidence for E to function as a neuroprotectant within the male (FIG. 2A), we were interested in determining whether this initial attenuation of the DA response was limited to the female and thereby account for this gender difference in neuroprotection. When CS tissue fragments from gonadectomized male mice were superfused in a manner identical to that performed in the female, we observed a very similar response. That is, DA output was substantially decreased in preparations in which E was included within the medium (FIG. 8B). These data suggest two interesting salient conclusions with regard to E/gender effects upon METH-induced NSDA neurotoxicity. First, this E-dependent decrease in the METH-evoked DA response does not appear to be gender specific, as both males and females are capable of showing similar attenuations to METH-induced DA in the presence of E. In this way, the CS DA response of the male is not incapable of responding to E. Therefore, if this response profile can be considered a component of neuroprotection, the female advantage could result from

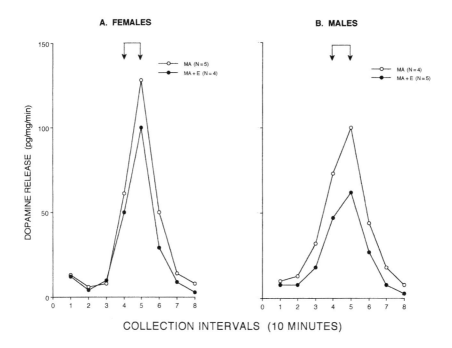

A. FEMALES   B. MALES

COLLECTION INTERVALS (10 MINUTES)

FIGURE 8. Summary of METH-evoked dopamine release *in vitro* (pg/mg/min) from superfused CS tissue fragments of gonadectomized female (**A**) and male (**B**) mice. Effluent samples were collected at 10-min intervals. During collection interval number four, superfusion medium containing METH (10 μM) in the presence or absence of E (300 nM) was infused into the chambers (*arrows*). For both gonadectomized female and male mice, the addition of E to the METH superfusion medium substantially diminished the amount of dopamine evoked by METH. These data suggest that E may contribute to the neuroprotectant effects observed by decreasing the initial efflux of extracellular dopamine evoked by METH. Although this effect is not gender specific, the presence of greater E concentrations in females would enable this effect to be better displayed in females. (Data adapted from Myers *et al.*[60])

the presence, and greater concentrations, of E in females. Second, these data make it somewhat problematic to explain how this similarity in the initial E-dependent reduction in METH-induced DA output (FIG. 8) may be related to the differences in CS DA concentrations at one week post-METH observed between gonadectomized males and females treated with E (FIG. 2). This follows because it would seem that similarities in reductions of initial METH-induced DA responses in females and males should result in equivalent NSDA neuroprotection. The data reveal that this is clearly not the case. Either this initial DA response is not illustrative of a parameter for NSDA neuroprotection or treatment with equivalent concentrations of systemic E *in vivo* does not produce equivalent effects localized within the NSDA system. In support of this latter possibility are data that show gonadectomized female and male rats treated with an identical systemic E regimen *in vivo* show markedly different serum E levels.[25] In this way, functional differences may exist in response to E admin-

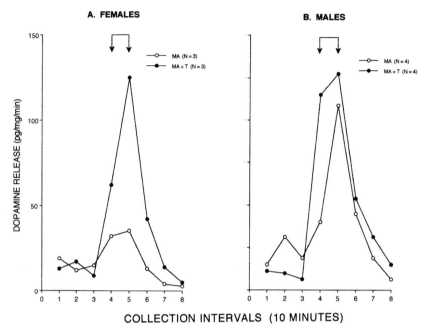

COLLECTION INTERVALS (10 MINUTES)

FIGURE 9. Summary of METH-evoked dopamine release *in vitro* (pg/mg/min) from superfused CS tissue fragments of gonadectomized female (**A**) and male (**B**) mice. The protocol for this experiment is similar to that described in FIGURE 8, with the exception that the METH was infused in the presence or absence of T (300 nM). The inclusion of T tended to increase the METH-evoked dopamine responses, an effect that was more prominent in gonadectomized females (FIG. 9A). These data suggest that unlike E (FIG. 8), T fails to reduce the METH-evoked dopamine responses and may increase the amount of dopamine evoked by METH. Such an effect may be related to the absence of a neuroprotective effect of T on METH-induced neurotoxicity and contribute to the greater degree of neurotoxicity observed in males. (Data adapted from Myers *et al.*[60])

istered *in vitro* or *in vivo* that are due to differences in effective concentrations acting on the NSDA system. Further work on this E effect on DA responses will be required to establish the meaning and implications of this phenomenon.

FIGURE 9 shows data from an analogous experiment in which the effects of T on METH-evoked DA release, as achieved by infusion of METH in the presence or absence of T (300 nM), were tested. Unlike that obtained with E, the co-infusion of T with METH did not reduce the METH-evoked DA responses. On the contrary, there was a tendency for T to increase these METH-evoked DA responses, particularly in females.[60] If one subscribes to the view that excess extracellular DA can produce damage to the NSDA system,[58,59] the presence of T in the male may exacerbate the neurotoxicity produced by METH as a result of this capacity for increasing extracellular DA levels. Gender differences reported for METH neurotoxicity may then involve the potential for a combination of neuroprotection by E along with potentiated neurotoxicity by T.

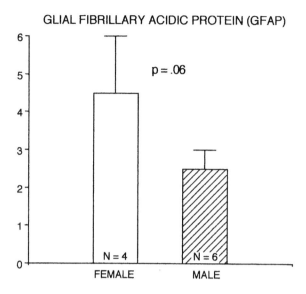

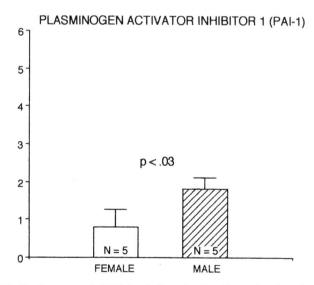

FIGURE 10. Summary of mRNA levels from the CS of intact female and male mice that tend to show discriminative responses to METH treatment. Glial fibrillary acidic protein (GFAP) tended to be increased in females, whereas plasminogen activator inhibitor-1 (PAI-1) was decreased in these females. These data suggest that the increased GFAP in females following METH may be involved with a capacity for greater wound healing or neuronal survival, which can contribute to the neuroprotective effects obtained in females. While PAI-1 levels are generally correlated with neuroprotection, this message has also been associated with impaired motor learning, suggesting the potential for reductions in this message to exert a positive effect upon neurode generative responses of the NSDA system. (Data adapted from Dluzen et al.[63])

Molecular Markers of Gender Differences to
METH-Induced NSDA Neurotoxicity

An additional approach we have employed to evaluate the bases for these gender differences in response to METH has involved determinations of mRNA levels in the CS of male and female mice following METH treatment. In collaboration with Nick Laping in the Department of Renal Pharmacology at Glaxo-SmithKline Laboratories, CS mRNA levels for fibronectin, activin-like kinase 5, transforming growth factor-B, glial fibrillary acid protein, and plasminogen-activator inhibitor-1 were measured in male and female mice at one week post-METH treatment.[63] Of these, two message levels emerged as showing a gender difference in response to METH. From these preliminary findings, we observed that levels of glial fibrillary acidic protein (GFAP) tended to be increased and plasminogen-activator inhibitor-1 (PAI-1) was decreased in female compared with male mice (FIG. 10). Because GFAP is generally thought to be associated with increased astrocyte activity, one interpretation for this tendency toward increased GFAP may be that it is involved with a greater ability for wound healing or neuronal survival in females.[64] Somewhat surprising was the reduction in PAI-1 in females. In general, PAI-1 has been associated with neuroprotection, so it would seem that a more consistent result would be for increased PAI-1 mRNA in females. It should be noted that the role of PAI-1 in neuroprotection can be quite complex. For example, PAI-1 has also been associated with impaired motor learning, which can be associated with degenerative effects in the NSDA system. Moreover, it appears that a critical interaction between PAI-1 and tPA exists that may be involved with the potential for a neuroprotective or neurodegenerative role of PAI-1.

CONCLUSIONS

It is clear that E can function as a powerful agent capable of diminishing NSDA neurotoxicity to the psychostimulant METH within the mouse model. The data reveal that this ability is confined to the female, but represents an effect that can be produced under physiological levels of E concentrations.[7,19] In contrast to this neuroprotective effect of E, the male gonadal steroid hormone T offers no neuroprotection to METH in either males or females. Although E can exert substantial effects on neuroprotection, we found no indication that E could restore CS DA levels within METH-treated mice, when administered one week post-METH. Whether E administration at earlier time periods following METH could act to restore or prevent this METH-induced neurodegeneration remains to be tested. When TMX is administered within gonadectomized+E–treated females, this anti-E exerts a classic antagonistic effect and abolishes the neuroprotective actions afforded by E. However, TMX appears to act as an agonist to E with regard to NSDA neuroprotection when administered to intact mice. Interestingly, unlike that observed for E, this capacity for TMX to act as a neuroprotectant is seen in both intact females and males.

The mechanisms by which E can function as a neuroprotectant of the NSDA system against METH-induced neurodegeneration are complex and multifarious, as summarized within FIGURE 6. One important action we have reviewed previously is the ability for E to inhibit DA transporter function.[22] Such an action has the potential for reducing the amount of uptake of neurotoxic agents like METH (MPTP and 6-OHDA) that will eventually produce neurodegeneration within the NSDA system. In this report we have presented data that expand upon this potential mechanism to show some complementary mechanisms by which E can be exerting these neuroprotectant effects. We have shown that E decreases body temperature when administered to gonadectomized females. No such effects were obtained when intact male mice were similarly treated. The putative effects for reductions in body temperature to decrease METH-induced neurotoxicity can, in part, be the result of E, thereby indicating an additional means by which E can act as a neuroprotectant. When E was co-infused with METH into CS tissue, a marked decrease in METH-evoked DA release was observed. Because increases in extracellular DA efflux can exert a neurodegenerative effect, the reduction in METH-evoked DA by E may indicate another neuroprotectant action of this gonadal steroid hormone. Finally, we have observed some relatively specific, discriminative changes in CS mRNA levels between male and female mice treated with METH. GFAP mRNA levels tended to be increased and PAI-1 levels decreased in females. The exact interpretations and involvement of E as related to these findings remain to be determined. However, data indicating a role for GFAP in wound healing/neuronal survival and an involvement of PAI-1 with impaired motor learning suggest that these message levels may be important components contributing to the gender differences in response to METH neurotoxicity of the NSDA system.

REFERENCES

1. ALI, S.F. & T. FREYALDENHOVEN. 1999. MPTP—a model of Parkinson's disease. *In* Chemicals and Neurodegenerative Disease. S.C. Bondy, Ed.: 161–188. Prominent Press. Scottsdale, AZ.
2. BROOKS, W.J., M.F. JARVIS & G.C. WAGNER. 1989. Influence of sex, age and strain of MPTP-induced neurotoxicity. Res. Comm. Subst. Abuse **10**: 181–184.
3. FREYALDENHOVEN, T.E., J.L. CADET & S.F. ALI. 1996. The dopamine depleting effect of 1-methyl-4-phenyl-1,2,3,6-tetrahydropyridine in CD-1 mice are gender dependent. Brain Res. **735**: 232–238.
4. HELLER, A. *et al.* 2001. Gender-dependent enhanced adult neurotoxic response to methamphetamine following fetal exposure to the drug. J. Pharmacol. Exp. Therap. **298**: 769–779.
5. MILLER, D.B., S.F. ALI, J.P. O'CALLAGHAN & S.C. LAWS. 1998. The impact of gender and estrogen on striatal dopamine neurotoxicity. Ann. N.Y. Acad. Sci. **844**: 153–165.
6. WAGNER, G.C., T.L. TEKIRIAN & C.T. CHEO. 1993. Sexual differences in sensitivity to methamphetamine toxicity. J. Neural Transm. Gen. Sect. **93**: 67–70.
7. YU, L. & P-C. LIAO. 2000. Sexual differences and estrous cycle in methamphetamine-induced dopamine and serotonin depletions in the striatum of mice. J. Neural Transm. **107**: 419–427.
8. YU, Y-L. & G.C. WAGNER. 1994. Influence of gonadal hormones on sexual differences in sensitivity to methamphetamine-induced neurotoxicity. J. Neural Transm. [P-D Sect] **8**: 215–221.
9. HALL, J.N. & P.M. BRODERICK. 1991. Community networks for response to abuse outbreaks of methamphetamine and its analogs. NIDA Res. Monogr. **115**: 109–120.
10. BALDERESCHI, M. *et al.* FOR THE ILSA WORKING GROUP. 2000. Parkinson's disease and parkinsonism in a longitudinal study two-fold higher incidence in men. Neurology **55**: 1358–1363.
11. BOWER, J.H., D.M. MARAGANORE, S.K. MCDONNELL & W.A. ROCCA. 2000. Influence of strict, intermediate, and broad diagnostic criteria on the age- and sex-specific incidence of Parkinson's disease. Move. Disord. **15**: 819–825.

12. DLUZEN, D.E., K.A. DISSHON & J.L. MCDERMOTT. 1998. Estrogen as a modulator of striatal dopaminergic neurotoxicity. *In* Recent Advances in Neurodegenerative Disorders. J. Marwah & H. Tietelbaum, Eds.: 149–192. Prominent Press. Scottsdale, AZ.
13. KUOPIO, A.M., R.J. MARTILLA, H. HELENIUS & U.K. RINNE. 1999. Changing epidemiology of Parkinson's disease in southwestern Finland. Neurology **52**: 302–308.
14. SCHRAG, A., Y. BEN-SHLOMO & N.P. QUINN. 2001. Cross sectional prevalence survey of idiopathic Parkinson's disease and parkinsonism in London. Br. J. Med. **321**: 21–22.
15. SWERDLOW, R.H. *et al.* 2001. Gender ratio differences between Parkinson's disease patients and their affected relatives. Parkinsonism Relat. Disord. **7**: 129–133.
16. DLUZEN, D.E., J.L. MCDERMOTT & B. LIU. 1996. Estrogen alters MPTP-induced neurotoxicity in female mice: effects of striatal dopamine concentrations and release. J. Neurochem. **66**: 658–666.
17. DLUZEN, D.E., J.L. MCDERMOTT & B. LIU. 1996. Estrogen as a neuroprotectant against MPTP-induced neurotoxicity in C57/Bl mice. Neurotox. Teratol. **18**: 603–606.
18. DLUZEN, D.E. 1997. Estrogen decreases corpus striatal neurotoxicity in response to 6-OHDA. Brain Res. **767**: 340–344.
19. GAO, X. & D.E. DLUZEN. 2001. Tamoxifen abolishes estrogen's neuroprotective effect upon methamphetamine neurotoxicity of the nigrostriatal dopaminergic system. Neuroscience **103**: 385–394.
20. GRANDBOIS, M., M. MORISSETTE, M. CALLIER & T. DI PAOLO. 2000. Ovarian steroids and raloxifene prevent MPTP-induced dopamine depletion in mice. NeuroReport **11**: 343–346.
21. DLUZEN, D.E. 2000. Neuroprotective effects of estrogen upon the nigrostriatal dopaminergic system. J. Neurocytol. **29**: 387–399.
22. DLUZEN, D.E. & J.L. MCDERMOTT. 2000. Neuroprotective role of estrogen upon methamphetamine and related neurotoxins within the nigrostriatal dopaminergic system. Ann. N.Y. Acad. Sci. **914**: 112–126.
23. DLUZEN, D.E. & J.L. MCDERMOTT. 2000. Gender differences in neurotoxicity of the nigrostriatal dopaminergic system: implications for Parkinson's disease. J. Gender Spec. Diff. **3**: 36–42.
24. HORSTINK, M.W.I.M., E. STRIJKS & D.E. DLUZEN. 2002. Estrogen and Parkinson's disease. Adv. Neurol. In press.
25. DISSHON, K.A. & D.E. DLUZEN. 2000. Estrogen reduces acute striatal dopamine responses in vivo to the neurotoxin MPP$^+$ in female, but not male rats. Brain Res. **868**: 95–104.
26. GAO, X. & D.E. DLUZEN. 2001. The effect of testosterone upon methamphetamine neurotoxicity of the nigrostriatal dopaminergic system. Brain Res. **892**: 63–69.
27. DLUZEN, D.E. 1996. The effects of testosterone upon MPTP-induced neurotoxicity of the nigrostriatal dopaminergic system in male C57/Bl mice. Brain Res. **715**: 113–118.
28. GRANDBOIS, M., B. TANGUAY & T. DI PAOLO. 1999. Estradiol and dehydroepiandrosterone but not dihydotestosterone protect against MPTP-induced dopamine depletion in mice (Miami, FL): No. 639.6. Society for Neuroscience. Washington, DC.
29. GREEN, P.S., J. BISHOP & J.W. SIMPKINS. 1997. 17 alpha-estradiol exerts neuroprotective effects on SK-N-SH cells. J. Neurosci. **17**: 511–515.
30. HAMMOND, J. *et al.* 2001. Testosterone-mediated neuroprotection through the androgen receptor in human primary neurons. J. Neurochem. **77**: 1319–1326.
31. YANG, S.H., J. SHI, A.L. DAY & J.W. SIMPKINS. 2000. Estradiol exerts neuroprotective effects when administered after ischemic insult. Stroke **31**: 745–755.
32. LINFORD, N., C. WADE & D. DORSA. 2000. The rapid effects of estrogen are implicated in estrogen-mediated neuroprotection. J. Neurocytol. **29**: 367–374.
33. JORDAN, V.G. & M. MORROW. 1999. Tamoxifen, raloxifene, and the prevention of breast cancer. Endo. Rev. **20**: 253–278.
34. STEPHENSON, J. 1999. Experts debate drugs for healthy women with breast cancer risk. JAMA **282**: 117.
35. DLUZEN, D.E., J.L. MCDERMOTT & L.I. ANDERSON. 2001. Tamoxifen eliminates estrogen's neuroprotective effect upon MPTP-induced neurotoxicity of the nigrostriatal dopaminergic system. Neurotox. Res. **3**: 291–300.

36. DLUZEN, D.E., J.L. McDERMOTT & L.I. ANDERSON. 2001. Tamoxifen diminishes methamphetamine-induced striatal dopamine depletion in intact female and male mice. J. Neuroendocrin. **13:** 618–624.

37. McDONNELL, D.P. 1999. The molecular pharmacology of SERMs. TEM **10:** 301–311.

38. BECKER, J.B. 1990. Direct effect of 17 beta-estradiol on striatum: sex differences in dopamine release. Synapse **5:** 157–164.

39. BECKER, J.B. & C.N. RUDICK. 1999. Rapid effects of estrogen or progesterone on the amphetamine-induced increase in striatal dopamine are enhanced by estrogen priming: a microdialysis study. Pharmacol. Biochem. Behav. **64:** 53–57.

40. McDERMOTT, J.L., B. LIU & D.E. DLUZEN. 1994. Sex differences and effects of estrogen on dopamine and DOPAC release from the striatum of male and female CD-1 mice. Exp. Neurol. **125:** 306–311.

41. ATTALI, G., A. WEIZMAN, I. GIL-AD & M. REHAVI. 1997. Opposite modulatory effects of ovarian hormones on rat brain dopamine and serotonin receptors. Brain Res. **756:** 153–159.

42. DISSHON, K.A., J.W. BOJA & D.E. DLUZEN. 1998. Inhibition of striatal dopamine transporter activity by 17β-estradiol. Eur. J. Pharmacol. **345:** 207–211.

43. ENERSBY, C.A. & C. WILSON. 1974. The effect of ovarian steroids on the accumulation of ^{3}H-labelled monoamines by hypothalamic tissue in vitro. Brain Res. **73:** 321–331.

44. FIGLEWICZ, D.P. *et al.* 1999. Neurotransmitter transporters: target for endocrine regulation. Horm. Metabol. Res. **31:** 335.

45. MICHEL, M.C., A. ROTHER, C. HIEMKE & R. GHRAF. 1987. Inhibition of synaptosomal high affinity uptake of dopamine and serotonin by estrogen agonists and antagonists. Biochem. Pharmacol. **36:** 3175–3180.

46. THOMPSON, T.L. 1999. Attenuation of DA uptake in vivo following priming with estradiol benzoate. Brain Res. **834:** 164–167.

47. THOMPSON, T.L., S.R. BRIDGES & W.J. WEIRS. 2001. Alteration of dopamine transport in the striatum and nucleus accumbens of ovariectomized and estrogen-primed rats following *N*-(*p*-isothiocyanatophenethyl) spiperone (NIPS) treatment. Brain Res. Bull. **54:** 631–638.

48. DI PAOLO, T., C. ROULLIARD & P. BEDARD. 1985. 17β-estradiol at a physiological dose acutely increases dopamine turnover in the rat brain. Eur. J. Pharmacol. **117:** 197–203.

49. PASQUALINI, C. *et al.* 1995. Acute stimulatory effect of estradiol on striatal dopamine synthesis. J. Neurochem. **65:** 1651–1657.

50. DI PAOLO, T., M. DAIGLE & F. LABRIE. 1984. Effect of estradiol and haloperidol on hypophysectomized rat brain dopamine receptors. Psychoneuroendocrinology **9:** 399–404.

51. LEVESQUE, D. & T. DI PAOLO. 1988. Rapid conversion of high into low striatal D2dopamine receptor agonist binding sites after an acute physiological dose of 17β-estradiol. Neurosci. Lett. **88:** 113–118.

52. CHEN, J.C. & V.D. RAMIREZ. 1988. Comparison of the effect of prolactin on dopamine release from the rat dorsal and ventral striatum and from the mediobasal hypothalamus *in vitro*. Eur. J. Pharmacol. **149:** 1–8.

53. BOWYER, J.F. *et al.* 1992. The influence of environmental temperature on the transient effects of methamphetamine on dopamine levels and dopamine release in the striatum. J. Pharmacol. Exp. Ther. **260:** 817–824.

54. MILLER, D.B. & J.P. O'CALLAGHAN. Environment-, drug- and stress-induced alterations in body temperature affect the neurotoxicity of substituted amphetamines in the C57BL/6J mouse. J. Pharmacol. Exp. Ther. **270:** 752–760.

55. ALI, S.F., G.D. NEWPORT & W. SLIKKER, JR. 1996. Methamphetamine-induced dopaminergic toxicity in mice. Role of environmental temperature and pharmacological agents. Ann. N.Y. Acad. Sci. **801:** 187–198.

56. KUPERMAN, D.I., T.E. FREYALDENHOVEN, L.C. SCHMUED & S.F. ALI. 1997. Methamphetamine-induced hyperthermia in mice: examination of dopamine depletion and heat-shock protein induction. Brain Res. **771:** 221–227.

57. YUAN, J., B.T. CALLAHAN, U.D. McCANN & G.A. RICAURTE. 2001. Evidence against an essential role of endogenous brain dopamine in methamphetamine-induced dopaminergic neurotoxicity. J. Neurochem. **77:** 1338–1347.

58. O'DELL, S.J., F.B. WEIHMULLER & J. MARSHALL. 1991. Multiple methamphetamine injections induce marked increases in extracellular striatal dopamine which correlate with subsequent neurotoxicity. Brain Res. **564:** 256–260.
59. WEIHMULLER, F.B., S.J. O'DELL & J.F. MARSHAL. 1992. MK-801 protection against methamphetamine-induced striatal dopamine terminal injury is associated with attenuated dopamine overflow. Synapse **11:** 155–163.
60. MYERS, R., L.I. ANDERSON & D.E. DLUZEN. 2002. Estrogen, but not testosterone,attenuates methamphetamine-evoked dopamine output from superfused striatal tissue fragments of female and male mice. In preparation.
61. DISSHON, K.A. & D.E. DLUZEN. 1997. Estrogen as a neuromodulator of MPTP-induced neurotoxicity: effects upon striatal dopamine release. Brain Res. **764:** 9–16.
62. ARVIN, M. *et al.* 2000. Estrogen modulates responses of striatal dopamine neurons to MPP$^+$: evaluations using in vitro and in vivo techniques. Brain Res. **872:** 160–171.
63. DLUZEN, D.E., C. TWEED & N.J. LAPING. 2001. Gender differences in methamphetamine (MA) induced mRNA levels associated with neurodegeneration in the mouse striatum (San Diego, CA): No. 971.9. Society for Neuroscience. Washington, D.C.
64. NICHOLS, N.R. 1999. Glial responses to steroids as markers of brain aging. J. Neurobiol. **40:** 585–601.

Effects of Cocaine Administration on VTA Cell Activity in Response to Prefrontal Cortex Stimulation

L.J. ALMODÓVAR-FÁBREGAS,[a] O. SEGARRA,[b] N. COLÓN,[b]
J.G. DONES,[c] M. MERCADO,[c] C.A. MEJÍAS-APONTE,[b] R. VÁZQUEZ,[a]
R. ABREU,[a] E. VÁZQUEZ,[a] J.T. WILLIAMS,[d] AND C.A. JIMÉNEZ-RIVERA[a]

[a]Department of Physiology, Universidad Central del Caribe, Bayamón,
Puerto Rico

[b]Department of Biological Sciences, University of Puerto Rico, Río Piedras,
Puerto Rico

[c]Section of Neurological Surgery, Department of Surgery, University of Puerto Rico,
Puerto Rico

[d]Vollum Institute, Oregon Health Sciences University, Portland, Oregon, USA

ABSTRACT: The repeated use of psychostimulants in humans has been associated with progressive enhancement of anxiety, panic attacks, and eventually paranoid psychosis. The appearance of such behaviors has been termed behavioral sensitization, which forms part of the basic pathological mechanisms involved in drug addiction. Psychostimulants act via a circuit involving the ventral tegmental area (VTA), prefrontal cortex (PFC), and nucleus accumbens. The PFC sends glutamatergic projections that activate dopaminergic neurons in the VTA. These projections provide an extremely important excitatory drive necessary for the development of sensitization. The effects of cocaine administration on the response of dopaminergic VTA cells to activation of the PFC have not been reported. Here the effects of acute cocaine administration on VTA cell response to PFC stimulation are examined. Statistical analysis of the changes in spontaneous activity and evoked response revealed a significant decrease in spontaneous activity at 1.0 mg/kg i.v. after cocaine treatment compared to baseline levels. The net effect was an increase in signal-to-noise ratio. Treatment with MK-801 at a dose of 2 mg/kg showed that the excitatory response was, at least partially, NMDA-mediated. Prazosin pretreatment (0.5 mg/kg i.p.) did not prevent a significant decrease in spontaneous activity brought about by cocaine (15 mg/kg, i.p.). Nonetheless, prazosin alone induced a significant decrease in the response to PFC stimulation when compared to baseline. In addition, iontophoretic application of norepinephrine (NE) onto VTA cells revealed that NE potentiated (19.2%), enhanced (26.9%), or suppressed (46.2%) the glutamate-evoked response in VTA cells. The results suggest that a possible role of cocaine in the process of sensitization might be to amplify the PFC-induced excitation at the VTA. Since the iontophoretic release of NE in almost half of the sampled cells produced similar effects to those of cocaine it may suggest a possible NE-mediated mechanism for cocaine actions.

Address for correspondence: C. A. Jiménez-Rivera, Department of Physiology, Universidad Central del Caribe, P.O. Box 60-327, Bayamon, Puerto Rico, 00960
cjimenez@uccaribe.edu

Ann. N.Y. Acad. Sci. 965: 157–171 (2002). © 2002 New York Academy of Sciences.

KEYWORDS: cocaine; norepinephrine; ventral tegmental area; prefrontal cortex; prazosin

INTRODUCTION

Cocaine is a potent central psychostimulant agent with well-known local anesthetic properties. It is one of the most widely used abuse drugs in the United States. Acute cocaine administration potentiates the effects of dopamine (DA), 5-hydroxytriptamine (5-HT), and norepinephrine (NE) in the central nervous system. This action of cocaine is achieved by binding to the transporter sites of neurotransmitters and blocking their reuptake into presynaptic terminals.[1,2]

Although increased dopaminergic transmission usually has been associated with cocaine-rewarding effects, other catecholamines can mediate cocaine's actions on sensory systems and on its discriminative stimulus properties. Several lines of investigation have shown that acute parenteral and locally administered cocaine can increase somatosensory cortical neuronal responsiveness to afferent excitatory synaptic inputs and iontophoretically applied glutamate.[3,4] These effects are similar to previously demonstrated facilitatory actions of NE on cell firing in cerebral cortex[5–7] and elsewhere.[8]

Repeated exposure to cocaine administration culminates in a progressive and lasting enhancement in the motor stimulant effect induced by a subsequent drug challenge.[9] This phenomenon is termed behavioral sensitization and forms part of the basic pathological mechanisms of cocaine addiction.[10,11]

The prefrontal cortex (PFC) is involved in cognitive processes such as attention, spatial learning, behavioral planning, and working memory.[12] This structure is also involved in the mediation of the primary rewarding effects of drugs of abuse. There is strong evidence implicating the PFC in the neural mechanism underlying drug addiction and craving.[13] It has been shown that the PFC sends glutamatergic projections to the ventral tegmental area (VTA).[14] The VTA is the source of dopaminergic projections that supply structures in the ventral forebrain and cortical areas, giving rise to a system collectively referred to as the mesocorticolimbic system.[15,16] This system has been implicated in motivated behavior as well as in mediating the reinforcing actions of drugs of abuse.[17,18]

Several lines of investigation demonstrate the crucial role that the PFC glutamatergic input to the VTA plays in the pathogenesis of drug addiction. Burst firing of VTA DA neurons is dependent, at least in part, on glutamatergic input. PFC stimulation increases burst firing of DA neurons.[19–21] Conversely, inactivation of the PFC brings about the opposite effect.[20,22] Investigations have shown that ibotenic acid lesions of the PFC completely prevented the development of cocaine sensitization.[23] Moreover, cutting the afferent projections arising from the PFC, which are excitatory to the VTA, abolished the development of sensitization induced by systemic injections of amphetamine but not stereotypy.[24]

Given the fundamental importance of the PFC input to the VTA, it is necessary to investigate the changes in the interaction between these two structures brought about by drugs of abuse such as cocaine. The effects of cocaine administration on the response of dopaminergic VTA cells to activation of the PFC have not yet been reported. In the present study, electrophysiological changes in VTA cell activity in the presence of cocaine were examined according to dose, route of administration, and coadministration with the noradrenergic alpha-1 receptor antagonist prazosin.

METHODS

Animals and Surgical Procedure

Male Sprague-Dawley rats (weight 275–400 g) were used in this study. Animals were initially anesthetized with chloral hydrate 400 mg/kg i.p., intubated, and allowed to breathe spontaneously. Additional anesthesia was administered at 100 mg/kg as needed. All animals used for intravenous cocaine injection study had a femoral vein catheter in place (PE 60, Intramedic, NJ). Once fully anesthetized, animals were mounted in a stereotaxic apparatus, and the skull and dura overlying the prefrontal cortex were clearly exposed. In experiments involving prefrontal cortex stimulation both bregma and the imaginary lambda were identified and their respective coordinates noted (see FIG. 1). The area overlying the prefrontal cortex was estimated to lie 3.2 mm anterior, 0.5 mm lateral to bregma, and 4.0 mm ventral to the skull surface.[25] A tungsten or stainless-steel monopolar stimulating electrode (Frederick Haer, ME) was inserted in the PFC through a small craniotomy and fixed to the skull. A reference electrode was placed just anterior to the stimulating electrode. The VTA was estimated to lie 3.2 mm anterior and 0.6–1.0 mm lateral to the imaginary lambda.[25] A second craniotomy, ipsilateral to the PFC electrode, was done overlying the

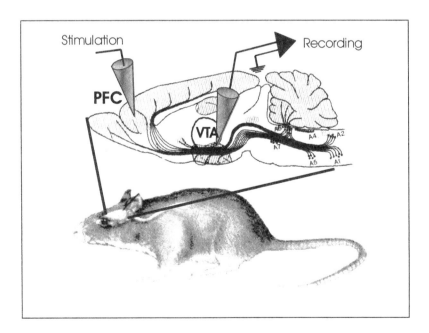

FIGURE 1. A picture depicting the position of the stimulating and recording electrodes used in the study of the VTA neuronal response to PFC stimulation.

VTA and the dura was retracted. In microiontophoretic studies, a single craniotomy was performed overlying the VTA. In all experiments the rats' body temperature was maintained at 37°C with a DC heating pad (Frederick Haer, ME). All animal experimentation was carried out in accordance with the Animal Welfare Act and the Guide for the Care and Use of Laboratory Animals. The procedures were approved by the Universidad Central del Caribe Institutional Animal Care and Use Committee.

Extracellular Single-Unit Recording and Data Acquisition

Single-barrel micropipettes filled with Pontamine Sky Blue (PSB) solution, tip diameter 3–6 mm, were used to record the spontaneous activity of VTA dopaminergic neurons and their response to prefrontal cortex stimulation. The recording micropipette was slowly advanced to 7–8 mm ventral from the cortical surface with a micromanipulator (Narishige, East Meadow, NY) until isolation of a single neuron was achieved. VTA dopaminergic neurons were identified using previously established electrophysiological criteria.[26] Briefly, DA neurons were identified by a wide action potential (>2.5 ms), biphasic or triphasic waveform, slow irregular firing pattern, and bursting activity (2–10 Hz). The prefrontal cortex was then stimulated (pulse width 500 ms, frequency 0.5 Hz, intensity 0.25–1.5 mA) and VTA cell response was recorded. Each recording session included one hundred stimuli. Neuronal activity was amplified (Dam80 amplifier, World Precision Instruments, Sarasota, FL) and sent to an interface for analog-to-digital signal conversion. The interface's output was fed to a computer for on-line window discrimination and wavemark display (Spike 2, Cambridge Electronic Design, UK). Poststimulus time histograms (PSTHs) were generated from each recording session. Both raw data and the PSTHs were stored for off-line analysis.

Parenteral Drug Administration

Acquisition of 2–3 baseline-recording sessions, a minimum of 7 min, was followed by parenteral drug administration. During intravenous injection experiments cocaine was administered via the femoral catheter (doses of 0.5, 1, or 2 mg/kg; Sigma, St. Louis, MO). Recordings were made at 5, 15, 25, 40, 50, and 60 min following cocaine injection. In experiments involving intraperitoneal injection cocaine was given at 15 mg/kg and recordings collected as just elucidated. During pharmacological studies, prazosin was administered at 0.5 mg/kg i.p., followed by cocaine at 15 mg/kg i.p. Recordings were taken at 5 and 10 min after the prazosin dose and as noted earlier after cocaine injection.

Microiontophoretic Studies

Five-barrel micropipettes, tip diameter 4–6 μm, were used to record spontaneous activity from individual VTA dopaminergic cells (as previously) and to apply chemical substances at the recording site by microiontophoresis. The center barrel was filled with PSB solution and used for recording (3–6-MΩ impedance) single-unit activity. Automatic current balancing was maintained via a side barrel filled with 3 M NaCl. The remaining barrels were filled with 1 M L-glutamate, pH 8.4 (Sigma), and norepinephrine (0.5 M) (Sigma). Neuronal activity was amplified (Dam80 amplifier, WPI) and conveyed to a window discriminator (Brainwave, Datawave Technology,

CO). The output of the discriminator was sent to a computer for on-line generation and display of continuous ratemeter records. Ratemeter records and raw spike-train data were also stored for off-line analysis. Regularly spaced iontophoretic pulses of glutamate (1–50 nA, 10-s duration every 40 s) were applied to individual VTA DA cells via a commercially available microiontophoresis machine (BH-2; Medical Systems, Great Neck, NY). Once a stable firing pattern was observed for a minimum of 5 min of glutamate-elicited excitation, NE was applied. NE was constantly released iontophoretically for 200 s while concurrently delivering glutamate pulses. Retaining currents (+10 nA for glutamate and −10 nA for NE) were applied routinely to drug barrels to prevent leakage of drug solutions into the surrounding tissue.

Data Analysis

Glutamate-induced and spontaneous discharge of individual neurons were quantified by averaging the firing rate of a cell during at least three transmitter applications for glutamate responses and by averaging the mean firing activity between drug pulses for spontaneous discharges. For each neuron, glutamate-evoked and spontaneous discharges were compared for a period of 200 s before, 200 s immediately following cocaine administration, and 200 s of recovery period.

The following operational definitions were employed as in previous reports[3,27] to assess the influence of NE on glutamate-induced excitation. "Enhancement" of the evoked response relative to background was declared when spontaneous firing was suppressed at least 15% more by NE application than was activity evoked by glutamate administration. "Potentiation" of evoked excitation was defined as an absolute increase in glutamate-induced response over control, together with an increase, decrease, or no change in the level of spontaneous discharge. Cocaine interactions with glutamate were termed "suppressive" when the evoked excitatory response was depressed proportionately more by NE application than was background discharge. Finally, it was assumed that NE had no net effect on excitatory responses when spontaneous, and evoked discharges were affected proportionately to the same extent during drug application. The latter case is represented by the dotted 45° "equivalence line" in the graph. It should be noted that these definitions, while providing a useful terminology, make no assumptions concerning linear or nonlinear summation effects.

Statistics

Statistical analyses were performed using *t*-tests for paired samples. A two-tailed *p* value of ≤0.05 was considered to be significant.

RESULTS

Data were collected from VTA cells that responded to electrical PFC stimulation. Based on the PSTHs, the spontaneous activity and the evoked response of the cell were measured and analyzed. The spontaneous activity (SA) was defined as the mean number of spikes per bin (bin size 5 ms) generated by a cell during the 500-ms period immediately preceding the PFC stimulation artifact. The evoked response

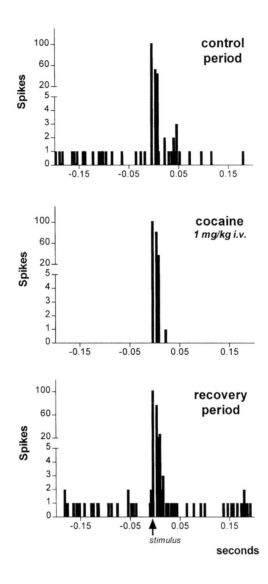

FIGURE 2. The figure shows a poststimulus time histogram (bin size 2 ms) of a representative cell in response to PFC stimulation, before and after an intravenous cocaine injection (1 mg/kg, i.v.). It can be observed that prefrontal cortex stimulation alone induces a sharp enhancement in firing, indicated by an increase in *spikes after the arrow* (stimulus artifact). After cocaine administration, both the spontaneous activity and the evoked excitation were diminished. However, the histogram reveals that cocaine was able to dramatically inhibit the spontaneous activity in comparison to the evoked excitation. The net effect of this action is an increase in the S/N. The recovery phase shows that the cells return to control-period levels after ~40 min postcocaine administration.

was defined as neuronal firing exceeding two standard deviations above the spontaneous activity. The beginning and ending of the evoked response were calculated using the time at which neuronal firing rose above or fell within two standard deviations above the SA, respectively. The magnitude of the evoked response was defined as the sum of spikes above the level of the SA. A total of 35 cells was analyzed. In the great majority of cases, only one cell was sampled from each animal. In four animals two cells were sampled. In these animals, successive treatments were spaced by at least 2 h.

Effects of Intravenous Cocaine Injection on VTA Cell Activity

FIGURE 2 illustrates a representative response from a VTA neuron to PFC stimulation before and after cocaine administration. In this particular case it can be seen that a cocaine injection (1 mg/kg, i.v.) was able to dramatically decrease the spontaneous activity, while the evoked-excitation remained practically unaffected. The net effect was an increase in the signal-to-noise ratio (S/N). Treatment of a cell with MK-801 at a dose of 2 mg/kg showed that the excitatory response was, at least partially, NMDA-mediated.

The effects of intravenous cocaine administration were analyzed for a total of 17 cells. Cells were divided into groups according to pharmacological treatment and dose. The results were expressed as mean percent change from baseline ± SEM for each of the parameters. FIGURE 3 illustrates the effects of cocaine injection at different doses. At a dose of 0.5 mg/kg ($n = 4$) all the cells showed a decrease in SA, which averaged $-36.0 \pm 15.6\%$ ($p = 0.076$), whereas the evoked response decreased by only $-6.5 \pm 2.5\%$ ($p = 0.219$). Although there is no statistically significant reduction in

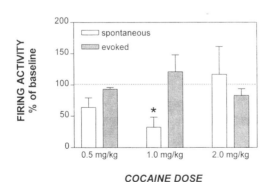

COCAINE DOSE

FIGURE 3. Effects of intravenous cocaine administration on VTA cell activity after PFC stimulation. The figure illustrates the changes observed in spontaneous activity and evoked response when compared to predrug levels (*dotted line*) following a cocaine injection. Note that 1 mg/kg cocaine administration caused a significant decrease in spontaneous activity compared to baseline levels ($p = 0.01$, paired-sample t-test, $n = 5$). At 0.5 mg/kg a strong tendency toward decreasing the spontaneous activity was seen, although it did not reach significance ($p = 0.08$, $n = 4$). At 2 mg/kg an appreciable yet very variable increase in spontaneous activity can be seen ($n = 9$). No significant effects were observed in the evoked response at all doses tested.

SA when compared to baseline, a strong tendency toward significance was observed. When the dose was increased to 1.0 mg/kg ($n = 5$), a statistically significant decrease in SA was noted when compared to predrug levels ($-72.0 \pm 28.0\%$, $p = 0.014$). There was a uniform decrease in spontaneous activity in all cells tested at 1.0 mg/kg; however, no clear effect was observed on the evoked response, with a mean increase of $20.5 \pm 27.1\%$ ($p = 0.641$). A further increase in dose to 2.0 mg/kg ($n = 8$) yielded a very variable effect in spontaneous activity ranging from an increase in 4 out of 8 cells (50%) to a decrease in the remaining 4 cells (50%). The magnitude of the increases was greater than that of the decreases, resulting in an average increase in SA ($29.3 \pm 47.3\%$, $p = 0.141$) for the entire group. A decrease in the response to PFC stimulation was observed in 6 out of 8 cells (75%), while an increase was seen in 2 out of 8 cells (25%). This resulted in a modest average decrease in evoked response ($-16.6 \pm 10.5\%$, $p = 0.376$) for the entire group. Statistical analysis did not reveal any significant changes in either of the two parameters analyzed. It is of interest to note, however, that the changes observed after intravenous cocaine injection appear to affect preferentially the spontaneous activity of the cell rather than the response to PFC stimulation.

Effects of Intraperitoneal Cocaine Injection on VTA Cell Activity

Cocaine was administered via the intraperitoneal route at a dose of 15 mg/kg ($n = 9$). A total of 8 out of 9 cells (88%) presented a decrease in SA following cocaine injection when compared with predrug levels. A strong tendency toward a significant decrease in spontaneous activity was observed ($-31.3 \pm 16.4\%$, $p = 0.078$). Cocaine's effects on the response to PFC stimulation were not as uniform. The evoked response increased in 5 out of 9 cells (55.5%), whereas a decrease was noted in 4 out of 9 cells (44.4%). Yet, the magnitude of the increases in evoked response was greater than that of the decreases, resulting in a visible average increase in the magnitude of the evoked response ($330.3 \pm 193.7\%$, $p = 0.738$) (figure not shown).

Effects of a Prazosin Injection Followed by Cocaine Administration on VTA Cell Activity

Prazosin was administered (0.5 mg/kg, i.p.) followed by cocaine (15 mg/kg, i.p.) 15 min later to a total of 9 cells (FIG. 4). When compared to predrug levels prazosin injection alone produced a statistically significant decrease in the response to PFC stimulation ($-33.1 \pm 13.4\%$, $p = 0.019$). This was accompanied by variable changes in the spontaneous activity ranging from marked increase (293.5%) to a marked decrease (-93.3%) in spontaneous activity. Nevertheless, there was a mean increase in the spontaneous activity ($34.5 \pm 34.7\%$, $p = 0.959$) after prazosin injection alone when compared to predrug levels. No significant increase in spontaneous activity could be observed after prazosin injection. Subsequent cocaine administration produced a statistically significant decrease in spontaneous activity when compared to the postprazosin levels ($-43.2 \pm 13.0\%$, $p = 0.011$) (see FIG. 4). However, when compared to predrug levels, this decrease in SA following cocaine injection was variable and did not reach statistical significance ($-19.8 \pm 22.6\%$, $p = 0.084$). Cocaine produced variable effects in the response to PFC stimulation. Four out of 9 cells (44.4%) increased the magnitude of the evoked response upon cocaine injection, whereas 5

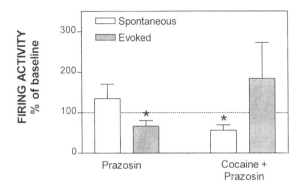

FIGURE 4. Effects of prazosin administration alone and after a subsequent cocaine injection on VTA cell activity in response to PFC stimulation. Prazosin (0.5 mg/kg i.p.) was injected 15 min before cocaine administration (15 mg/kg, i.p.). The graph illustrates the changes in spontaneous activity and evoked response observed after prazosin administration alone (*left side*) and after cocaine (*right side*). A significant decrease in the evoked response can be observed after a prazosin injection ($p = 0.02$, $n = 9$, paired-sample t-test) when compared to predrug levels (*dotted line*). Subsequent administration of cocaine causes a significant decrease in the spontaneous activity when compared to postprazosin levels ($p = 0.01$, $n = 9$). This is accompanied by a variable increase in evoked response.

out of 9 cells (55.5%) decreased the magnitude of the evoked response. Nonetheless, a mean increase of $84.3 \pm 89.1\%$ ($p = 0.803$) in evoked response was observed after cocaine injection when compared to postprazosin levels. This change was not statistically significant.

Effects of Microiontophoretic NE Application on Glutamate-Evoked VTA Cell Excitation

The effects of norepinephrine on glutamate-evoked excitation were observed in a total of 26 cells. All drugs were microiontophoretically applied, as explained in the Materials and Methods section. As can be seen in the 45° equivalence line graph, two distinct cell responses to NE application could be identified (see FIG. 5). Norepinephrine was found to increase the S/N in a group of 12 out of 26 cells (46.2%). Of these, NE absolutely potentiated the excitation induced by glutamate pulses in 5 out of 12 cells (41.6%) (see FIG. 6). In the remaining seven cells within this group (58.3%) application of NE enhanced the glutamate-evoked excitation by decreasing the spontaneous activity of the cell while having no observable effect on the glutamate-induced excitation. Norepinephrine was found to suppress the excitation elicited by glutamate pulses on 12 out of 26 cells (46.2%). No differential effect could be observed in 2 out of 26 cells (7.6%).

DISCUSSION

The goal of the present study was to examine the effects of acute cocaine administration on VTA cell response to PFC stimulation. The results revealed that cocaine

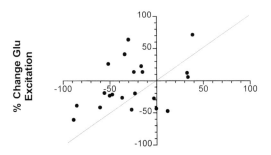

% Change Spontaneous Activity

CATEGORIES	Number of cells (n = 26)
Suppression	12 (46.15%)
Enhancement	7 (26.92%)
Absolute Potentiation	5 (19.23%)
No differential effect	2 (7.69%)

FIGURE 5. A summary of the population results for the iontophoretic studies. The *dotted 45°-equivalence line* represents a proportional change in spontaneous and evoked discharges. Points lying near or within that line indicate no significant net effect on the excitatory response during drug administration. Points that lie below the 45°-equivalence line indicate cases where NE-suppressed glutamate evoked responses more than spontaneous activity, thus yielding a net reduction in cell responsiveness to glutamate. Points above the line in the left lower quadrant represent a greater decrease in spontaneous discharge compared to evoked excitation. Points in the left upper quadrant demonstrate absolute increases of the excitatory response or potentiation. The table under the graph shows that there are two major effects. One group of cells exhibited suppression of the glutamate-evoked response, whereas another group showed an increase in the S/N expressed either as filter effect (or enhancement) or an absolute potentiation.

administration (1.0 mg/kg i.v.) produced a significant decrease in the SA of VTA neurons without changing the stimulus-evoked excitation. The net effect was an enhancement of stimulus-evoked discharges, thus producing an increase in the S/N. It was shown that the administration of an alpha-1 adrenoceptor antagonist does not block the inhibition in SA induced by cocaine injections. However, in the presence of prazosin alone, there was a significant reduction in the stimulus-induced excitation, suggesting a possible modulatory role of NE in this excitatory connection. For the first time it was found that NE iontophoretically released into the VTA can have facilitatory actions on neuronal responsiveness to glutamate-induced excitations. Intravenous cocaine administration mimicked some of these noradrenergic modulatory effects in the VTA. The results suggest that a possible role of cocaine in the process of sensitization might be to amplify the PFC-induced excitation at the VTA.

Studies have demonstrated two separate and distinct processes in sensitization: initiation and expression. Initiation of sensitization refers to the immediate molecular and/or cellular effects that induce behavioral sensitization. Expression indicates the long-term consequences of these effects.[28] Numerous studies have shown that the VTA is the site where the processes responsible for the initiation of sensitization occur[29] (reviewed in Ref. 30).

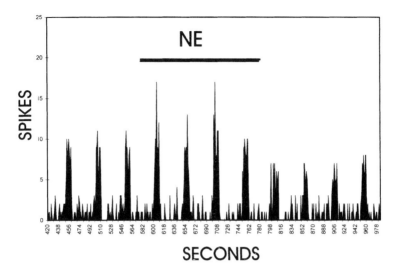

FIGURE 6. The figure illustrates a VTA's neuronal response to uniform glutamate iontophoretic pulses (5 nA, 10-s duration, every 40 s) before, during, and after NE microiontophoretic application (7 nA). NE could produce a net potentiation of glutamate-induced excitation in the VTA by increasing the glutamate-evoked response and decreasing the spontaneous activity of the cell.

The PFC and its excitatory afferents play an important role in the process of sensitization. Cuts of the afferent projections from the PFC, which are excitatory to the VTA, abolished the development of sensitization induced by systemic injections of amphetamine but not stereotypy[24] (see review in Ref. 31). Moreover, it was further demonstrated that these projections from the prefrontal cortex were not important for the expression of amphetamine-induced sensitization.[32] Ibotenic acid lesions of the PFC before the induction of sensitization by intra-VTA amphetamine injections completely abolished the development of sensitization.[33] In addition, ibotenic acid lesions of the PFC clearly prevented the development of cocaine sensitization.[23] Taken together, these studies indicate that PFC projections into the VTA are necessary for the development of sensitization to both amphetamine and cocaine.

How does the PFC interact with the VTA to enable the development of cocaine sensitization? It has been demonstrated that the PFC provides monosynaptic EAA inputs to the cells in the VTA.[14] These projections are essential in regulating the dopaminergic cell activity of this structure.[19–21] Furthermore, ibotenic acid lesions of the PFC diminish the number of spontaneously active DA cells in the VTA, although no effects were seen on firing rate or bursting activity.[34] Thus, the PFC projection provides an extremely important excitatory drive to the VTA necessary for the development of sensitization. Our findings demonstrating that acute cocaine administration enhanced the stimulus-bound excitation over background activity in the VTA could be one of those crucial changes in the initiation of behavioral sensitization.

Recent studies have placed a new emphasis on excitatory neurotransmitters in the initiation of behavioral sensitization. Several investigations have demonstrated that NMDA receptor blockade inhibits the development of sensitization when coadministered repeatedly with cocaine or amphetamine.[24,35–44] Not only does NMDA receptor inhibition block cocaine sensitization, but also the neuroadaptations that usually accompany it.[45,46] In addition, NMDA administration into the VTA induced sensitization to the locomotor activating effects of NMDA. However, the animals were not sensitized to the activating actions of systemically administered cocaine, suggesting that other excitatory receptors might be involved in the development of cocaine sensitization.[47] Although NMDA receptors do play a significant role in the development of sensitization, recent discoveries also attribute an important part in these phenomena to AMPA receptors.[48,49]

It has long been demonstrated that NE plays an important role as a neuromodulatory transmitter in the CNS (see reviews in Refs. 8, 50, 51). Furthermore, NE-induced enhancement of excitability in the somatosensory cortex for long periods of time suggests long-lasting effects of noradrenergic transmission in neuronal activity.[52] An alpha-1 receptor antagonist blocked these long-acting actions. The effect of NE in increasing glutamatergic transmission has been carefully characterized in Ref. 6. It was demonstrated that NE enhance glutamate excitation in the cortex by an alpha-1-mediated receptor mechanism. In addition, activation of protein kinase C mimicked the potentiating effects of NE on glutamate-induced excitation. A recent study found that in the somatosensory cortex, NE exerted a current-dependent facilitation of glutamate-evoked discharge, followed by suppression of the maximal facilitated response. The data indicated that the facilitating and suppressant actions of NE were mediated by an alpha-1 and beta receptors, respectively.[7] Thus, an extensive body of work exists demonstrating the role of NE as a modulator of glutamatergic excitatory transmission in the CNS. The results of the present study demonstrating that prazosin by itself blocks the stimulus-evoked excitation provide further evidence for a NE modulatory role in the VTA.

On the other hand, similar facilitatory actions on glutamate-evoked excitation have been demonstrated after acute cocaine administration. Parenteral and locally applied cocaine can increase cortical cell responsiveness to afferent excitatory synaptic inputs and iontophoretically released glutamate.[3,4] The results indicated that while high doses of cocaine can suppress both evoked and spontaneous activity of cortical neurons (local anesthetic actions), low doses can selectively enhance stimulus-evoked discharge. These facilitating effects could also be observed during iontophoretic interaction of cocaine with glutamate-induced excitation in the somatosensory cortex.[3] A recent study in the cerebellum demonstrated that acute cocaine administration inhibits spontaneous Purkinje cell activity and have a differential effect on glutamate-evoked excitation.[27] At lower doses (0.25 mg/kg. i.v.), 42% of the cells showed facilitatory actions and 63% had either no differential changes or a suppression (9%) of evoked-excitation. It was found that the decreases in spontaneous Purkinje cell activity and glutamate-evoked discharges after cocaine injections were mediated by a mechanism involving alpha-2 adrenoceptor activation. Since in our study cocaine can still suppress the SA of VTA cells in the presence of prazosin, it suggests that the inhibition is not mediated by an alpha-1 noradrenergic receptor. Further investigations should explore a possible involvement of alpha-2 receptors in this cocaine-induced inhibition. On the other hand, the possibility that dopamine D2 receptors are involved in this suppression cannot be ruled out. Indeed, a recent study has shown that amphetamine can produce two types of responses in the VTA:[53] one is to inhibit DA cell activity (via D2 receptors), and the other, an excitatory effect on DA cells, which is masked by the inhibitory actions.

Finally, further studies should be conducted to assess whether NE facilitatory actions in the VTA are enhanced or still present in animals subjected to a process of cocaine sensitization.

ACKNOWLEDGMENTS

This work was supported by the NINDS and NCRR (RCMI) SNPR Program, grant #NS39408, and GM 50695 to C.A.J.R. The authors thank Dr. Priscilla Sanabria for her great help in editing and figure preparation of the manuscript.

REFERENCES

1. RITZ, M.C., R.J. LAMB, S.R. GOLDBERG & M.J. KUHAR. 1987. Cocaine receptors on dopamine transporters are related to self-administration of cocaine. Science **237:** 1219–1223.
2. RITZ, M.C., E.J. CONE & M.J. KUHAR. 1990. Cocaine inhibition of ligand binding at dopamine, norepinephrine and serotonin transporters: a structure-activity study. Life Sci. **46:** 635–645.
3. JIMÉNEZ-RIVERA, C.A. & B.D. WATERHOUSE. 1991. Effects of systemically and locally applied cocaine on cerebrocortical neuron reponsiveness to afferent synaptic inputs and glutamate. Brain Res. **546:** 287–296.
4. WATERHOUSE, B.D., E.M. GOULD & I. BEKAVAC. 1996. Monoaminergic substrates underlying cocaine-induced enhancement of somatosensory-evoked discharges in rat barrel field cortical neurons. J. Pharmacol. Exp. Ther. **279:** 582–592.
5. WATERHOUSE, B.D., H.C. MOISES & D.J. WOODWARD. 1981. Alpha-receptor-mediated facilitation of somatosensory cortical neuronal responses to excitatory synaptic inputs and iontophoretically applied acetylcholine. Neuropharmacology **20:** 907–920.
6. MOURADIAN, R.D., F.M. SESSLER & B.D. WATERHOUSE. 1991. Noradrenergic potentiation of excitatory transmitter action in cerebrocortical slices: evidence for mediation by an alpha 1 receptor-linked second messenger pathway. Brain Res. **546:** 83–95.
7. DEVILBISS, D.M. & B.D. WATERHOUSE. 2000. Norepinephrine exhibits two distinct profiles of action on sensory cortical neuron responses of excitatory synaptic stimuli. Synapse **37**(4): 273–282.
8. WOODWARD, D.J. *et al.* 1991, Modulatory actions of norepinephrine on neural circuits. Adv. Exp. Med. Biol. **287:** 193–208.
9. ROBINSON, T.E. & K.C. BERRIDGE. 1993. The neural basis of drug craving: an incentive-sensitization theory of addiction [Rev.]. Brain Res. Brain Res. Rev. **18:** 247–291.
10. KOOB, G.F. & M. LE MOAL. 1997. Drug abuse: hedonic homeostatic dysregulation. Science **278:** 52–58.
11. ROBINSON, T.E. & K.C. BERRIDGE. 2000. The psychology and neurobiology of addiction: an incentive-sensitization view. Addiction **95**(Suppl. 2): S91–S117.
12. FUSTER, J.M. 2001. The prefrontal cortex—An update: time is of the essence. Neuron **30**(2): 319–333.
13. TZSCHENTKE, T.M. 2001. Pharmacology and behavioral pharmacology of the mesocortical dopamine system. Prog. Neurobiol. **63**(3): 241–320.

14. SESACK, S.R. & V.M. PICKEL. 1992. Prefrontal cortical efferents in the rat synapse on unlabeled neuronal targets of catecholamine terminals in the nucleus accumbens septi and on dopamine neurons in the ventral tegmental area. J. Comp. Neurol. **320:** 145–160.
15. DAHLSTROM, A. & K. FUXE. 1964. Evidence for the existence of monoamine-containing neurons in the central nervous system. I. Demostration of monoamines in the cell bodies of brain stem neurones. Acta Physiol. Scand. **62:** 1–55.
16. UNGERSTEDT, U. 1971. Stereotaxic mapping of the monoamine pathways in the rat brain. Acta Physiol. Scand. **367**(Suppl.): 1–48.
17. KOSOBUD, A.E., G.C. HARRIS & J.K. CHAPIN. 1994. Behavioral associations of neuronal activity in the ventral tegmental area of the rat. J. Neurosci. **14:** 7117–7129.
18. WHITE, F.J. 1996. Synaptic regulation of mesocorticolimbic dopamine neurons. Annu. Rev. Neurosci. **19:** 405–436.
19. GARIANO, R.F. & P.M. GROVES. 1988. Burst firing induced in midbrain dopamine neurons by stimulation of the medial prefrontal and anterior cingulate cortices. Brain Res. **462:** 194–198.
20. MURASE, S. *et al.* 1993. Prefrontal cortex regulates burst firing and transmitter release in rat mesolimbic dopamine neurons studied in vivo. Neurosci. Lett. **157:** 53–56.
21. TONG, Z.Y., P.G. OVERTON & D. CLARK. 1996. Stimulation of the prefrontal cortex in the rat induces patterns of activity in midbrain dopaminergic neurons which resemble natural burst events. Synapse **22:** 195–208.
22. SVENSSON, T.H. & C.S. TUNG. 1989. Local cooling of pre-frontal cortex induces pacemaker-like firing of dopamine neurons in rat ventral tegmental area in vivo. Acta Physiol. Scand. **136:** 135–136.
23. LI, Y. *et al.* 1997. Effects of the AMPA receptor antagonist NBQX on the development and expression of behavioral sensitization to cocaine and amphetamine. Psychopharmacology (Berl.) **134:** 266–276.
24. WOLF, M.E. *et al.* 1995. Effects of lesions of prefrontal cortex, amygdala, or fornix on behavioral sensitization to amphetamine: comparison with N-methyl- D-aspartate antagonists. Neuroscience **69:** 417–439.
25. PAXINOS, G. AND C. WATSON. 1986. The Brain in Stereotaxic Coordinates. Academic Press. San Diego.
26. GRACE, A.A. & B.S. BUNNEY. 1983. Intracellular and extracellular electrophysiology of nigral dopaminergic neurons—1. Identification and characterization. Neuroscience **10:** 301–315.
27. JIMÉNEZ-RIVERA, C.A., O. SEGARRA, Z. JIMENEZ & B.D. WATERHOUSE. 2000. Effects of intravenous cocaine administration on cerebellar Purkinje cell activity. Eur. J. Pharmacol. **407:** 91–100.
28. KALIVAS, P.W. 1995. Interactions between dopamine and excitatory amino acids in behavioral sensitization to psychostimulants [Rev.]. Drug Alcohol Depend. **37:** 95–100.
29. VANDERSCHUREN, L.J. & P.W. KALIVAS. 2000. Alterations in dopaminergic and glutamatergic transmission in the induction and expression of behavioral sensitization: a critical review of preclinical studies. Psychopharmacology (Berl.) **151:** 99–120.
30. KALIVAS, P.W. & J. STEWART. 1991. Dopamine transmission in the initiation and expression of drug- and stress-induced sensitization of motor activity [Rev.]. Brain Res. Brain Res. Rev. **16:** 223–244.
31. WOLF, M.E. 1998. The role of excitatory amino acids in behavioral sensitization to psychomotor stimulants. Prog. Neurobiol. **54:** 679–720.
32. LI, Y. & M.E. WOLF. 1997. Ibotenic acid lesions of prefrontal cortex do not prevent expression of behavioral sensitization to amphetamine. Behav. Brain Res. **84:** 285–289.
33. CADOR, M., Y. BJIJOU, S. CAIHOL & L. STINUS. 1997. D-Amphetamine-induced behavioral sensitization: implication of a glutamatergic medical prefrontal cortex-ventral tegmental area innervation. Neuroscience **94:** 705–721.
34. SHIM, S.S., B.S. BUNNEY & W.X. SHI. 1996. Effects of lesions in the medial prefrontal cortex on the activity of midbrain dopamine neurons. Neuropsychopharmacology **15:** 437–441.

35. KARLER, R., L.D. CALDER & S.A. TURKANIS. 1991. DNQX blockade of amphetamine behavioral sensitization. Brain Res. **552:** 295–300.
36. KARLER, R., L.D. CALDER & J.B. BEDINGFIELD. 1994. Cocaine behavioral sensitization and the excitatory amino acids. Psychopharmacology (Berl.) **115:** 305–310.
37. WOLF, M.E. & M.R. KHANSA. 1991. Repeated administration of MK-801 produces sensitization to its own locomotor stimulant effects but blocks sensitization to amphetamine. Brain Res. **562:** 164–168.
38. KALIVAS, P.W. & J.E. ALESDATTER. 1993. Involvement of N-methyl-D-aspartate receptor stimulation in the ventral tegmental area and amygdala in behavioral sensitization to cocaine. J. Pharmacol. Exp. Ther. **267:** 486–495.
39. STEWART, J. & J.P. DRUHAN. 1993. Development of both conditioning and sensitization of the behavioral activating effects of amphetamine is blocked by the non-competitive NMDA receptor antagonist, MK-801. Psychopharmacology **110:** 125–132.
40. WOLF, M.E. & M. JEZIORSKI. 1993. Coadministration of MK-801 with amphetamine, cocaine or morphine prevents rather than transiently masks the development of behavioral sensitization. Brain Res. **613:** 291–294.
41. HARACZ, J.L., S.A. BELANGER, J.S. MACDONALL & R. SIRCAR. 1995. Antagonist of N-methyl-D-aspartate receptors partially prevent the development of cocaine sensitization. Life Sci. **57:** 2347–2357.
42. IDA, I., T. ASAMI & H. KURIBARA. 1995. Inhibition of cocaine sensitization by MK-801, a noncompetitive N-methyl-D-aspartate (NMDA) receptor antagonist: evaluation by ambulatory activity in mice. Jpn. J. Pharmacol. **69:** 83–90.
43. SHOAIB, M., R. SPANAGEL, T. STOHR & T.S. SHIPPENBERG. 1995. Strain differences in the rewarding and dopamine-releasing effects of morphine in rats. Psychopharmacology (Berl.) **117:** 240–247.
44. KIM, H.S., W.K. PARK, C.G. JANG & S. OH. 1996. Inhibition by MK-801 of cocaine-induced sensitization, conditioned place preference, and dopamine-receptor supersensitivity in mice. Brain Res. Bull. **40:** 201–207.
45. WOLF, M.E., C.J. XUE, F.J. WHITE & S.L. DAHLIN. 1994. MK-801 does not prevent acute stimulatory effects of amphetamine or cocaine on locomotor activity or extracellular dopamine levels in rat nucleus accumbens. Brain Res. **666:** 223–231.
46. WHITE, F.J., X.T. HU, X.F. ZHANG & M.E. WOLF. 1995. Repeated administration of cocaine or amphetamine alters neuronal responses to glutamate in the mesoaccumbens dopamine system. J. Pharmacol. Exp. Ther. **273:** 445–454.
47. SCHENK, S. & B. PARTRIDGE. 1997. Effects of acute and repeated administration of N-methyl-D-aspartate (NMDA) into the ventral tegmental area: locomotor activating effects of NMDA and cocaine. Brain Res. **769:** 225–232.
48. ZHANG, X.F., X.T. HU, F.J. WHITE & M.E. WOLF. 1997. Increased responsiveness of ventral tegmental area dopamine neurons to glutamate after repeated administration of cocaine or amphetamine is transient and selectively involves AMPA receptors. J. Pharmacol. Exp. Ther. **281:** 699–706.
49. CARLEZON, W.A., JR., *et al.* 1997. Sensitization to morphine induced by viral-mediated gene transfer. Science **277:** 812–814.
50. WATERHOUSE, B.D. *et al.* 1988. New evidence for a gating action of norepinephrine in central circuits of mammalian brain. Brain Res. Bull. **21:** 425–432.
51. WOODWARD, D.J. *et al.* 1979. Modulatory actions of norepinephrine in the central nervous system. Fed. Proc. **38:** 2109–2116.
52. WARREN, R.A. & R.W. DYKES. 1996. Transient and long-lasting effects of iontophoretically administered norepinephrine on somatosensory cortical neurons in halothane-anesthetized cats. Can. J. Physiol. Pharmacol. **74:** 38–57.
53. SHI, W.X. *et al.* 2000. Dual effects of D-amphetamine on dopamine neurons mediated by dopamine and nondopamine receptors. J. Neurosci. **20:** 3504–3511.

Adaptation to Repeated Cocaine Administration in Rats

ZBIGNIEW K. BINIENDA,[a] FREDERICO PEREIRA,[a,c]
KENNETH ALPER,[b] WILLIAM SLIKKER, JR.,[a] AND
SYED F. ALI[a]

[a]Division of Neurotoxicology, NCTR/FDA, Jefferson,
Arkansas 72029, USA

[b]Brain Research Laboratories, New York University
Medical Center, New York, New York 10016, USA

[c]Instituto de Farmacologia e Terapeutica Experimental,
University of Coimbra Medical School, Coimbra, Portugal

ABSTRACT: Quantitative electroencephalogram (EEG) studies in cocaine-dependent human patients show deficits in slow-wave brain activity, reflected in diminished EEG power in the delta and theta frequency bands. In the present study, electrophysiological measures were monitored in 10 nonanesthetized, adult male Sprague-Dawley rats via bipolar, epidural electrodes implanted over the somatosensory cortex. Control electrocorticograms (ECoG) were recorded twice within a two-week interval to establish a baseline. Rats were subsequently injected daily with cocaine HCl at 15 mg/kg, i.p., for two weeks. The ECoG was recorded during a 1-h session one day after the last injection. Total concentrations of dopamine (DA) and its metabolites were assayed in caudate nucleus (CN) and frontal cortex (FC) using HPLC/EC. Compared with controls, marked increases in DA concentrations were observed in both regions. The DA turnover decreased significantly. The power spectra, obtained by use of a fast Fourier transformation, revealed a significant decrease in slow-wave delta frequency bands following repeated exposure to cocaine. These data are consistent with reported findings in humans that repeated exposures to cocaine result in a decrease in slow-wave brain activity. Further studies are necessary to establish whether regional alterations in blood flow and metabolic activity may underlie such observations.

KEYWORDS: rat; brain; cocaine; EEG; slow wave; delta frequency

INTRODUCTION

Repeated exposure to cocaine (COC) has been shown to sensitize animals to the locomotor-activating effects of this agent, leading to hyperactivity and stereotypy.[1,2] Behavioral sensitization to psychostimulants including COC is thought to involve

Address for correspondence: Dr. Zbigniew K. Binienda, Division of Neurotoxicology, HFT-132, FDA/NCTR, Jefferson, AR 72079-9502. Voice: 870-543-7920; fax: 870-543-7745.
zbinienda@nctr.fda.gov

Ann. N.Y. Acad. Sci. 965: 172–179 (2002). © 2002 New York Academy of Sciences.

increased dopamine (DA) neurotransmission in nigrostriatal and mesolimbic pathways.[3] Alterations of the gamma-aminobutyric acid (GABA) receptor system may contribute to those behavioral changes as well, since repeated injections of COC decrease GABA receptor in the striatum.[4] In addition, it was shown that the increased responsiveness of dopaminergic neurons to glutamate in the ventral tegmental area, after chronic exposure to COC, selectively involved ionotropic glutamate receptors AMPA.[5] Recently, an increase in glutamate receptor subunit levels (GluR2/3) was observed in rats that developed behavioral sensitization to repeated COC exposure.[6]

Quantitative electroencephalogram (EEG) studies in COC-dependent human patients show deficits in slow-wave brain activity, reflected by diminished EEG power in the delta and theta bands.[7,8] A decrease in low-frequency electrocorticograms (ECoG) after chronic or repeated COC exposure may be associated with reduced metabolic activity in the frontal cortex,[9] and could be related to alterations in cortical processing modulated by DA.[10] Experimental induction of addiction to COC in human subjects is impossible due to ethical constraints, necessitating a need for a relevant animal model. The aim of this study was to evaluate alterations in dopaminergic neurotransmission and ECoG following repeated COC administration in rats.

MATERIAL AND METHODS

Animals

Adult, male CD strain, Sprague-Dawley rats from the FDA/NCTR breeding colony were used for this study. Animals were kept under controlled environmental conditions (temperature 22°C, relative humidity 45–55%, 12-h light/dark cycle) and housed individually with food and water supplied ad libitum. Animal care and use procedures were in accordance with the American Association for Accreditation of Laboratory Animal Care (AAALAC) guidelines and approved by the Institutional Animal Care and Use Committee (IACUC).

Instrumentation

Rats in the COC group were instrumented under general isoflurane anesthesia. Upon placing the animal's head in the stereotaxic apparatus, the skin and muscle tissue on the upper cranium were incised and tissues reflected to expose the skull. Five stainless-steel screws (size No. 0-80 × 1/8-in. length) were installed as epidural electrodes in the undersized holes drilled in the scull above the somatosensory cortex (3 mm laterally from the sagittal fissure and 1 and 4 mm posterior to bregma). The screws were soldered to the connector via stainless-steel wires. The connector was attached to the skull using dental cement, and a ground wire was implanted under the skin in the dorsal neck, as previously described.[11]

ECoG Recording and Cocaine Administration

The baseline ECoG was recorded twice at a seven-day interval during a 1-h session (reference run) after a seven-day postsurgical recovery. The ECoG was recorded via a tether and swivel system. During recording, animals remained in a microdialysis bowl placed inside a Faraday cage. The signals were amplified using BioAmp 100 differential amplifiers and a CyberAmp 380 signal conditioner (Axon Instruments, Inc., Union City, CA) to pass frequencies of 1–40 Hz and processed with LabView software (National Instruments, Austin, TX). The power spectra obtained by use of fast Fourier transform (FFT) were divided into 1.25–4.50 Hz (delta), 4.75–6.75 Hz (theta), 7.00–9.50 Hz (alpha-1), 9.75–12.50 Hz (alpha-2), 12.75–18.50 Hz (beta-1), and 18.75–35.00 Hz (beta-2) frequency bands. Following the baseline ECoG recording, rats were injected (i.p.) daily with cocaine hydrochloride obtained from the Research Triangle Institute (Research Triangle Park, NC) at 15 mg/kg for two weeks. The ECoG signals were recorded again during a 1-h session approximately 24 h following the last COC injection.

Neurochemical Analysis

Neurochemical assessments were performed in the COC-treated rats and a separate group of rats ($n = 5$) used as control for this analysis. All rats were sacrificed by decapitation upon completion of the EEG recording. Their brains were removed, frozen on dry ice, and stored at $-80°C$ until dissection of the caudate nucleus (CN) and frontal cortex (FC) according to Glowinski and Iversen.[12] Concentrations of DA and its metabolites, 3,4-dihydroxyphenylacetic acid (DOPAC) and homovanillic acid (HVA), were assayed using a high-performance liquid chromatography method coupled with electrochemical detection (HPLC/EC) according to Ali et al.[13]

Statistical Analysis

After scanning for noise (time points where all signals were outside the first or 99th percentiles of the entire run), data for each animal at a given frequency band were adjusted to the reference run in that band. Each power measurement during treatment was divided by the median power in the reference run (baseline or reference level). In this way, all animals were placed on a similar scale despite factors that made the absolute power different between animals. Once all the animals were adjusted to similar scales, a log-transform was used to normalize the data. Power difference between a given interval (5 or 30 min) and the reference-level period was tested against zero using the Student's t-test at the significance level $p < 0.05$.

The two-sample Student's t-test was applied to compare monoamine levels between control and treated rats at $p < 0.05$.

RESULTS AND DISCUSSION

Repeated administration of COC produced enhancement of locomotor activity and stereotyped behavior (pronounced sniffing) observed by the first week of treatment within less than 20 min after the injection. The COC was administered to rats using a paradigm that produces sensitization, as reported in other studies.[1,6,14] No significant changes in power spectra were observed when comparing the baseline ECoG recordings during the two sessions recorded at a seven-day interval. However, compared with the baseline obtained from the reference-run recording, the power spectra analyzed in rats treated with COC for two weeks revealed a significant de-

TABLE 1. Concentrations of dopamine (DA) and its metabolites DOPAC and HVA (ng/100-mg wet weight of tissue) in the caudate nucleus and frontal cortex of rats injected i.p. with cocaine daily at 15 mg/kg, i.p., for a 14-day period

Region		DA	DOPAC	HVA	Turnover	Region
Caudate Nucleus	Control	1085.8 ± 27.7	137.3 ± 8.1	81.5 ± 7.1	0.20 ± 0.01	
	Cocaine	1696.8* ± 174.5	112.0 ± 26.7	71.0 ± 10.5	0.12* ± 0.02	
Frontal Cortex	Control	78.3 ± 8.3	60.3 ± 3.9	62.0 ± 4.6	1.57 ± 0.12	
	Cocaine	197.0* ± 9.5	37.7 ± 19.5	76.8 ± 23.6	0.57* ± 0.20	

NOTE: Turnover calculated as DOPAC + HVA/DA. Data are expressed as mean ± SEM; $n = 5$ rats; *$p < 0.05$ significantly different from control.

crease in slow-wave frequency bands, lasting until 30 min after the beginning of recording (FIG. 1). There was also a decrease of power observed in alpha-1, alpha-2, and beta-1 frequency bands, but much less pronounced and lasting only about 15 min (FIG. 2). The values recovered near baseline after approximately 30 min of recording (FIGS. 1 and 2). The recovery of the EEG signals observed during recording may be related to the resting-state animals assumed with time, compared to the initial alertness related to the initiation of the recording procedure.

Ferger and his collaborators reported that rats injected daily for 10 days with COC at 10 mg/kg, but not 20 mg/kg, led to a decrease in all spectral EEG frequency bands.[14] The effect lasted until 45 min after COC administration. In contrast, an increase in the alpha-1 power was observed following repeated COC injections at 20 mg/kg. In the present study, the reduction in slow-wave activity was observed 24 h after the last COC injection. A decrease in low-frequency brain activity has been associated with reduced metabolic activity in the frontal cortex, as shown by positron emission tomography and EEG correlation analyses.[9]

TABLE 1 shows the effect of repeated COC administration on the levels of DA and its metabolites in CN and FC. The concentration of DA increased significantly in both regions, suggesting that this COC treatment regimen increased the tyrosine hydroxylase (TH) activity. Compared with controls, the levels of DA metabolites decreased concomitantly with a significant decrease in DA turnover, calculated as DOPAC + HVA/DA ratio. Attenuation of DA levels in medial prefrontal cortex observed with increasing DA in the nucleus accumbens has been reported in rats treated with COC at 15 mg/kg for five days. Those observations were made using microdialysis techniques that determine extracellular DA concentrations.[16] An increase in the extracellular DA concentration in the axon terminals of striatum and nucleus accumbens has been reported in association with sensitization to amphetamine and cocaine,[17,18] and is consistent with sensitization to cocaine, inducing an increase in total content of striatal DA. The ECoG findings in the present study resemble the outcome of studies of COC-dependent human subjects. In human studies, a marked deficit in slow-wave brain activity, along with an enhancement of activity in beta power band, was frequently observed (see Ref. 10). The animal model presented here may prove to be useful in the study of human COC dependence.

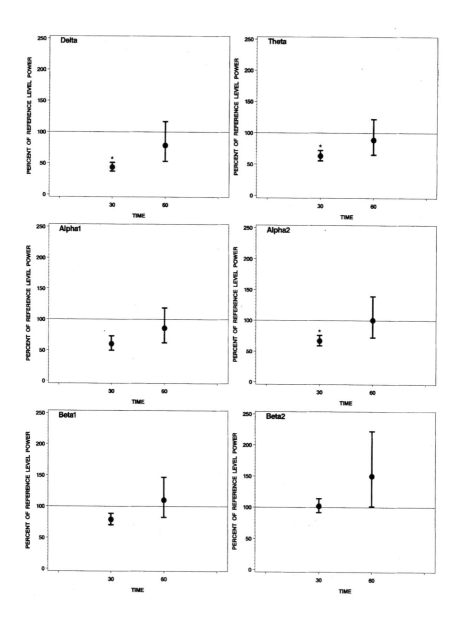

FIGURE 1. Brain activity in rats injected with cocaine daily at 15 kg/day, i.p., for a 14-day period. Power values calculated in 30-min time intervals as percent of the 1-h reference-level power assigned as a value of 100% in each band. Mean ± SEM; $n = 5$. *$p < 0.05$ significantly different from reference level (baseline). Frequency waves: delta (1.25–4.50 Hz); theta (4.75–6.75 Hz); alpha-1 (7.00–9.50 Hz); alpha-2 (9.75–12.50 Hz); beta-1 (12.75–18.50 Hz); beta-2 (18.75–35.00 Hz).

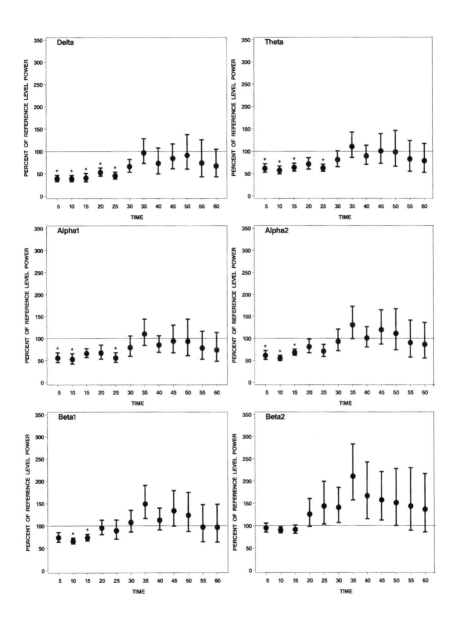

FIGURE 2. Brain activity in rats injected with cocaine daily at 15 kg/day, i.p., for a 14-day period. Power values calculated in 5-min time intervals as percent of the 1-h reference-level power assigned as a value of 100% in each band. Mean ± SEM; $n = 5$. *$p < 0.05$ significantly different from reference level (baseline). Frequency waves: delta (1.25–4.50 Hz); theta (4.75–6.75 Hz); alpha-1 (7.00–9.50 Hz); alpha-2 (9.75–12.50 Hz); beta-1 (12.75–18.50 Hz); beta-2 (18.75–35.00 Hz).

CONCLUSIONS

Data gathered in the present study are consistent with reported findings in humans that repeated exposures to COC result in a decrease in slow-wave brain activity. A decrease in DA metabolism and increase in total DA concentration in CN and FC was also observed. Further studies are necessary to establish whether regional alterations in blood flow and metabolic activity may underlie such observations.

ACKNOWLEDGMENTS

The authors thank Brett Thorn (R.O.W. Sciences) for the statistical analysis of the EEG data.

REFERENCES

1. POST, R.M. & H. ROSE. 1976. Increasing effects of repetitive cocaine administration in the rat. Nature **260:** 731–732.
2. KALIVAS, P.W. *et al.* 1988. Neurochemical and behavioral effects of acute and daily cocaine administration in rats. J. Pharmacol. Exp. Ther. **245:** 485–492.
3. GRACE, A.A. 1995. The tonic/phasic model of dopamine system regulation: its relevance for understanding how stimulant abuse alter basal ganglia function. Drug Alcohol Depend. **37:** 111–129.
4. GALE, K. *et al.* 1981. Effects of chronic cocaine administration on nigrostriatal function: neurochemical and behavioral changes in rats. Fed. Proc. **40:** 291.
5. ZHANG, X.-F., X.-T. HU & F.J. WHITE 1997. Increased responsiveness of dopamine neurons in ventral tegmental area to glutamate after repeated administration of cocaine or amphetamine is transient and selectively involves AMPA receptors. J. Pharm. Exp. Ther. **281:** 699–706.
6. CHURCHILL, L. *et al.* 1999. Repeated cocaine alters glutamate receptor subunit levels in the nucleus accumbens and ventral tegmental area of rats that develop behavioral sensitization. J. Neurochem. **72:** 2397–2403.
7. HERNING, R.I. *et al.* 1997. Neurophysiological signs of cocaine dependence: increased electroencephalogram beta during withdrawal. Biol. Psychiatry **41:** 1087–1094.
8. ALPER, K.R. *et al.* 1990. Quantitative EEG correlates of crack cocaine dependence. Psychiatry Res. **35:** 95–105.
9. ALPER, K.R. 1999. The EEG and cocaine sensitization: a hypothesis. J. Neuropsychiatry Clin. Neurosci. **11:** 209–221.
10. ALPER, K. *et al.* 1998. Correlation of qEEG with PET in schizophrenia. Neuropsychobiology **38:** 50–56.
11. BINIENDA, Z. *et al.* 2000. Application of electrophysiological method to study interactions between ibogaine and cocaine. Ann. NY Acad. Sci. **914:** 387–393.
12. GLOWINSKI, J. & L.L. IVERSEN. 1966. Regional studies of catecholamines in the rat brain. I. The disposition of ^{3}H-dopamine, ^{3}H-dopa in various regions of the brain. J. Neurochem. **13:** 655–669.
13. ALI, S.F. *et al.* 1994. Low environmental temperatures or pharmacologic agents that produce hypothermia decrease methamphetamine toxicity in mice. Brain Res. **658:** 33–38.
14. FERGER B., D. STAHL & K. KUSCHINSKY. 1996. Effects of cocaine on the EEG power spectrum of rats are significantly altered after its repeated administration: Do they reflect sensitization phenomena? Naunyn-Schmiedeberg's Arch. Pharmacol. **353:** 545–551.
15. PRASAD, B.M., T. HOCHSTATTER & B.A. SORG. 1999. Expression of cocaine sensitization: regulation by the medial prefrontal cortex. Neurosci. **88:** 765–774.

16. ROBINSON, T.E. *et al.* 1988. Persistent sensitization of dopamine neurotransmission in ventral striatum (nucleus accumbens) produced by prior experience with (+)-amphetamine: a microdialysis study in freely moving rats. Brain Res. **462:** 211–222.

17. KALIVAS, P.W. & P. DUFFY. 1990. The effect of acute and daily cocaine treatment on extracellular dopamine in the nucleus accumbens. Synapse **5:** 48–58.

18. LIVEZEY, G.T. & S.B. SPARBER. 1990. Hyperthermia sensitizes rats to cocaine's proconvulsive effects and unmasks EEG evidence of kindling after chronic cocaine. Pharm. Biochem. Behav. **37:** 761–767.

Neurochemical Changes and Neurotoxic Effects of an Acute Treatment with Sydnocarb, A Novel Psychostimulant

Comparison with D-Amphetamine

V. BASHKATOVA,[a] A.-M. MATHIEU-KIA,[b] C. DURAND,[b]
AND J. PENIT-SORIA[b]

[a]Institute of Pharmacology RAMS, Moscow, Russia

[b]FRE–CNRS 2371, Neurobiologie des Processus Adaptatifs, Université P et M Curie,
9, Quai Saint-Bernard, 75005, Paris, France

ABSTRACT: Sydnocarb [(phenylisopropyl)N-phenylcarbamoylsydnonimine; SYD] was introduced to clinical practice in Russia as a psychostimulant drug used for the treatment of asthenia and apathy, which accompany schizophrenia and manic depression. It has been described as a psychostimulant with addiction liability and toxicity less than amphetamine (AMPH). The precise cellular mechanisms by which sydnocarb elicits its psychostimulant effect are still unclear. At present its neurochemical and neurotoxic effects are compared to those of AMPH in the striatum, the main input structure of the basal ganglia. The expression of c-fos protein in striatal neurons was much more increased after a single injection of D-AMPH (5 mg/kg) than after an equimolar concentration of SYD (23.8 mg/kg) in both the anterior and the posterior part of the striatum. Using *in situ* hybridization on striatal slices, we observed that AMPH increased the striatal levels of preprodynorphin (PPDYN) mRNAs in both parts of the striatum, while SYD did not affect basal levels of PPDYN mRNAs. Furthermore, AMPH and SYD increased striatal preprotachykinin (PPT-A) and preproenkephalin (PPE) mRNA levels. The effects of AMPH and SYD on PPT-A–mRNA levels were similar. A differential effect of AMPH and SYD was observed only on the PPE–mRNA levels measured in the anterior striatum where SYD increased these levels more than AMPH. The acute neurotoxicity of these two psychostimulants was analyzed by measuring their effects on the parameters of oxidative stress, such as nitric oxide (NO) generation, as well as specific indices of lipid peroxidation (i.e., thiobarbituric acid reactive substances; TBARS), while, on the other hand, the alpha-tocopherol level was taken as an index of antioxidant defense processes. Measuring generation of NO directly by electron paramagnetic resonance, it was observed that AMPH shows a more pronouced increase in comparison to SYD, in the striatum and in cortex. TBARS levels in the striatum and cortex were significantly less enhanced than AMPH after a single injection of SYD. Similarly, the alpha-tocopherol level was decreased only by AMPH in the striatum, and neither AMPH nor SYD had

Address for correspondence: Dr. V. Bashkatova, Institute of Pharmacology RAMS, Baltiyskaya, 8, 125315, Moscow, Russia. Fax: 007095 151-1261.
vata@rinet.ru

Ann. N.Y. Acad. Sci. 965: 180–192 (2002). © 2002 New York Academy of Sciences.

any effect in the cortex. Results show that a single injection of a high dose of AMPH is able to induce several neurotoxic effects. The study also demonstrates that SYD has mild neurochemical effects as well as fewer neurotoxic properties than AMPH.

KEYWORDS: sydnocarb; amphetamine; D-amphetamine; neurotoxicity; schizophrenia; psychostimulant drugs

INTRODUCTION

Sydnocarb [(phenylisopropyl)*N*-phenylcarbamoylsydnonimine; SYD] (Chemical-Pharmaceutical Institute, Moscow) was introduced in clinical practice in Russia as a psychostimulant drug, and has been used as an adjunct therapy of several clinical aspects of schizophrenia and manic depression, such as asthenia, apathy, and adynamia. Compared with the stimulating effect of amphetamine in clinical trials, sydnocarb has activating effects that develop more gradually and lead to a final stimulatory effect that is smaller, lasts longer (6–8 h),[1] and does not induce the peripheral sympatomimetic effects induced by amphetamine (AMPH).

The precise mechanisms by which SYD induces its psychostimulant effects are not well understood. Animal studies indicate that the main behavioral effects of SYD are the consequence of the activation of the dopaminergic (DA) systems. Nevertheless, the locomotor hyperactivity and the stereotypies elicited by SYD are less important than those observed with AMPH or metamphetamine (METH).[2,3] Using microdialysis in the dorsal striatum and the nucleus accumbens of freely moving rats, SYD induced a relatively modest but long-lasting increase in extracellular DA in the dorsal striatum.[3] In contrast with AMPH, no decrease in extracellular DOPAC was observed with SYD. Altogether these results have suggested that the neurochemical profile of SYD might be that of a DA uptake inhibitor rather than that of a DA.[2] Anyhow, as far as we know, the precise neurochemical effects induced by this novel psychostimulant have not been studied. Striatal neurons are known to be under the modulation of DA. They include two major types of neurons identified on the basis of their axonal projections and their neuropeptide contents. The striatonigral neurons express substance P, while the striatopallidal neurons express enkephalin. In addition, part of both populations synthesize dynorphin (see Ref. 4 for review). The synthesis of these neuropeptides is under dopaminergic control. Numerous studies have shown that DA agonists and antagonists, disruption of DA transmission, but also psychostimulants, can modulate striatal peptide at the level of their mRNA synthesis.[5–7] Indeed, the acute administration of AMPH is able to induce the acute reinforcing actions of the psychostimulant and is accompanied by an increase of the mRNA levels of the three striatal neuropeptides [preproenkephalin (PPE), preprotachykinin-A (PPT-A), and preprodynorphin (PPDYN)].

In the striatum, the basal level of c-fos expression is very low, but increases dramatically after acute treatment with AMPH.[8,9] Fos is an immediately early gene (IEG) product that, after dimerization with Jun, forms a transcriptional activating factor that binds to an AP1 site at consensus DNA sequences. So, it regulates initial events leading to long-lasting alterations in various gene expressions following acute extracellular signals. Some striatal neuropeptide genes, such as those encoding for dynorphin and perhaps enkephalin, have AP1 sites and are regulated by these IEGs.

The clinical use of psychomotor stimulants is restricted by their side effects. Neurotoxicity is one of the most important among them. While the neurotoxic effects of substituted amphetamines are well documented, the possible toxicity of AMPH itself is poorly documented. Nevertheless, several studies have shown that AMPH also is able, after repeated injections, to induce several toxic effects, such as behavioral evidence of DA dysfunction and enhanced generation of reactive oxygen species (ROS) following depletion of endogenous DA.[10–12] In addition, a few years ago it was shown that a single high dose of AMPH also induces the production of ROS such as hydroxyl radicals (•OH) and also that of nitric oxide (NO).[13,14] Moreover, it was shown recently that acute administration of SYD increases the parameters of DA dysfunction, such as behavioral stereotypies, but only after a very high dose (30 mg/kg), suggesting that SYD has a mild neurotoxicity.[3] It was also found that SYD increased (•OH) generation to a lesser degree than D-AMPH.[15] Although ROS may induce neuronal damage by their own action, they may also induce neurotoxicity by their interaction with NO. Indeed, peroxynitrite, a highly reactive toxic compound, is formed during this reaction. Thus, in the brain, neurotoxicity induced by amphetamines may involve NO and ROS generation.

In the present study, in order to better understand the neurochemical effects of SYD, we compared its acute effects on c-fos expression and striatal neuropeptide mRNA levels to those of an equimolar concentration of AMPH. The acute neurotoxic effects of these psychostimulants were studied by analyzing their effect on NO generation, lipid peroxidation production in the rat striatum and the cerebral cortex, while alpha-tocopherol levels were used as good antioxidant defense indices.

MATERIALS AND METHODS

Acute Psychostimulant Treatment

Male Sprague-Dawley rats (180–210 g) were used in these experiments. All animal experiments were carried out in accordance with French decree No. 87848/19 October 1987 and associated guidelines and European Community Council directive 86/609/ EEC/ November 1986. Rats were housed for at least five days under standard conditions before use. Rats were kept on a 12-h light/dark cycle, maintained at 20–22°C with water and food *ad libitum*. The day of the experiment, the animals were injected in a quiet (low-stress) homeroom. The rats received a single injection of D-AMPH (Sigma Chemical Co.), 5 mg/kg, i.p., dissolved in isotonic 0.9% sodium or a single injection of SYD at equimolar dose 23.8 mg/kg, i.p., dissolved in Tween 80 and then diluted in isotonic 0.9% NaCl, as required. Similarly, control animals were injected with either the saline alone or the same saline containing Tween 80. Rats were returned to their cages for a 2-h period. Then they were sacrificed.

Neuropeptide mRNA In Situ Hybridization and c-fos Immunocytochemistry Procedures

In these types of experiments, rats were deeply anesthetized with pentobarbital (200 mg/kg) and intracardially perfused with 0.9% saline (100 mL) followed by a 0.1-M phosphate buffer solution (pH = 7.4; 500 mL) containing 4% paraformaldehyde (PFA). Brains were removed and following a 2-h postfixation in a 4% PFA phosphate-buffered solution, they were stored for 48 h in a 20% phosphate-buffered sucrose. Frontal sections (20 μm) were cut using a freezing microtome at various rostrocaudal levels of the striatum: according to the rat brain atlas of Paxinos and Watson,[16] $A = +2.2, +1.7$, and $+1.2$ mm from bregma for the anterior part and $A = -0.2$, -0.9, and -1.6 mm for the posterior part of the striatum. They were kept at $-20°C$ in a cryoprotecting medium (30% ethylene glycol, 30% glycerol, and 0.1% diethylpyrocarbonate (Sigma) in 0.1-M phosphate buffer) until use. The day of the experiment, the slices were rinsed in a 0.1-M phosphate buffer, thaw mounted, and dried. Sections were then used for *in situ* hybridization (ISH) of striatal neuropeptide mRNAs and c-fos immunocytochemistry using techniques identical to those already described in previous studies.[17,18]

Briefly, synthetic DNA oligonucleotide probes were used. Oligonucleotide probes were labeled with [^{35}S] dATP (1.000 Ci/mmol; Amersham) by terminal deoxynucleotide terminal transferase. The specific activity of the probes was $5–8 \cdot 10^8$ dpm/mg. The radiolabeled DNA probes were precipitated in 75% ethanol and 0.4 M NaCl at $-30°C$. After centrifugation, the pellet was dissolved in 50% deionized formamide and in 50% stock hybridization buffer.[17] The mixture (30 mL/section) was set over sections and the slides were incubated for 17–18 h at 48°C in humid chambers. Slides were apposed to β max Hyperfilm (Amersham) for 7 to 15 days. For each peptide mRNA, quantitative analysis of hybridization signals was performed using a computerized image analyzer. Assessment of neuropeptide mRNA levels were performed on autoradiographic films at the six rostrocaudal levels selected in both parts of the striatum, as described earlier. All optical density measurements were done on both sides of each section. With regard to both parts of the striatum, data were averaged for each rat and the mean ± SEM of these values was calculated (six rats per group). Results were expressed in each region in percent of the optical density measured in the corresponding striatum of control rats treated with the corresponding vehicle (saline for AMPH and saline + Tween for SYD.

c-Fos immunocytochemistry was achieved on striatal sections obtained as described earlier, by using a basic procedure already described in Ref. 18 and modified as follows: the sections were incubated during 2 h with each antibody, the first being diluted 1:500.

Determination of NO

For NO determination diethyldithiocarbamate (DETC; Sigma) 500 mg/kg, i.p., and a mixture of $FeSO_4$ (37.5 mg/kg, s.c.) and sodium citrate (165 mg/kg, s.c.) were simultaneously injected 1.5 h after a single injection of isotonic saline or drugs (AMPH, 5 mg/kg or SYD, 23.8 mg/kg). DETC penetrates the blood-brain barrier and forms a complex with intracellular nonheme iron. The scavenger traps NO in the tissue, thereby generating a paramagnetic mononitrosyl–iron DETC complex.[10] Animals were decapitated 30 min after DETC injection. The brains were rapidly removed, and cerebral cortices as well as striatal were immediately dissected and frozen in liquid nitrogen. The electron paramagnetic resonance (EPR) spectra were recorded at 77 K using a Brucker ESR 300E spectrometer at a frequency of 9.33 kHz, H.F.-modulation frequency 0.5 mT, microwave power 20 mW, and time constant 0.05 s.[19] The concentration of trapped NO was calculated from the intensity of the third ultrafine splitting line of the resonance at 2.035 g of the NO–Fe $(DETC)_2$ complex. For all the experiments concerning the neurotoxic effects, it was previously verified that the vehicle used had no effect, and control rats were treated with normal saline.

Determination of LPO Processes

Determination of LPO processes in brain tissue was performed by measuring thiobarbituric acid reactive substances (TBARS).[20] Briefly, 10% (w/w) tissue homogenate was mixed with sodium dodecyl sulfate, acetate buffer (pH 3.5), and aqueous solution of thiobarbituric acid. After heating at 95°C for 60 min, the red pigment was extracted with *n*-butanolpyridine mixture and absorbance was determined at 532 nm.

Determination of Alpha-Tocopherol Levels

Determination of alpha-tocopherol in brain tissue was performed, following Ref. 21. Briefly, α-tocopherol was extracted from tissue homogenate with a mixture of ethanol and hexane, and determined in hexane extract at 290-nm excitation and 330-nm emission range. Concentration of α-tocopherol was calculated according to the reference curve using standard α-tocopherol ("Calbiohem," USA).

Statistical Analysis

Data are expressed as mean ± SEM. All data were analyzed for statistical significance using unpaired Student's *t*-test. The significance at the $p < 0.05$ level and below is reported.

RESULTS

Effects of AMPH and SYD on c-fos Immunoreactivity of Striatal Neurons

AMPH and SYD acute treatments induced the appearance of fos-immunoreactive (fos-IR) neurons in both parts of the striatum. Very few fos-IR neurons were observed in control rats. Following acute injection of AMPH, the density of fos-IR neurons was 6-fold higher than that observed after an equimolar dose of SYD (TABLE 1). Furthermore, a patchy pattern was observed in the anterior striatum after AMPH treatment, an effect that was not observed after SYD treatment.

Effects of AMPH and SYD on mRNA Levels of Striatal Neuropeptides

In both parts of the striatum, a single injection of AMPH increased significantly the levels of PPDYN mRNA, while the injection of SYD had no effect (FIG.1). Indeed, the acute treatment with AMPH increased by +12% ± 5% and by +13% ± 5%, in the anterior and the posterior part of the striatum, respectively, when compared to the basal levels measured in the corresponding control group of rats treated with saline only. In contrast, an equimolar dose of SYD had no significant effect in the anterior or in any part of the striatum. In contrast, both psychostimulants increased the levels of striatal PPT-A and PPE mRNAs. The effects of AMPH and SYD on PPT-A–mRNA levels were identical. Indeed, AMPH increased PPT–mRNA levels by

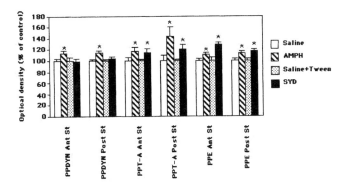

FIGURE 1. Compared effects of acute administration of AMPH (5 mg/kg) and SYD (23.8 mg/kg) on the levels of neuropeptide: PPDYN, PPT-A, and PPE mRNAs in the anterior (Ant St) and the posterior part (Post St) of the dorsal striatum. Each experimental group contained 6 animals. Statistical comparisons showed that AMPH and SYD had significant stimulatory effects on neuropeptide mRNAs levels, except SYD for PPDYN mRNA in both parts of the striatum (*$p < 0.05$, unpaired Student's *t*-test).

TABLE 1. Comparison of the density of fos immunoreactive neurons in the anterior and the posterior parts of the dorsal striatum, after acute treatment with amphetamine (5 mg/kg) and sydnocarb (23.8 mg/kg)

	AMPH (cells/mm^2)	SYD (cells/mm^2)
Anterior striatum	605 ± 50	100 ± 9
	$p < 0.001$	
Posterior striatum	800 ± 75	120 ± 11
	$p < 0.001$	

NOTE: Results are expressed as numbers of labeled fos-IR neurons/mm^2, and were obtained by counting positive neurons on both sides of striatal slices corresponding to several anteroposterior levels in both parts of the striatum, as described in the Materials and Methods section. In every control rat, the total number of c-fos positive neurons, counted in six striatal sections, was less than 50. So, the basal density was considered as negligible and was not quantified.

+16% ± 7% and by +43% ± 17%, in the anterior and posterior striatum, respectively, while SYD increased these levels by +15% ± 6% and by +20% ± 8%, respectively. Significant differences in the effects of AMPH and SYD were observed only when the PPE–mRNA levels were measured in the anterior striatum. In this region, AMPH induced a +11% ± 4% increase, while SYD increased these levels by +28% ± 4%. Finally, in the posterior striatum, AMPH and SYD increased PPE–mRNA levels identically (+12% ± 4% and by 15% ± 4%, respectively).

Effects of AMPH and SYD on the Generation of NO

The basal levels of NO measured in control rats were 1.90 ± 0.04 nmol/mg and 1.79 ± 0.03 nmol/mg in the striatum and the cortex, respectively (FIG. 2). Two hours

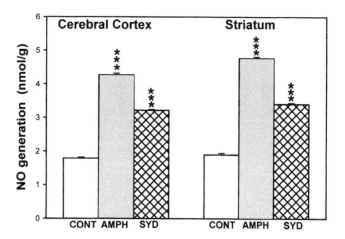

FIGURE 2. Compared effects of an acute treatment with AMPH and SYD on the generation of NO in the striatum and in the cortex. Each experimental group contained 10 animals. Statistical comparisons with control levels measured in vehicle-treated animals were done using unpaired Student's t-test (***$p < 0.001$).

after the AMPH injection, NO levels were increased by ±150% ± 3% in the striatum and by ± 138% ± 3% in the cortex (FIG. 2). An equimolar dose of SYD also enhanced NO generation, but to a lesser extent, since NO levels were increased by ±79% ± 2% in the striatum as well as in the cortex.

Effects of AMPH and SYD on Lipid Peroxidation: TBARS Levels

The basal level of TBARS in the striatum (74 ± 3 nmol/g) was similar to that measured in the cortex (69 ± 2.0 nmol/g). In the striatum, the formation of TBARS measured 2 h after AMPH administration were increased by +279% ± 13% when compared to the corresponding basal level (FIG. 3). When an equimolar dose of SYD was acutely administrated, the level of TBARS was enhanced by +111% ± 13%. The cortical levels of TBARS were also affected by the two psychostimulants. Indeed, the concentration of TBARS measured after AMPH injection dramatically increased (+253% ± 10%) in comparison to the control level (FIG. 3). Here again, SYD induced a smaller effect on TBARS (+120% ± 11%).

Effects of AMPH and SYD on the Levels of Alpha-Tocopherol

The basal levels of α-tocopherol measured in control rats were 2.55 ± 0.12 and 2.25 ± 0.13 mg/kg, in the striatum and the cortex, respectively (FIG. 4). Two hours after the AMPH injection, the striatal tocopherol levels were slightly decreased (−18% ± 6%), while SYD had no effect. In the cortex, no effect at all was observed with any of these two psychostimulants.

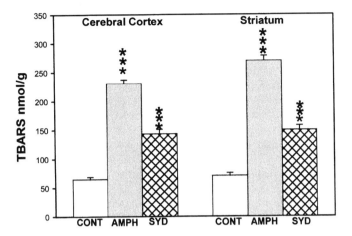

FIGURE 3. Compared effects of an acute treatment with AMPH and SYD on the level of TBARS: specific indices of lipid peroxidation in the striatum and the cortex. Each experimental group contained 10 animals. Statistical comparisons with control levels measured in vehicle-treated animals were done using unpaired Student's t-test (***$p < 0.001$).

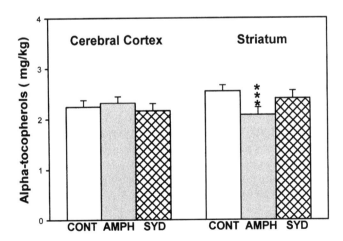

FIGURE 4. Compared effects of an acute treatment with AMPH and SYD on the level of α-tocopherols: indices of antioxidant defense. Each experimental group contained 10 animals. Statistical comparisons with control levels measured in vehicle-treated animals were done using unpaired Student's t-test (***$p < 0.001$).

DISCUSSION

The results of our study show that SYD increased the density of c-fos immunoreactive neurons in the rat striatum weakly, when compared with the very large increase observed after AMPH administration. SYD remains without any effect on the levels of striatal PPDYN mRNAs, while AMPH increased these levels in the striatum. Both psychostimulants increased PPT-A–mRNA levels as well as PPE–mRNA levels, and no differences could be measured between the effects of the two drugs. The neurotoxic effects of SYD measured in the striatum and the cerebral cortex by the generation of NO and TBARS levels, were less developed under SYD administration than that of AMPH. Finally, the level of antioxidant defense measured by α-tocopherol tissue content was not affected by either of the two drugs, except by AMPH in the striatum.

The effect on c-fos striatal expression we measured after an acute administration of AMPH is in good agreement with that previously described by others.[8] SYD had less of an effect on the striatal expression of c-fos; this is most probably due to the smaller increase in DA release induced by this drug, as previously measured by others.[2] Furthermore, SYD did not induce a clear patchy pattern of c-fos expression in the striatum, as we could observe in that of AMPH-treated rats. It was previously shown that AMPH and cocaine induced strikingly different patterns of c-fos expression in the striosome-matrix compartments of the striatum. Indeed, while AMPH-treated animals showed a patchy pattern of fos expression, the cocaine-treated animals showed a more homogenous fos pattern of expression.[22]

The small but significant increases in the striatal neuropeptide mRNA levels induced by the acute administration of AMPH are in total agreement with previous results obtained by others.[8] The effects induced by SYD were not completely identical to those induced by AMPH. Indeed, SYD was not able to induce any effect on PP-DYN–mRNA levels. It is possible that a small effect of SYD might not have been seen. Indeed, our measurements were only done 2 h after drug administration. This time was chosen in order to ensure the best measurement of c-fos protein expression. However, this does not mean that this time is not sufficient to reach the maximal increase in PPDYN–mRNA levels, which have often been observed 3–4 h after the psychostimulant injection. It also might be possible that the increase in DA release evoked by SYD is not sufficient to induce an effect on PPDYN–mRNA levels, while it is sufficient to induce effects on PPT-A– and PPE–mRNA levels. Finally, an increase in the PPE–mRNA level was induced by AMPH, a rather surprising result, since striatopallidal neurons, which synthesize this neuropeptide, are thought to be under the inhibitory control by DA. Results similar to ours showing the opposite effect have been previously obtained by others,[8] and suggest that, in fact, D1 and D2 –DA receptors act synergistically to regulate gene expression in the striatum

Effects of AMPH and SYD in Parameters of Oxidative Stress

The exact mechanisms by which AMPH and several AMPHs, such as METH, elicit neurotoxic effects are still not well understood. The mechanism of dopaminergic toxicity has been mainly studied using a model where repeated injections of a high dose of METH or AMPH were done, the former inducing larger neurotoxicity. In this model it has been shown that the excessive increase in acute DA release produced by the AMPH seems to be the first step of the cascade of reactions underlying this neurotoxicity.[23] Indeed, DA by itself can produce neurotoxicity[24] and generate hydroxyl radicals.[25,26] The enzymatic degradation or the auto-oxidation of DA result in the formation of •OH and superoxide radicals. Finally, •OH is susceptible to iron-catalyzed formation of hydroxyl free radicals via the Fenton reaction.[27]

During the last few years, it has been shown that glutamate (GLU) also plays a role in this neurotoxicity. Indeed, GLU antagonists block the METH-induced decrease in striatal DA content.[23,28] Furthermore, METH increases GLU extracellular concentrations. DA antagonists block this increase in GLU, as well as the decrease in DA content produced by METH.[29] Recently it has been proposed that AMPHs increase brain energy utilization, leading to a state of metabolic stress. Moreover, a direct inhibition of Na-K ATPase by DA might lead to the disruption of the ionic gradients necessary for the inward transport of GLU, leading, in fact, to a net efflux of GLU. Nevertheless, a direct increase in striatal GLU release most probably also occurs, since activation of the thalamocortical and corticostriatal pathways underlie the behavioral activation due to AMPHs.

The production of ROS induced by the increased GLU transmission is now well documented. Indeed, ROS can be released through the production of NO. This effect is in fact initiated by the opening of the NMDA receptor channels, which allows the influx of calcium in the cytoplasmic compartment, which in turn induces the activation of the brain nitric oxide synthase (NOS) by a Ca-calmoduline. NO-mediated neurotoxicity may arise from the formation of free radicals (peroxynitrite and breakdown products)[30–32] and activation of the nuclear enzyme poly *n* (ADP-ribose) synthase that leads to energy depletion and cell death.[33] Several studies have clearly shown that inhibitors of NOS, such as selective neuronal NOS inhibitor 7-nitroindazole, protected against METH neurotoxicity and that NOS knockout mice were resistant to METH neurotoxicity.[34,35] Recently it was found that even a single injection of METH produced a significant increase in the formation of 3-nitrotyrosine, a biomarker of peroxynitrite production in the striatum.[31] Moreover, METH induced alterations in the expression of p53 and bcl-2 protein in the striatum of wild-type and nNOS knockout mice.[32] The authors suggest that METH might cause its neurotoxic effects via the production of free radicals and secondary perturbations in the expression of genes known to be involved in apoptosis and cell death machinery.[32]

In summary, after repeated injections of AMPHs, an increased production of free radicals such as (•OH) and peroxynitrite is elicited consecutively by the large and repeated increases in DA release.[36] It was recently shown that intrastriatal injection of AMPH elevates (•OH) formation.[12] It was also demonstrated that repeated injections of a high dose of AMPH and SYD (identical to that we used in the present study for the acute treatment), were able to induce a significant increase in (•OH) generation after the second injection.[15] An increased formation of free radicals induces a lipid peroxidation measured by the TBARS level, which is thus considered to be an index of neurotoxicity. Interestingly, we have recently shown that repeated injections of AMPH increase TBARS in the cerebral cortex. We also observed that cortical generation of NO was increased. The last effect might induce an additional neurotoxicity since NO can interact with (•OH), leading to the formation of peroxinitrite, a highly reactive toxic product.[37]

Until now, few data concerning the neurotoxic effects of an acute AMPH treatment were available. However, it has been shown that a single injection of AMPH in disimipramine-treated rats induced (•OH) formation, enhanced NO formation (measured as content of nitrate/nitrite), and induced a concomitant DA loss in the striatum.[13,14] Interestingly, the last study shows that these effects were all blocked by nonselective NOS inhibitor (L-NAME) or by an antagonist of NMDA glutamate receptor (MK-801).

Our results show that a single injection of a high dose of AMPH, without any blockade of amphetamine metabolism, such as that used in Refs. 13 and 14, is even sufficient to affect the parameters of oxidative stress, which are currently considered as markers of cellular neurotoxicity such as the intensity of lipid peroxydation and NO generation. Here again, SYD had a smaller effect than AMPH. These data are consistent with recent studies using the same doses of AMPH and SYD and demonstrating a less significant increase in (•OH) generation after repeated administration of SYD when compared to AMPH.[15] Interestingly, no effect of these two drugs on α-tocopherol levels could be detected, except for AMPH in the striatum where its effect is rather small. It might be suggested that perhaps this pathway is switched on only after repeated injections of psychostimulants. Such biochemical adaptations, which counteract the primary effects of psychostimulants, have already been observed. For example, a gradual increase in PPDYN–mRNA synthesis was observed, and this effect slows down the enhancement of DA release.

Finally, our results suggest that in the cerebral cortex, AMPH and to a lesser degree SYD also seem to have a neurotoxic effect. Such an effect has been described already using repeated injections of METH.[38] In this study, it was shown that this cortical neurotoxicity is mainly due to the AMPH activation of the thalamocortical pathway, which induces the hyperactivity of cortical neurons, leading to an increase in extracellular GLU.

In conclusion, our results indicate that a single injection of AMPH drastically enhanced the expression of c-fos protein in both the anterior and the posterior parts of the striatum, while SYD produced only a small increase in this parameter. PPDYN–mRNA striatal levels were weakly increased by AMPH, but were not affected by SYD. The gene-encoding expressions for PPE and PPT-A were increased in a similar manner by both psychostimulants, except PPE gene expression in the posterior striatum, on which SYD exerted a greater effect. Our results demonstrate that NO generation and TBARS levels are significantly increased in the striatum and in the cortex of rats after acute treatment with these psychostimulants. Nevertheless, in this acute model, the antioxidant defense measured by α-tocopherol did not seem to be switched on. Moreover, our results provide the first direct evidence that the Russian-made psychostimulant SYD increases the NO tissue level. Our data strongly suggest that ROS and NO are involved in AMPH- and SYD-induced neurotoxicity.

ACKNOWLEDGMENTS

This work was supported by CNRS Convention d'Echanges Franco-Russe No. 6527 and RFBR grant. The authors are grateful to Dr. Varsak Mikoyan for his assistance with EPR determination of NO.

REFERENCES

1. RUDENKO, G.M. & R.A. ALTSHULER. 1979. Peculiarities of clinical activity and phar-macokinetics of sydnocarb (sydnocarbum) and original pshychodtimulant. Agressologie **20:** 265–270.
2. GAINETDINOV, R.R., T.D. SOTNIKOVA, T.V. GREHKOVA & K.S. RAYEVSKY. 1997. Effects of a psychostimulant drug sydnocarb on rat brain dopaminergic transmission in vivo. Eur. J. Pharmacol. **340:** 53–58.
3. WITKIN, J.M. *et al.* 1999. Behavioral, toxic, and neurochemical effects of sydnocarb, a novel psychomotor stimulant: comparisons with methamphetamine. J Pharmacol. Exp. Ther. Mar. **288:** 1298–1310.
4. REINER, A. & K.D. ANDERSON. 1990. The patterns of neurotransmitter and neuropeptide co-occurrence among striatal projection neurons: conclusions based on recent findings. Brain Res. Rev. **15:** 251–265.
5. YOUNG, S.W., III, T. BONNER & M.R. BRANN. 1986. Mesencephalic dopamine neurons regulate the expression of neuropeptide mRNA in the rat forebrain. Proc. Natl. Acad. Sci. USA **88:** 1291–1295.
6. LINDERFORS, N. 1992. Amphetamine and haloperidol modulate preprotacchykinin A mRNA expression in rat nucleus accumbens and caudate-putamen. Mol. Brain Res. **13:** 151–154.
7. JABER, M., F. TISON, M.C. FOURNIER & B. BLOCH. 1994. Differential influence of halo-peridol and sulpiride on dopamine receptors and peptide mRNAs levels in the rat striatum and pituotary. Mol. Brain Res. **23:** 14–20.
8. JABER, M. *et al.* 1995. Acute and chronic treatments differentially regulate neuropep-tide messenger RNA levels and Fos immunoreacitivity in ray striatal neurons. Neuroscience **65:** 1041–1050.
9. COLE, R.L., C. KONRADI, J. DOUGLASS & S.E. HYMAN. 1995. Neuronal adaptation to amphetamine and dopamine: molecular mechanisms of prodynorphin gene regulation in rat striatum. Neuron **14:** 813–823.
10. GIBB, J.W., M. JOHNSON & G.R. HANSON. 1990. Neurochemical basis of neurotoxicity. Neurotoxicology **11:** 317–321.
11. BOWYER, J.F. *et al.* 1998. Long-term effects in aged rats of amphetamine neurotoxicity on tyrosine hydroxylase mRNA and protein. J. Pharmacol. Exp. Ther. **286:**1074–1085.
12. WAN, F.J., H.C. LIN, Y.S. LIN & C.J. TSENG. 2000. Intra-striatal infusion of D-amphet-amine induces hydroxyl radical formation: inhibition by MK-801. Pretreatment. Neuropharmacology **28:** 419–426.
13. HUANG, N.K., F.J. WAN, C.J. TSENG & C.S. TUNG. 1997. Amphetamine induces hydroxyl radical formation in the striatum of rats. Life Sci. **61:** 2219–2229.
14. LIN, H.-G. *et al.* 1999. Systemic administration of D-amphetamine induced a delayed production of nitric oxide in the striatum of rats. Neurosci. Lett. **276:** 141–144.
15. ANDRERZHANOVA, E.A., I.I. AFAN,AS'EV, V.S. KUDRIN & K.S. RAYESKY. 2000. Effect of D-amphetamine and psychostimulant drug sydnocarb on dopamine, 3,4 dihydrox-yphenylacetic acid extracellular concentration and generation of hydroxyl radicals in rat striatum. Ann. N.Y. Acad. Sci. **914:** 137–146.
16. PAXINOS, G. & C. WATSON. 1986. The Rat Brain in Stereotaxic Coordinates, 2nd ed. Academic Press. Orlando.
17. MATHIEU, A.M., J. CABOCHE & M.J. BESSON. 1996. Distribution of preproenkephalin, preprotachykinin A, and preprodynorphin mRNAs in the rat nucleus accumbens: effect of repeated administration of nicotine. Synapse **23:** 94–106.
18. SGAMBATO, V. *et al.* 1997. Effect of electrical stimulation of the cerebral cortex on the expression of the fos protein in the basal ganglia. Neuroscience **81:** 93–112.
19. MIKOYAN, V.D. *et al.* 1995. The influence of antioxidants and cycloheximide on the level of nitric oxide in the livers of mice in vivo. Biochim. Biophys. Acta **1269**(1): 19–24.
20. OHKAWA, H., N. OHISHI & K. YAGI. 1979. Assay for lipid peroxides in animal tissues by thiobarbituric acid reaction. Anal. Biochem. **95:** 351–358.

21. Duggan, D. 1959. Spectrofluorimetric determination of tocopherols. Arch. Biochem. Biophys. **84**(1): 116–119.
22. Graybiel, A.M., R. Moratalla & H.A. Robertson. 1990. Amphetamine and cocaine induce drug specific activation of the c-fos gene in striosomes-matrix compartments and limbic subdivisions of the striatum. Proc. Natl. Acad. Sci. USA **87**: 6912–6916.
23. Abekawa, T., T. Ohmori & T. Koyama. 1994. Effects of repeated administration of a high dose of methamphetamine on dopamine and glutamate release in rat striatum and nucleus cumbers. Brain Res. **643**: 276–281.
24. Filloux, F. & J.J. Townsend. 1993. Pre and post synaptic neurotoxic effects of dopamine demonstrated by intrastriatal injection. Exp. Neurol. **119**: 79–88.
25. Michel, P.P. & F. Hefti. 1990. Toxicity of 6-hydroxydopamine and dopamine for dopaminergic neurons in culture. J. Neurosci. Res. **26**: 428–435.
26. Tanaka, M., A. Sotomatsu, H. Kanai & S. Hirai. 1991. Dopa and dopamine cause culture neuronal death in the presence of iron. J. Neurol. Sci. **101**: 198–203.
27. Olanow, C.F. An introduction to the free radical hypothesis in Parkinson's disease. Ann. Neurol. **32**: S2–S9.
28. Sonsalla, P.K., D.E. Riordan & R.E. Heikkila. 1991. Competitive and non competitive antagonists at NMDA receptors protect against methamphetamine-induced dopaminergic damage in mice. J. Pharmacol. Exp. Ther. **256**: 506–512.
29. Stephans, S.E. & B.K. Yamamoto. 1994. Methamphetamine neurotoxicity: roles for glutamate and dopamine efflux. Synapse **17**: 203–209.
30. Beckman, J.S. et al. 1990. Apparent hydroxy radical production by peroxinitrite: implication for endothelial injury from nitric oxide and superoxide. Proc. Natl. Acad. Sci. USA **87**: 1621–1624.
31. Imam, S.Z. et al. 2001. Methamphetamine-induced alteration in striatal p53 and bcl-2 expressions in mice. Brain Res. Mol. Brain Res. **91**: 174–178.
32. Imam, S.Z. et al. 2001. Methamphetamine-induced dopaminergic neurotoxicity: role of peroxynitrite and neuroprotective role of antioxidants and peroxynitrite decomposition catalysts. Ann. N.Y. Acad. Sci. **939**: 366–880.
33. Zhang, J., V.L. Dawson, D.M. Dawson & S.H. Snyser. 1994. Nitric oxid activation of poly (ADP-ribose) synthetase in neurotoxicity. Science. **263**: 687–689.
34. Itzhak, Y. & S.F. Ali. 1996. The neuronal nitric oxide syntheses inhibitor, 7-nitroindazole, protects against methamphetamine-induced neurotoxicity. J. Neurochem. **67**: 1770–1773.
35. Itzhak, Y., J. Martin & S.F. Ali. 1999. Methamphetamine and methyl-4-phenyl-1,2,3,4-tetrahydropyridine-induced dopaminergic neurotoxicity in inducible nitric oxide synthase-deficient mice. Synapse **34**: 305–312.
36. Yamamoto, B.K. & W. Zhu. 1998. The effects of methamphetamine on the production of free radicals and oxidative stress. J. Pharmacol. Exp. Ther. **287**: 107–114.
37. Bashkatova, V. et al. 1999. Influence of NOS inhibitors on changes in ACH release and NO level in the brain elicited by amphetamine neurotoxicity. Neuroreport **10**: 3155–3158.
38. Eisch, A.J. & J.F. Marshall. 1998. Methamphetamine neiurotoxicity: dissociation between striatal dopamine terminal damage from parietal cortical cell body injury. Synapse **30**: 433–445.

Effects of Acute Toxic Doses of Psychostimulants on Extracellular Levels of Excitatory Amino Acids and Taurine in Rats

Comparison of *d*-Amphetamine and Sydnocarb

E. ANDERZHANOVA,[a,c] K.S. RAYEVSKY,[c] P. SARANSAARI,[a]
E. RIITAMAA,[a] AND S.S. OJA[a,b]

[a]*Brain Research Center, University of Tampere, Medical School, Tampere, Finland*

[b]*Department of Clinical Physiology, Tampere University Hospital, Tampere, Finland*

[c]*Laboratory of Neurochemical Pharmacology, Institute of Pharmacology, Russian Academy of Medical Sciences, Moscow, Russia*

ABSTRACT: We used microdialysis to study how acute toxic doses of *d*-amphetamine and sydnocarb [3-(β-phenylisopropyl)-*N*-phenylcarbamoylsydnonimine], an original Russian psychostimulant, affect extracellular levels of glutamate, aspartate, and taurine in the neostriatum of halothane-anesthetized male Sprague-Dawley rats. The administration of *d*-amphetamine (5.0 mg/kg × 4 ip) caused gradual fivefold increases in the extracellular glutamate and taurine levels and moderate increases in the extracellular aspartate level. Sydnocarb administration (23.8 mg/kg × 4 ip, a dose equimolar to 5.0 mg/kg *d*-amphetamine) elicited a marked increase in the extracellular aspartate level and a small increase in the extracellular level of glutamate. The extracellular taurine level increased only after the last (fourth) injection. We conclude that a massive increase in extracellular taurine reflects hyperactivation of glutamatergic neurotransmission elicited by acute toxic dose of *d*-amphetamine. Sydnocarb seems to be less neurotoxic than *d*-amphetamine, because it elicits lesser changes in the extracellular levels of glutamate and taurine.

KEYWORDS: *d*-amphetamine; sydnocarb; amino acids; neurotoxicity; striatum; microdialysis

INTRODUCTION

Amphetamines produce substantial psychostimulation through activation of the mesolimbic and mesocortical dopaminergic systems. The primary reasons for the reduced clinical use of psychostimulant drugs are profound neurotoxic effects and the tolerance and dependence that develop with repeated administrations.

Address for correspondence: Elmira Anderzhanova, Ph.D., Brain Research Center, Medical School, FIN-33014 University of Tampere, Tampere, Finland. Voice: 358-3-215-6869; fax: 358-3-215-6170.

anderzhanova@hotmail.com

Ann. N.Y. Acad. Sci. 965: 193–203 (2002). © 2002 New York Academy of Sciences.

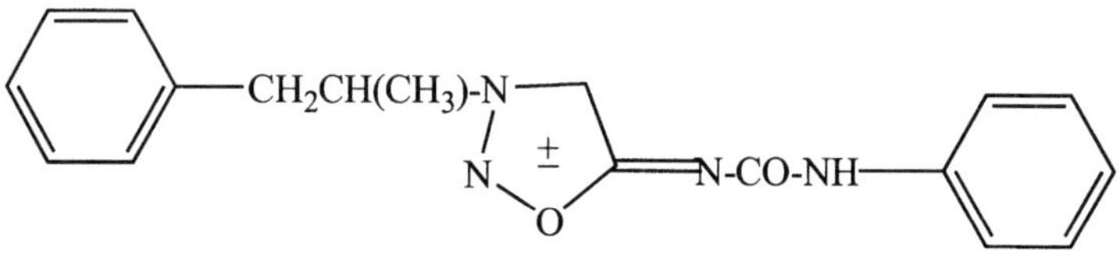

sydnocarb=3-(β-phenylisopropyl)-N-phenylcarbamoylsydnonimine

FIGURE 1. Structural formula of sydnocarb.

Relatively moderate doses of amphetamine increase the extracellular levels of excitatory amino acids in the striatum, but the mechanism by which endogenous glutamate enhances the stimulatory action of amphetamines is still a matter of debate. On the other hand, dopaminergic and glutamatergic neurons are reciprocally excited in the caudate putamen upon methamphetamine exposure, and this interplay exacerbates oxidative stress and results in damage to dopaminergic synaptic terminals. Suggestive evidence for the involvement of glutamate in the neurotoxicity of systemically administered amphetamines is afforded by the association of monoaminergic neuronal impairment with an increased extracellular level of glutamate.[1–5] In addition to the stimulation of locomotor activity and euphoria, systemic administration of psychostimulants increases the core body temperature.[6–9] Glutamate release and hyperthermia both contribute to metabolic stress and may be key factors in amphetamine neurotoxicity. They may not be independently involved in the mechanisms of neurotoxicity. N-Methyl-D-aspartate (NMDA) receptor antagonists counteract the elevation in temperature and attenuate methamphetamine-induced toxicity in mice.[10–13] However, the degree of suppression of methamphetamine-induced hyperthermia does not correlate with the extent of protection afforded by this pharmacologic treatment.[12] Methamphetamine-induced neurotoxicity can occur in the absence of any essential change in temperature.[12,14] In addition to the significant release of glutamate and hyperthermia, other factors such as increased dopamine oxidation may also be involved.[15]

Sydnocarb [3-(β-phenylisopropyl)-N-phenylcarbamoylsydnonimine], synthesized in the Russian Center for Drug Chemistry (Moscow), is a psychostimulant used in clinical practice in Russia (FIG. 1). Compared to the stimulatory effects of amphetamines, the activating effects of sydnocarb develop more gradually, last longer, and are less frequently accompanied by stereotypy. There are no peripheral sympatomimetic effects, pronounced euphoria, or motor excitation. Sydnocarb has also been characterized as a stimulant with a weak ability for addiction to develop. Neither behavioral nor physical dependence on sydnocarb has been noted.[16,17] Comparison of the behavioral and toxic effects indicate that sydnocarb is less neurotoxic than methamphetamine. It has been suggested that the mechanism of the sydnocarb-induced increase in the extracellular dopamine level is, in part, independent of extracellular Ca^{2+}.[18] Sydnocarb produces a slow and gradual increase in the parameters indicative of dopaminergic dysfunction when administered at a dose of 30 mg/ kg.[19] In contrast to *d*-amphetamine, sydnocarb does not induce any dramatic increase in the formation of hydroxyl radicals in the rat caudate putamen on subchronic treatment.[20]

The present study compares the effects of *d*-amphetamine and sydnocarb on the extracellular levels of excitatory amino acids and taurine in the rat neostriatum measured by microdialysis.

MATERIAL AND METHODS

Animal Preparation. Adult male Sprague-Dawley rats weighing 200–250 g (Orion, Espoo, Finland) were given food and water ad libitum and maintained in a temperature-controlled room (22 ± 1°C) and constant relative humidity (50%) under a 12-hour light/dark cycle. Procedures were followed in accordance with the European Community Directive for the ethical use of experimental animals. All efforts were made to minimize both the suffering and the number of animals used.

Rats were anesthetized with 4% halothane in air within 2 minutes and then maintained under anesthesia with 1% halothane in air delivered at 1.2 L/min. Microdialysis probes were stereotaxically implanted into the left and right neostriata (coordinates from bregma, AP = 0.5, ML = ±0.3, DV = −6.5 according to the atlas of Paxinos and Watson[21]).

Pharmacologic Treatment. Sydnocarb was administered in a dose (23.8 mg/kg) equimolar to those of *d*-amphetamine (5.0 mg/kg). *d*-Amphetamine (Sigma, St. Louis, MO, USA) was dissolved in 0.85% NaCl, sydnocarb (Russian Center for Drug Chemistry, Moscow, Russia) in 0.85% NaCl-propyleneglycol mixture (50/50, v/v).[19] Both drugs were administered to the rats by intraperitoneal injection. In a series of control experiments the possible effects of both vehicle solutions were tested.

Microdialysis Procedure. Microdialysis probes of a concentric design (0.5-mm outer diameter, a 2-mm dialyzing membrane) were used (CMA 12, CMA/Microdialysis AB, Sweden). The probes were perfused with artificial cerebrospinal fluid containing (in mM): Na^+ 150; K^+ 3.0; Ca^{2+} 1.2, Mg^{2+} 0.8; $H_2PO_4^-$ 31.0; Cl^- 155; pH 7.4. All probes were perfused at 2 µL/min for 1–2 hours before samples were collected, and the same constant flow rate was maintained with a microdialysis pump (CMA/Microdialysis AB, Sweden) throughout the experiment.

High-Pressure Liquid Chromatography of Amino Acids. Amino acids were assayed in dialysates kept frozen at −70°C and thawed immediately prior to analysis. The concentrations of glutamate, aspartate, and taurine were measured by high-pressure liquid chromatography with fluorescence detection (Shimadzu Scientific Instruments, Kyoto, Japan) after precolumn derivatization with *o*-phthaldialdehyde (Sigma, St. Louis, MO, USA). Derivatization was performed by an autoinjector SIL-10AD (Shimadzu Scientific Instruments, Kyoto, Japan). Samples in the autoinjector were maintained at 4°C by a Peltier thermoelectric sample cooler. Samples and reagent were allowed to react for 2 minutes, after which a portion of the mixture was injected onto a C18-HC column (ODS, 5 µm packing, 4.6 mm internal diameter × 25 cm, Waters, UK) equipped with a guard column (4 × 20 mm). The mobile phase was 0.075 M phosphate buffer (pH 6.5); methanol and acetonitrile were used as organic eluents with gradient profiles of 14–25% and 0–10%, respectively. The amino

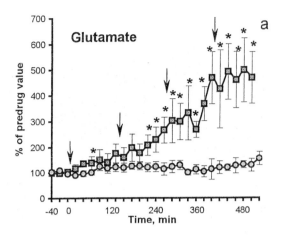

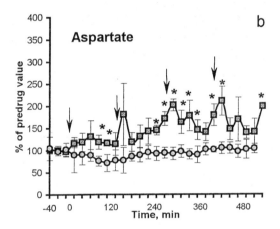

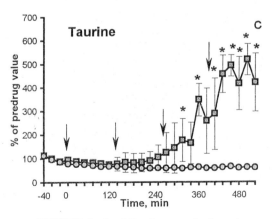

FIGURE 2. *See following page for legend.*

acid derivatives were assayed using an RF-10A fluorescence detector (Shimadzu Scientific Instruments, Kyoto, Japan) with excitation and emission wavelengths set at 340 and 450 nm, respectively. Data were analyzed by PC using VPclass5 software and quantified by comparing the peak areas to those of standards.

Data Analysis. The relative magnitudes of the evoked effects of different treatments were estimated by expressing them as percentage changes from baseline (100%). Basal levels of amino acids for each rat were defined as the mean of three successive baseline values obtained prior to injection of drugs or vehicle. Statistical analysis was made with Excel2000 software (Microsoft, USA). Comparisons of different groups were done using two-way analysis of variance (ANOVA), group × time, with the repeated measures as one variable. In all cases, the limit of significance was set at $p < 0.05$.

RESULTS

Basal Extracellular Levels of Amino Acids. Basal extracellular levels of amino acids measured in 69 rats were, in the caudate putamen, 0.384 ± 0.142 µM for glutamate, 0.241 ± 0.094 µM for aspartate, and 1.214 ± 0.218 µM for taurine. These values are not corrected for recovery in the dialysate samples.

Effects of an Acute Toxic Dose of d-Amphetamine. Subchronic *d*-amphetamine administration (5.0 mg/kg × 4, $n = 8$) caused a marked gradual increase in extracellular levels of glutamate and taurine up to 400–550% and 480–580% of controls, respectively (FIG. 2a and 2c) and a moderate increase in the level up to 170–200% (FIG. 2b). The effect was already discernible in the case of glutamate, in aspartate after the first injection of *d*-amphetamine, whereas with taurine only after the third administration.

Effects of an Acute Toxic Dose of Sydnocarb. The level of glutamate was practically unaffected when compared to that of the control group (FIG. 3a). Sydnocarb administration (23.8 mg/kg × 4, $n = 6$) elicited marked increases in the aspartate level after the second and fourth injections (up to 250–350% in both cases) (FIG. 3b). The taurine level was not altered within the first 6 hours and significantly increased only after the last (fourth) injection. The final extracellular level of taurine attained after sydnocarb treatment was three times less than that after *d*-amphetamine administration (FIG. 3c).

FIGURE 2. Effects of *d*-amphetamine administration (5.0 mg/kg × 4 ip) on extracellular levels of (**a**) glutamate, (**b**) aspartate, and (**c**) taurine in the neostriatum in halothane-anesthetized rats (–○– 0.85% NaCl × 4 ip; –□– *d*-amphetamine). *Significant difference from the saline-treated group, ANOVA, $p < 0.05$, $n = 8$. *Arrows* indicate moments of drug administration.

FIGURE 3. Effects of sydnocarb administration (23.8 mg/kg × 4 ip) on extracellular levels of (**a**) glutamate, (**b**) aspartate, and (**c**) taurine in the neostriatum in halothane-anesthetized rats (–○– propyleneglycol/0.85% NaCl × 4 ip; –□– sydnocarb). *Significant difference from the saline-treated group, ANOVA, $p < 0.05$, $n = 6$. *Arrows* indicate moments of drug administration.

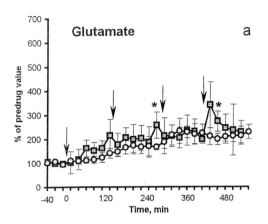

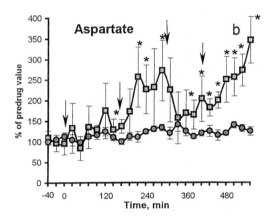

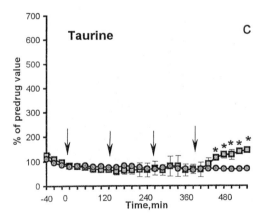

FIGURE 3. *See previous page for legend.*

DISCUSSION

The neurotoxic consequences of methamphetamine have been associated with an increase in the core temperature,[22] metabolic and oxidative stress,[5,23] and excessive glutamate release.[1,3,24] Repeated, but not single, systemic administration of amphetamine or methamphetamine led to monoamine depletion in the rat and monkey striatum, frontal cortex, and amygdala,[25,26] to a decline in the number of high-affinity uptake sites for dopamine, and to inhibition of tyrosine and tryptophan hydroxylase in the rat striatum and hippocampus.[27–29] One current hypothesis is that the excessive release of dopamine from nerve endings mediates the neurotoxic action of amphetamines. Catecholamines were found to be toxic *in vivo* and *in vitro*.[30–32] However, microdialysis experiments have shown that the reduced toxicity of methamphetamine at low environmental temperature (5°C) is not the result of decreased dopamine release.[15] The competitive and noncompetitive NMDA receptor antagonists attenuate amphetamine- and methamphetamine-induced neurotoxicity, whereas they do not block the increase in dopamine efflux.[10,33] Both local and systemic administration of amphetamines acutely enhances dopamine release, but only systemic administration results in neurotoxicity and increases the extracellular concentration of glutamate.[1–5,34]

The mechanism by which amphetamines increase extracellular glutamate is poorly understood. Clearly, the release as well as the uptake systems have to be affected but not necessarily in a direct fashion. The increase in dopamine efflux produces an activation of dopaminergic neurotransmission in the neostriatum. It has been suggested that stimulation of both dopamine D_1 and D_2 receptors enhances the release of intracellular glutamate in the striata of freely moving rats.[35,36] However, the ability of local or systemic administrations of moderate doses of amphetamine to markedly elevate extracellular glutamate and aspartate seems to depend on the degree of activation of basal ganglia circuits.[5,34,37,38] In our previous study,[39] this indirect effect was thus a likely cause for the elevation of extracellular glutamate after single systemic *d*-amphetamine administration. This assumption is also consistent with the partial neuroprotective effects of the dopamine receptor antagonists eticlopride, haloperidol, and SCH23390 and underlies the importance of the dopamine receptor in amphetamine-induced neurotoxicity.[12,40]

Several additional mechanisms may explain the gradual increase in extracellular glutamate in different brain structures under toxic *d*-amphetamine exposure.[3,24,34] One current theory is that the excessive release of dopamine triggers an accumulation of reactive dopamine metabolites and hyperproduction of hydroxyl radicals. We have indeed shown that the production of hydroxyl radicals is intensified by the acute toxic dose of *d*-amphetamine.[20] It has been suggested that glutamate uptake is inhibited (or reversed) by oxygen radicals,[41,42] nitric oxide,[43] or arachidonic acid[44] on *d*-amphetamine administration. The slowly incurring effects of these agents could underlie the delayed increase in extracellular glutamate in the present experiments.

The energy consumption of the brain is increased after systemic methamphetamine administration, as evidenced by an immediate and sustained increase in extracellular lactate in the striatum. ATP is depleted in brain regions susceptible to amphetamines.[45,46] The increase in glutamate release and the methamphetamine-induced depletion of energy stores are thus positively correlated. The activation of NMDA receptors by glutamate activates nitric oxide synthase. The subsequent enhanced generation of nitric oxide is followed by the formation of reactive oxygen species and mitochondrial dysfunction due to direct inhibition of complex IV in the electron transport chain, cytochrome c oxidase.[47,48] On the other hand, under experimentally induced metabolic stress (e.g., glucose deprivation), NMDA receptors are activated more readily, and even normally nontoxic concentrations of glutamate can produce NMDA-receptor–mediated toxicity.[49,50] Hyperthermia can foment enzymatic and nonenzymatic degradation of dopamine and exitatory amino acid-dependent formation of reactive oxygen species. Indeed, when the incubation temperature is lowered in *in vitro* toxicity models (e.g., cortical cultures of the chick retina), damage produced by excitotoxins or oxygen-glucose deprivation is reduced.[51,52]

The increase in extracellular glutamate after *d*-amphetamine administration was now largely paralleled by a similar increase in extracellular taurine, a general modulator of neural excitability and regulator of cell volumes.[53] It was previously demonstrated that taurine release both *in vivo* and *in vitro* is markedly enhanced by glutamate and its agonists.[54] The released taurine is believed to originate from both neurons and glial cells[55] and to act neuroprotective and osmoregulatory,[56] counteracting the harmful metabolic cascades initiated by an excess of extracellular glutamate. The level of extracellular taurine would also appear to be a good indicator of the extent of neural damage under various cell-damaging conditions.[57,58]

The mechanisms of sydnocarb's actions have been only partially studied hitherto.[18–20] In the present experiments, sydnocarb affected the extracellular levels of glutamate and taurine markedly less than did *d*-amphetamine at equimolar doses. The elevation in extracellular aspartate on sydnocarb administration was relatively more pronounced that the increase in glutamate, whereas the effects of *d*-amphetamine were precisely the opposite. Furthermore, Witkin and colleagues[19] showed that the convulsive effects of cocaine are significantly aggravated by methamphetamine but not by sydnocarb.

In conclusion, the increase in the extracellular level of glutamate contributes to excitotoxic damage to neurons caused by *d*-amphetamine. A massive increase in extracellular taurine reflects hyperactivation of glutamatergic neurotransmission elicited by *d*-amphetamine. Extracellular taurine could be a useful biochemical marker of neurotoxicity. Sydnocarb may be less neurotoxic than *d*-amphetamine, because it elicits less marked changes in extracellular glutamate and taurine.

ACKNOWLEDGMENTS

This work was supported by grants from the Center for International Mobility (CIMO), Finland, the Medical Research Fund of Tampere University Hospital, Finland, and the Russian Foundation for Basic Research.

REFERENCES

1. NASH, J.F. & B.K. YAMAMOTO. 1992. Methamphetamine neurotoxicity and striatal glutamate release: comparison to 3,4-methylenedioxymethamphetamine. Brain Res. **581:** 237–243.

2. ABEKAWA, T. *et al.* 1994. Effects of repeated administration of a high dose of methamphetamine on dopamine and glutamate release in rat striatum and nucleus accumbens. Brain Res. **643:** 276–281.
3. STEPHANS, S. & B.K. YAMAMOTO. 1994. Methamphetamine-induced neurotoxicity: role for glutamate and dopamine efflux. Synapse **17:** 203–209.
4. WOLF, M.E. & C.-J. XUE. 1998. Amphetamine and D1 dopamine receptor agonists produce biphasic effects on glutamate efflux in rat ventral tegmentum area: modification by repeated amphetamine administration. J. Neurochem. **70:** 198–209.
5. BURROWS, K.B. *et al.* 2000. Central administration of methamphetamine synergizes with metabolic inhibition to deplete striatal monoamines. J. Pharmacol. Exp. Ther. **292:** 853–860.
6. BOWYER, J.F. *et al.* 1992. The influence of environmental temperature on the transient effects of methamphetamine on dopamine levels and dopamine release in rat striatum. J. Pharmacol. Exp. Ther. **260:** 817–824.
7. BOWYER, J. *et al.* 1993. Effects of the cool environment or age on methamphetamine-induced dopamine release in the caudate-putamen of female rats. Pharmacol. Biochem. Behav. **44:** 87–98.
8. BOWYER, J.F. *et al.* 1994. Futher studies of the role of hyperthermia in methamphetamine neurotoxicity. J. Pharmacol. Exp. Ther. **268:** 1571–1580.
9. COLADO, M.L. *et al.* 1998. Role of hyperthermia in the protective action of clomethiazole against MDMA ('ecstasy')-induced neurodegeneration: comparison with the novel NMDA channel blocker AR-R15896AR. Br. J. Pharmacol. **124:** 479–484.
10. SONSALLA, P.K. 1995. The role of *N*-methyl-D-aspartate receptors in dopaminergic neuropathology produced by the amphetamines. Drug Alcohol Depend. **37:** 101–105.
11. WEIHMULLER, F.B. *et al.* 1992. MK-801 protection against methamphetamine-induced striatal dopamine terminal injury is associated with attenuated dopamine overflow. Synapse **11:** 155–163.
12. ALBERS, D.S. & P.K. SONSALLA. 1995. Methamphetamine-induced hyperthermia and dopaminergic neurotoxicity in mice: pharmacological profile of protective and non-protective agents. J. Pharmacol. Exp. Ther. **275:** 1104–1114.
13. FARFEL, G.M. & L.S. SEIDEN. 1995. Role of hypothermia in the mechanism of protection against serotonergic toxicity. II. Experiments with methamphetamine, *p*-chloroamphetamine, fenfluramine, dizocilpine and dextromethorphan. J. Pharmacol. Exp. Ther. **272:** 868–875.
14. MILLER, D.B. & J.P. O'CALLAGHAN. 1994. Environment-, drug- and stress-induced alterations in body temperature affect the neurotoxicity of substituted amphetamines in the C57BL/6J mouse. J. Pharmacol. Exp. Ther. **270:** 752–760.
15. LAVOIE, M.J. & T.G. HASTINGS. 1999. Dopamine quinone formation and protein modification associated with the striatal neurotoxicity of methamphetamine: evidence against a role for extracellular dopamine. J. Neurosci. **19:** 1484–1491.
16. MASHKOVSKY, M.D. *et al.* 1971. Experimental and clinical study on new psychostimulator sydnocarb. Korsakov's J. Neuropathol. Psychiat. **71:** 1704–1709.
17. RUDENKO, G.M. & R.A. ALTSHULER. 1978. Experimental and clinical study of sydnocarb. Hung. Pharmacother. **124:** 150–154.
18. GAINETDINOV, R.R. *et al.* 1997. Effects of a psychostimulant drug sydnocarb on rat brain dopaminergic transmission *in vivo*. Eur. J. Pharmacol. **340:** 53–58.
19. WITKIN, J.M. *et al.* 1999. Behavioural, toxic, and neurochemical effects of sydnocarb, a novel psychomotor stimulant: comparisons with methamphetamine. J. Pharmacol. Exp. Ther. **288:** 1298–1310.
20. ANDERZHANOVA, E.A. *et al.* 2000. Effect of d-amphetamine and sydnocarb on the extracellular level of dopamine, 3,4-dihydroxyphenylacetic acid and hydroxyl radicals generation in rat striatum. Ann. N.Y. Acad. Sci. USA **914:** 137–145.
21. PAXINOS, G. & C. WATSON. 1996. The Rat Brain Sterotaxic Coordinates, 2nd Ed. Academic Press. Sydney.
22. ASKEW, B.M. 1962. Hyperpyrexia as a contributing factor in the toxicity of amphetamine in aggregated mice. Br. J. Pharmacol. **19:** 245–257.
23. CADET, J.L. & C. BRANNOCK. 1998. Free radicals and the pathology of the brain dopamine systems. Neurochem. Int. **32:** 117–131.

24. OHMORI, T. *et al.* 1996. The role of glutamate in behavioral and neurotoxic effects of methamphetamine. Neurochem. Int. **29:** 301–307.
25. RICAURTE, G.A. *et al.* 1980. Long term effects of repeated methylamphetamine administration on dopamine and serotonin neurons in rat brains: a regional study. Brain Res. **193:** 153–163.
26. RICAURTE, G.A. *et al.* 1982. Dopamine nerve terminals degeneration produced by high doses of methylamphetamine in the rat brain. Brain Res. **235:** 93–103.
27. FIBIGER, H.C. & E.G. MCGEER. 1971. Effect of acute and chronic methamphetamine treatment on tyrosine hydroxylase activity in brain and adrenal medulla. Eur. J. Pharmacol. **16:** 176–180.
28. HOTCHKISS, A.J. & J.W. GIBB. 1980. Long-term effects of multiple doses of methamphetamine on tryptophan hydroxylase and tyrosine hydroxylase activity in rat brain. J. Pharmacol. Exp. Ther. **214:** 257–262.
29. WAGNER, G.C. *et al.* 1980. Long lasting depletion of striatal dopamine and loss of dopamine uptake sites following repeated administration of methamphetamine. Brain Res. **181:** 1151–1160.
30. FILLOUX, F. & J.J TOWNSEND. 1993. Pre- and postsynaptic neurotoxic effects of dopamine demonstrated by intrastriatal injections. Exp. Neurol. **119:** 79–88.
31. HASTINGS, T.G. *et al.* 1996. Role of oxidation in the neurotoxic effect of the intrastriatal dopamine injection. Proc. Natl. Acad. Sci. USA **93:** 1956–1961.
32. STOKES, A.H. *et al.* 1999. Cytotoxic and genotoxic potential of dopamine. J. Neurosci. Res. **55:** 659–665.
33. MILLER, D.W. & E.D. ABERCROMBIE. 1996. Effects of MK-801 on spontaneous and amphetamine-stimulated dopamine release in striatum measured with *in vivo* microdialysis in awake rats. Brain Res. Bull. **40:** 57–62.
34. WOLF, M.E. & C.-J. XUE. 1999. Amphetamine-induced glutamate efflux in the rat ventral tegmental area is prevented by MK-801, SCH 23390, and ibotenic acid lesion of the prefrontal cortex. J. Neurochem. **73:** 1529–1538.
35. CEPEDA, C. & M.S. LEVINE. 1998. Dopamine and *N*-methyl-D-aspartate receptor interaction in the neostriatum. Dev. Neurosci. **20:** 1–18.
36. EXPOSITO, I. *et al.* 1999. Endogenous dopamine increases extracellular concentrations of glutamate and GABA in striatum of the freely moving rat: involvement of D1 and D2 dopamine receptors. Neurochem. Res. **24:** 849–856.
37. O'DELL, S.J. *et al.* 1994. Excitotoxic striatal lesions protect against subsequent methamphetamine-induced dopamine depletions. J. Pharmacol. Exp. Ther. **269:** 1319–1325.
38. ABARCA, J. & G. BUSTOS. 1999. Differential regulation of glutamate, aspartate and γ-amino-butyrate release by N-methyl-D-aspartate receptors in rat striatum after partial and extensive lesions to the nigro-striatal dopamine pathway. Neurochem. Int. **35:** 19–33.
39. ANDERZHANOVA, E.A. *et al.* 2001. Effect of sydnocarb and d-amphetamine on the extracellular level of amino acids in the rat caudate-putamen. Eur. J. Pharmacol. **428:** 87–95.
40. O'DELL, S.J. *et al.* 1993. Methamphetamine-induced dopamine overflow and injury to striatal dopamine terminals: attenuation by dopamine D_1 and D_2 antagonists. J. Neurochem. **60:** 1792–1799.
41. TROTTI, D. *et al.* 1998. Glutamate transporters are oxidant-vulnerable: a molecular link between oxidative and excitotoxic neurodegeneration. Trends Pharmacol. Sci. **19:** 328–334.
42. WOLF, M.E. *et al.* 2000. Amphetamine increases glutamate efflux in the rat ventral tegmental area by a mechanism involving glutamate transporters and reactive oxygen species. J. Neurochem. **75:** 1634–1644.
43. YE, Z.-C. & H. SONTHEIMER. 1996. Cytokine modulation of glial glutamate uptake: a possible involvement of nitric oxide. Neuroreport **7:** 2181–2185.
44. VOLTERRA, A. *et al.* 1994. Glutamate uptake is inhibited by arachidonic acid and oxygen radicals via two distinct and additive mechanisms. Mol. Pharmacol. **46:** 986–992.
45. CHAN, P. *et al.* 1994. Rapid ATP loss caused by methamphetamine in the mouse striatum: relationship between energy impairment and dopaminergic neurotoxicity. J. Neurochem. **62:** 2484–2487.

46. STEPHANS, S.E. *et al.* 1998. Substrates of energy metabolism attenuate methamphetamine-induced neurotoxicity in striatum. J. Neurochem. **71:** 613–621.
47. LIZASOAIN, I. *et al.* 1996. Nitric oxide and peroxynitrite exert distinct effect on the mitochondrial respiration which are differentially blocked by glutathione or glucose. Biochem. J. **314:** 877–880.
48. CLEETER, M.W. *et al.* 1994. Reversible inhibition of cytochrome c oxidase, the terminal enzyme of the mitochondrial respiratory chain, by nitric oxide. Implication for neurodegenerative disorders. FEBS Lett. **345:** 50–54.
49. ZEEVALK, G.D. & W.J. NICKLAS. 1992. Evidence that the loss of the voltage-dependent Mg^{2+} block at the *N*-methyl-D-aspartate receptors underlies receptor activation during inhibition of neuronal metabolism. J. Neurochem. **59:** 1211–1220.
50. ZEEVALK, G.D. & W.J. NICKLAS. 1993. Hypothermia, metabolic stress, and NMDA-mediated excitotoxicity. J. Neurochem. **61:** 1445–1453
51. ZEEVALK, G.D. *et al.* 1995. NMDA receptor involvement in toxicity to dopamine neurons *in vitro* caused by the succinate dehydrogenase inhibitor 3-nitropropionic acid. J. Neurochem. **61:** 455–458.
52. BRUNO, V.M.G. *et al.* 1994. Neuroprotective effect of hypothermia in cortical cultures exposed to oxygen-glucose deprivation or excitatory amino acids. J. Neurochem. **63:** 1398–1406.
53. OJA, S.S. & P. SARANSAARI. 1996. Taurine as osmoregulator and neuromodulator in the brain. Metab. Brain Dis. **11:** 153–164.
54. OJA, S.S. & P. SARANSAARI. 2000. Modulation of taurine release by glutamate receptors and nitric oxide. Prog. Neurobiol. **62:** 407–425.
55. SARANSAARI, P. & S.S. OJA. 1992. Release of GABA and taurine from brain slices. Prog. Neurobiol. **38:** 455–482.
56. SARANSAARI, P. & S.S. OJA. 2000. Taurine and neural cell damage. Amino Acids **19:** 509–526.
57. SARANSAARI, P. & S.S. OJA. 1997. Enhanced taurine release in cell-damaging conditions in the developing and ageing mouse hippocampus. Neuroscience **79:** 847–854.
58. SARANSAARI, P. & S.S. OJA. 1998. Release of endogenous glutamate, aspartate, GABA, and taurine from hippocampal slices from adult and developing mice under cell-damaging conditions. Neurochem. Res. **23:** 563–570.

Methamphetamine-Induced Dopaminergic Neurotoxicity and Production of Peroxynitrite Are Potentiated in Nerve Growth Factor Differentiated Pheochromocytoma 12 Cells

SYED Z. IMAM,[a,b] GLENN D. NEWPORT,[a] HELEN M. DUHART,[a]
FAKHRUL ISLAM,[b] WILLIAM SLIKKER, JR.,[a] AND SYED F. ALI[a]

[a]Neurochemistry Laboratory, Division of Neurotoxicology, National Center for Toxicological Resarch/US FDA, Jefferson, Arkansas 72079, USA

[b]Neurotoxicology Laboratory, Department of Medical Elementology and Toxicology, Jamia Hamdard (Hamdard University), New Delhi 110 062, India

ABSTRACT: Methamphetamine (METH) is a widely abused psychomotor stimulant known to cause dopaminergic neurotoxicity in rodents, nonhuman primates, and humans. METH administration selectively damages the dopaminergic nerve terminals, which is hypothesized to be due to release of dopamine from synaptic vesicles within the terminals. This process is believed to be mediated by the production of free radicals. The current study evaluates METH-induced dopaminergic toxicity in pheochromocytoma 12 (PC12) cells cultured in the presence or absence of nerve growth factor (NGF). Dopaminergic changes and the formation of 3-nitrotyrosine (3-NT), a marker for peroxynitrite production, were studied in PC12 cell cultures grown in the presence or absence of NGF after different doses of METH (100–1,000 μM). METH exposure did not cause significant alterations in cell viability and did not produce significant dopaminergic changes or 3-NT production in PC12 cells grown in NGF-negative media after 24 hours. However, cell viability of PC12 cells grown in NGF-positive media was decreased by 45%, and significant dose-dependent dopaminergic alteration and 3-NT production were observed 24 hours after exposure to METH. The current study supports the hypothesis that METH acts at the dopaminergic nerve terminals and produces dopaminergic damage by the production of free radical peroxynitrite.

KEYWORDS: methamphetamine; peroxynitrite; oxidative stress; nerve growth factor; dopaminergic neurotoxicity

Address for correspondence: Syed F. Ali, Ph.D., Head, Neurochemistry Laboratory, HFT-132, Division of Neurotoxicology, National Center for Toxicological Research/US FDA, 3900 NCTR Rd., Jefferson, AR 72079. Voice: 870-543-7123; fax: 870-543-7745.
sali@nctr.fda.gov

Ann. N.Y. Acad. Sci. 965: 204–213 (2002). © 2002 New York Academy of Sciences.

INTRODUCTION

A variable class of neurotoxins that give rise to specific degeneration of the dopaminergic nervous system is postulated to elicit their detrimental effects, at least in part, through oxidative stress. Methamphetamine (METH), a widely abused potent psychostimulant drug, has the potential to selectively damage the brain dopamine (DA) system. Laboratory animals given repeated doses of METH show large, long-lasting depletion of brain DA and its metabolites[1,2] and a decrease in the number of DA transporters.[3] These dopaminergic damages are thought to be produced by the generation of reactive oxygen (ROS) and nitrogen (RNS) species. The role of nitric oxide (NO) and superoxide (O_2^-) radicals in METH-induced neurotoxicity is well documented. The protection of METH-induced dopaminergic neurotoxicity by a selective neuronal nitric oxide synthase (nNOS) inhibitor, 7-nitroindazole, implicates the role of NO radicals in METH neurotoxicity.[4,5] nNOS knockout mice, being protected against METH-induced dopaminergic neurotoxicity, provided further insight into the role of NO in METH-induced neurotoxicity.[3] Several published reports discuss the involvement of O_2^- radicals in METH-induced neurotoxicity. (For a review, see Ref. 6.) METH-induced dopaminergic depletion is reported to be attenuated in copper-zinc superoxide dismutase (CuZn-SOD) overexpressed transgenic mice.[7,8] Therefore, the possibility of the interaction between O_2^- and NO may not be ruled out in METH-induced neurotoxicity.

Peroxynitrite ($OONO^-$), the reaction product of O_2^- and NO, is a potent oxidant. It has now been demonstrated clearly that $OONO^-$ can oxidize lipid membranes[9] and sulfhydryl moities[10] as well as hydroxylating and nitrating aromatics.[11] $OONO^-$ crosses the lipid membranes at a rate significantly faster than those of its known decomposition pathways,[12] indicating that this oxidant, unlike reactive radicals such as O_2^-· or ·OH, can travel distances of cellular dimensions.

METH was also reported to affect dopaminergic nerve terminals and cause selective degeneration of these neurons.[13] PC12 cells are pheochromocytoma cells, which are catecholamine-containing cell lines derived from rat medulla and have dopamine synthesizing, storing, and releasing properties similar to those of neurons.[14] They also produce neurites in response to the nerve growth factor (NGF).[15] These cells have also been extensively and suitably used to study the effects of various dopaminergic neurotoxins.[28] Therefore, NGF-treated PC12 cells may constitute a useful model to investigate features of the mechanism of METH cytotoxicity on nerve terminals. In the current study, we initially examined the cytotoxicity of METH on cultures of PC12 cells grown in media either with or without NGF. To evaluate whether the toxicity of METH is site specific at terminals, the presence of NGF in growth media served as a factor for neurite outgrowth and the viability of cells provided information about METH-induced cytotoxicity. To further elucidate the role of ROS- and RNS-based oxidative stress in METH-induced dopaminergic toxicity, the generation of $OONO^-$ was studied in cultures of PC12 cells grown in the media with or without NGF, and production of 3-NT was monitored as a marker for $OONO^-$ generation.

MATERIAL AND METHODS

Drugs and Chemicals. Methamphetamine-HCl, DA, DOPAC, HVA, and NGF were purchased from Sigma (St. Louis, MO, USA). Tyrosine and 3-nitrotyrosine were purchased from Calbiochem (La Jolla, CA, USA). METH-HCl solution was prepared in deionized water.

Cell Cultures. For cell culture studies, rat pheochromocytoma (PC12) cells were grown in 75-cm^2 tissue culture flasks at 37°C in an atmosphere of 5% CO_2/95% air in RPMI 1640 medium (Sigma) containing 10% horse serum and 5% fetal bovine serum. The growth medium contained 50 ng/ml nerve growth factor (NGF). The medium was changed every 3 days, and cells were subcultured once a week. In experiments in which toxicity was assessed, cells were plated in 24-well trays at a concentration of 100,000 cells/well, and the almost confluent cells were used 3 days later for the experiment. Cells were exposed to different doses of METH (100–1,000 μM) for 24 hours.

Assessment of Cell Viability. After each experiment, culture medium was removed from culture plates. Cells were then washed with Hank's balanced salt solution (HBSS). During washing, cells that were not attached to culture plates were eliminated. The attached cells, which represent survived cells, were harvested with trypsin (1%). The number of cells were counted with a Coulter Counter (Channelyzer 256). The percentage of survival versus METH concentration was used to assess cytotoxcity.

Determination of 3-NT and Tyrosine (TYR). 3-NT and TYR in cell cultures were determined by high-performance liquid chromatography (HPLC)-CoulArray electrochemical detection method[16] with slight modifications.[17] In brief, cell cultures were sonicated in 400 μl of 10 mM sodium acetate (NaOAc), pH 6.5. A 50-μl aliquot of the homogenate was used to determine protein concentration.[18] Remaining homogenate was centrifuged at $14,000 \times g$ for 10 minutes at 4°C. The supernatant was removed and treated with 100 μl of 1 mg/ml pronase for 18 hours at 50°C. Enzymatic digests were then treated with 0.5 ml of 10% TCA and centrifuged at $14,000 \times g$ for 10 minutes at 4°C, and supernatants were passed through a 0.2-μm PVDF filter before injection onto the HPLC instrument. All samples were analyzed on an ESA (Cambridge, MA) CoulArray HPLC equipped with eight electrochemical channels using platinum electrodes arranged in line and set to increasing specified potentials [channel(potential): 1(180 mV); 2(240 mV); 3(350 mV); 4(500 mV); 5(550 mV); 6(690 mV); 7(875 mV); and 8(900 mV)]. The analytic column was a TSK-GEL ODS 80-TM reverse-phase column with a column size of 4.6 mm × 25.0 cm (TOSO-HAAS, Mongtomeryville, PA). The mobile phase was 50 mM NaOAc/5% (v/v) methanol, pH 4.8. HPLC was performed under isocratic conditions. 3-NT and TYR were quantified relative to known standards. 3-NT values were represented as 3-NT per 100 TYR. 3-NT and TYR were quantified relative to known standards.

Determination of Dopamine Concentration. Concentrations of DA were quantified by a modified HPLC method combined with electrochemical detection.[1] Cell cultures were collected in a measured volume of 0.2 M perchloric acid containing internal standard 3,4-dihydroxybenzylamine, 100 ng/ml. Cells were disrupted by ultrasonication and centrifuged at 4°C ($15,000 \times g$; 7 minutes), and 150 μl of the supernatant was removed and filtered through a Nylon-66 microfilter (pore size, 0.2 μm; MF-1 centrifugal filter; Bioanalytical Systems, West Lafayette, IN, USA). Aliquots of 25 μl representing 2.5 mg of brain tissue were injected directly onto the HPLC/electrochemical detection system for separation of analytes. The amount of DA was calculated using standard curves that were generated by determining in trip-

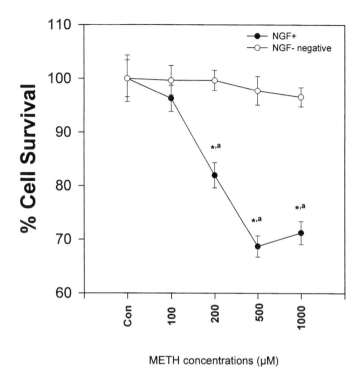

FIGURE 1. Effects of various doses of METH (100–1,000 μM) on the cell viability of PC12 cells grown in the presence or absence of NGF after 24 hours of treatment. *$p < 0.05$, significantly different from control group, [a]$p < 0.05$, significantly different from respective NGF-negative groups.

licate the ratio between three different known amounts of the amine and a constant amount of internal standard.

RESULTS

The viability of the PC12 cells grown in the presence or absence of NGF 24 hours after treatment with various doses of METH is presented in FIGURE 1. A dose-dependent decrease in the cell viability of NGF-differentiated PC12 cells was observed, whereas cell viability was negligible in cells grown in the absence of NGF. METH 500 μM caused the maximum decrease in cell viability (45%).

FIGURE 2 represents the effect of METH on DA content in cell lysates of NGF-differentiated PC12 cells after 24 hours. A significant dose-dependent decrease in DA content was observed after various doses of METH ranging from 100-1,000 μM.

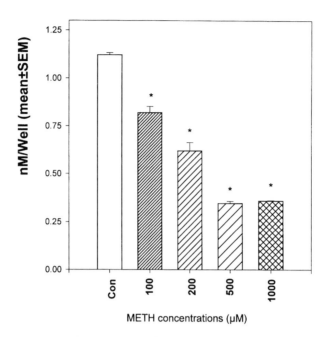

FIGURE 2. Effects of various doses of METH (100–1,000 µM) on the DA content in NGF-differentiated PC12 cells after 24 hours of treatment. Each value is mean ± SEM derived from three different sets of experiments. *$p < 0.05$, significantly different from control group.

FIGURE 3 presents the effect of METH on DA content in cell lysates of PC12 cells grown in the absence of NGF. No significant depletion was observed 24 hours after any dose of METH.

The effect of varying doses of METH (100–1,000 µM) on the production of 3-NT in the cell lysates of NGF-differentiated PC12 cells is represented in FIGURE 4. Exposure to METH resulted in a significant dose-dependent increase in the production of 3-NT 24 hours after METH exposure.

FIGURE 5 presents the effect of varying concentrations of METH (100–1,000 µM) on the production of 3-NT in the cell lysates of PC12 cells grown in the absence of NGF. No significant production of 3-NT was observed at any dose of METH.

DISCUSSION

The current study demonstrates that NGF-differentiated PC12 cells are more susceptible to METH-induced dopaminergic toxicity and the production of free radicals. This study also demonstrates that METH might produce dopaminergic toxicity by acting on cell terminals and producing peroxynitrite, which results in the depletion of DA from the cell terminals.

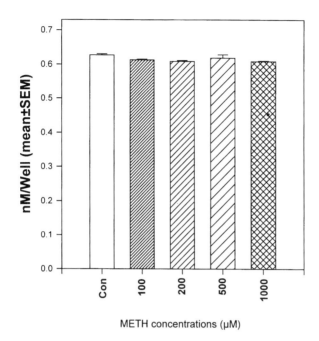

FIGURE 3. Effects of various doses of METH (100–1,000 μM) on the DA content of PC12 cells grown in the absence of NGF after 24 h of treatment. Each value is mean ± SEM derived from three different sets of experiments.

Dopaminergic neurons appear more prone to oxidative damage than do other neuronal cell types in brain.[19,20] Neurotoxins with specific detrimental toxic effects on the dopaminergic system, such as METH, appear to act in part by the production of either ROS or RNS species. Various data suggest the role of both superoxide (O_2^-) (see Ref. 6 for a review) and nitric oxide (NO)[3–5] in METH-induced dopaminergic neurotoxicity. Superoxide and NO produced by different cellular sources can react in the extracellular environment to produce peroxynitrite.[9] OONO⁻ has been reported to be involved in various kinds of oxidative damage.[9,10] It has also been implicated in a host of disease states, including various neurodegenerative disorders such as Alzheimer's disease, amyotrophic lateral sclerosis, and Huntington's disease.[21,22,23]

PC12 cells are a catecholamine-containing cell line derived from the rat adrenal medulla and have dopamine synthesizing, storing, and releasing properties similar to those of neurons, and they produce neurites in response to nerve growth factor.[24,25] Downregulation of copper zinc superoxide dismutase (Cu/Zn SOD) activity in PC12 cells by exposure to an appropriate antisense oligonucleotide has been reported to lead them to cell death via a NO/OONO⁻ pathway.[26] Exposure of PC12 cells to OONO⁻ has been reported to inhibit the synthesis of DOPA, and this inhibition has been thought to be due to inactivation of tyrosine hydroxylase by OONO⁻ exposure.[27] Recent evidence suggests that tyrosine hydroxylase is a selective target for nitration after exposure of PC12 cells to either OONO⁻ or 1-methyl-4-phenyl-

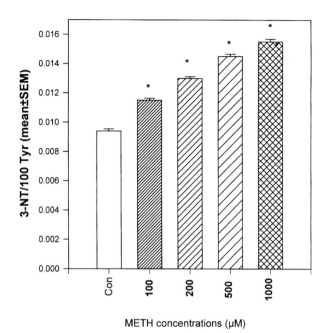

FIGURE 4. Effects of various doses of METH (100–1,000 μM) on 3-NT production in NGF-differentiated PC12 cells after 24 hours of treatment. Each value is mean ± SEM derived from three different sets of experiments. *$p < 0.05$, significantly different from control group.

pyridinium ion (MPP[+]).[28] Therefore, PC12 cells are a suitable model to study and to understand the role of OONO[−] in METH-induced neurotoxicity.

In the current study, we first demonstrated that exposure to METH can result in significant loss of cell survival in a dose-dependent manner in NGF-differentiated PC12 cells. METH exposure (500 μM) resulted in a 45% decrease in cell viability. The presence of NGF in the media, which resulted in neurite growth in PC12 cells, provided increased susceptibility of NGF-differentiated PC12 cells to METH. This increased susceptibility of NGF-differentiated PC12 cells to METH can be attributed to the fact that METH tends to act more at the nerve terminals than at the cell body. To further confirm the susceptibility of NGF-differentiated PC12 cells to METH exposure, we studied the METH-induced depletion of DA. Our results showed a significant dose-dependent decrease in DA in both cell lysates as well as the media 24 hours after exposure of the cells to different concentrations of METH.

It is evident from the literature that METH produces dopaminergic neurotoxicity by the generation of free radicals.[6] METH appears to elicit its effects by acting as a weak base and collapsing the pH gradients of acidic DA-containing synaptic vesicles, resulting in the redistribution of DA to the cytoplasm where it may undergo either auto-oxidation to produce superoxide radicals or metabolism by monoamine oxidase.[2,13,29,30] Both inhibition of DA synthesis and treatment with antioxidants ascorbate and vitamin E appear to reduce METH toxicity in dopaminergic nerve ter-

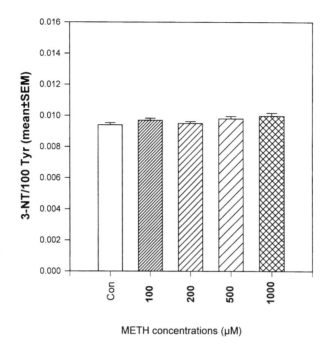

FIGURE 5. Effects of various doses of METH (100–1,000 μM) on 3-NT production in PC12 cells grown in the absence of NGF after 24 hours of treatment. Each value is mean ± SEM derived from three different sets of experiments.

minals,[31–33] suggesting that DA oxidation and superoxide production may be involved in the degenerative effects of METH at dopaminergic nerve terminals. PC12 cells overexpressing glutathione peroxidase enzyme have also been reported to be protected against METH-induced free-radical mediated toxicity and dopaminergic damage.[14]

The role of nitric oxide has also been well documented in METH-induced dopaminergic neurotoxicity. Blockade of NO formation with several NO synthase inhibitors attenuated METH-mediated cell death in primary mesencephalic cultures exposed to various concentrations of METH.[34] Therefore, the possible interaction of superoxide and NO during METH exposure is very likely.

In the current study, for the first time, we reported that METH exposure resulted in the generation of OONO⁻ in NGF-differentiated PC12 cells. Dose-dependent formation of 3-nitrotyrosine was observed 24 hours after exposure of NGF-differentiated PC12 cells to various concentrations of METH. The dopaminergic toxicity induced by METH exposure might be attributed to this METH-induced generation of OONO⁻. In summary, we conclude that METH causes cell death and dopaminergic toxicity in NGF-differentiated PC12 cells by the generation of peroxynitrite. Further studies are needed to clarify the role of peroxynitrite in mediating METH-induced dopaminergic neurotoxicity both *in vitro* and *in vivo*.

ACKNOWLEDGMENTS

This research was supported in part by an appointment (S.Z.I) to the Research Participation Program at the National Center for Toxicological Research administered by the Oak Ridge Institute of Science and Education through an interagency agreement between the U.S. Department of Energy and the U.S. Food and Drug Administration.

REFERENCES

1. ALI, S.F. *et al.* 1994. Low environmental temperature or pharmacologic agents that produce hypothermia decrease methamphetamine neurotoxicity in mice. Brain Res. **658:** 33–38.
2. SIEDEN, L.S. & G.A. RICUARTE. 1987. Neurotoxicity of methamphetamine and related drugs. *In* Psychopharmacology: The Third Generation of Progress. H.Y. Meltzer, ed.: 359–366. Raven Press. New York.
3. ITZHAK, Y., C. GANDIA, P.L. HAUNG & S.F. ALI. 1998. Resistance to neuronal nitric oxide synthase deficient mice to methamphetamine-induced dopaminergic neurotoxicity *in vivo*. J. Pharmacol. Exp. Ther. **284:** 1040–1047.
4. DI MONTE, D.A., J.E. ROYLAND, M.W. JAKOWEC & J.W. LANGSTON. 1996. Role of nitric oxide in methamphetamine neurotoxicity: protection by 7-nitroindazole, an inhibitor of neuronal nitric oxide synthase. J. Neurochem. **67:** 2443–2450.
5. ITZHAK, Y. & S.F. ALI. 1996. The neuronal nitric oxide synthase inhibitor, 7-nitroindazole, protect against methamphetamine-induced neurotoxicity *in vivo*. J. Neurochem. **67:** 1770–1773.
6. CADET, J.L. & C. BRANNOCK. 1998. Free radicals and pathobiology of brain dopamine systems. Neurochem. Int. **32:** 117–131.
7. CADET, J.L. *et al.* 1994. Attenuation of methamphetamine-induced neurotoxicity in copper/zinc superoxide dismutase in transgenic mice. J. Neurochem. **62:** 380–383.
8. CADET, J.L., S.F. ALI, R.B. ROTHMAN & C.J. EPSTIEN. 1995. Neurotoxicity, drugs of abuse, and the cuzn-superoxide dismutase in transgenic mice. Mol. Neurobiol. **11:** 155–163.
9. RADI, R., J.S. BECKMAN, K.M. BUSH & B.A. FREEMAN. 1991. Peroxynitrite-induced membrane lipid peroxidation: the cytotoxic potential of superoxide and nitric oxide. Arch. Biochem. Biophys. **288:** 481–487.
10. RUBBO, H. *et al.* 1994. Nitric oxide regulation of superoxide and peroxynitrite-dependent lipid peroxidation: formation of novel nitrogen-containing lipid derivatives. J. Biol. Chem. **269:** 26066–26075.
11. VAN DER VLIET, A. *et al.* 1994. Aromatic hydroxylation and nitration of phenylalanine and tyrosine by peroxynitrite: evidence for hydroxyl radical production from peroxynitrite. FEBS Lett. **339:** 89–92.
12. MARLA, S.S., J. LEE & J.T. GROVES. 1994. Peroxynitrite rapidly permeates phospholipid membranes. Proc. Natl. Acad. Sci. USA **94:** 14243–14248.
13. CUBELLS, J. F., S. RAYPORT, G. RAYNDRION & D. SULZER. 1994. Methamphetamine neurotoxicity involves vacuolation of endocytic organelles and dopamine-dependent intracellular oxidative stress. J. Neurosci. **14:** 2260–2271.
14. HOM, D.G. *et al.* 1997. Elevated expression of glutathione peroxidase in PC12 cells results in protection against methamphetamine but not MPTP toxicity. Mol. Brain Res. **46:** 154–160.
15. RONG, P., A.M. BENNIE, W.R. EPA & G.L. Barrett. 1999. Nerve growth factor determines survival and death of PC12 cells by regulation of the bcl-x, bax, and caspase-3 genes. J. Neurochem. **72:** 2294–2300.
16. HENSLEY, K. *et al.* 1996. Quantitation of protein-bound 3-nitrotyrosine and 3,4-dihydroxyphenylalanine by high-performance liquid chromatography with electrochemical detection. Anal. Biochem. **251:** 187–195.

17. IMAM, S.Z. & S.F. ALI. 2000. SF (2000) Selenium, an antioxidant, attenuates metham-phetamine-induced dopaminergic-neurotoxicity and peroxynitrite generation. Brain Res. **855:** 186–191.
18. LOWRY, O.H., N.J. ROSEBROUGH, A.L. FARR & R.J. RANDALL. 1951. Protein measure-ment with the folin phenol reagent. J. Biol. Chem. **193:** 265–275.
19. ANDERSEN, J.K., D.M. FRIM, O. ISACSON & X.O. BREAKFIELD. 1994. Catecholaminergic cell atrophy in a transgenic mouse aberrantly overexpressing MAO-B in neurons. Neurodegeneration **3:** 97–109.
20. HIRSCH, E.C. 1992. Why are nigral catecholaminergic neurons more vulnerable than other cells in Parkinson's disease. Ann. Neurol. **32** (Suppl): S88–S93.
21. BECKMAN, J.S., M. CARSON, C.D. SMITH & W.H. Koppenol. 1993. ALS, SOD and per-oxynitrite. Nature **364:** 584.
22. LIPTON, S.A. P.A. ROSENBERG. 1994. Excitatory amino acids as a final common path-way for neurologic disorders. N. Engl. J. Med. **330:** 613–622.
23. PRYOR, W.A., X. JIN & G.L. SQUADRITO. 1994. One- and two-electron oxidations of methionine by peroxynitrite. Proc. Natl. Acad. Sci. USA **91:** 11173–11177.
24. GREEN, L.A. & G. REIN. 1977. Release, storage, and uptake of catecholamines by a clonal cell line of nerve growth factor responsive pheochromocytoma cells. Brain Res. **129:** 247–263.
25. REBOIS, R.V., E.E. REYNOLDS, L. TOLL & B.D. HOWARD. 1980. Storage of dopamine and acetylcholine in granules of PC12, a clonal pheochromocytoma cell line. Bio-chemistry **19:** 1240–1248.
26. SULTZER, D. 1992. Weak base model of amphetamine action. Ann. N.Y. Acad. Sci. **654:** 525–528.
27. ISCHIROPOULOS, H., D. DURAN & J. HORWITZ. 1995. Peroxynitrite-mediated inhibition of DOPA synthesis in PC12 cells. J. Neurochem. **65:** 2366–2372.
28. ARA, J. *et al.* 1998. H. Inactivation of tyrosine hydroxylase by nitration following exposure to peroxynitrite and 1-methyl-4-phenyl-1,2,3,6-tetrahydropyridine (MPTP). Proc. Natl. Acad. Sci. USA **95:** 7659–7663.
29. SIEDEN, L.S., M.W. FISCHMAN & C.R. SCHUSTER. 1975. Long-term methamphetamine induced changes in brain catecholamines in tolerant rhesus monkeys. Drug Alcohol Depend. **1:** 215–219.
30. SULTZER, D., N.T. MAIDMENT & S. RAYPORT. 1993. Amphetamine and other weak bases act to promote reverse transport of dopamine in ventral midbrain neurons. J. Neurochem. **60:** 527–535.
31. FULLER, R.W. & S.K. HEMRICK-LUECKE. 1982. Further studies on the long-term deple-tion of striatal dopamine in iprindole-treated rats by amphetamine. Neuropharmacol-ogy **21:** 433–438.
32. GIBB, J.W. & F.J. KOGAN 1979. Influence of dopamine synthesis on methamphetamine-induced changes in striatal and adrenal tyrosine hydroxylase activity. Naunyn Schmiedeberg's Arch Pharmacol. **310:** 185–187.
33. SCHMIDT, C.J. *et al.* 1985. Role of dopamine in the neurotoxic effects of methamphet-amine. J. Pharmacol. Exp. Ther. **233:** 539–544.
34. SHENG, P., C. CERRUTI, S.F. ALI & J.L. CADET. 1996. Nitric oxide is a mediator of methamphetamine-induced neurotoxicity: *in vitro* evidence from primary cultures of mesencephalic cells, Ann. N.Y. Acad. Sci. **801:** 174–187.

Neurotoxicity of Diethylpropion

Neurochemical and Behavioral Findings in Rats

SONIA GALVAN-ARZATE AND ABEL SANTAMARIA

Departamento de Neuroquímica, Instituto Nacional de Neurología y Neurocirugía Manuel Velasco Suárez, S.S.A. México D.F. 14269, México

ABSTRACT: The effects of diethylpropion (DEP), an amphetamine derivative and a well-known anorectic agent, on different neurochemical and behavioral markers of toxicity in rats were evaluated. Animals received a daily dose of DEP (5 mg/kg po) for 15 days, and all tests were performed 24 hours after the last DEP administration. As neurochemical markers, the brain regional levels of some amino acids, such as aspartate (Asp), glutamate (Glu), gamma-aminobutyric acid (GABA), and glutamine (Gln), as well as the brain regional rates of lipid peroxidation as a current index of oxidative stress were measured. As behavioral markers, the actions of DEP on both mercaptopropionic acid (MPA)-induced seizures and kainic acid (KA)-induced wet-dog body shakes were explored to investigate whether DEP induces behavioral sensitization to the effects of agents affecting the central activity of neuroactive amino acids. Treatment with DEP produced significant changes in the levels of Asp in the hypothalamus (Ht) and cortex (Cx); Glu in the Ht, Cx, midbrain (Mb), and striatum (S); and Gln in the Cx. The regional levels of GABA remain unchanged. Lipid peroxidation was increased in the hippocampus (Hc), Mb, and S. Also, latency to the first seizure induced by MPA (1.2 mmol/kg ip) and the total number of wet-dog body shakes induced by KA (10 mg/kg ip) were significantly affected by DEP treatment. These findings suggest that low doses of DEP may affect different neurochemical substrates, inducing changes in neuroactive amino acids along the brain regions, probably involving dopamine release. Consequently, behavioral changes could be the result of excitotoxic events related to excessive Glu or lack of an inhibitory process. Also, DEP is thought to involve free radical formation and oxidative stress as potential features of its regional pattern of neurotoxicity, as evidenced by lipid peroxidation.

KEYWORDS: diethylpropion; neurotoxicity; brain regions; amino acids; oxidative damage; behavioral changes

INTRODUCTION

As well-known sympathomimetic drugs, amphetamine and derivatives may produce severe neurologic alterations, such as intracerebral vasculitis, ischemic stroke,

Address for correspondence: Abel Santamaría, Departamento de Neuroquímica, Instituto Nacional de Neurología y Neurocirugía Manuel Velasco Suárez, S.S.A. Insurgentes Sur # 3877, México D.F. 14269, México. Voice: (+525)606-3822; fax: (+525)528-0095.
absada@yahoo.com

Ann. N.Y. Acad. Sci. 965: 214–224 (2002). © 2002 New York Academy of Sciences.

and cerebral hemorrhage.[1] Because some neurochemical features of amphetamine toxicity include the release of newly synthesized dopamine (DA)[2,3] and increased extracellular levels of other neurotransmitters and neuromodulators, such as serotonin,[4] acetylcholine,[5] and excitatory and inhibitory amino acids,[6,7] it is likely that substituted amphetamines might evoke similar actions in the brain.

Diethylpropion (DEP), also known as amfepramone, is an amphetamine-like anorectic drug and psychostimulant.[8] It has been suggested that DEP may exert its effects in the brain through both catecholamine pathways[9] and dopamine and/or opioid receptor stimulation.[10] Moreover, as a centrally acting appetite-suppressing agent, DEP has frequently been employed to treat obesity.[10,11] DEP has been also tested, unsuccessfully, as an alternative therapeutic drug to attenuate cocaine cue-induced craving and as a potential drug to develop medication with cocaine-agonist properties.[12] However, despite its many clinical applications and its apparent lack of toxic neuropsychological actions,[8] still only limited information is available on its side effects and its pattern of toxicity in the brain at experimental level.

In a previous study by our group, we addressed preliminary findings on some neurochemical and behavioral markers of toxicity induced by DEP in rats.[13] To provide further information on the possible mechanisms of neurotoxicity elicited by DEP on different neurochemical substrates in the brain, we exposed rats to a subchronic daily dose of DEP to investigate its effects on regional brain levels of neuroactive amino acids such as aspartate (Asp), glutamate (Glu), gamma-aminobutyric acid (GABA), and glutamine (Gln), measured by HPLC. Additionally, since free radical formation and oxidative stress have currently been associated with cytotoxicity[14,15] and excitotoxic events,[16,17] we also evaluated whether DEP can induce lipid peroxidation as an index of oxidative stress probably associated with its general pattern of toxicity. The actions of DEP on different behavioral parameters of excitotoxic injury induced by either kainic acid (a well-known glutamate agonist and excitotoxin able to produce wet-dog body shakes and prolonged convulsive stages in rats)[18] or mercaptopropionic acid (an excitotoxic compound able to depress synthesis of the inhibitory neurotransmitter GABA by blocking the activity of glutamate decarboxylase)[19] were also studied, because both of these molecules are useful experimental tools to indicate excitotoxicity.

MATERIAL AND METHODS

Animals. Adult male Wistar rats (200–250 g) were used throughout the study. Animals were housed five per cage in acrylic cages and provided with water and food *ad libitum.* The room was maintained under constant conditions of temperature (25 ± 3°C), humidity (50 ± 10%), and light (12:12 light:dark cycles).

Reagents and Experimental Procedures. Deionized water was used for preparation of all reagents and solutions, except for DEP, which was prepared in drinking water. DEP was purchased from Neobes Medix (Mexico). Kainic acid (KA), 3-mercaptopropionic acid (MPA), 2-mercaptoethanol, *o*-phthaldialdehyde (OPA), and a kit of HPLC-grade L-amino acids were all obtained from Sigma Chemical Co. (St. Louis, MO). Rats (10 per experimental group) received either water by mouth or an oral daily dose of DEP 5 mg/kg for 15 days. Body weight was recorded every day.

Twenty-four hours after the last DEP dose, behavioral and biochemical tests were applied to all groups.

Measurement of Amino Acids. The brain regional content of neuroactive amino acids was measured using HPLC with fluorometric detection, according to reported methods.[20–22] Twenty-four hours after the last DEP dose, animals from two groups (controls and DEP-treated animals) were injected with MPA (1.2 mmol/kg iv) to prevent a postmortem increase in GABA.[19] Two minutes later, rats were sacrificed by decapitation, their brains dissected out, and the following regions separated: hypothalamus (Ht), medulla oblongata (Mo), hippocampus (Hc), pons (P), cortex (Cx), midbrain (Mb), and striatum (S). Tissue samples were then weighed, immediately sonicated in 15 volumes of a methanol:water mixture (85%), and centrifuged (3000 g for 15 minutes). Aliquots of the supernatants were stored at −65°C until the corresponding chromatographic analysis was performed. For the precolumn derivatization procedure, volumes of 100 µl of samples were added with 100 µl of the *o*-phthalaldehyde (OPA) reagent (containing 5 mg OPA + 625 µl methanol + 5.6 ml borate buffer 0.4 M, pH 9.5 + 25 µl 2-mercaptoethanol). After stirring for 1 minute, 20 µl of the mixture were injected with a 25-µl Hamilton microsyringe into a Perkin-Elmer Series 3B chromatograph with a Beckman 157 fluorescence detector. An OPA-HS Alltech reversed-phase column with a 3-µm particle size was employed. Linear gradient programming was used to elute OPA-amino acids from 10–65% methanol. The gradient mixture consisted of (a) 50 mM sodium acetate aqueous buffer solution (pH 5.9) containing 1.5% v/v of tetrahydrofuran, and (b) HPLC-grade methanol as solvent. Amino acids analyzed by this method were Asp, Glu, GABA, and Gln.

Assay of Lipid Peroxidation. Lipid peroxidation (LP), a current index of oxidative stress, was measured in brain tissue samples 24 hours after the last DEP dose using a modified method of chloroform extraction based on the detection of fluorescent pigments derived from peroxidized lipids.[23] After sacrifice by decapitation and dissection of brains, aliquots of rat brain tissue samples (1 ml) were added with 4 ml of a chloroform-methanol mixture (2:1, v:v). After phase separation, luminescence of the chloroform layer was measured in a Perkin-Elmer LS50B luminescence spectrophotometer at 370 nm of excitation and 430 nm of emission wave lengths. Results were expressed as relative fluorescence units (FU) per gram of wet tissue.

Behavioral Tests. Twenty-four hours after the last DEP dose was administered, animals from two independent groups (controls and DEP-treated animals) were injected either with KA (10 mg/kg ip)[18] or MPA (1.2 mmol/kg ip).[19,22] Because KA can produce wet-dog body shakes in rats after excitotoxic injury and MPA may induce seizures by a mechanism related to brain GABA depletion, in this study both reagents were employed to evaluate possible sensitization of either KA-induced body shakes or MPA-induced seizures after DEP administration. For these purposes, the latency of onset to the first wet-dog body shake and the total number of body shakes over 120 minutes were recorded in KA-treated rats; for MPA treatment, the latency of onset to the first seizure and the duration of seizures were recorded. Other general aspects, such as mortality and body weight gain of DEP-treated rats, were also recorded.

Statistical Analysis. Statistical analysis was performed using Student's t test for comparison of both amino acid contents and levels of lipid peroxidation between

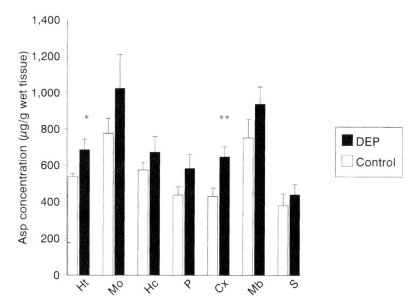

FIGURE 1. Effect of diethylpropion (DEP) on brain regional levels of aspartate (Asp) in rats. Animals received a daily dose of 5 mg/kg DEP orally for 15 days. Twenty-four hours later, the following brain regions were dissected out: hypothalamus (Ht), medulla oblongata (Mo), hippocampus (Hc), pons (P), cortex (Cx), midbrain (Mb), and striatum (S). Levels of Asp were measured in all regions by HPLC with fluorometric detection. Results are expressed as μg per gram of wet tissue. Mean values ± SEM of 10 rats/group. *$p < 0.05$ and **$p < 0.01$, statistical differences from control group; Student's t test.

DEP-treated rats and control animals. For behavioral data analysis we used Mann-Whitney's U test. P values less than 0.05 were considered statistically significant.

RESULTS

Effect of DEP on Brain Regional Content of Amino Acids. FIGURE 1 shows the effect of DEP on brain regional levels of aspartate in rats. Aspartate concentrations were significantly increased in Ht (27%) and Cx (50%) as compared to control values. Brain regional levels of glutamate after DEP administration to rats are shown in FIGURE 2. Glutamate was significantly increased in Ht (47%), Cx (73%), Mb (56%), and S (29%). FIGURE 3 shows brain levels of GABA from DEP-treated rats. No significant changes were found in GABA concentrations along all regions analyzed. Finally, glutamine contents in brain regions (FIG. 4) were significantly increased after DEP treatment only in the Cx (75%).

Effect of DEP on Brain Regional Lipid Peroxidation. The action of DEP on brain regional lipid peroxidation is shown in FIGURE 5. Among brain regions, Cx exhibited lower basal levels of lipid peroxidation (8.79 FU/g tissue), whereas Ht exhibited

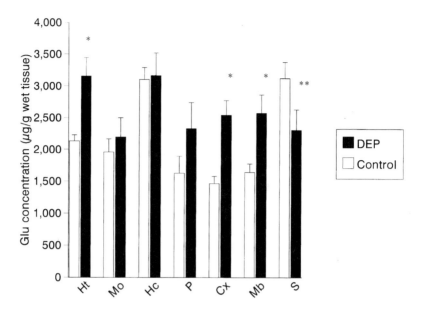

FIGURE 2. Effect of diethylpropion (DEP) on brain regional levels of glutamate (Glu) in rats. Levels of Glu were measured in all regions by HPLC with fluorometric detection. Results are expressed as μg per gram of wet tissue. Mean values ± SEM of 10 rats/group. $*p < 0.05$ and $**p < 0.01$, statistical differences from control group; Student's t test. Data were partially presented as preliminary results in the *Proceedings of the Western Pharmacology Society.*[13]

TABLE 1. Behavioral parameters of diethylpropion toxicity in rats

Treatment	Mortality	Body weight gain (g)	Latency to first MPA-induced seizure	Latency to first KA-induced shake (min)[a]	Duration of seizures (min)	Total number of shakes (in 120 min)
Contro	0/10	25.41 ± 6.62	4.00 ± 0.75	22.02 ± 6.31	17.50 ± 1.04	38.33 ± 7.79
DEP	1/10	21.83 ± 9.38	2.79 ± 0.32*	23.90 ± 4.27	16.02 ± 2.12	50.06 ± 10.67*

NOTE: Mean values ± SEM of 10 animals per group. Rats received either water by mouth (control) or a daily dose of diethylpropion (DEP) 5 mg/kg for 15 days. Body weight gain was recorded at the end of treatment. Mercaptopropionic acid (MPA; 1.2 mmol/kg ip) and kainic acid (KA; 10 mg/kg ip) were administered to animals on day 16. Duration of MPA-induced seizures and the total number of KA-induced wet-dog body shakes were both recorded for 120 minutes starting immediately after toxin injection.

$*p < 0.05$, significantly different from control group; U of Mann-Whitney's test.
[a]Data partially presented as preliminary results in the *Proceedings of the Western Pharmacology Society.*[13]

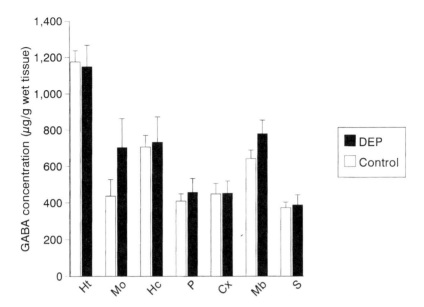

FIGURE 3. Effect of diethylpropion (DEP) on brain regional levels of gamma-aminobutyric acid (GABA) in rats. Levels of GABA were measured in all regions by HPLC with fluorometric detection. Results are expressed as μg per gram of wet tissue. Mean values ± SEM of 10 rats/group. Data were partially presented as preliminary results in the *Proceedings of the Western Pharmacology Society*.[13]

higher basal levels (259.26 FU/g tissue). Lipid peroxidation was significantly increased in Hc (75%), Mb (37%), and S (30%), compared with control values.

Effect of DEP on Behavioral Markers. Mortality, body weight gain, and some behavioral markers of toxicity after DEP administration to rats are all shown in TABLE 1. Exploratory behavior was slightly increased in DEP-treated animals. The control group exhibited no mortality throughout the experiments, whereas 1 rat of 10 die in the DEP-treated group. Although the DEP-treated group exhibited an average tendency to decrease body weight gain, as compared with the control group (−15%), no significant differences were found. In the groups treated with MPA, we found a significant decrease in the latency to the first seizure (−30%) after DEP treatment. The total number of wet-dog body shakes induced by KA was also increased in DEP-treated animals compared with the control group (31%), whereas the duration of MPA-induced seizures and the latency to the first KA-induced shake both remain unchanged.

DISCUSSION

The major findings in this work were the enhanced levels of two excitatory amino acids, Asp and Glu, in the hypothalamus, cortex, and midbrain as well as the increased rates of lipid peroxidation in the hippocampus, midbrain, and striatum after

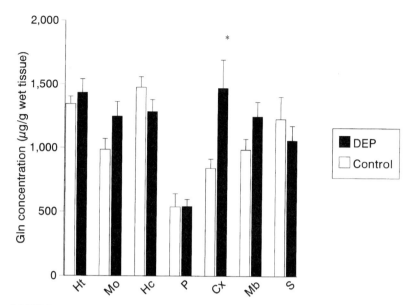

FIGURE 4. Effect of diethylpropion (DEP) on brain regional levels of glutamine (Gln) in rats. Levels of Gln were measured in all regions by HPLC with fluorometric detection. Results are expressed as μg per gram of wet tissue. Mean values ± SEM of 10 rats/group. *$p < 0.01$, statistical differences from control group; Student's t test.

the exposure of rats to subchronic administration of DEP. These results suggest primary release of dopamine in the brain, which in turn might mediate the release of amino acids in remote areas, as has been reported for amphetamine.[4,6] We also suggest an active role of free radicals and oxidative stress in DEP toxicity, as evidenced by lipid peroxidation. The behavioral sensitization induced by DEP on both the latency to the first MPA-induced seizure and the total number of KA-induced wet-dog body shakes was also considered a remarkable finding and evidence of potential excitotoxicity.

The psychostimulant DEP has commonly been employed as a "short-term use" treatment in the management of obesity because of its well-known anorectic effects.[11,24] Despite the suggestion by some investigators that the lack of neurotoxic effects can be detected with standardized neuropsychological tests,[8] DEP is not lacking in neurotoxic effects at all, as evidenced by this study and others.[9,25] Moreover, DEP has become a major public health problem in countries such as Brazil, where combined anorectic-alcohol misuse leads to severe stimulating effects on the nervous system.[10]

DEP has been reported to exert its effects on the brain mainly through dopaminergic[25] and catecholaminergic pathways,[9] although the opioid system was also recently implicated in combined DEP-ethanol toxicity.[10] Recently, Reimer and coworkers[9] described the ability of DEP, as a psychomotor stimulant, to induce conditional place preferences, conditional behaviors, and behavioral sensitization in

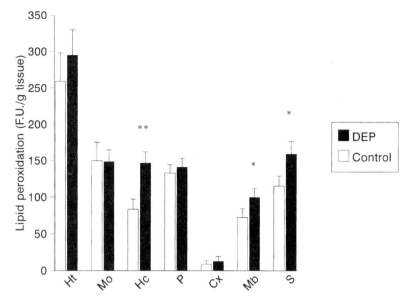

FIGURE 5. Effect of diethylpropion (DEP) on brain regional lipid peroxidation in rats. Animals received a daily dose of 5 mg/kg DEP orally for 15 days. Twenty-four hours later, the following brain regions were dissected out: hypothalamus (Ht), medulla oblongata (Mo), hippocampus (Hc), pons (P), cortex (Cx), midbrain (Mb), and striatum (S). Lipid peroxidation was measured by detection of fluorescent pigments derived from peroxidized lipids and expressed as relative fluorescence units (FU) per gram of wet tissue. Mean values ± SEM of 10 rats/group. $*p < 0.05$ and $**p < 0.01$, statistical differences from control group; Student's t test.

rats. They tested different doses of DEP (10, 20, and 40 mg/kg ip) for 36 days and found that 10 mg/kg produced conditional locomotion, place preferences, and rearing. These investigators also found changes in the levels of some monoamines and metabolites. Shortly thereafter, Planeta and coworkers[25] reported again the conditioning place preference after DEP treatment in rats to evaluate the reinforcing properties of this drug. On testing doses of 10, 15, and 20 mg/kg, they found that only a 15-mg/kg dose produced significant place preferences. Also, the use of SCH 23,390, a D1 antagonist, but not D2 antagonists, blocked DEP-induced conditioned place preferences, pointing out the participation of selective dopaminergic pathways in DEP effects. In 1999, Gevaerd and coworkers[10] demonstrated the participation of dopaminergic and/or opioid pathways in the locomotor activity produced by the combination of DEP-ethanol, when DEP was administered at 5 mg/kg. It is important to note that higher doses of DEP or doses similar to those employed in this work produce behavioral alterations involving different neurochemical substrates and, therefore, several possible mechanisms of toxicity.

This is, to our knowledge, the first study suggesting a potential role of excitotoxic effects induced by DEP and mediated by excitatory amino acids, as evidenced by increased levels of aspartate and glutamate in some brain regions as well as sensitization of KA-induced behavior, or lack of inhibitory events, as evidenced by sensitization of MPA-induced behavior. It is known that any excess of excitatory amino acids in the brain, particularly glutamate, represents a potential risk for excitotoxic events and neurodegenerative processes,[16,17] and so the enhanced levels of these two amino acids in some brain regions could be mediating biochemical and behavioral alterations in DEP-treated rats. These considerations are reinforced by our own behavioral findings, because KA, an excitotoxic molecule, is acting through the direct activation of glutamate receptors,[18] eventually involving this pathway. Moreover, the assumed decreased levels of GABA induced by MPA[19] and the corresponding effect of DEP on MPA-induced behavior could also suggest the lack of inhibitory effects and the possible implication of the GABAergic pathway in DEP toxicity. Furthermore, it has been shown that MK-801, an N-methyl-D-aspartate (NMDA) subtype of glutamate of receptor antagonist, can attenuate the methamphetamine-induced[26] and amphetamine-induced[27] dopamine depletion; consequently, as an amphetamine-like drug, it is likely that DEP might be evoking the same effects in the brain. However, with the actual results, we are unable to reject the possibility that our observations could merely be a secondary effect derived from the primary release of dopamine with the subsequent remote release of amino acids, as occurs during amphetamine administration.[6] Therefore, the question of whether DEP toxicity involves direct excitotoxic processes mediated by glutamatergic and/or GABAergic pathways remains to be tested in further studies.

On the other hand, our findings also suggest that DEP can induce oxidative stress and free radical formation as part of its pattern of neurotoxicity. Oxidative stress is a complex of deleterious events, leading to cell death preceded by a cascade of toxic insults. Lipid peroxidation, a current expression of oxidative stress, involves the direct reaction of oxygen-derived and nitrogen-derived radicals with membrane lipids to form free radical intermediates and semistable peroxides.[28] Lipid peroxidation is damaging to cells because of the subsequent chain reactions produced by free radicals, such as peroxyl and hydroxyl radicals, in biologic substrates. Thus, it was not surprising at all to find increased rates of lipid peroxidation in some brain regions after DEP administration, because it has been demonstrated that other amphetamine derivatives, such as methamphetamine, involve free radical-mediated mechanisms as part of their toxicity and such an oxidative insult is thought to occur before the dopaminergic toxicity. Therefore, it is likely that chemically related drugs, such as DEP, might share similar mechanisms of injury, but this consideration must be supported by further studies. Moreover, the susceptibility exhibited by the hippocampus and striatum to DEP-induced lipid peroxidation seems to have no direct relation to the levels of aspartate or glutamate in the same brain regions, because the latter remain unchanged. This agrees with the aforementioned observations[29,30] that methamphetamine-induced oxidative stress occurs even before dopaminergic toxicity and other events, suggesting that during amphetamine toxicity, free radical production and oxidative damage can trigger processes of general damage. However, evidence in this work is insufficient to reject the possibility that early dopamine-mediated excitatory amino acid release during the first stages of DEP toxicity might partially account for the observed behavioral excitotoxicity and lipid peroxidation. These considerations deserve further investigation.

In summary, whatever mechanisms are involved in DEP toxicity, it is clear, in light of our findings, that potential excitotoxic events as well as oxidative stress both actively participate in DEP actions on the central nervous system. More studies employing higher doses or longer periods of exposure would help to support or discard these observations.

ACKNOWLEDGMENTS

This work was supported by the Consejo Nacional de Ciencia y Tecnología (CONACyT), Grant J28612-M, México. The authors wish to express gratitude to Dr. Syed F. Ali for helpful discussion.

REFERENCES

1. AASLY, J. *et al.* 1993. Minor structural brain changes in young drug abusers. Acta Neurol. Scand. **87:** 210–214.
2. CALDWELL, J. 1980. Amphetamines and related stimulants: some introductory remarks. *In* Amphetamines and Related Stimulants: Chemical, Biological and Sociological Aspects. J. Caldwell, Ed. :1–12. CRC Press. Boca Raton, FL.
3. BUTCHER, S.P., I.S. FAIRBROTHER, J.S. KELLY, *et al.* 1988. Amphetamine-induced dopamine release in the rat striatum: an *in vivo* microdialysis study. J. Neurochem. **50:** 346–355.
4. KUCZENSKI, R. & D. SEGAL. 1989. Concomitant characterization of behavioral and striatal neurotransmitters response to amphetamine using *in vivo* microdialysis. J. Neurosci. **9:** 2051–2065.
5. GUIX, T., Y.L. HURD & U. UNGERSTEDT. 1992. Amphetamine enhances extracellular concentrations of dopamine and acetylcholine in dorsolateral striatum and nucleus accumbens of freely moving rats. Neurosci. Lett. **138:** 137–140.
6. PORRAS, A. & F. MORA. 1993. Dopamine receptor antagonist blocks the release of glycine, GABA, and taurine produced by amphetamine. Brain Res. Bull. **31:** 305–310.
7. XUE, CH.-J. *et al.* 1996. Acute and repeated systemic amphetamine administration: effects on extracellular glutamate, aspartate, and serine levels in rat ventral tegmental area and nucleus accumbens. J. Neurochem. **67:** 352–363.
8. OLLO, C. *et al.* 1996. Lack of neurotoxic effect of diethylpropion in crack-cocaine abusers. Clin. Neuropharmacol. **19:** 52–58.
9. REIMER, A.R. *et al.* 1995. Conditioned place preferences, conditioned locomotion, and behavioral sensitization occur in rats treated with diethylpropion. Pharmacol. Biochem. Behav. **51:** 89–96.
10. GEVAERD, M.S., E.T. SULTOWSKI & R.N. TAKAHASHI. 1999. Combined effects of diethylpropion and alcohol on locomotor activity of mice: participation of the dopaminergic and opioid systems. Braz. J. Med. Biol. Res. **32:** 1545–1550.
11. POSTON, W.S. *et al.* 1998. Challenges in obesity management. South. Med. J. **91:** 710–720.
12. ALIM, T.N. *et al.* 1995. Diethylpropion pharmacotherapeutic adjuvant therapy for inpatient treatment of cocaine dependence: a test of the cocaine-agonist hypothesis. Clin. Neuropharmacol. **18:** 183–195.
13. MARTÍNEZ, M. *et al.* 1998. The action of anfepramone on neurochemical and behavioral markers in rats. *In* Proceedings of the Western Pharmacology Society. Vol. 41: 125. The Western Pharmacology Society. Mazatlán, México.
14. KEHRER, J.P. 1993. Free radicals as mediators of tissue injury and disease. Crit. Rev. Toxicol. **23:** 21–48.
15. NAKAZAWA, H., C. GENKA & M. FUJISHIMA. 1996. Pathological aspects of active oxygens/free radicals. Jap. J. Physiol. **46:** 15–32.

16. BONDY, S.C. & D.K. LEE. 1993. Oxidative stress induced by glutamate receptor agonists. Brain Res. **610:** 229–233.
17. COYLE, J.T. & P. PUTTFARCKEN. 1993. Oxidative stress, glutamate, and neurodegenerative disorders. Science **262:** 689–694.
18. SPERK, G. *et al.* 1983. Kainic acid-induced seizures: neurochemical and histopathological changes. Neuroscience **10:** 1301–1315.
19. VAN DER HEYDEN, J.A.M. & J. KORF. 1978. Regional levels of GABA in the brain: rapid semiautomated assay and prevention of postmortem increase by 3-marcaptopropionic acid. J. Neurochem. **31:** 197–203.
20. FLEURY, M.O. & D.V. ASHLEY. 1983. High-performance liquid chromatography analysis of amino acids in physiological fluids: on line precolumn derivatization with o-phthaldialdehyde. Anal. Biochem. **133:** 330–335.
21. SMITH, R.J. & K.A. PANICO. 1985. Automated analysis of o-phthalaldehyde derivatives of amino acids in physiological fluids by reverse phase high performance liquid chromatography. J. Liquid Chromatogr. **8:** 1783–1795.
22. SANTAMARÍA, A. *et al.* 1996. Systemic DL-kynurenine and probenecid pretreatment attenuates quinolinic acid-induced neurotoxicity in rats. Neuropharmacology **35:** 23–28.
23. SANTAMARÍA, A. & C. RÍOS. 1993. MK-801, an *N*-methyl-D-aspartate receptor antagonist, blocks quinolinic acid-induced lipid peroxidation in rat corpus striatum. Neurosci. Lett. **159:** 51–54.
24. DONNA, R.H. 2000. Use of sibutramine and other noradrenergic and serotonergic drugs in the management of obesity. Endocrine **13:** 193–199.
25. PLANETA, C.S. & R. DE LUCIA. 1998. Involvement of dopamine receptors in diethylpropion-induced conditioning place preference. Braz. J. Med. Biol. Res. **31:** 561–564.
26. SONSALLA, P.K., W.J. NICKLAS & R.E. HEIKKILA. 1989. Role of excitatory amino acids in methamphetamine-induced nigrostriatal dopaminergic toxicity. Science **243:** 398–400.
27. HENDERSON, M.G., S. HEMRICK-LUECKE & R.W. FULLER. 1992. MK-801 protects against amphetamine-induced striatal dopamine depletion in iprindole-treated rats, but not against brain serotonin depletion after p-chloroamphetamine administration. Ann. N.Y. Acad. Sci. **648:** 286–288.
28. GUTTERIDGE, J.M.C. & B. HALLIWELL. 1990. The measurement and mechanism of lipid peroxidation in biological systems. TIBS **15:** 129–135.
29. CADET, J.L. *et al.* 1994. Attenuation of methamphetamine-induced neurotoxicity in copper/zinc superoxide dismutase transgenic mice. J. Neurochem. **62:** 380–383.
30. IMAM, S.Z. *et al.* 1999. Methamphetamine generates peroxynitrite and produces dopaminergic neurotoxicity in mice: protective effects of peroxynitirte decomposition catalyst. Brain Res. **837:** 15–21.

The Protective Role of L-Carnitine against Neurotoxicity Evoked by Drug of Abuse, Methamphetamine, Could Be Related to Mitochondrial Dysfunction

ASHRAF VIRMANI,[a] FRANCO GAETANI,[a] SYED IMAM,[b]
ZBIGNIEW BINIENDA,[b] AND SYED ALI[b]

[a]*Research and Development, Sigma tau–HealthScience, Pomezia 00040, Italy*

[b]*Neurochemistry Laboratory, Division of Neurotoxicology, National Center for Toxicological Research, Food and Drug Administration, Jefferson, Arkansas, USA*

ABSTRACT: There is growing evidence that suggests that brain injury after amphetamine and methamphetamine (METH) administration is due to an increase in free radical formation and mitochondrial damage, which leads to a failure of cellular energy metabolism followed by a secondary excitotoxicity. Neuronal degeneration caused by drugs of abuse is also associated with decreased ATP synthesis. Defective mitochondrial oxidative phosphorylation and metabolic compromise also play an important role in atherogenesis, in the pathogenesis of Alzheimer's disease, Parkinson's disease, diabetes, and aging. The energy deficits in the central nervous system can lead to the generation of reactive oxygen and nitrogen species as indicated by increased activity of the free radical scavenging enzymes like catalase and superoxide dismutase. The METH-induced dopaminergic neurotoxicity may be mediated by the generation of peroxynitrite and can be protected by antioxidants selenium, melatonin, and selective nNOS inhibitor, 7-nitroindazole. L-Carnitine (LC) is well known to carry long-chain fatty acyl groups into mitochondria for β-oxidation. It also plays a protective role in 3-nitropropioinc acid (3-NPA)-induced neurotoxicity as demonstrated *in vitro* and *in vivo*. LC has also been utilized in detoxification efforts in fatty acid–related metabolic disorders.
    In this study we have tested the hypothesis that enhancement of mitochondrial energy metabolism by LC could prevent the generation of peroxynitrite and free radicals produced by METH. Adult male C57BL/6N mice were divided into four groups. Group I served as control. Groups III and IV received LC (100 mg/kg, orally) for one week. Groups II and IV received 4 × 10 mg/kg METH i.p. at 2-h intervals after one week of LC administration. LC treatment continued for one more week to groups III and IV. One week after METH administration, mice were sacrificed by decapitation, and striatum was dissected to measure the formation of 3-nitrotyrosine (3-NT) by HPLC/Coularry system. METH treatment produced significant formation of 3-NT, a marker of peroxynitrite generation, in mice striatum.

Address for correspondence: Ashraf Virmani, Sigma tau-HealthScience, Pomezia 00040, Italy.

Ann. N.Y. Acad. Sci. 965: 225–232 (2002). © 2002 New York Academy of Sciences.

The pre- and post-treatment of mice with LC significantly attenuated the production of 3-NT in the striatum resulting from METH treatment. The protective effects by the compound LC in this study could be related to the prevention of the possible metabolic compromise by METH and the resulting energy deficits that lead to the generation of reactive oxygen and nitrogen species. These data further confirm our hypothesis that METH-induced neurotoxicity is mediated by the production of peroxynitrite, and LC may reduce the peroxynitrite levels and protect against the underlying mechanism of METH toxicity, which are models for several neurodegenerative disorders like Parkinson's disease.

KEYWORDS: L-carnitine; methamphetamine; neurotoxicity

INTRODUCTION

There is a growing body of evidence suggesting that brain injury observed after amphetamine and methamphetamine (METH) administration is due to an increase in free radical formation and mitochondrial damage, which leads to a failure of cellular energy metabolism followed by a secondary excitotoxicity.[10,11,17,20] Neuronal degeneration is also associated with decreased ATP synthesis. The energy deficits in the central nervous system can lead to the generation of reactive oxygen and nitrogen species as indicated by increased activity of the free radical scavenging enzymes like catalase and superoxide dismutase.[1,4]

Recently, we have reported that METH-induced dopaminergic neurotoxicity may be mediated by the generation of peroxynitrite and can be protected by antioxidants selenium, melatonin, and selective nNOS inhibitor, 7-nitroindazole.[2,10,11,13,14] L-Carnitine (LC) is a well-known molecule that carries long-chain fatty acyl groups into mitochondria for β-oxidation (FIG. 1). It also plays a protective role in 3-nitropropionic acid (3-NPA)-induced neurotoxicity as demonstrated *in vitro*[18] and *in vivo*.[3,5] In addition, LC has been utilized in detoxification efforts in

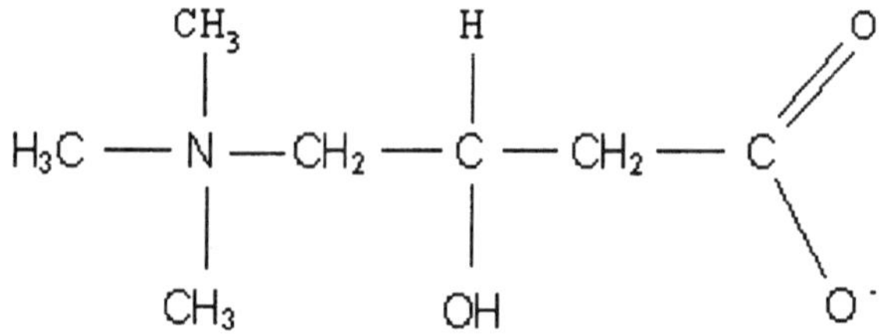

FIGURE 1. Structure of L-carnitine.

fatty acid–related metabolic disorders.[10] It has been shown to prevent mitochondrial damage induced in the rat choroid plexus by medium-chain fatty acid.[15]

In this study we have tested the hypothesis that enhancement of mitochondrial energy metabolism by LC could prevent the generation of peroxynitrite and free radicals produced by METH.

METHOD

Adult male C57BL/6N mice were divided into four groups:
- Group I served as control.
- Groups III and IV received LC (100 mg/kg, orally) for one week.
- Groups II and IV received 4 × 10 mg/kg METH i.p. at 2-h intervals after one week of LC administration.

LC treatment continued for one more week to groups III and IV.

One week after the METH administration, mice were sacrificed by decapitation, and striatum was dissected to measure the formation of 3-nitrotyrosine (3-NT) by HPLC/Coularry system.

RESULTS

The toxicity of METH has been shown previously to increase the production of 3-nitrotyrosine (3-NT) *in vitro,* for example, in cultured PC12 cells (FIG. 2) and also *in vivo,* as shown in the striatum of adult male mice (FIG. 3).

In the present experiment, METH treatment also produced significant formation of 3-NT, a marker of peroxynitrite generation, in the mice striatum (FIG. 4). The pre- and post-treatment of mice with LC significantly attenuated the production of 3-NT in the striatum resulting from METH treatment.

DISCUSSION

The *in vivo* toxicity of METH as manifested by the increase in the production of 3-NT in the striatum of mice was reduced by the pretreatment of the animals with LC. The METH-induced dopaminergic neurotoxicity is thought to be mediated by the generation of peroxynitrite radicals and can be protected by antioxidants selenium, melatonin, and selective nNOS inhibitor, 7-nitroindazole.[11,12] The protective effects by the compound LC in this study could be related to the prevention of the possible metabolic compromise by METH and the resulting energy deficits that lead to the generation of reactive oxygen and nitrogen species.

LC is required for the transport of activated acyls, namely, acyl-CoAs, across the inner mitochondrial membrane (FIG. 5). The LC requirement is related to the fact that fatty acids activated in the form of acyl-CoA outside the mitochondria cannot be imported into the mitochondrial matrix where the β-oxidation enzymes are located. In addition, by interacting with coenzyme A (CoA), LC exerts a role in any CoA-

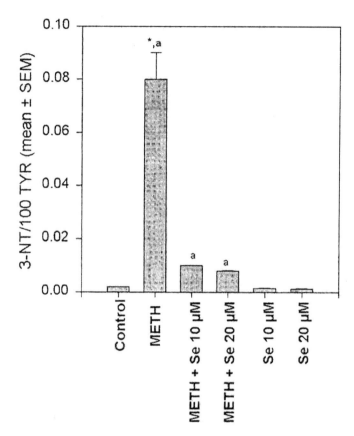

FIGURE 2. Methamphetamine-evoked (200 μM) production of 3-nitrotyrosine (3-NT) in PC 12 cells after 24 h in culture. (Adapted from Imam and Ali.[10])

dependent process. An increase in CoASH availability or a decrease in acyl CoA levels expands the roles of LC to substrate choice, removal of inhibitory metabolites, and modulation of key enzymatic steps.

Defective mitochondrial oxidative phosphorylation and metabolic compromise play an important role in atherogenesis, in the pathogenesis of Alzheimer's disease, Parkinson's disease, diabetes, and aging.[7] Various compounds, known to be detrimental, act on the respiratory chain. Thus, cholic acid in experimental atherogenic diets inhibits Complex IV; cocaine inhibits Complex I; the poliovirus inhibits Complex II; ceramide inhibits Complex III; azide, cyanide, chloroform, and methamphetamine inhibit Complex IV.[6,21] The METH-evoked toxicity has been shown to be attenuated by substrates of energy metabolism such as with decylubiquinone or

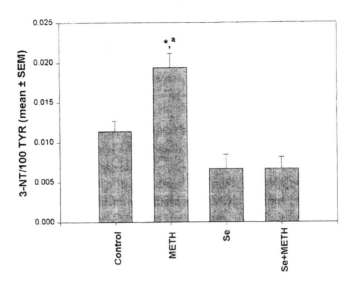

FIGURE 3. Methamphetamine-evoked (4 × 100 mg/kg i.p.) production of 3-nitrotyrosine in the striatum of adult male mice. (Adapted from Imam and Ali.[10])

3-NT in Mice Striatum

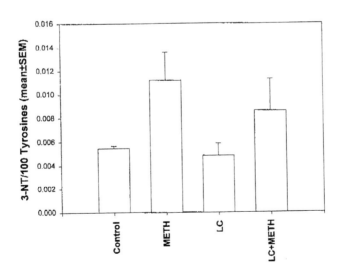

FIGURE 4. Protective effect of L-carnitine on the methamphetamine-evoked toxicity in mice striatum.

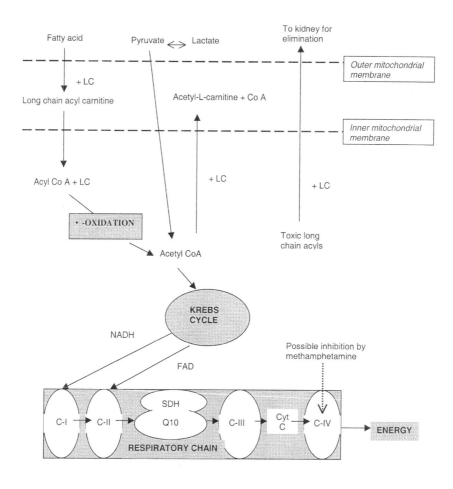

FIGURE 5. Schematic representation of the role of L-carnitine in mitochondrial metabolism. Cell toxicity and damage can be attenuated by energy substrates such as L-carnitine (LC). LC enhances fatty-acid metabolism and allows the transport of acetyl groups and coenzyme A (CoA) out of the mitochondria because the inner membrane is impermeable. LC would also enhance pyruvate metabolism by maintaining appropriate levels of acetyl CoA. In addition, LC removes toxic long-chain acyl groups from the mitochondria. The Krebs cycle feeds reducing energy in the form of nicotineamide adenine dinucleotide (NADH) and flavin adenine dinucleotide (FAD) into the respiratory chain. Coenzyme Q10 (Q10) is located in the electron transport system of the mitochondria, linking complexes I (C-I) and II (C-II) with complex III (C-III) of the respiratory chain. Cytochrome c (Cyt C) links complex III to complex IV (C-IV). Methamphetamine is thought to inhibit C-IV activity.

nicotinamide.[9,17] A similar mechanism probably underlies the protective efficacy of the carnitines.[18,19] The protective effect of LC against METH-neurotoxicity may be through effects on mitochondrial oxidative phosphorylation and reduced formation of free radical species.

In summary, these data further confirm our hypothesis that METH-induced neurotoxicity is mediated by the production of peroxynitrite, and LC may improve the mitochondrial oxidative phosphorylation and/or scavenge the peroxynitrite and protect against the underlying mechanisms of METH toxicity, which are models for several neurodegenerative disorders such as Parkinson's disease.

REFERENCES

1. ACIKGOZ, O., S. GONENC, B.M. KAYATEKIN, *et al.* 1998. Methamphetamine causes lipid peroxidation and an increase in superoxide dismutase activity in the rat striatum. Brain Res. **813**(1): 200–202.
2. ALI, S.F. & Y. ITZHAK. 1998. Effects of 7-nitroindazole, an NOS inhibitor on methamphetamine-induced dopaminergic and serotonergic neurotoxicity in mice. Ann. N.Y. Acad. Sci. **844**: 122–130.
3. BINIENDA, Z.K. & S.F. ALI. 2001. Neuroprotective role of L-carnitine in the 3-nitropropionic acid induced neurotoxicity. Toxicol. Lett. **125**(1–3): 67–73.
4. BINIENDA, Z., C.E. SIMMONS, S.M. HUSSAIN, *et al.* 1998. Effect of acute exposure to 3-nitropropionic acid on activities of endogenous antioxidants in the rat brain. Neurosci. Lett. **251**: 173–176.
5. BINIENDA, Z., J.R. JOHNSON, A.A. TYLER-HASHEMI, *et al.* 1999. Protective effect of L-carnitine in the neurotoxicity induced by the mitochondrial inhibitor 3-nitropropionic acid (3-NPA). Ann. N.Y. Acad. Sci. **890**: 173–178.
6. BURROWS, K.B., W.L. NIXDORF & B.K. YAMAMOTO. 2000. Central administration of methamphetamine synergizes with metabolic inhibition to deplete striatal monoamines. J. Pharmacol. Exp. Ther. **292**(3): 853–860.
7. FOSSLIEN, E. 2001. Mitochondrial medicine—molecular pathology of defective oxidative phosphorylation. Ann. Clin. Lab. Sci. **31**(1): 25–67.
8. GUTIERREZ-RIVAS, E., A. RUEDA, R. RAMOS, *et al.* 1989. Improvement of deglutition in amyotrophic lateral sclerosis after L-carnitine treatment. Neurologia **4**(10): 358.
9. HUANG, N.K., F.J. WAN, C.J. TSENG & C.S. TUNG. 1997. Nicotinamide attenuates methamphetamine-induced striatal dopamine depletion in rats. Neuroreport **8**(8): 1883–1885.
10. IMAM, S.Z. & S.F. ALI. 2000. Selenium, an antioxidant, attenuates methamphetamine-induced dopaminergic toxicity and peroxynitrite generation. Brain Res. **855**: 186–191.
11. IMAM, S.Z. & S.F. ALI. 2001. Aging increases the susceptiblity to methamphetamine-induced dopaminergic neurotoxicity in rats: correlation with peroxynitrite production and hyperthermia. J. Neurochem. **78**(5): 952–959.
12. IMAM, S.Z., J. EL-YAZAL, G.D. NEWPORT, *et al.* 2001. Methamphetamine-induced dopaminergic neurotoxicity: role of peroxynitrite and neuroprotective role of antioxidants and peroxynitrite decomposition catalysts. Ann. N.Y. Acad. Sci. **939**: 366–380.
13. ITZHAK, Y. & S.F. ALI. 1996. The neuronal nitric oxide synthase inhibitor, 7-nitroindazole, protects against methamphetamine-induced neurotoxicity *in vivo*. J. Neurochem. **67**: 1770–1773.
14. ITZHAK, Y., J.L. MARTIN, M.D. BLACK & S.F. ALI. 1998. Effects of melatonin on methamphetamine- and MPTP-induced dopaminergic neurotoxicity and methamphetamine-induced behavioral sensitization. Neurophramacology **37**: 781–791.
15. KIM, C.S., C.R. ROE & W.W. AMBROSE. 1990. L-Carnitine prevents mitochondrial damage induced by octanoic acid in the rat choroid plexus. Brain Res. **536**: 335–338.

16. ROE, C.R., D.S. MILLINGTON, D.A. MALTBY & T.P. BOHAN. 1983. Status and function of L-carnitine in Reye's syndrome (RS) and related metabolic disorders. J. Natl. Reye's Syndrome Foundat. **4:** 58–59.
17. STEPHANS, S.E., T.S. WHITTINGHAM, A.J. DOUGLAS, *et al.* 1998. Substrates of energy metabolism attenuate methamphetamine-induced neurotoxicity in striatum. J. Neurochem. **71**(2): 613–621.
18. VIRMANI, M.A., R. BISELLI, A. SPADONI, *et al.* 1995. Protective actions of L-carnitine and acetyl-L-carnitine on the neurotoxicity evoked by mitochondrial uncoupling or inhibitors. Pharmacol. Res. **32:** 383–389.
19. VIRMANI, M.A., V. CASO, A. SPADONI, *et al.* 2001. The action of acetyl-L-carnitine on the neurotoxicity evoked by amyloid fragments and peroxide on primary rat cortical neurones. Ann. N.Y. Acad. Sci. **939:** 162–178.
20. YAMAMOTO, B.K. & W. ZHU. 1998. The effects of methamphetamine on the production of free radicals and oxidative stress. J. Pharmacol. Exp. Ther. **287**(1): 107–114.
21. YUAN, C. & D. ACOSTA, JR. 2000. Effect of cocaine on mitochondrial electron transport chain evaluated in primary cultures of neonatal rat myocardial cells and in isolated mitochondrial preparations. Drug Chem. Toxicol. **23**(2): 339–348.

A Single Exposure to Restraint Stress Induces Behavioral and Neurochemical Sensitization to Stimulating Effects of Amphetamine

Involvement of NMDA Receptors

A.M. PACCHIONI, G. GIOINO, A. ASSIS, AND L.M. CANCELA

Departamento de Farmacología, Facultad de Ciencias Químicas,
Universidad Nacional de Córdoba, 5000 Córdoba, Argentina

ABSTRACT: Evidence indicates that repeated exposure to stressful events sensitizes the motor and addictive effects of drugs of abuse in rats. Regarding a single exposure to one restraint stress, previous findings have shown that it is sufficient to induce behavioral sensitization to stimulating and reinforcing properties of abuse drugs (e.g., amphetamine and morphine), as measured by locomotor activity and conditioned place preference, respectively. It is well known that enhanced dopaminergic neurotransmission in the nucleus accumbens and striatum plays a critical role in the development and/or expression of repeated stress-induced or drug-induced sensitization. In addition, involvement of NMDA receptors has been implicated in its development. However, whether sensitization induced by a single restraint stress exposure represents the same neurobiologic phenomenon is unknown. We studied the following issues: (a) influence of a single restraint exposure on the stimulating effects of amphetamine on dopamine release by microdialysis from striatum and (b) involvement of glutamatergic pathways, specifically those innervating striatum, on stress-induced sensitization to amphetamine, by administering MK-801 ip (0.1 mg/kg) or intrastriatally (1 µg/0.5 µL) previous to an acute restraint stress. For microdialysis studies (a) or intrastriatal administration of MK-801 (b), Wistar rats (250–330 g) were implanted stereotactically under anesthesia with a guide cannula in the striatum. After 2 days, animals were immobilized for 2 hours in a Plexiglas device. Control animals remained in their home cages. The following day we evaluated the stimulating effect of amphetamine on (a) dopamine release from striatum or (b) locomotor activity. In studies (a), dialysis probes were inserted into the guide cannula, and baseline dopamine levels were collected for 2 hours before a challenge of amphetamine (1.5 mg/kg ip). Dialysates were then collected by 3 hours. Amphetamine challenge induced a significantly higher increase in dopamine release and locomotor activity in animals previously subjected to one restraint stress exposure, relative to that observed in the no-restraint stress group. MK-801 administered ip or intrastriatally blocked the restraint stress-induced sensitization to amphetamine. First, our results point out that a single restraint stress exposure is a pertinent stimulus to induce sensitization of amphetamine's stimulating effects

Address for correspondence: Dr. Liliana M. Cancela, Departamento de Farmacología, Facultad de Ciencias Químicas, Universidad Nacional de Córdoba, 5000 Córdoba, Argentina. Voice: 54-351-4334437; fax: 54-351-4334420.
lcancela@fcq.unc.edu.ar

Ann. N.Y. Acad. Sci. 965: 233–246 (2002). © 2002 New York Academy of Sciences.

on dopaminergic neurotransmission in the striatum. Secondly, NMDA-glutamatergic receptors, specifically those placed in the striatum, are implicated in the development of stress restraint-induced sensitization.

KEYWORDS: restraint stress; dopamine release; microdialysis; striatum; sensitization; NMDA receptors; locomotor activity

INTRODUCTION

Evidence indicates that repeated exposure to stressful events sensitizes the motor and addictive effects of drugs of abuse in rats. Repeated stress not only increases the propensity for drug-taking, but also augments the psychomotor effects of psychostimulants and opioids.[1–11] After the acute application of stress, there is evidence that the stimulant effects of amphetamine on motor activity are not modified,[4,5] that heroin-seeking in drug-free animals is reinstated,[10] and that the stimulating and reinforcing properties of amphetamine and morphine, as measured by locomotor activity and conditioned place preference, respectively, are enhanced.[12,13]

Behavioral sensitization is defined as a potentiated behavioral response to a drug after prior chronic treatment with the drug or stress[6,14,15] and is thought to underlie certain aspects of drug addiction and drug-induced psychosis.[15,16]

Numerous efforts have been made to investigate the neural mechanisms underlying the sensitization phenomenon. Among these neuroadaptive phenomena, long-lasting hyperreactivity of the mesolimbic and striatal dopaminergic pathways has been addressed.[17] (For a review, see Pierce and Kalivas.[14]) Also, it has been demonstrated that sensitization to the locomotor-stimulating effect of cocaine, amphetamine, or morphine can be blocked by NMDA receptor antagonists.[18–20] The noncompetitive NMDA antagonist MK-801 also blocks the cellular changes in the mesoaccumbens dopamine system that normally accompany the development of behavioral sensitization.[21]

It has been proposed that similar neural mechanisms act in drug- and stress-induced sensitization. Exposure to pharmacologic and aversive stimuli induces dopamine (DA) release from neurons arising in the ventral tegmental area, and both repeated stress and drug administration persistently augment mesocorticolimbic and striatal dopaminergic transmission.[6,15,22–25] Evidence indicates interactions occur between glutamatergic and dopaminergic systems in the development of stimulant sensitization as well as in the neurochemical responses to different stressors.[26] Notwithstanding all of this evidence, there are no studies to indicate that the sensitization induced by a single restraint stress exposure represents the same neurobiologic phenomenon as those described for treatment with drugs and/or repeated stress.

Thus, our experimental approaches were oriented to study the following issues: (a) the influence of a single restraint exposure on the stimulating effects of amphetamine on DA release by microdialysis in the striatum, and (b) involvement of NMDA receptors, specifically those located in the striatum, on acute restraint stress-induced sensitization to stimulating effects of amphetamine on locomotor activity, by administering MK-801 (systemically or intrastriatally) before restraint stress.

MATERIAL AND METHODS

Animals

Adult male inbred Wistar rats weighing 250–330 g were used. They were maintained at 20–24°C under a 12-hour light-dark cycle (lights on at 7:00 AM) with free access to food and water. Rats were housed in a nursery of four per box and placed in the experimental room for at least 7 days before trials.

Surgery

Animals were anesthetized with chloral hydrate (400 mg/kg ip) and placed in a Koopf stereotaxic instrument with the incisor bar at −3.3 mm above the interaural line. The skull was exposed, and a hole was drilled to allow implantation of a bilateral stainless steel guide cannula (23 gauge) 2.0 mm above the final injection site or a microdialysis guide cannula (21 gauge). The microinjection cannulas were positioned to aim at the caudate putamen (CPu) at the coordinates (in mm) AP + 1.2 from bregma, ML ± 2.5, and DV −4.5 from the skull. The coordinates for the microdialysis cannulas in the CPu were AP + 1.2 , ML ± 2.5, and DV −6.0. The cannulas were secured in place with one stainless steel screw and dental cement. Animals were allowed to recover for 48–72 hours before the start of behavioral or microdialysis testing.

Drugs

D-amphetamine sulfate was purchased from Sigma Chemical Co., St. Louis, MO, USA, and (+)–MK-801 hydrogen maleate from Research Biochemical International, Natick, MA, USA. Drugs were dissolved in saline solution immediately before use.

Microinfusions

Bilateral intracerebral microinjections of MK-801 and saline were made through a 30-gauge stainless steel cannula which extended 2 mm beyond the tip of the guide cannula. The injection cannula was connected to a 10-µL Hamilton syringe via a length of polyethylene tubing (PE-10). Injections were made using a syringe pump (Harvard 22 syringe pump). The solution was infused in a volume of 0.5 µL/side and delivered over 93 seconds followed by a 60-second diffusion time.

Stress

Rats were immobilized for 2 hours in a Plexiglas restraining device. The Plexiglas cylinders were devised so that the rats' tails emerged from the rear. All animals were stressed from 10:00 AM and 2:00 PM.

All procedures were conducted in accordance with the National Institutes of Health Guide for the Care and Use of Laboratory Animals as approved by the Animal Care and Use Committee of the Facultad de Ciencias Químicas, Universidad Nacional de Córdoba.

Locomotor Activity

The testing apparatus consisted of a circular (60-cm diameter) cage equipped with two perpendicular infrared photocell beams located 3 cm above the floor. Interruption of either beam resulted in a photocell count. The testing apparatus was placed in a room different from the one where restraint was applied to check for possible conditioning effects. All animals were tested between 9:00 AM and 6:00 PM, only once, under white light in a quiet room. Animals were placed individually in the testing apparatus for a 1-hour habituation period. Animals were then injected with amphetamine (0.5 mg/kg ip), and motor activity counts were determined at 10-minute intervals for 2 hours after the injection.

Microdialysis Procedure

Probes. A concentric design like that of Lavicky and Dunn,[27] with little modifications, was used (FIG. 1). The microdialysis probes consisted of an outer cannula of 26-gauge stainless steel tubing (Small Parts Inc., Miami, FL, USA) and an inner silica tube (Polymicro Technologies, Phoenix, AZ, USA). The tubes were assembled concentrically, and the stainless steel tube was inserted into a holder made from a tip of a Beckman tube. Polyethylene tubing (PE-20, Clay Adams) was attached to both tubes to serve as inlet and outlet tubes (FIG. 1), and the whole assembly was fixed with epoxy glue. The dialysis membrane 250-330-μm tube with a molecular weight cutoff of 5000–6000 (Spectra Por Fiber, Spectron Medical, Los Angeles, CA, USA) was attached to the end of the stainless steel tube and closed at the tip with epoxy cement. The active length of the dialysis membrane was 3.0 mm.

Microdialysis. On the day of the experiment, a dialysis probe was inserted through the guide cannula, and the animals were transferred to the dialysis cage (40 × 34 cm). The probe was connected to the Bioanalytical Systems (BAS) syringe pump via peek tubing connected to a two-channel swivel, and the perfusion was started immediately (1 μL/min). The perfusion fluid was a modified artificial cerebrospinal fluid (aCSF) composed of 145 mM NaCl, 1.2 mM $CaCl_2$, 2.7 mM KCl, 1.0 mM $MgCl_2$, 2 mM Na_2HPO_4, and ascorbate 0.01 mM, pH 6.8. Samples were collected every 30 minutes and immediately injected onto an HPLC column.

HPLC Analysis of Dopamine. The DA content of dialysate was measured by HPLC with electrochemical detection. In summary, this system consisted of a reverse-phase column (RP 18, 125 × 4.6 mm, 5 μm) coupled to an LC-4C potentiostat (BAS). Samples were injected via a 20 μL injection loop. The composition of the mobile phase was 50 mM NaH_2PO_4/5 mM Na_2HPO_4, 0.1 mM EDTA-Na_2, 0.5 mM *n*-octyl sodium sulfate, and 9% methanol, with pH was adjusted to 5.4, as previously described by Di Chiara *et al.*[28] with little modification. The mobile phase was pumped (Spectra Series P200-SP Thermo Separations Products) at a flow rate of 1.0 mL/min. The sensitivity of the assay for DA was 10 fmol per sample.

In Vitro *Recovery.* The probe was prepared with 3 mm of dialyzing surface, immersed in aCSF at room temperature, and perfused at 1 mL/min for 30 minutes. Subsequently, the external aCSF was exchanged for one containing 72 nM DA in aCSF, while normal aCSF was pumped through the probe. After 30 minutes, two 30-minute samples were collected and analyzed for DA. Recovery was calculated as a percentage of the amount present in the same volume of the external aCSF.

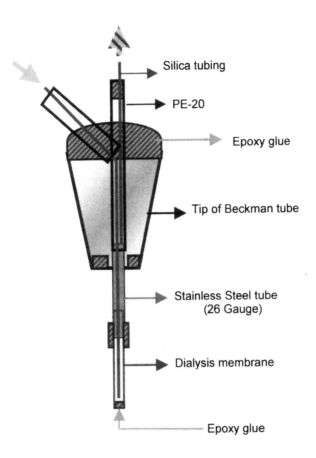

FIGURE 1. Schematic diagram of the microdialysis probe. For details, see Material and Methods.

Statistics

In experiment 1, data were analyzed by one-way ANOVA for repeated measures, with the following factors: treatment (0 or 1 restraint stress session) and time as the repeated measure (30-minute blocks for 180 minutes).

Data from experiments 2 and 3 were analyzed by two-way ANOVA for repeated measures, with the following factors: treatment (0 or 1 restraint stress session), drug (MK-801 or vehicle) and time as the repeated measure (10-minute blocks for 120 minutes). In both experiments, data expressed as the total cumulative counts were analyzed with two-way ANOVA.

All ANOVAs were followed by a post hoc Fisher test.

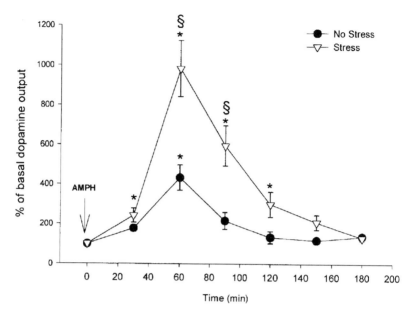

FIGURE 2. Effects of amphetamine (1.5 mg/kg ip) on dopamine output in dialysates from CPu 24 hours after the restraint stress session. Data are means ± SEM of 11 rats and are expressed as a percentage of basal values. The location of these probes is shown in Fig-URE 3. *Significantly different from baseline samples, $p < 0.05$. §Significantly different compared to the corresponding time-point in the no-stress group, $p < 0.0005$.

Histology

At the end of the experiments, to assess cannula and probe placement in the CPu, animals were deeply anesthetized with choral hydrate (400 mg/kg ip) and perfused transcardially with a solution of formaldehyde (10%). The brains were stored in 10% formaldehyde until sectioning. Following fixation, coronal sections 60 μm in thickness were cut on a cryostat, and each section was stained with thionin. Cannula placements were determined according to the atlas of Paxinos and Watson[29] with a light microscope.

Experimental Design

Experiment 1. Influence of a single exposure to restraint stress on DA release from CPu after a challenge with amphetamine.

Eleven rats were randomly assigned to one of two conditions defined by treatment: 0 or 1 restraint sessions. Animals assigned to the no-stress group (0 restraint session) were left undisturbed in their home cages. The day before the microdialysis experiment, animals assigned to the stress group (one restraint session) were immobilized for 2 hours. Twenty-four hours after restraint, a dialysis probe was inserted through the guide cannula and the perfusion of aCSF started immediately (1 μL/min). After 1 hour, baseline samples were collected every 30 minutes. Two hours later, an-

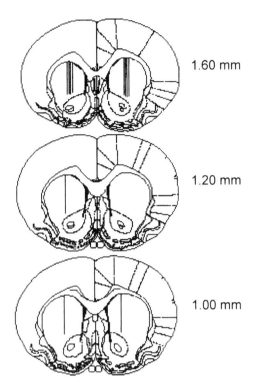

1.60 mm

1.20 mm

1.00 mm

FIGURE 3. Schematic sections of the rat brain, adapted from the stereotactic atlas of Paxinos and Watson,[29] showing the location of microdialysis probes in the caudate putamen. For details and exact coordinates, see Material and Methods.

imals received an injection of amphetamine (1.5 mg/kg ip), and samples were collected every 30 minutes for 180 minutes.

Experiment 2. Effect of MK-801 pretreatment on acute restraint stress-induced sensitization to the locomotor-activating effect of amphetamine.

Thirty-four rats were randomly assigned to one of four conditions defined by treatment (0 or 1 restraint stress session) and drug (saline [1 mL/kg ip] and MK-801 [0.1 mg/kg ip]). Rats were immobilized 30 minutes after drug administration. Control rats received drug or saline solution, were returned to their home cages, and were left undisturbed. Twenty-four hours after restraint and/or drug administration, all animals received a challenge injection of amphetamine, and locomotor activity was evaluated for 120 minutes after injection.

Experiment 3. Effect of MK-801 pretreatment intra-CPu on stress-induced sensitization to the locomotor-activating effect of amphetamine.

Thirty-two rats were randomly assigned to one of four conditions defined by treatment (0 or 1 restraint sessions) and drug (MK-801 [1 µg/0.5 µL/side] or saline [0.5 µL/side]). Animals assigned to the no-stress group (0 restraint session) received the infusion of MK-801 or saline and were then left undisturbed in their home cages. Animals assigned to the stress group (one restraint session) received the infusion of MK-801 or saline before they were immobilized for 2 hours. Twenty-four hours after restraint and/or drug administration, all animals were administered amphetamine (0.5 mg/kg ip) and locomotor activity was evaluated for 120 minutes after the injection.

RESULTS

Experiment 1. Influence of a single exposure to restraint stress on DA release from the CPu following a challenge with amphetamine.

Baseline levels of DA in the CPu were: 94.0 ± 20.2 fmol/sample for the no-stress group and 72.6 ± 3.4 fmol/sample for the stress group; there was no difference between these groups. Probe recovery of DA was $16 \pm 4\%$.

After the challenge of amphetamine (1.5 mg/kg ip) in the stress and the no-stress group, an increase in DA levels in the CPu was observed, expressed as a percentage of the mean of the four baseline samples. A one-way ANOVA for repeated measures showed a significant effect of treatment ($F(1,9) = 17.67, p < 0.005$) and time ($F(6,54) = 42.15, p < 0.0001$) as well as a significant interaction between treatment and time ($F(6,54) = 10.12, p < 0.0001$). Post hoc comparisons indicated that in the stress group, a significant increase in the percentage of basal DA output was observed after 30, 60, 90, and 120 minutes of amphetamine challenge, meanwhile in the no-stress group such an increase occurred at 30 and 60 minutes, with respect to baseline levels. Post hoc comparison also showed that at 60 and 90 minutes, the stress group showed a significant increase in the percentage of basal DA output as compared to the values of the no-stress group at those time-points (FIG. 2).

Experiment 2. Effect of NMDA receptor antagonist pretreatment on acute restraint stress-induced sensitization to the locomotor-activating effect of amphetamine.

FIGURE 4A and 4B shows that MK-801 pretreatment blocked the restraint stress-induced sensitization to amphetamine compared to that obtained in the saline-restraint stress group. A two-way ANOVA for repeated measures showed a significant effect of treatment ($F(1,30) = 13.27, p < 0.005$), drug ($F(1,30) = 7.96, p < 0.01$), and time ($F(11,330) = 3.14, p < 0.0005$) as well as a significant interaction between treatment x drug ($F(1,30) = 7.22, p < 0.05$). Post hoc comparisons indicated that photocell counts at 10 minutes, in saline-restraint stress, were significantly different from those obtained in MK-801–restraint stress groups; at 20 minutes, the values observed in saline-restraint stress were significantly higher than those obtained in MK-801 no-stress and stress groups; at 60 and 70 minutes in saline-restraint stress they were significantly higher than those obtained in all no-stress groups; and at 80 minutes in saline-restraint stress they were significantly higher than those obtained in MK-801–restraint stress and all no-stress groups.

FIGURE 4A and 4B also shows the total photocell counts over 120 minutes in saline and MK-801–restraint stress and no-stress groups challenged with amphetamine. A two-way ANOVA applied to the total cumulative counts over 120 minutes indicated a significant effect of treatment ($F(1,30) = 13.27, p < 0.005$) and drug ($F(1,30) = 7.95, p < 0.01$) as well as a significant interaction between treatment x

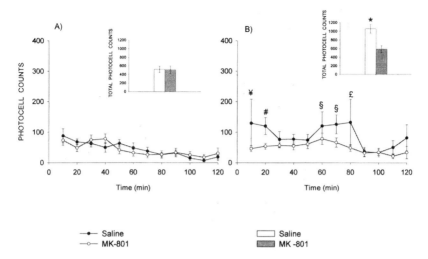

FIGURE 4. Reversal by MK-801 of the restraint stress-induced sensitization to the locomotor-activating effects of amphetamine. (**A**) No stressed animals were injected with their respective drugs or saline solution and were then placed in their home cages. (**B**) Animals were administered with vehicle or MK-801 (0.1 mg/kg ip) 30 minutes prior to the stress session. After 24 hours, the locomotor response to amphetamine was measured. Values represent the means (±SEM) of photocell counts over 10-minute periods, $n = 8$–10. At the top of both figures (**A** and **B**), the total photocell counts over 120 minutes were shown as means (±SEM). *Significantly different from all the no-stress groups and MK-801–stress group, $p < 0.001$. ¥Significantly different from MK-801–stress group, $p < 0.01$. #Significantly different from the MK-801 no-stress and stress group, $p < 0.05$. §Significantly different from all the no-stress groups, $p < 0.05$. £Significantly different from all the no-stress groups and MK-801–stress group, $p < 0.01$.

drug ($F(1,30) = 7.22$, $p < 0.05$). Post hoc comparisons indicated that the total cumulative counts in the saline-restraint stress group were significantly increased over those of the MK-801– restraint stress and all no-stress groups.

Experiment 3. Effect of MK-801 pretreatment intra-CPu on stress-induced sensitization to the locomotor-activating effect of amphetamine.

FIGURE 5A and 5B shows that MK-801 pretreatment intra-CPu prevented the restraint stress-induced sensitization to amphetamine seen in the saline-restraint stress group. A two-way ANOVA for repeated measures showed a significant effect of treatment ($F(1,28) = 6.17$, $p < 0.05$), drug ($F(1,28) = 8.30$, $p < 0.01$), and time ($F(11,308) = 7.05$, $p < 0.0001$) as well as a significant interaction between treatment x drug ($F(1,28) = 5.83$, $p < 0.05$). Post hoc comparisons indicated that photocell counts at 30, 40, 60, and 80 minutes in saline-restraint stress were significantly different from those obtained in MK-801–restraint stress and all no-stress groups; at 50 minutes in saline-restraint stress they were significantly higher than those obtained in MK-801 no-stress and stress groups; at 70 minutes in saline-restraint stress they were significantly higher than those obtained in all no-stress groups; and at 20 and 100 minutes in saline-restraint stress they were significantly higher than those obtained in MK-801 no-stress groups.

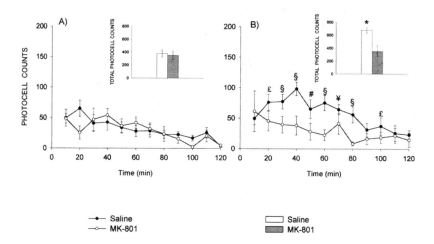

FIGURE 5. MK-801 pretreatment intra-CPu blocked the stress-induced sensitization to the locomotor-activating effect of amphetamine. (**A**) No stressed animals were injected with their respective drugs or saline solution and were then placed in their home cages. (**B**) Animals were administered with saline (0.5 µL) or MK-801 (1 µg/0.5 µL) immediately before the stress session. After 24 hours, the locomotor response to amphetamine was measured. Values represent the means (±SEM) of photocell counts over 10-minute periods, $n = 6–11$. In the left corner of both figures (**A** and **B**) the total photocell counts over 120 minutes were shown as means (±SEM). *Significantly different from all the no-stress groups and MK-801–stress group, $p < 0.001$. #Significantly different from the saline no-stress and MK-801 stress group, $p < 0.05$. §Significantly different from all the no-stress groups and MK-801–stress group, $p < 0.05$. £Significantly different from MK-801 no-stress group, $p < 0.05$. ¥Significantly different from all the no-stress groups, $p < 0.05$.

FIGURE 5A and 5B also shows the total photocell counts over 120 minutes in saline and MK-801–restraint stress and no-stress groups challenged with amphetamine. A two-way ANOVA applied to the total cumulative counts over 120 minutes indicated a significant effect of treatment ($F(1,28) = 6.13$, $p < 0.05$) and drug ($F(1,28) = 8.36$, $p < 0.01$) as well as a significant interaction between treatment x drug ($F(1,28) = 5.82$, $p < 0.05$). Post hoc comparisons indicated that the total cumulative counts in the saline-restraint stress group was significantly increased with respect to those of the MK-801–restraint stress and all no-stress groups.

Assessment of Cannula Placement. Animals with traces of injection cannulas or probes outside the CPu and animals showing an important gliosis level at those levels were eliminated from the experiments. Probe placement is illustrated in FIGURE 3, and microinjection cannula placements are shown in FIGURE 6.

DISCUSSION

This study showed that a single restraint stress was sufficient to cause sensitization to amphetamine-induced striatal DA release. Among others, neuroadaptive phe-

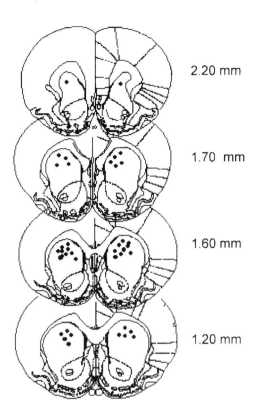

2.20 mm

1.70 mm

1.60 mm

1.20 mm

FIGURE 6. Schematic sections of the rat brain, adapted from the stereotactic atlas of Paxinos and Watson,[29] showing the placements of the CPu injection cannula. For details and exact coordinates, see Material and Methods.

nomena, an enhanced dopaminergic neurotransmission in the striatum, has been proposed to underlie the sensitization process to chronic treatment with psychostimulants or repeated stress.[6,15] Because common neural pathways are activated by drugs or stress,[1,6] it is important to point out that a single exposure to amphetamine also causes long-lasting behavioral sensitization associated with neurochemical and neuroendocrine adaptations.[30] Our results indicate that the restraint stress-induced sensitization was expressed in a context-independent manner, as observed in the sensitization induced by a single dose of amphetamine.[30] Previous studies from our laboratory have pointed out that the behavioral sensitization to amphetamine's stimulating effects was observed at least 1 week after a single restraint exposure.[3] However, further studies are necessary to confirm the long-lasting hiperresponsiveness of the striatal system to amphetamine's activating effects.

The present findings agree with those pointing out that full stimulation of D_1 and D_2 dopaminergic receptors seems to be necessary for the restraint stress-induced sensitization to amphetamine and morphine's stimulating and reinforcing properties.[3,12,13,31] Furthermore, unpublished results from our laboratory indicate that intrastriatal administration of the D_2/D_1 dopamine receptor antagonist haloperidol abrogated the sensitizing effects of restraint stress on the stimulating and reinforcing properties of amphetamine, as measured by locomotor activity and conditioned place preference.[32]

Several studies have implicated interactions between glutamatergic and dopaminergic systems in the development of behavioral sensitization to amphetamine, cocaine, and morphine.[18–20] Previously, we found that pretreatment with a noncompetitive NMDA antagonist, MK-801, blocked the restraint stress-induced enhancement on morphine-induced locomotion.[13] Coincidently, in the present study, we also found involvement of NMDA receptors in the development of stress-induced sensitization to amphetamine's stimulating effects. The noncompetitive NMDA antagonist MK-801 also blocks cellular changes in the mesoaccumbens DA system that normally accompany the development of behavioral sensitization.[21] This blockade has usually been interpreted as evidence that stimulation of NMDA receptors is required for the long-term neuronal changes responsible for the development of behavioral sensitization. Glutamatergic neurotransmission exerts its influence on mesolimbic dopaminergic pathways directly or throughout gabaergic interneurons.[33,34] The striatum receives glutamatergic input from all cortical areas. Neocortical areas project mainly to more dorsal parts of the striatum, whereas other regions such as hippocampus and amygdala project mainly to ventral parts of the striatum.[35] On striatal dopaminergic nerve terminals, it has been shown that NMDA receptors located in the presynapsis[36,37] are involved in the control of DA release.[37] Furthermore, the development of cocaine and amphetamine sensitization is prevented by the coadministration of NMDA/AMPA antagonist as well as by prior ibotenic acid lesions of the medial prefrontal cortex.[20,21] In the present study, the intrastriatal administration of a noncompetitive NMDA antagonist, MK-801, blocked the restraint stress-induced sensitization on amphetamine's stimulating properties on locomotor activity. Thus, a link between glutamate and DA can be established at neural circuits implicated in the sensitization process. Hence, it is apparently MK-801 acting at this level to block the restraint stress-induced sensitization to amphetamine.

Summing up, our results indicate that a single restraint stress exposure is a pertinent stimulus to inducing sensitization of amphetamine's stimulating effects on dopaminergic neurotransmission in the striatum. Also, NMDA-glutamatergic receptors, specifically those placed in the striatum, are implicated in the development of restraint stress-induced sensitization. Further experiments will be carried out to elucidate the neural basis of this glutamatergic-dopaminergic interaction.

This present study helps to identify the factors that contribute to enhance the stimulating properties of d-amphetamine as well as its possible mechanism. Finally, these results could be relevant to the study of drug abuse and other psychiatric disorders.

ACKNOWLEDGMENTS

This work was supported by grants from Agencia Córdoba Ciencia, SECyT, and Ministerio de Salud de la Nación Argentina. The authors thank Paul David Hobson, Ph.D., for English technical assistance.

The authors are recipients of fellowships from FOMEC (A.M. Pacchioni), Agencia Córdoba Ciencia (G. Gioino), and Ramón Carrillo-Oñativia (Ministerio de Salud de la Nación Argentina, A. Assis).

REFERENCES

1. ANTELMAN, S.M., A.J. EICHLER, C.A. BLACK & D. KOCAN. 1980. Interchangeability of stress and amphetamine in sensitization. Science 207: 329–330.
2. DEROCHE, V., P.V. PIAZZA, M. LE MOAL & H. SIMON. 1994. Social isolation-induced enhancement of the psychomotor effects of morphine depends on corticosterone secretion. Brain Res. 640: 136–139.
3. DÍAZ-OTAÑEZ, C.S., N.R. CAPRILES & L.M. CANCELA. 1997. D_1 and D_2 dopamine and opiate receptors are involved in the restraint stress-induced sensitization to the psychostimulant effects of amphetamine. Pharmacol. Biochem. Behav. 58: 9–14.
4. HAHN, B., R.M. ZACHARKO & H. ANISMAN. 1986. Alterations of amphetamine elicited preservation and locomotor excitation following acute and repeated stressor application. Pharmacol. Biochem. Behav. 25: 29–33.
5. HERMAN, J.P., L. STINUS & M. LE MOAL. 1984. Repeated stress increases locomotor response to amphetamine. Psychopharmacology 84: 431–435.
6. KALIVAS, P.W. & J. STEWART. 1991. Dopamine transmission in the initiation and expression of drug-and stress-induced sensitization of motor activity. Brain Res. Rev. 16: 223–244.
7. LEYTON, M. & J. STEWART. 1990. Preexposure to foot-shock sensitizes the locomotor response to subsequent systemic morphine and intra-nucleus accumbens amphetamine. Pharmacol. Biochem. Behav. 37: 303–310.
8. MOLINA, V.A, C.J. HEYSER & L.P. SPEAR. 1994. Chronic variable stress enhances the stimulatory action of a low dose of morphine: reversal by desipramine. Eur. J. Pharmacol. 260: 57–64.
9. ROBINSON, T.E., A.L. ANGUS & J.B. BECKER. 1985. The enduring effects of prior stress on amphetamine-induced rotational behavior. Life Sci. 37: 1039–1042.
10. SHAHAM, Y., J.E. KELSEY & J. STEWART. 1995. Temporal factors in the effect of restraint stress on morphine-induced behavioral sensitization in the rat. Psychopharmacology 117: 102–109.
11. STÖHR, T. *et al.* 1999. Stress and corticosteroid-induce modulation of the locomotor response to morphine in rats. Behav. Brain Res. 103: 85–93.
12. CAPRILES, N.R. & L.M. CANCELA. 2002. Motivational effects of μ and k opioid agonists following acute and chronic restraint stress: involvement of dopamine D_1 and D_2 receptors. Behav. Brain Res. In press.
13. CAPRILES, N.R., A.M. PACCHIONI & L.M. CANCELA. 2002. Influence of acute or repeated restraint stress on morphine-induced locomotion: involvement of dopamine, opiate and glutamate receptors. In press.
14. PIERCE, R.C. & P.W. KALIVAS. 1997. A circuit model of the expression of behavioral sensitization of amphetamine-like psychostimulants. Brain Res. Rev. 25: 192–216.
15. ROBINSON, T.E. & K.C. BERRIDGE. 1993. The neural basis of drug craving: an incentive-sensitization theory of addiction. Brain Res. Rev. 18: 247–291.
16. ROBINSON, T.E. & J.B. BECKER. 1986. Enduring changes in brain and behavior produced by chronic amphetamine administration: a review and evaluation of animal models of amphetamine psychosis. Brain Res. Rev. 11: 157–198.
17. ROBINSON, T.E., P.A. JURSON, J.A. BENNETT & K.M. BENTGEN. 1988. Persistent sensitization of dopamine transmission in the ventral striatum (nucleus accumbens) produced by a previous experience with (+)-amphetamine: a microdialysis study in freely moving rats. Brain Res. 462: 211–222.
18. JEZIORSKI, M., F. WHITE & M. WOLF. 1994. MK-801 prevents the development of behavioral sensitization during repeated morphine administration. Synapse 16: 137–147.
19. WOLF, M.E. & M. JEZIORSKI. 1993. Coadministration of MK-801 with amphetamine, cocaine or morphine prevents rather than transiently masks the development of behavioral sensitization. Brain Res. 613: 291–294.

20. WOLF, M.E. *et al.* 1995. Effects of lesions of prefrontal cortex, amygdala, or fornix on behavioral sensitization to amphetamine: comparison with N-methyl-D-aspartate antagonist. Neuroscience **69:** 417–439.
21. LI, Y. *et al.* 1999. Both glutamate receptors antagonists and prefrontal cortex lesions prevent induction of cocaine sensitization and associated neurodaptations. Synapse **34:** 169–180.
22. CADONI, C. & G. DI CHIARA. 1999. Reciprocal changes in dopamine responsiveness in the nucleus accumbens shell and core and in the dorsal caudate-putamen in rats sensitized to morphine. Neuroscience **90:** 447–455.
23. IMPERATO, A. *et al.* 1992. Repeated stressful experiences differently affect limbic dopamine release during and following stress. Brain Res. **577:** 194–199.
24. IMPERATO, A., S. CABIB & S. PUGLISI-ALLEGRA. 1993. Repeated stressful experiences differently affect the time-dependent responses of mesolimbic dopamine system to the stressor. Brain Res. **601:** 333–336.
25. PONTIERI, F.E., G. TANDA & G. DI CHIARA. 1995. Intravenous cocaine, morphine, and amphetamine preferentially increase extracellular dopamine in the "shell" as compared with the "core" of the rat nucleus accumbens. Proc. Natl. Acad. Sci. USA **92:** 12304–12308.
26. TAKAHATA, R. & B. MOGHADDAM. 1998. Glutamatergic regulation of basal and stimulus-activated dopamine release in the prefrontal cortex. J. Neurochem. **71:** 1443–1449.
27. LAVICKY, J. & A.J. DUNN. 1993. Corticotropin-releasing factor stimulates catecholamine release in hypothalamus and prefrontal cortex in freely moving rats as assessed by microdialysis. J. Neurochem. **60:** 602–612.
28. DI CHIARA, G., G. TANDA, R. FRAU & E. CARBONI. 1993. On the preferential release of dopamine in the nucleus accumbens by amphetamine: further evidence obtained by vertically implanted concentric dialysis probes. Psychopharmacology **112:** 398–402.
29. PAXINOS, G. & C. WATSON. 1997. The Rat Brain in Stereotaxic Coordinates, 2nd Ed. Academic Press. New York.
30. VANDERSCHUREN, L.J.M. *et al.* 1999. A single exposure to amphetamine is sufficient to induce long-term behavioral, neuroendocrine, and neurochemical sensitization in rats. J. Neurosci. **19:** 9579–9586.
31. CAPRILES, N.R. & L.M. CANCELA. 1999. Effect of acute and chronic restraint stress on amphetamine-associated place preference: involvement of dopamine D_1 and D_2 receptors. Eur. J. Pharmacol. **3866:** 127–134.
32. CAPRILES, N., A. PACCHIONI, L. PONCE & L.M. CANCELA. 1999. Effects of haloperidol pretreatment in dopamine mesocorticolimbic areas on restraint stress-induced sensitization to reinforcing and locomotor stimulating properties of d-amphetamine. 21st International Summer School of Brain Research: Cognition, Emotion and Autonomic Responses: The Integrative Role of Prefrontal Cortex and Limbic Structures. Amsterdam.
33. NARAYANAN, S. *et al.* 1996. Role of dopaminergic mechanism in the stimulatory effects of MK-801 injected into the ventral tegmental area and the nucleus accumbens. Pharmacol. Biochem. Behav. **54:** 565–573.
34. SEUTIN, V., S.W. JOHNSON & R.A. NORTH. 1994. Effect of dopamine and baclofen on N-methyl-D-aspartate-induced burst firing in rat ventral tegmental neurons. Neuroscience **58:** 201–206.
35. MCGEORGE, A.J. & R.L. FAULL. 1989. The organization of the projections from the cerebral cortex to the striatum in the rat. Neuroscience **29:** 503–537.
36. BOUYER, J.J., D.H. PARK, T.H. JOH & V.M. PICKEL. 1984. Chemical and structural analysis of the relation between cortical inputs and tyrosine hydroxylase-containing terminal in rat neostriatum. Brain Res. **302:** 267–275.
37. KREBS, M.O. *et al.* 1991. Glutamtergic control of dopamine release in the rat striatum: evidence for presynaptic NMDA receptors on dopaminergic terminals. J. Neurochem. **56:** 81–85.

Ontogeny of Neurokinin-1 Receptor Mediation of Methamphetamine Neurotoxicity in the Striatum of the Mouse Brain

JING YU,[a] SIMONE ALLISON,[a] DINA IBRAHIM,[a] JEAN LUD CADET,[b] AND JESUS A. ANGULO[a]

[a]Department of Biological Sciences, Hunter College of the City University of New York, New York, New York 10021, USA

[b]Molecular Neuropsychiatry Section, Division of Intramural Research, NIH/NIDA, Baltimore, Maryland, USA

ABSTRACT: We studied the role of the peptide substance P, signaling through the neurokinin-1 (NK-1) receptor, on methamphetamine-induced loss of dopamine transporter sites, a well-documented marker of toxicity in the striatum of the mouse brain, because this peptide is under dynamic regulation by the neurotransmitter dopamine. Methamphetamine is a psychostimulant that induces dopamine overflow from dopamine terminals of the striatum. Mice were given four injections of methamphetamine (7.5 mg/kg of body weight) at two-hour intervals and were sacrificed three days after the treatment. Dopamine transporter levels in the striatum were assessed by receptor autoradiography with [^{125}I]RTI-121. Exposure to methamphetamine resulted in significant loss of dopamine transporters in the caudate-putamen. This loss was prevented by preexposure (30 min before the first injection of methamphetamine) of the neurokinin-1 receptor antagonist L-733,060. The inactive enantiomer of L-733,060 (L-733,061) failed to protect dopamine transporter sites from methamphetamine, suggesting specificity for the neurokinin-1 receptor. Moreover, the protective effect of L-733,060 was observed in mice that were 10 weeks of age or older (dopamine transporter sites in mice six and eight weeks old were not protected from methamphetamine by the neurokinin-1 receptor antagonist). The results demonstrate that the deleterious effect of methamphetamine on dopamine transporter sites of the striatum is mediated via the neurokinin-1 receptor. The involvement of the NK-1 receptor appears after the eighth week of postnatal life, suggesting that the link between dopamine transporters and the neurokinin-1 receptor becomes functional at approximately the time when the mouse reaches reproductive age.

KEYWORDS: dopamine transporter; methamphetamine; neurokinin-1 receptor; L-733,060; striatum; neurotoxicity; substance P

Address for correspondence: Dr. Jesus A. Angulo, Hunter College of CUNY, Department of Biological Sciences, 695 Park Avenue, Room 927 North, New York, NY 10021. Voice: 212-772-5232; fax. 212-772-5230.
angulo@genectr.hunter.cuny.edu

Ann. N.Y. Acad. Sci. 965: 247–253 (2002). © 2002 New York Academy of Sciences.

INTRODUCTION

Methamphetamine (METH) is a long-acting derivative of d-amphetamine that displays addictive properties in laboratory animals and humans. Methamphetamine alters behavior and neurochemistry by increasing the activity of monoamines (serotonin, adrenalin, noradrenalin, and dopamine) in the brain.[1,2] METH is a potent indirect dopamine agonist that releases vesicular dopamine in the cytoplasm of terminals of nigrostriatal and mesolimbic neurons.[3] The elevated concentration of dopamine in the presynaptic terminal is dissipated by the dopamine transporter, resulting in elevation of extracellular dopamine in the striatum.[4] Exposure to METH causes behavioral and neurochemical alterations that persist for a long time after termination of drug exposure. Some of these alterations include decrements in dopamine transporter sites, tyrosine hydroxylase, and dopamine levels.[5,6] Even doses of METH within the recreational range have been shown to elicit deficits of dopamine transporter sites in baboons.[7] In the light of these findings, it is clear that METH exposure is highly toxic to neurons, resulting in observable neurochemical deficits. This is becoming a serious health hazard because METH usage in on a steep rise in the United States and other parts of the world.

Although the preponderance of published studies demonstrates that the adverse effects of METH on striatal neurons and terminals is due to the excess release of dopamine evoked by this drug, it is also possible for neuropeptides to modulate the effects of METH on striatal markers such as dopamine transporter sites. Striatal neurons express moderate to high levels of various neuropeptides, among them substance P, neurokinin A, dynorphin, and enkephalins. The latter peptide is expressed by striatal neurons that project to the globus pallidum, and the first three are coexpressed by striatonigral neurons.[8] Direct application of these neuropeptides into the brain has been shown to alter behaviors as well as neurotransmitter release.[9,10] For example, the *delta* opioid receptor agonist DADLE blocks METH-induced loss of DAT binding sites and TH protein levels in the striatum.[11,12] Similarly, the κ-opioid receptor agonist U69593 was shown to attenuate METH-induced long-term depletion of DA levels.[13] Exposure to METH causes elevation of substance P and neurokinin A in striatonigral neurons due to the excess of synaptic dopamine evoked by METH.[8,14]

In this study we demonstrate that the nonpeptide neurokinin-1 receptor antagonist L-733,060 attenuates the loss of dopamine transporter sites in the striatum of mice exposed to a neurotoxic regimen of METH. We also demonstrate that the ability of the NK-1 antagonist to protect the dopamine transporter depends on the age of the animal.

METHODS

Animal Treatment

Six-, eight-, and ten-week-old-male ICR mice weighing 36–44 mg (Taconic, Germantown, NY) were used in these studies. Mice were single housed on a 12-h light/dark cycle with food and water available *ad libitum* and were habituated for two weeks before commencement of drug treatments. Methamphetamine (Sigma, St.

Louis, MO) was dissolved in saline, and four injections (7.5 mg/kg of body weight) were administered at 2-h intervals intraperitoneally for one day. L-733,060 was dissolved in 45% 2-hydroxypropyl-β-cyclodextrin (RBI/Sigma, Natick, MA) and given 30 min before the first injection of METH, and then once in the morning on the second and third days posttreatment. We have found that this paradigm is most effective in preventing the neurotoxic changes induced by multiple administrations of METH (data not shown). Animals were sacrificed by decapitation on day 3 posttreatment (day of treatment is taken as day 0). All animal use procedures were according to the *National Institutes of Health Guide for the Care and Use of Laboratory Animals* and were approved by the Institutional Animal Care and Use Committee at Hunter College of the City University of New York.

Autoradiography of Dopamine Transporter Sites

The autoradiographic assays were performed as previously described[6,11] with minor modifications. Briefly, after decapitation the brains were rapidly removed and frozen on dry ice. Twenty-micrometer-thick coronal sections of the brain regions encompassing the nucleus accumbens and caudate-putamen were cut on a cryostat. Typically four slides with 6–8 sections each from every mouse brain were used. Sections were vacuum-dried and incubated with 0.073 nM [^{125}I]RTI-121 (3β-(4-[^{125}I]iodophenyl)tropame-2β-carboxylic acid isopropyl ester, 2200 Ci/mmol; New England Nuclear, Boston, MA) in assay buffer (137 mM NaCl, 2.7 mM KCl, 10.14 mM Na_2HPO_4, 1.76 mM KH_2PO_4, 10 mM NaI) at room temperature for 60 min. Nonspecific binding was determined with 10 μM GBR-12909. After incubation, the slides were washed in ice-cold assay buffer twice for 20 min to remove free radioactive ligand. The slides were then quickly dipped into ice-cold distilled water to remove salts and immediately dried under a fan. The slides were apposed to Hyperfilm MP (Amersham Pharmacia Biotech, Piscataway, NJ) for 51–53 h together with [^{125}I]microscales. The binding of [^{125}I]RTI-121 to the brain was quantified by densitometry using a computer-based NIH image analysis system.

RESULTS

We assessed dopamine transporter levels in coronal sections of striatal brain tissue from vehicle-injected control mice as well as mice treated with 7.5 mg/kg of METH four times at 2-hour intervals. Dopamine transporter sites were markedly reduced in the caudate-putamen and the nucleus accumbens three days after the treatment (FIG. 1). Dopamine transporter sites of the nucleus accumbens are more refractory to the neurotoxic impact of METH (FIG. 1B). In a separate group of animals, Western blotting was used to assess dopamine transporter protein levels. METH-induced reductions in dopamine transporter protein or binding sites in the caudate-putamen and the nucleus accumbens were equivalent (data not shown), demonstrating that the reductions observed three days after METH treatment are due to decrements of transporter protein levels on the membrane of the dopamine terminals.

The loss of striatal dopamine transporter sites induced by treatment with METH can be effectively attenuated by coadministration of a nonpeptide neurokinin-1 re-

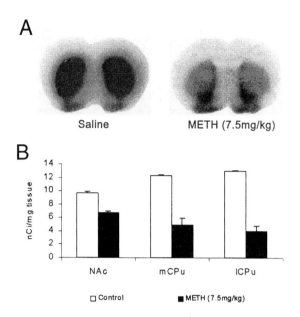

FIGURE 1. Effect of methamphetamine on dopamine transporter (DAT) sites of the caudate-putamen and the nucleus accumbens of the mouse brain. Dopamine transporter sites were assessed with the specific ligand $[^{125}I]$RTI-121 in coronal sections of brain tissue (8 animals per group) as shown **(A)**. METH-induced (7.5 mg/kg 4x at 2-h intervals) loss of DAT sites in medial and lateral aspects of the caudate-putamen and the nucleus accumbens at day three posttreatment **(B)**. Note that dopamine transporter sites of the nucleus accumbens are less affected by multiple injections of METH **(B)**. Symbols over the bars indicate standard error of the mean values. Nac, mCPu, and lCPu represent the nucleus accumbens, medial, and lateral aspects of the caudate-putamen, respectively. *$p < 0.05$ (Student's t-test).

ceptor antagonist. Administration of L733,060 30 min before the first injection of METH prevents the loss of dopamine transporter sites in the striatum (FIG. 2). Interestingly, the ability of L733,060 to protect dopamine transporter sites from METH is not observable before 10 weeks of age (FIG. 2). Moreover, the severity of METH toxicity on the dopamine transporter sites increases between weeks 6 and 10 (FIG. 2). The severity of depletion of dopamine transporter sites between the lateral and medial aspects of the caudate-putamen is of comparable magnitude.

DISCUSSION

This study demonstrates that the loss of striatal dopamine transporter sites observed three days after exposure to a neurotoxic dose of methamphetamine can be effectively prevented by preexposure to a nonpeptide neurokinin-1 receptor antagonist. The protection afforded by the NK-1 antagonist is at the level of transporter molecules on dopaminergic terminals of the striatum. An additional interesting finding of this study is that the protection afforded by neurokinin-1 receptor antagonists

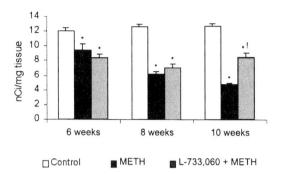

FIGURE 2. Protection of dopamine transporter sites from methamphetamine by neuro-kinin-1 receptor antagonist in the medial (**A**) and lateral (**B**) aspects of the caudate-putamen (CPu). Mice (8 per group) were treated with METH (7.5 mg/kg 4x at 2-h intervals and sac-rificed three days after the treatment) or METH plus L-733,060 (2 mg/kg; *gray bar*) given 30 min before METH. DAT sites were assessed by autoradiographic methods as described. The neurokinin-1 receptor antagonist fails to prevent the loss of DAT sites at six and eight weeks of age. The *y*-axis represents the binding of $[^{125}I]RTI$-121 to dopamine transporter sites. Symbols over the bars represent standard error of the mean values. $*p < 0.05$ (ANOVA) as compared to control; $^!p < 0.05$ as compared to METH-treated group.

is not present in mice tested at six or eight weeks of age, suggesting that the pepti-dergic system signaling through this receptor (namely substance P) reaches full cou-pling to intracellular components and perhaps ion channels after the eighth week of postnatal life. In both lateral and medial aspects of the caudate-putamen, the loss of dopamine transporter sites increases with age between weeks six and ten, and sub-sequently the NK-1 antagonist displays protection at the 10th week when the loss of dopamine transporter sites reaches adult levels. It appears that the mechanism by which METH causes the loss of dopamine transporter sites in the striatum during the first eight weeks of life is independent of substance P signaling through the neuro-kinin-1 receptor. We are currently measuring neurokinin-1 receptor levels in the stri-atum in mice six, eight, and ten weeks old in order to compare this to tissue dopamine levels. It is also conceivable that METH fails to release robust levels of dopamine in preadolescent mice.

The protective properties of the L-733,060 neurokinin-1 receptor antagonist on dopamine transporter sites of the neostriatum is also duplicated by other neurokinin-1 receptor antagonists. For example, the nonpeptide neurokinin-1 receptor antago-nist WIN-51,708 confers nearly 100% protection from METH on the dopamine transporter sites of the striatum assessed by receptor autoradiography as well as by Western blotting.[15] These results strongly suggest that signaling through the NK-1 receptors of the striatum by the neuropeptide substance P in the presence of METH leads to a cascade of neurotoxic reactions that compromise the dopamine transporter sites on the presynaptic terminals of dopamine neurons.

Neurochemical studies demonstrate that the neurotoxic effects of methamphet-amine are mediated in part by the production of free radicals in striatal tissue. For example, 7-nitroindazole, a selective inhibitor of neuronal nitric oxide synthase pro-tects against METH-induced neurotoxicity.[16] Neuronal nitric oxide synthase knockout mice are resistant to METH-induced dopaminergic neurotoxicity.[17] Exposure to METH increases striatal levels of peroxynitrite, an oxidant that appears to mediate the damaging effects of METH in this part of the mouse brain.[18] In the light of these studies, it is imperative to investigate a possible connection between the striatal neurokinin-1 receptor and oxidative stress.

Our data provide the first pharmacological evidence that tachykinins, particularly substance P, work through NK-1 receptors in the pathogenesis of neurochemical deficits produced by multiple exposures to METH. For the future, it will be essential to demonstrate protection against toxin-induced death of dopamine cell bodies located in the substantia nigra and the ventral tegmental area. Because METH can also cause apoptosis in various brain regions,[19] it will also be important to investigate the role of NK-1 receptors in METH-induced cell death by using similar pharmacological manipulations. Future studies are planned to characterize the exact neural locations of NK-1 receptor in the striatum and the underlying mechanisms by which they mediate neurotoxicity to METH. The identification of the role of NK-1 receptors in the production of METH-induced toxicity may lead to a new approach in the pharmacological treatment, not only for drug addictions but also for a number of diseases caused by excitatory neurotransmission or oxidative stress, including Parkinson's and Huntington's diseases.

REFERENCES

1. KUCZENSKI, R., D.S. SEGAL, A.K. CHO & W. MELEGA. 1995. Hippocampus norepinephrine, caudate dopamine and serotonin, and behavioral responses to the stereoisomers of amphetamine and methamphetamine. J. Neurosci. **15:** 1308–1317.
2. LESHNER, A.I. & G.F. KOOB. 1999. Drugs of abuse and the brain. Proc. Assoc. Am. Physicians **111:** 99–108.
3. SULZER, D. et al. 1995. Amphetamine redistributes dopamine from synaptic vesicles to the cytosol and promotes reverse transport. J. Neurosci. **15:** 4102–4108.
4. JONES, S.R., R.R. GAINETDINOV, R.M. WIGHTMAN & M.G. CARON. 1998. Mechanisms of amphetamine action revealed in mice lacking the dopamine transporter. J. Neurosci. **18:** 1979–1986.
5. CHAPMAN, D.E., G.R. HANSON, R.P. KESNER & K.A. KEEFE. 2001. Long-term changes in basal ganglia function after a neurotoxic regimen of methamphetamine. J. Pharmacol. Exp. Ther. **296:** 520–527.
6. HIRATA, H. et al. 1996. Autoradiographic evidence for methamphetamine-induced striatal dopaminergic loss in mouse brain: attenuation in CuZn-superoxide dismutase transgenic mice. Brain Res. **714:** 95–103.
7. VILLEMAGNE, V. et al. 1998. Brain dopamine neurotoxicity in baboons treated with doses of methamphetamine comparable to those recreationally abused by humans: evidence from [11C]WIN-35,428 positron emission tomography studies and direct in vitro determinations. J. Neurosci. **18:** 419–427.
8. ANGULO, J.A. & B.S. MCEWEN. 1994. Molecular aspects of neuropeptide regulation and function in the corpus striatum and nucleus accumbens. Brain Res. Rev. **19:** 1–28.
9. KHAN, S., N. BROOKS, R. WHELPTON & A.T. MICHAEL-TITUS. 1995. Substance P-(1-7) and substance P-(5-11) locally modulate dopamine release in rat striatum. Eur. J. Pharmacol. **282:** 229–233.
10. REID, M.S. et al. 1990. Effects of intranigral substance P and neurokinin A on striatal dopamine release—I. Interactions with substance P antagonists. Neuroscience **36:** 643–658.
11. TSAO, L.I. et al. 1998. Delta opioid peptide [D-Ala2,D-leu5]enkephalin blocks the long-term loss of dopamine transporters induced by multiple administrations of

methamphetamine: involvement of opioid receptors and reactive oxygen species. J. Pharmacol. Exp. Ther. **287:** 322–331.

12. TSAO, L.I., T. HAYASHI & T.P. SU. 2000. Blockade of dopamine transporter and tyrosine hydroxylase activity loss by [D-Ala(2), D-Leu(5)]enkephalin in methamphetamine-treated CD-1 mice. Eur. J. Pharmacol. **404:** 89–93.

13. EL DALY, E., V. CHEFER, S. SANDILL & T.S. SHIPPENBERG. 2000. Modulation of the neurotoxic effects of methamphetamine by the selective kappa-opioid receptor agonist U69593. J. Neurochem. **74:** 1553–1562.

14. SONSALLA, P.K., J.W. GIBB & G.R. HANSON. 1986. Nigrostriatal dopamine actions on the D2 receptors mediate methamphetamine effects on the striatonigral substance P system. Neuropharmacology **25:** 1221–1230.

15. YU, J., J.L. CADET & J.A. ANGULO. 2001. The role of neurokinin-1 receptor in methamphetamine-induced dopaminergic terminal toxicity. Soc. Neurosci. Abstr. **27:** 445.11.

16. ITZHAK, Y. & S.F. ALI. 1996. The neuronal nitric oxide synthase inhibitor, 7-nitroindazole, protects against methamphetamine-induced neurotoxicity in vivo. J. Neurochem. **67:** 1770–1773.

17. ITZHAK, Y., C. GANDIA, P.L. HUANG & S.F. ALI. 1998. Resistance to neuronal nitric oxide synthase deficient mice to methamphetamine-induced dopaminergic neurotoxicity in vivo. J. Pharmacol. Exp. Ther. **284:** 1040–1047.

18. IMAM, S.Z. *et al.* 2001. Peroxynitrite plays a role in methamphetamine-induced dopaminergic neurotoxicity: evidence from mice lacking neuronal nitric oxide synthase gene or overexpressing copper-zinc superoxide dismutase. J. Neurochem. **76:** 745–749.

19. DENG, X., B. LADENHEIM, L.I. TSAO & J.L. CADET. 1999. Null mutation of *c-fos* causes exacerbation of methamphetamine-induced neurotoxicity. J. Neurosci. **19:** 10107–10115.

Morphological and Biochemical Evidence that Apomorphine Rescues Striatal Dopamine Terminals and Prevents Methamphetamine Toxicity

G. BATTAGLIA,[a] M. GESI,[b] P. LENZI,[b] C.L. BUSCETI,[a] P. SOLDANI,[b] F. ORZI,[a,c] L. RAMPELLO,[d] F. NICOLETTI,[a,e] S. RUGGIERI,[a,c] AND F. FORNAI[b]

[a]I.R.C.C.S., I.N.M., Neuromed, Pozzilli, Italy

[b]Department of Human Morphology and Applied Biology, University of Pisa, Pisa, Italy

[c]Departments of Neurological Sciences, University of Rome "La Sapienza," Rome, Italy

[d]Department of Neurological Sciences, University of Catania, Catania, Italy

[e]Human Physiology and Pharmacology, University of Rome "La Sapienza," Rome, Italy

ABSTRACT: Apomorphine, given by a single injection, repeated injections, or by continuous infusion, was tested for neuroprotective effects in mice administered methamphetamine or N-methyl-4-phenyl-1,2,3,6-tetrahydropyridine (MPTP) in order to induce striatal dopamine (DA) depletion. In the first part of the study, the DA agonist (R)-apomorphine was administered at various doses (1, 5, and 10 mg/kg), 15 min before methamphetamine (5 mg/kg × 3, 2 h apart). Mice were sacrificed 5 days later. In the second part, apomorphine was administered either continuously by subcutaneous minipump (cumulative daily dose of 0.5, 1, and 3.15 mg/kg), or as single, repeated daily injections (up to 5 mg/kg) starting 40 h after an acute administration of MPTP (30 mg/kg). Mice were sacrificed at different time intervals (up to 1 month) following MPTP injection. In all the animals, the integrity of striatal DA terminals was evaluated by measuring striatal DA levels and TH immunohistochemistry. Apomorphine dose-dependently prevented methamphetamine toxicity. These effects were neither due to a decrease in the amount of striatal methamphetamine nor to the hypothermia, and they were not reversed by the DA antagonist haloperidol. Moreover, chronic, continuous (but not pulsatile) administration of apomorphine rescued damaged striatal dopaminergic terminals. These findings confirm a protective effect of apomorphine that also consists of a neurorescue of damaged striatal DA terminals. This suggests a new hypothesis about the long-term benefits observed during continuous apomorphine administration in Parkinson's disease patients.

KEYWORDS: methamphetamine; apomorphine; MPTP; dopaminergic neurons; neuroprotection; neurorescue

Address for correspondence: Francesco Fornai, Department of Human Morphology and Applied Biology, University of Pisa, Pisa, Italy. Voice: +39-050-835927; fax: +39-050-835925.
f.fornai@med.unipi.it

Ann. N.Y. Acad. Sci. 965: 254–266 (2002). © 2002 New York Academy of Sciences.

INTRODUCTION

Substituted amphetamines are drugs of abuse that are neurotoxic on cerebral monoamine systems of various animal species,[1] including nonhuman[2,3] and human[4] primates. In the rat, methamphetamine induces chronic dopamine (DA) and serotonin (5HT) depletion associated with terminal loss,[5–7] whereas in the mouse the effect is prevalent in the nigrostriatal DA terminals.[8,9] The mechanism of methamphetamine toxicity seems to be related to the property of increasing intra- and extracellular DA levels. The increase occurs immediately following a single administration by means of various concomitant effects, including inhibition of monoamine oxidase A (MAO-A) activity,[10] reversal of the action of the DA transporter,[11] and increasing intracellular DA release from newly synthesized vesicles.[12] A role for DA in methamphetamine toxicity is strongly suggested by the close correlation between methamphetamine-induced extracellular striatal DA release and the subsequent terminal loss,[13] as well as by the protective effects of DA synthesis inhibitors. To date, strong evidence indicates that DA itself, when present within the DA terminal in concentrations far exceeding physiological levels, induces marked oxidative stress,[14–17] as a result of auto-oxidative mechanisms[18] and production of H_2O_2 associated with DA catabolism.

Parkinson's disease (PD) is a neurodegenerative disorder whose motor symptoms are closely related to degeneration of dopaminergic neurons of the pars compacta of the substantia nigra,[19,20] and methamphetamine is widely employed to induce experimental parkinsonism, because it mimics both the selectivity of the neurodegeneration of the PD and the role of the oxidative stress on the progression of the disease.[21]

Since the late 1960s, the gold standard in the therapy of PD has been L-dihydroxyphenylalanine (L-DOPA). The direct DA precursor is rapidly converted into DA by spared surviving nigrostriatal terminals, glial cells, and serotonergic neurons.[22] Chronic administration of L-DOPA is complicated, however, by fluctuations in its therapeutic efficacy (such as wearing off and drug-resistant off and on–off phenomena) and by late-onset dyskinesias. In order to reduce L-DOPA-induced dyskinesia, DA receptor agonists have been recently employed. Among them, apomorphine, a mixed DA agonist, when continuously infused s.c. produces a dramatic relief in motor fluctuations in patients receiving L-DOPA.[23] A number of findings indicate that discontinuous DA stimulation is a trigger for L-DOPA-induced dyskinesia, which, however, depends on the degree of nigro-striatal dopaminergic degeneration.[24,25] It is, therefore, a question of whether apomorphine is effective because of the continuous (as opposed to pulsatile) DA stimulation and/or because of a putative neurorescue effect of striatal DA terminals. Recent studies do in fact demonstrate that apomorphine possesses strong antioxidant effects, both in vitro[26–28] and in vivo (see below). In particular, high doses of apomorphine (10 mg/kg) prevent the dopaminergic neurotoxicity induced by N-methyl-4-phenyl-1,2,3,6-tetrahydropyridine (MPTP).[29] It is a substantial question, however, whether continuous apomorphine administration rescues DA axons once the lesion is already established. Such a hypothesized neurorescue might account for the reduction of dyskinesias observed in parkinsonian subjects undergoing continuous subcutaneous delivery of apomorphine.[30,31]

Therefore, in the first part of this study, we investigated the protective effects of apomorphine against the nigrostriatal DA toxicity induced by methamphetamine, whereas in the second part we tested whether chronic apomorphine administration rescues the nigrostriatal pathway once a lesion has occurred. We chose MPTP because it induces highly reproducible DA lesions in mice.[32] Moreover, since its toxic metabolite MPP$^+$ is cleared from the neostriatum within 12 h of systemic administration,[33] starting apomorphine infusions 40 hours after acute MPTP injection represents a safe procedure to avoid pharmacokinetic/pharmacodynamic interactions.

MATERIALS AND METHODS

Animals

Male C57/6N black mice (Charles River, Calco, CO, Italy), 10 weeks old and weighing 22–24 g, were kept under environmentally controlled conditions (ambient temperature = 21 ± 1°C) with food and water *ad libitum*. Given the dependency of methamphetamine toxicity on the aggregation of the animals,[34] they were housed 10 per cage in small cages (38 × 22 cm wide and 15 cm high). Every effort was made to reduce the animals' suffering and to minimize the number of animals. Experiments were performed following the Guidelines for Animal Care and Use of the National Institutes of Health.

Experimental Design

Effects of Apomorphine on Methamphetamine Neurotoxicity

Given the high variability of methamphetamine toxicity, the dose of methamphetamine (5 mg/kg × 3, 2 h apart) was selected in order to produce a consistent degree of striatal DA depletion.[35]

To measure effects induced by systemic administration of (R)-apomorphine on methamphetamine toxicity, mice were divided into eight groups, each composed of 10 animals. Three groups were treated intraperitoneally (i.p.) with different doses of (R)-apomorphine (1, 5, and 10 mg/kg; Chiesi, Parma, Italy), 15 min before methamphetamine (5 mg/kg × 3, 2 h apart, i.p; Sigma Chemical Co., Saint Louis, MO). Control groups received either saline, methamphetamine, or (R)-apomorphine, at the same doses and times used for the groups given the combined treatments. Five days after methamphetamine administration, the animals were sacrificed, and the striatum was dissected and processed for monoamine levels and tyrosine hydroxylase (TH) activity. In order to evaluate the role of DA receptors on the effects of apomorphine on methamphetamine toxicity, additional groups of mice received haloperidol either alone or in combination with methamphetamine and/or apomorphine; haloperidol (5 mg/kg; RBI, Natick, MA) was injected 30 min before methamphetamine (15 min before apomorphine).

Additional animals were divided in all the above-mentioned groups, in order to measure effects on body temperature at various time intervals (30 min, 1 h, and 3 h) after drug administration.

Finally, we measured striatal methamphetamine levels at three different time intervals (1, 2, and 4 h) after administration of a single dose (5 mg/kg) of methamphetamine to exclude potential effects of apomorphine on striatal availability of systemically injected methamphetamine. For this experiment additional animals were divided into two groups. Both groups received methamphetamine (5 mg/kg).

Animals belonging to the first group were previously injected (15 min before meth-amphetamine) with saline, whereas animals belonging to the second group received the highest dose (10 mg/kg) of apomorphine. From each group of animals, six mice were sacrificed at each time interval (1, 2, and 4 h after methamphetamine administration), and striata were dissected to measure methamphetamine levels.

Chronic Effects of Apomorphine after DA Lesion with MPTP

Mice were treated as follows. On day 1, all animals received a single i.p. injection of either saline or MPTP (30 mg/kg; Sigma). Afterwards, both saline or MPTP-injected animals were subjected to a continuous subcutaneous infusion with either saline or (*R*)-apomorphine for 28 days by means of an osmotic pump (Alzet). The nominal delivery of the pump was 0.25 μl/h, corresponding to a cumulative daily dose of 3.15 mg/kg apomorphine. The original solution was employed or further diluted (1:3 and 1:6 to achieve a daily delivery of 1.05 and 0.525 mg/kg, respectively; subsequently referred to as 1 and 0.5 mg/kg). Control animals received an equivalent volume of saline. The delivery of apomorphine or saline was started 40 h after the injection of MPTP. The size of each group ranged from 8 to 10 animals. All mice were killed by decapitation 30 days after the injection of saline or MPTP. In most animals the striata were dissected and used for the determination of monoamine levels; in some animals from each group, brains were processed for TH, DAT, or GFAP immunostaining.

Assay of Catecholamines

The striatum was sonicated in 0.6 ml of ice-cold 0.1 M perchloric acid. An aliquot of the homogenate (50 μl) was assayed for protein.[36] After centrifugation at $8,000 \times g$ for 10 min, 20 μl of the clear supernatant was injected into an HPLC system where norepinephrine (NE), DA, 5HT, and metabolites were analyzed as previously described.[37]

Assay of TH Activity

The striatum was homogenized in 600 μl of deionized water. Aliquots of the tissue homogenate were then incubated in PBS containing L-[^{14}C]tyrosine (540 mCi/mmol). TH activity was measured as previously described.[38]

Assay of Methamphetamine

The striatum was sonicated in 0.2 ml of ice-cold 0.1 M perchloric acid. An aliquot of the homogenate (50 μl) was assayed for protein. After centrifugation at $8,000 \times g$ for 10 min in an ALC microcentrifugette (Milan, Italy), 100 μl of the clear supernatant was used for methamphetamine assay as previously described.[37]

Measurement of Body Temperature

Because previous studies have shown that apomorphine produces hypothermia,[39–41] we measured body temperature at 30 min and 1, 3, and 12 h after beginning pharmacological treatments. Measurements were carried out at constant daytime intervals starting at 9:00 A.M. as previously described.[42]

Immunostaining

Brains were immediately frozen and stored at −80°C. For TH immunostaining, 10-μm sections were incubated overnight with primary antibodies, and then for 1 hour with secondary antibodies. 3,3′-diaminobenzidine (DAB) immunostaining was used for the detection of TH (ABC Elite Kit, Vector Laboratories, Burlingame, California). The primary antibodies were monoclonal mouse antibodies against TH (1:2000; Sigma). TH immunoreactivity was quantified by measuring the relative optical densities.

For glial fibrillary acidic protein (GFAP) immunostaining, 10-μm sections were incubated overnight with monoclonal mouse antibodies against GFAP (1:500), and then for 1 hour against fluorescein-bound rabbit anti-mouse antibodies (1:200). Slides were rapidly photographed by a camera mounted on fluorescence microscope (Leica).

Data Analysis

Results are expressed as the mean ± SEM. For each experiment the effects of different treatments on striatal catecholamine levels were evaluated using analysis of variance (ANOVA) with Sheffé's *post hoc* analysis. The null hypothesis was rejected when $p < 0.05$.

RESULTS

Effects of Apomorphine on Methamphetamine Toxicity

Apomorphine administration did not modify striatal DA (FIG. 1A) nor dihydroxyphenylacetic acid (DOPAC) (FIG. 1B) levels at any dose. In contrast, methamphetamine produced an intermediate degree of striatal DA depletion (FIG. 1A) and DOPAC reduction (FIG. 1B). In animals receiving the combined treatment, (R)-apomorphine produced dose-dependent protection against methamphetamine-induced striatal DA toxicity. In particular, while animals administered apomorphine at the lowest dose (1 mg/kg) had striatal DA levels and TH activity comparable with those of mice injected with methamphetamine alone, mice receiving apomorphine at 5 mg/kg were significantly protected against methamphetamine-induced striatal DA depletion (FIG. 1A). Similarly, mice administered 10 mg/kg apomorphine had DA levels comparable with those of controls, and there was significant protection against DOPAC loss as well (FIG. 1). TH levels were similarly affected by the various treatments. In contrast, 5HT levels were not affected by any treatment (data not shown).

Effects of Haloperidol on Apomorphine-Induced Protection of Methamphetamine Toxicity

As shown in FIGURE 2, haloperidol (5 mg/kg) alone did not modify striatal DA levels. In contrast, when haloperidol was combined with methamphetamine (5 mg/kg × 3, 2 h apart), full protection against striatal DA depletion was obtained. Again, in animals receiving the combined treatment with haloperidol + (R)-apomorphine, methamphetamine-induced striatal DA toxicity was completely prevented (FIG. 2).

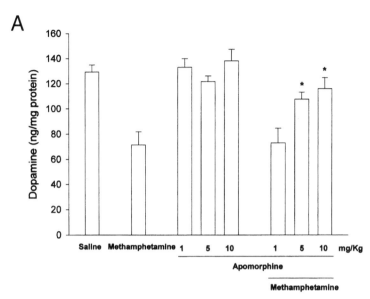

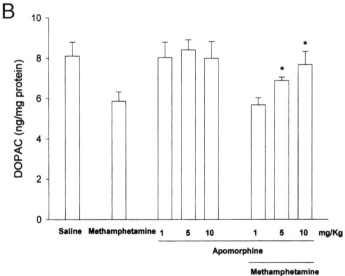

FIGURE 1. Effects of apomorphine on methamphetamine-induced striatal DA (**A**) and DOPAC (**B**) loss. Apomorphine dose-dependently prevents methamphetamine-induced striatal DA loss. Apomorphine *per se* does not change striatal DA levels. Values are given as the mean ± SEM. Data analysis was carried out by using analysis of variance. *$p < 0.05$ compared with mice administered methamphetamine alone.

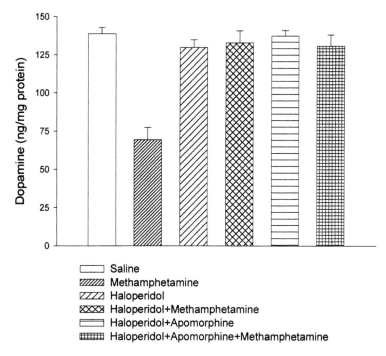

FIGURE 2. Effects of haloperidol on apomorphine-induced protection against meth-amphetamine-induced decrease of striatal DA levels. Haloperidol does not modify striatal DA levels but prevents methamphetamine-induced striatal DA loss. Preadministration of ha-loperidol does not modify neuroprotective activity of apomorphine. Values are given as the mean ± SEM. Data analysis was carried out by using analysis of variance.

In particular, there was no statistical difference (ANOVA) among animals receiving either saline, apomorphine plus methamphetamine, haloperidol plus methamphet-amine, or apomorphine plus haloperidol plus methamphetamine. A similar effect was obtained by measuring striatal DOPAC levels (data not shown). These data in-dicate that protective effects of apomorphine are neither antagonized nor reversed by administration of a DA antagonist.

Methamphetamine Levels

Despite a clear neuroprotective effect, apomorphine did not modify the peak of striatal methamphetamine levels measured 1 h after administration (0.065 ± 0.003 g/ mg of protein and 0.062 ± 0.007 μg/mg of protein). Also, the area under the curve (AUC) was not significantly different compared with that obtained in mice injected with methamphetamine alone. Despite that, we measured a paradoxical, delayed clearance of methamphetamine from the striatum of apomorphine-pretreated com-pared with saline-pretreated mice at 4 h after methamphetamine injection (0.022 ± 0.003 μg/mg of protein and 0.007 ± 0.002 ∝g/mg of protein, respectively).

TABLE 1. Effects of apomorphine on methamphetamine-induced hyperthermia

	Body temperature (°C)		
Treatment	30 min	1 h	3 h
Saline ($n = 7$)	38.0 ± 0.4	37.7 ± 0.2	37.8 ± 0.3
Apo (5 mg/kg) + saline ($n = 7$)	35.3 ± 0.7*	35.8 ± 0.3*	35.8 ± 0.5*
Apo (10 mg/kg) + saline ($n = 7$)	33.9 ± 1.1*	35.9 ± 0.5*	33.3 ± 0.6*
Saline + Meth ($n = 5$)	39.4 ± 1.1**	39.4 ± 0.3**	39.8 ± 0.4**
Apo (5 mg/kg)+ Meth ($n = 5$)	39.2 ± 0.2**	39.5 ± 0.6**	39.6 ± 0.1**
Apo (10 mg/kg) + Meth ($n = 6$)	39.6 ± 0.9**	39.3 ± 0.3**	39.0 ± 1.2**

NOTE: Body temperature was measured only for those doses of apomorphine that provided neuroprotection against methamphetamine toxicity. Apomorphine alone induced hypothermia, although it was not effective when given in combination with methamphetamine.
*$p < 0.05$ compared with saline.
**$p < 0.05$ compared with both saline and apomorphine alone.

Effects on Body Temperature

Apomorphine (1 mg/kg) induced a significant hypothermic effect compared with control mice (TABLE 1). Higher doses of apomorphine (5 and 10 mg/kg) did not further decrease body temperature. In contrast, methamphetamine produced significant hyperthermia that was not antagonized by any dose of apomorphine (TABLE 1).

Effects of Prolonged Apomorphine Administration on Chronic MPTP Toxicity

One day after MPTP administration, a marked reduction in striatal DA and DOPAC levels (nearly 80%) was observed. A substantial reduction in the striatal levels of DA and DOPAC was observed in mice 30 days after a single i.p. injection of 30 mg/kg of MPTP followed by a 28-day infusion with saline, although DA levels partially recovered from the massive acute depletion (day 1) induced by MPTP (FIG. 3). A 28-day s.c. infusion with apomorphine (3.15 mg/kg per day, starting 40 hours after MPTP injection) markedly attenuated the drop in DA levels induced by MPTP and brought DOPAC and homovanillic acid (HVA) levels back to the control values. Conversely, apomorphine administered as a single daily bolus for 28 days (1 or 5 mg/ kg) did not increase DA and DOPAC levels compared with the MPTP plus saline group (data not shown).

Immunostaining

The neurorescue effect of apomorphine against MPTP neurotoxicity was confirmed by TH (FIG. 4) immunostaining in the corpus striatum. MPTP injection dramatically reduced the intensity of striatal TH staining 30 days later. This reduction was markedly attenuated when MPTP injection was followed by a 28-day s.c. infusion with apomorphine (FIG. 4). Conversely, loss of TH immunostaining in the substantia nigra pars compacta (SNpc) of MPTP-treated animals was not rescued by the prolonged s.c. infusion of apomorphine (not shown). GFAP immunostaining, an index of gliosis, was markedly increased both in striatum and SNpc 30 days after

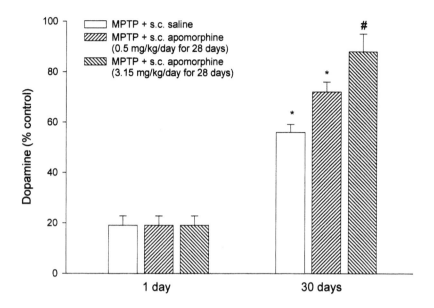

FIGURE 3. Effects of continuous subcutaneous infusion of apomorphine on striatal DA levels after MPTP. Continuous apomorphine administration dose-dependently reverses the MPTP-induced striatal DA depletion. Values are given as the mean ± SEM. Data analysis was carried out by using analysis of variance. $*p < 0.05$ compared with early (1-day) striatal DA loss. $\#p < 0.05$ compared with early (1-day) striatal DA loss and late (30-day) striatal DA levels in mice receiving continuous saline or a lower dose of apomorphine.

MPTP administration. A 28-day s.c. infusion with apomorphine did not modify either the striatal or the nigral MPTP-induced gliosis.

DISCUSSION

We show here that the nonselective agonist apomorphine dose-dependently protects nigrostriatal DA terminals against methamphetamine-induced neurotoxicity. These effects are not associated either with alterations in pharmacokinetics of striatal methamphetamine or with changes in body temperature.

Although a dose of 1 mg/kg was ineffective, apomorphine at 5 mg/kg significantly prevented methamphetamine-induced neurotoxicity, and the highest dose (10 mg/kg) provided full protection. The protective effect is unlikely to be dependent on DA receptor agonism for a number of reasons: (1) protective effects occur at doses higher than those required to stimulate DA receptors[43] (see also the present results); (2) protective effects are produced by only a few DA agonists[44,45]; (3) protective effects are neither antagonized nor reversed following single or combined administration of DA antagonists[46,47] (see also the present results); (4) protective effects are not related to DA receptor–dependent hypothermic effects; (5) free radical scavenging properties of apomorphine are similar for other apomorphine enantiomers that do not

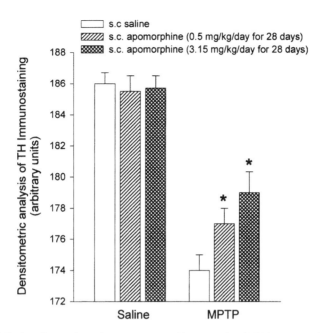

FIGURE 4. Effects of continuous apomorphine on striatal TH immunostaining. Apomorphine dose-dependently rescues MPTP-induced loss of striatal TH immunostaining. Values are given as semiquantitative densitometry and represent mean ± SEM values from different animals (see methods section). Data analysis was carried out by using analysis of variance. *$p < 0.05$ compared with mice administered saline following MPTP.

possess DA agonist properties, for the reason that the S enantiomer is even more powerful than the R in preventing DA toxicity.[48]

In particular, haloperidol, a potent, nonselective DA antagonist, did not reverse the neuroprotective effects induced by apomorphine. These data are in line with what has recently been published on apomorphine enantiomers. The S enantiomer, which is virtually ineffective in stimulating DA receptors, is even more powerful than the R enantiomer in protecting against MPTP toxicity.[48]

These data relate both to drugs of abuse and the treatment of PD. Concerning drugs of abuse, neuroprotection by apomorphine against methamphetamine toxicity configures as a potential means of managing methamphetamine-addicted patients. Under these conditions, chronic treatment with apomorphine should attenuate potential methamphetamine-induced neurodegeneration and, at the same time, continuous DA stimulation might modulate methamphetamine craving as a result of continuous DA receptor activation in the nucleus accumbens.

Concerning PD, these data offer new vistas for the treatment of the progression of PD. An elegant clinical study performed within the last decade[24] suggested that abnormal involuntary movements (AIMs) occurring in PD are related to the progression of the disease. In particular, whereas L-DOPA as well as noncontinuous administration of other DA agents can functionally elicit AIMs, the onset of the phenomenon is directly related to the degree of damage within the basal ganglia.[24,25,49] Reduction of dyskinesia achieved by continuous apomorphine administration might therefore be the effect of two coexisting phenomena: (1) symptomatic improvement resulting from continuous versus intermittent DA receptor stimulation and (2) the slowing of the disease process and/or a combined improved recovery of striatal DA function. However, the data presented here are also intriguing for their potential in the future therapy of PD and deserve further, more extensive studies performed at the clinical level as well as using animal models. In particular, long time course analyses in humans and chronic animal models need to be carried out.

We found that apomorphine rescues striatal DA terminals when administered by continuous subcutaneous infusion at doses that approximate those administered to humans. This effect specifically targets striatal dopaminergic axon terminals, and it occurs once the lesion is established. The infusion of apomorphine does not in fact prevent the nigral cell loss induced by MPTP, whereas the toxin modifies both the nigral and striatal GFAP immunoreactivity, suggesting a similar neurotoxic insult in both areas. Therefore, it is the striatal dopaminergic innervation that recovers under apomorphine administration, as witnessed by specific markers for DA axon terminals (DA and metabolites levels; TH immunohistochemistry).

Subcutaneous infusion of apomorphine in parkinsonian patients represents a useful tool in the treatment of severe on–off fluctuations and also in the control of certain L-DOPA-related off-period disabilities, such as pain, bladder dysfunction, dystonia, and gastrointestinal symptoms.[23,50] In patients treated by continuous subcutaneous infusion, apomorphine is delivered at a maximal daily dose of 4 mg/kg,[51] which is beyond the range of doses delivered to mice daily (0.5–3.15 mg/kg) in this study.

In conclusion, the protective activity of continuous subcutaneous infusion of apomorphine is particularly promising from a clinical standpoint and encourages the use of the drug to prevent or delay the onset of the "long-term L-DOPA syndrome," which is believed to result from the ongoing degeneration of nigrostriatal dopaminergic neurons.

REFERENCES

1. SEIDEN, L.S. & K.E. SABOL. 2001. Methamphetamine and methilenedioxymethamphetamine neurotoxicity: possible mechanisms of cell destruction. NIDA Monogr. **163:** 251–276.
2. VILLEMAGNE, V. et al. 1998. Brain dopamine neurotoxicity in baboons treated with doses of methamphetamine comparable to those recreationally abused by humans: evidence from [^{11}C]WIN-35,428 positron emission tomography studies and direct in vitro determinations. J. Neurosci. **18:** 419–427.
3. SEIDEN, L.S., M.W. FISCHMAN & C.R. SCHUSTER. 1975. Long-term methamphetamine-induced changes in brain catecholamine in tolerant rhesus monkeys. Drug Alcohol Depend. **1:** 215–219.
4. WILSON, J.M. et al. 1996. Striatal dopamine nerve terminal markers in human, chronic methamphetamine users. Nat. Med. **2:** 699–703.
5. ELLISON, G., M.S. EISON, H.S. HUBERMAN & F. DANIEL. 1978. Long-term changes in dopaminergic innervation of caudate nucleus after continuous amphetamine administration. Science **201:** 276–278.
6. RICAURTE, G.A., C.R. SCHUSTER & L.S. SEIDEN. 1980. Long-term effects of repeated metylamphetamine administration on dopamine and serotonin neurons in the rat brain: regional study. Brain Res. **193:** 153–163.

7. AXT, K.J. & M.E. MOLLIVER. 1991. Immunocytochemical evidence for methamphetamine-induced serotonergic axon loss in the rat brain. Synapse **9:** 304–313.
8. SONSALLA, P.K., W.J. NICKLAS & R.E. HEIKKILA. 1989. Role for excitatory amino acids in methamphetamine-induced nigro-striatal dopaminergic toxicity. Science **243:** 398–400.
9. SONSALLA, P.K. *et al.* 1996. Treatment of mice with methamphetamine produces cell loss in the substantia nigra. Brain Res. **738:** 172–175.
10. SUZUKI, O. *et al.* 1980. Inhibition of monoamine oxidase by *d*-methamphetamine. Biochem. Pharmacol. **29:** 2071–2073.
11. LIANG, N.Y. & C.O. RUTLEDGE. 1982. Comparison of the release of [^{3}H]dopamine from isolated corpus striatum by amphetamine, fenfluramine and unlabelled dopamine. Biochem. Behav. **31:** 983–992.
12. SULZER, D. *et al.* 1995. Amphetamine redistributes dopamine from synaptic vescicles to the cytosol and promotes reverse transport. J. Neurosci. **15:** 4102–4108.
13. O'DELL, S.J., F.B. WEIHMULLER & J.F. MARSHALL. 1991. Multiple methamphetamine injections induced marked increases in extracellular striatal dopamine which correlate with subsequent neurotoxicity. Brain Res. **564:** 256–260.
14. CUBELLS, J.F., S. RAYPORT, G. RAJENDRAN & D. SULZER. 1994. Methamphetamine neurotoxicity involves vacuolation of endocytic organelles and dopamine-dependent intracellular stress. J. Neurosci. **14:** 2260–2271.
15. GIOVANNI, A., L.P. LIANG, T.G. HASTINGS & M.J. ZIGMOND. 1995. Estimating hydroxyl radical content in rat brain using systemic and intraventricular salicylate: impact of methamphetamine. J. Neurochem. **64:** 1819–1825.
16. MILLER, G.W., R.R. GAINETDINOV, A.I. LEVEY & M.G. CARON. 1999. Dopamine transporters and neuronal injury. Trends Pharmacol. Sci. **20:** 424–429.
17. YAMAMOTO, B.K. & W. ZHU. 1998. The effects of methamphetamine on the production of free radicals and oxidative stress. J. Pharmacol. Exp. Ther. **287:** 107–114.
18. GRAHAM, D.G. 1978. Oxydative pathway for catecholamines in the genesis of neuromelanin and cytotoxic quinones. Mol. Pharmacol. **14:** 633–643.
19. TRETIAKOFF, C. 1919. Contribution à l'ètude de l'Anatomie pathologique du Locus Niger de Sommering avec quelques dèductions relatives à la pathogènie des troubles du tonus muscolaire de la maladie de Parkinson. Thèse de Paris, Paris, France.
20. EHRINGER, H. & O. HORNYKIEWICZ. 1960. Distribution of noradrenaline and dopamine (3-hydroxytyramine) in the human brain and their behavior in diseases of the extrapyramidal system. Klin. Wochenschr. **38:** 1236–1239.
21. MIZUNO, Y., N. HATTORI & H. MATSUMINE. 1998. Neurochemical and neurogenetic correlates of Parkinson's disease. J. Neurochem. **71:** 893–902.
22. HEFTI, F., E. MELAMED & R.J. WURTMAN. 1981. The site of dopamine formation in rat striatum after L-DOPA administration. J. Pharmacol. Exp. Ther. **217:** 189–197.
23. LEES, A.J. 1993. Dopamine agonists in Parkinson's disease: a look at apomorphine. Fundam. Clin. Pharmacol. **7:** 121–128.
24. BLIN, A.J., M. BONNET & Y. AGID. 1988. Does levodopa aggravate Parkinson's disease? Neurology **38:** 1410–1416.
25. BEDARD, P.J. *et al.* 1999. Pathophysiology of L-DOPA induced dyskinesia. Mov. Dis. **14:** 4–8.
26. GASSEN, M., Y. GLINKA, B. PINCHASI & M.B. YOUDIM. 1996. Apomorphine is a highly potent free radical scavenger in rat brain mitochondrial fraction. Eur. J. Pharmacol. **308:** 219–225.
27. UBEDA, A., C. MONTESINOS, M. PAYA & M.J. ALCARAZ. 1993. Iron-reducing and free-radical-scavenging properties of apomorphine and some related benzylisoquinolines. Free Radic. Biol. Med. **15:** 159–167.
28. YOUDIM, M.B.H., E. GRUNBLATT & S. MANDEL. 1999. The pivotal role of iron in NF-kappa B activation and nigrostriatal dopaminergic neurodegeneration. Prospects for neuroprotection in Parkinson's disease with iron chelators. Ann. N.Y. Acad. Sci. **890:** 7–25.
29. GRUNBLATT, E., S. MANDEL, T. BERKUZKI & M.B. YOUDIM. 1999. Apomorphine protects against MPTP-induced neurotoxicity in mice. Mov. Disord. **14:** 612–618.
30. GANCHER, S.T., J.G. NUTT & W.R. WOODWARD. 1995. Apomorphine infusional therapy in Parkinson's disease: clinical utility and lack of tolerance. Mov. Disord. **10:** 37–43.

31. COLZI, A., K. TURNER & A.J. LEES. 1998. Continuous subcutaneous waking day apomorphine in the long-term treatment of levodopa-induced interdose dyskinesias in Parkinson's disease. J. Neurol. Neurosurg. Psychiatry **64:** 573–576.
32. GIOVANNI, A., B.A. SIEBER, R.E. HEIKKILA & P.K. SONSALLA. 1994. Studies on species sensitivity to the dopaminergic neurotoxin 1-methyl-4-phenyl-1,2,3,6-tetrahydropyridine. Part I: systemic administration. J. Pharmacol. Exp. Ther. **270:** 1000–1007.
33. FORNAI, F. et al. 1997. Effects of noradrenergic lesions on MPTP/MPP$^+$ kinetics and MPTP-induced nigrostriatal dopamine depletions. J. Pharmacol. Exp. Ther. **283:** 100–107.
34. WAGNER, G.C., J.B. LUCOT, C.R. SCHUSTER & L.S. SEIDEN. 1981. The ontogeny of aggregation-enhanced toxicity. Psychopharmacology **75:** 92–93.
35. GESI, M. et al. 2000. The role of locus coeruleus in the development of Parkinson's disease. Neurosci. Biobehav. Rev. **24:** 655–668.
36. LOWRY, O.H., N.J. ROSEBROUGH, A.L. FARR & R.J. RANDALL. 1951. Protein measurement with the Folin phenol reagent. J. Biol. Chem. **193:** 265–275.
37. FORNAI, F. et al. 1999. Effects of pretreatment with DSP-4 on methamphetamine-induced striatal dopamine loss and pharmacokinetics. J. Neurochem. **72:** 777–784.
38. FORNAI, F. et al. 1995. Clonidine suppresses 1-methyl-4-phenyl-1,2,3,6-tetrahydropyridine-induced reductions of striatal dopamine and tyrosine hydroxylase activity in mice. J. Neurochem. **65:** 704–709.
39. CUSACK, B. et al. 2000. Effects of a novel neurotensin peptide analog given extracranially on CNS behaviors mediated by apomorphine and haloperidol. Brain Res. **856:** 48–54.
40. SANCHEZ, C. & J. ARNT. 1992. Effects on body temperature in mice differentiate between dopamine D_2 receptor agonists with high and low efficacies. Eur. J. Pharmacol. **211:** 9–14.
41. USUDA, S. 1981. Neuroleptic properties of cis-N-(1-benzyl-2-methylpyrrolidin-3-yl)-5-chloro-2-methoxy-4-methylaminobenzamide (YM-09151-2) with selective antidopaminergic activity. Psychopharmacology **73:** 103–109.
42. FORNAI, F. et al. 2001. Dose-dependent protective effects of apomorphine against methamphetamine-induced nigrostriatal damage. Brain Res. **898:** 27–35.
43. GASSEN, M., Y. GLINKA, B. PINCHASI & M.B. YOUDIM. 1996. Apomorphine is a highly potent free radical scavenger in rat brain mitochondrial fraction. Eur. J. Pharmacol. **308:** 219–225.
44. HALL, E.D. et al. 1996. Neuroprotective effects of the dopamine D2/D3 agonist pramipexole against postischemic or methamphetamine-induced degeneration of nigrostriatal neurons. Brain Res. **742:** 80–88.
45. MENA, M.A., V. DAVILA, J. BOGALUVSKY & D. SULZER. 1998. A synergistic neurotrophic response to l-dihydroxyphenylalanine and nerve growth factor. Mol. Pharmacol. **54:** 678–686.
46. BUENING, M.K. & J.W. GIBB. 1974. Influence of methamphetamine and neuroleptic drugs on tyrosine hydroxilase activity. Eur. J. Pharmacol. **26:** 30–34.
47. SONSALLA, P.K., J.W. GIBB & G.R. HANSON. 1986. Role of D1 and D2 dopamine receptor subtypes in mediating the methamphetamine-induced changes in monoamine system. J. Pharmacol. Exp. Ther. **238:** 932–937.
48. GRUNBLATT, E., S. MANDELL & M.B.H. YOUDIM. 2001. Effects of R- and S-apomorphine on MPTP-induced nigro-striatal dopamine neuronal loss. J. Neurochem. **77:** 146–156.
49. BALLARD, P.A., J.W. TETRUD & J.W. LANGSTON. 1985. Permanent human parkinsonism due to 1-methyl-4-phenyl-1,2,3,6-tetrahydropyridine (MPTP): seven cases. Neurology **35:** 949–956.
50. HUGHES, A.J. et al. 1993. Subcutaneous apomorphine in Parkinson's disease: response to chronic administration for up to five years. Mov. Disord. **8:** 165–170.
51. WENNING, G.K. et al. 1999. Effects of long-term, continuous subcutaneous apomorphine infusions on motor complications in advanced Parkinson's disease. Adv. Neurol. **80:** 545–548.

Neurokinin Receptors Modulate the Neurochemical Actions of Cocaine

P.-A.H. NOAILLES AND J.A. ANGULO

Department of Biological Sciences, Hunter College of the City University of New York, New York, New York 10021, USA

ABSTRACT: The psychostimulant cocaine is an indirect agonist that increases synaptic dopamine (DA) by binding with high affinity to the DA transporter (DAT) and blocking the active transport of synaptic DA back into the terminal. The resulting increase in extracellular DA alters postsynaptic activity in the circuitry of the basal ganglia. This study examines the role of neurokinin receptors on cocaine-evoked DA overflow in the striatum. Male Sprague-Dawley rats (n = 8) were treated with cocaine (10 mg/kg body weight i.p.) acutely or chronically. The pattern of DA release was assessed using *in vivo* microdialysis. In separate experiments two different neurokinin-1 (NK-1) receptor antagonists (D-Arg^1, D-Pro^2, D-Trp^{7,9}, Leu^{11}, or L-733,060) were perfused via the microdialysis probe for one hour in awake and freely moving animals that were subsequently injected i.p. with cocaine. Throughout the procedure, DA release was monitored at 1/2-hour intervals at a flow rate of 1 μl/min. In the groups of rats preperfused with NK-1 antagonists into the striatum, the cocaine-evoked release of DA was significantly reduced. This result suggests a significant role for the NK-1 receptor in the striatal response to acute and chronic cocaine administration.

KEYWORDS: neurokinin receptors; cocaine; dopamine; dopamine transporter; psychostimulants

INTRODUCTION

Psychostimulants such as cocaine are known to affect reward mechanisms in the brain in such a way as to increase the likelihood of self-administration and are known to have addictive properties in humans.[1,2] Our current understanding of the biological basis of drug-induced neurochemical plasticity implicates in part the activity of the mesolimbic system.[3] The mesolimbic pathway emanates from dopamine cell bodies of the ventral tegmental area and projects to the nucleus accumbens and prefrontal cortex. The mesolimbic pathway has been implicated in drug reinforcement and reward.[4] The nigrostriatal dopaminergic neurons and their targets in the forebrain (neurons projecting from the substantia nigra to the striatum) are also involved in reward but have a larger role in the phenomenon of locomotor sensitization to cocaine.[5] Pharmacological and behavioral studies have demonstrated that cocaine ad-

Address for correspondence: Dr. Jesus A. Angulo, Department of Biological Sciences, Hunter College of the City University of New York, 695 Park Ave., Rm. 927HN, New York, NY 10021. Voice: 212-772-5232; fax: 212-772-5230.
angulo@genectr.hunter.cuny.edu

Ann. N.Y. Acad. Sci. 965: 267–273 (2002). © 2002 New York Academy of Sciences.

ministration affects both nigrostriatal and mesocorticolimbic systems.[6] Sensitization to psychostimulants develops with intermittent or repeated treatment but not with continuous exposure to some drugs of abuse.[7] Intermittent treatment with psychostimulants causes a progressive increase in drug-elicited locomotion that can be long lasting.[5]

Acute cocaine administration causes an increase in dopamine release that can be measured by *in vivo* microdialysis. We administered NK-1 receptor antagonists into the striatum and the nucleus accumbens concomitant with systemic cocaine administration to evaluate the effects of blockade of NK-1 receptors on cocaine-evoked dopamine release. Three types of neurokinin receptors—neurokinin-1 (NK-1), neurokinin-2 (NK-2), and neurokinin-3 (NK-3)—have been characterized.[8,9] Based on the binding affinity, substance P, neurokinin A, and neurokinin B selectively bind to NK-1, NK-2, and NK-3, respectively. Affinity for substance P is 100 times higher for the NK-1 receptor than for NKA. At the NK-3 receptor affinity for NKA is twice that of SP, although the highest affinity is for NKB. Receptor autoradiography and lesion studies indicate that both neurokinin-1 and neurokinin-3 receptors are located in intrinsic striatal neurons, whereas in the substantia nigra neurokinin-3 receptors are located on dopaminergic projection neurons.[10] NK-2 receptors are widely distributed in the peripheral nervous system.[11,12] In the striatum, substance P (NK-1) receptors are expressed by a large percentage of cholinergic interneurons;[13] activation of NK-1 receptors in the striatum elicits a dose-dependent increase in acetylcholine (Ach)m release.[14]

This study focuses on investigating the role of the NK-1 receptor on cocaine-evoked dopamine release in the striatum, because our previous data demonstrate that these receptors play a critical role in the observed dopamine-dependent increase in locomotor behaviors resulting from administration of this psychostimulant.[15] Our aim is to determine whether the augmentation of dopamine release in the striatum resulting from acute administration of cocaine is dependent on neurokinin-1 receptor activity. We examined the effects of coadministration of cocaine with peptide or nonpeptide antagonists ([D-Arg^1, D-Pro^2, D-Trp^{7,9}, Leu^{11}] and L-733,060) on dopamine overflow.

METHODS AND MATERIALS

Stereotaxy and in Vivo Microdialysis

Dopamine release was determined by microdialysis in freely moving rats. Rats were anesthetized with isoflourane and placed in a Kopf stereotaxic apparatus. The plastic outer housing of the cannula containing a stainless steel post was affixed to the skull with two screws and dental cement. Subsequent to implantation of the guide cannula, animals were single housed. The animals were allowed to recover from surgery for seven days before psychostimulant treatment.

Approximately 18 hours before treatment, the rats were housed in a modified operant conditioning chamber, with food and water, and attached to a swivel arm assembly that carried a tube from an infusion pump connected to an INSTECH double-channel fluid swivel that permitted unrestricted movement. Artificial CSF (145 mM NaCl/2.7 mM KCl/1.2 mM CaCl$_2$/1 mM MgCl$_2$, pH 5.2) was perfused through the

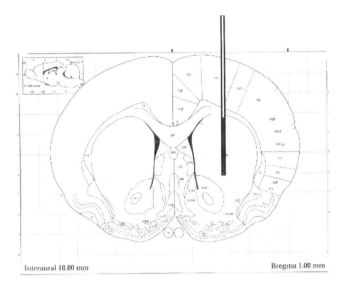

FIGURE 1. Anatomical placement of microdialysis probes is shown in schematic form in a coronal section through the striatum. *Black area* indicates the active portion of the microdialysis membrane.[17]

CMA 12/03 microdialysis (20 kDa) probe at a rate of one µl/min. Fractions of the dialysate were collected every 30 minutes in a plastic tube. Dopamine was measured by high-performance liquid chromatography (HPLC) with electrochemical detection using an ESA Choulochem II with a reversed-phase ESA microbore column. The mobile phase consists of 9 g/l NaH_2PO_4, 520 mg/l octane sulfonic acid, 8% (vol/vol) acetonitrile, 250 mg/l EDTA, and 175 µl/l triethylamine (adapted from Jedema and Moghaddam[16]). Quantification of the peaks is performed using Millennium computer chromatography enhancement program. Efficiency of recovery of the probes for dopamine recovery ranges from 9 to 24%. Probe placement verified in coronal sections of brain tissue (20 µm) stained with Cresyl violet. Brain dialysate fluid obtained from caudate putamen coordinates: A = 1.6 mm, L = 2.5 mm, D = 2.8 mm (see FIG. 1).[17]

Statistical Analysis

Analysis of variance (ANOVA) was used to analyze effects of drug treatment. The Newman-Keuls test was used for post hoc analysis. Neurotransmitter release was expressed as percent change relative to baseline. This was necessitated by the observation that baseline values are highly variable between animals. However, percent differences in neurotransmitter release relative to baseline are highly comparable. Thus, we averaged percent values from 10 animals and performed a paired Student's t-test and obtained p values smaller than 0.05. In order to perform comparisons between neurotransmitter levels at different time points and between different treatment groups, we utilized percent changes from individual subjects and performed a bifactorial analysis.

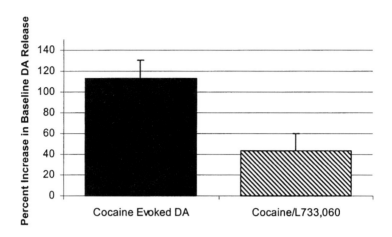

FIGURE 2. Effect of neurokinin-1 receptor antagonist on cocaine-evoked dopamine overflow in the striatum. Coadministration of the NK-1 receptor peptide antagonist (D-Arg[1], D-Pro[2], D-Trp[7,9], Leu[11]) through the microdialysis probe suppresses dopamine release in rats treated acutely with cocaine. The peptide NK-1 receptor antagonist (1 mM in artificial CSF) was perfused 60 minutes before the systemic injection of cocaine. The level of dopamine shown represents overflow during the first 30 minutes of sampling. $*p < 0.05$ (Newman-Keuls test).

RESULTS

Dopamine overflow was measured one-half hour post cocaine injection. It was found that in the animals perfused for one hour before injection with the NK-1 receptor peptide antagonist D-Arg[1], D-Pro[2], D-Trp[7,9], Leu[11] at a concentration of 10^{-3} M, the evoked release of dopamine was reduced by approximately 90% in the striatum in the first half-hour after systemic cocaine administration (FIG. 2). D-Arg[1], D-Pro[2], D-Trp[7,9], Leu[11] is a high-affinity (~10^{-9} M IC$_{50}$) competitive antagonist. This decrease in cocaine-evoked dopamine overflow was observed at every half-hour time point for two hours post injection (data not shown). Interestingly, in the one-hour period before cocaine administration when animals were perfused with D-Arg[1], D-Pro[2], D-Trp[7,9], Leu[11], there was no change in basal dopamine overflow, suggesting that NK-1 receptors do not affect basal levels of dopamine. To assure that the effect was specific to the activity of the NK-1 receptor, we employed the high-affinity nonpeptide NK-1 receptor antagonist L-733,060 (administered at a concentration of 10^{-4} M via the microdialysis probe 60 min before systemic cocaine administration). The effects of this nonpeptide antagonist were similar to those we found with D-Arg[1], D-Pro[2], D-Trp[7,9], Leu[11]. L-733,050 resulted in an approximately 80% decrease in cocaine-evoked dopamine overflow in the striatum (FIG. 3). In addition, we found that, as with D-Arg[1], D-Pro[2], D-Trp[7,9], Leu[11], L-733,050 had no specific effect on the basal release of dopamine in the striatum. When rats were treated chronically with cocaine (one daily injection of 10 mg/kg for six consecutive days) and then one final injection on the seventh day, it was found that D-Arg[1], D-Pro[2], D-Trp[7,9], Leu[11] had

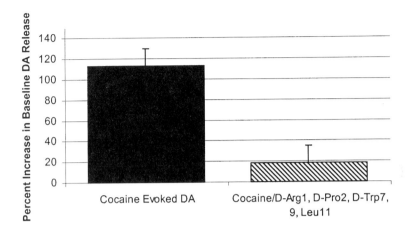

FIGURE 3. Effect of the nonpeptide neurokinin-1 receptor antagonist L-733,050 on cocaine-evoked dopamine overflow in the striatum. The L-733,050 was perfused through the microdialysis probe (100 μM in artificial CSF) for one hour before the systemic injection of cocaine. Cocaine-evoked dopamine overflow was significantly reduced with coadministration of the NK-1 receptor nonpeptide antagonist. The level of dopamine shown represents overflow during the first 30 minutes of sampling. $*p < 0.05$ (Newman-Keuls test).

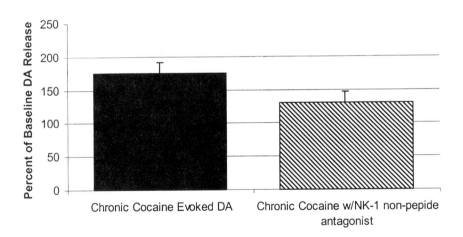

FIGURE 4. Lack of modulation of cocaine-evoked dopamine overflow by the neurokinin-1 receptor antagonist in the striatum of rats chronically treated with cocaine for seven consecutive days. The antagonist was infused through the microdialysis probe (1 mM in artificial CSF) for 60 minutes before the systemic injection of cocaine on day seven of chronic treatment. The level of dopamine shown represents overflow during the first 30 minutes of sampling.

no significant effect on cocaine-evoked dopamine overflow (FIG. 4). Therefore, chronic exposure to cocaine abrogates the modulatory actions of substance P on cocaine-evoked dopamine overflow in the striatum.

DISCUSSION

The results demonstrate that striatal neurokinin-1 receptors can modulate cocaine-evoked dopamine overflow without affecting the basal levels of release of this neurotransmitter. Chronic cocaine exposure abrogates this modulation of dopamine release. The neurokinin peptides substance P and NKA are expressed by the projection neurons of the direct striatonigral pathway. Both *in vivo* and *in vitro* studies indicate that exogenous substance P and NKA can elicit dopamine release from substantia nigra and striatum,[18,19] suggesting that both neuropeptides may act as neuromodulators in the direct striatonigral pathway. We infused the neurokinin-1 receptor antagonists through the microdialysis probe, thus eliminating the possibility of distant effects in the motor circuits that might influence the release of dopamine in the presence of cocaine. Our results are consistent with the hypothesis that augmented dopamine overflow in response to cocaine releases substance P in the striatum, which then acts through the neurokinin-1 receptor to boost dopamine overflow. We have unpublished observations that demonstrate that injection of cocaine releases substance P and that this peptide is then internalized with its receptor into endosomes in cholinergic interneurons of the striatum.[20] The effects of substance P on cocaine-evoked dopamine overflow have consequences on the output of the dopamine network. We have observed that systemic injection of a neurokinin-1 receptor antagonist inhibits cocaine-evoked locomotion in rats that are naive to the psychostimulant but has no effect in rats that have received chronic cocaine treatment.[15] Taken together, these observations suggest that the neurokinin-1 receptor of the striatum modulates cocaine-evoked dopamine overflow and that its ability to increase dopamine release is diminished with increasing exposure to cocaine. This finding has relevance to the mechanism of development of tolerance to cocaine. Characterizing the role of neurokinin receptors in the basal ganglia will aid in defining therapeutic targets in the treatment of substance abuse as well as in understanding the mechanisms involved in neurochemical plasticity in the central nervous system.

REFERENCES

1. PIAZZA, P.V. *et al.* 1991. Corticosterone levels determine individual vulnerability to amphetamine self-administration. Proc. Natl. Acad. Sci. USA **88:** 2088–2092.
2. PIAZZA, P.V. *et al.* 1991. Dopaminergic activity is reduced in the prefrontal cortex and increased in the nucleus accumbens of rats predisposed to develop amphetamine self-administration. Brain Res. **567:** 169–174.
3. RITZ, M.C. & M.J. KUHAR. 1993. Psychostimulant drugs and a dopamine hypothesis regarding addiction: update on recent research. Biochem. Soc. Symp. **59:** 51–64.
4. SELF, D.W. *et al.* 1995. Biochemical adaptations in the mesolimbic dopamine system in response to heroin self-administration. Synapse **21:** 312–318.
5. YI, S.J. & K.M. JOHNSON. 1990. Effects of acute and chronic administration of cocaine on striatal uptake, compartmentalization and release of [^{3}H]dopamine. Neuropharmacology **29:** 475–486.

6. KALIVAS, P.W. & J.E. ALESDATTER. 1993. Involvement of N-methyl-D-aspartate receptor stimulation in the ventral tegmental area and amygdala in behavioral sensitization to cocaine. J. Pharmacol. Exp. Ther. **267:** 486–495.
7. POST, R.M. 1980. Intermittent versus continuous stimulation: effect of time interval on the development of sensitization or tolerance. Life Sci. **26:** 1275–1282.
8. LEE, C.M. *et al.* 1986. Multiple tachykinin binding sites in peripheral tissues and in brain. Eur. J. Pharmacol. **130:** 209–217.
9. HELKE, C.J. *et al.* 1990. Diversity in mammalian tachykinin peptidergic neurons: multiple peptides, receptors, and regulatory mechanisms. FASEB J. **4:** 1606–1615.
10. STOESSL, A.J. 1994. Localization of striatal and nigral tachykinin receptors in the rat. Brain Res. **646:** 13–18.
11. YASHPAL, K., T.V. DAM & R. QUIRION. 1990. Quantitative autoradiographic distribution of multiple neurokinin binding sites in rat spinal cord. Brain Res. **506:** 259–266.
12. DAM, T.V., E. ESCHER & R. QUIRION. 1988. Evidence for the existence of three classes of neurokinin receptors in brain. Differential ontogeny of neurokinin-1, neurokinin-2 and neurokinin-3 binding sites in rat cerebral cortex. Brain Res. **453:** 372–376.
13. KAWAGUCHI, Y., T. AOSAKI & Y. KUBOTA. 1997. Cholinergic and GABAergic interneurons in the striatum. Nihon Shinkei Seishin Yakurigaku Zasshi **17:** 87–90.
14. GUZMAN, R.G., K.M. KENDRICK & P.C. EMSON. 1993. Effect of substance P on acetylcholine and dopamine release in the rat striatum: a microdialysis study. Brain Res. **622:** 147–154.
15. KRAFT, M., P. NOAILLES & J.A. ANGULO. 2001. Substance P modulates cocaine-evoked dopamine overflow in the striatum of the rat brain. Ann. N.Y. Acad. Sci. **937:** 121–131.
16. JEDEMA, H.P. & B. MOGHADDAM. 1994. Glutamatergic control of dopamine release during stress in the rat prefrontal cortex. J. Neurochem. **63:** 785–788.
17. PAXINOS, G.A.W. 1986. The Rat Brain in Stereotaxic Coordinates. Harcourt Brace Javanovich. New York.
18. PETIT, F. & J. GLOWINSKI. 1986. Stimulatory effect of substance P on the spontaneous release of newly synthesized [^{3}H]dopamine from rat striatal slices: a tetrodotoxin-sensitive process. Neuropharmacology **25:** 1015–1021.
19. HOKFELT, T. *et al.* 1991. Tachykinins and related peptides in the substantia nigra and neostriatum. Ann. N.Y. Acad. Sci. **632:** 192–197.
20. NOAILLES, P.-A.H. *et al.* 2000. Cocaine-evoked release of substance P and signaling through the NK-1 receptor in the neostriatum. Presented at the Society for Neuroscience Meeting.

Calpain Upregulation and Neuron Death in Spinal Cord of MPTP-Induced Parkinsonism in Mice

BHISHAM CHERA,[a] KURT E. SCHAECHER,[a,b] ANNE ROCCHINI,[a]
SYED Z. IMAM,[c] SWAPAN K. RAY,[a] SYED F. ALI,[c] AND NAREN L. BANIK[a]

[a]Department of Neurology, Medical University of South Carolina, Charleston, South Carolina 29425, USA

[c]Neurochemistry Laboratory, Division of Neurotoxicology, National Center for Toxicological Research-FDA, Jefferson, Arkansas 72079, USA

ABSTRACT: Parkinson's disease (PD) is a neurodegenerative disorder resulting in slowness, tremors, and imbalance. Treatment of mice with 1-methyl-4-phenyl-1,2,3,6 tetrahydropyridine (MPTP) is one of several models used to mimic PD in humans. Administration of MPTP leads to the production of 1-methyl-4-phenyl-2,3 dihydropyridinium (MPP^+). MPP^+ is taken up by dopaminergic neurons, causing mitochondrial dysfunction and cell death. Because calpain is involved in neuronal cell death and mitochondrial dysfunction, we examined the level of calpain in neurons in the substantia nigra (SN) and hippocampus of MPTP-treated C57BL/6 mice. Because of the interconnections between spinal cord and upper central nervous system neurons, we examined morphology, calpain activity, and calpain expression in neurons by double immunofluorescence using calpain and neuron marker (NeuN) antibodies. In controls, calpain expression was low in SN, hippocampus, and spinal cord $NeuN^+$ cells, and the NeuN stain was concentrated around the nucleus. In mice sacrificed 24 h after administration of three 20 mg/kg doses of MPTP, calpain expression was slightly increased in SN and hippocampal neurons and moderately increased in spinal cord neurons. In these animals, the NeuN stain was less concentrated around the nuclear membrane. One week after MPTP treatment, calpain content in $NeuN^+$ cells was greatly increased in SN, hippocampus, and spinal cord. Morphologically, SN and spinal cord neurons, treated for one week, were necrotic with a granular cytoplasmic NeuN content. Also, MPTP treatment upregulated calpain activity and mRNA level in spinal cord. These data suggest that following MPTP treatment, calpain causes neuronal death in SN as well as in spinal cord.

KEYWORDS: substantia nigra; dopaminergic neurons; apoptosis; astrocyte; motor neuron

Address for correspondence: Naren L. Banik, Department of Neurology, P.O. Box 250606, Suite 307, 96 Jonathan Lucas St., Charleston, SC 29425. Voice: 843-792-3946; fax: 843-792-8626.

baniknl@musc.edu

[b]Present address: Dr. Kurt Schaecher, Department of Microbiology and Immunology, Walter Reed Memorial Institute, Baltimore, Maryland.

Ann. N.Y. Acad. Sci. 965: 274–280 (2002). © 2002 New York Academy of Sciences.

INTRODUCTION

Parkinson's disease (PD) is a debilitating movement disorder associated with characteristic clinical symptoms of tremor, rigidity, bradykinesia, imbalance, and dementia.[1] The etiology of PD is largely unknown and thought to be of idiopathic and sporadic type. Nevertheless, several causes or factors have been recently implicated in the pathogenesis of PD. These include vascular disease, environmental toxins, drugs (MPTP, metamphetamine), and genetic factors.[1–3] Early onset of this disease has been recently described as mutations in the α-synuclein, parkin, and ubiquitin genes.[4–6] PD affects catecholaminergic and primarily dopaminergic neurons in the central nervous system (CNS) with occasional inclusion of Lewy bodies.[7–9] In brain, it primarily affects substantia nigra (SN), locus coeruleus (LC), and other areas with resultant motor dysfunction. Although the pathophysiological mechanism of neuronal loss in neurodegenerative diseases is poorly understood, the loss of dopaminergic neurons, particularly in SN in PD, is thought to be a predominant feature and apoptotic in nature.[7,8]

To understand the mechanisms by which the dopaminergic neurons may be dying in SN, investigators have utilized an animal model of parkinsonism induced by the heroin analogue 1-methyl-4-phenyl-1,2,3,6-tetrahydropyridine (MPTP) in primates and mice.[10–13] Following administration, MPTP becomes concentrated in dopaminergic neurons where it is oxidized by monoamine oxidase (MAO-B) to neurotoxic 1-methyl-4-pheynlypyridinium ion (MPP^+).[14,15] The neurotoxic effects of MPP^+, which readily crosses the blood–brain barrier (BBB), have been suggested to be due to several mechanisms. It has been found to irreversibly inhibit complex 1 of the mitochondrial respiratory chain, leading to depletion of ATP synthesis in MPTP-induced mice as well as in PD patients.[16–19] Depletion of ATP synthesis and disruption of oxidative phosphorylation by MPP^+ lead to release of toxic free radicals which are detrimental to cell survival.[20–22] Thus, dopaminergic neurons under oxidative stress in SN become vulnerable and succumb to apoptotic death. Apoptosis of dopaminergic neurons in SN in PD mice as well as in PD patients with mitochondrial complex 1 defect has been associated with increased caspase activity.[16,18,23] Cell death due to oxidative stress has been demonstrated *in vitro* in the presence of MPP^+.[24]

In addition to inhibition of mitochondria complex 1, MPP^+ has been implicated in the activation of N-methyl-D-aspartate (NMDA) receptors. Thus, MPP^+ plays an important role in inducing excitotoxicity which causes Ca^{2+}-influx leading to activation of many Ca^{2+}-dependent events, including proteases and lipases.[25] Activation of both lipase (e.g., phospholipase A_2) and the calcium-activated proteinase calpain is known to mediate formation of free radicals (via arachidonic acid and its cascades) and degradation of cytoskeletal proteins, respectively, and these may participate in dopaminergic neuron death in SN in PD mice. Recent reports suggest that catecholaminergic and cholinergic neurons in brain are also affected by MPTP neurotoxicity.[26–28]

Although most of the PD-related work has been directed to dopaminergic neurons in SN and other areas of brain, such studies on spinal cord lagged behind. Because one of the normal functions of spinal cord is to coordinate movements and sensation in the body, and because PD is characterized as a movement disorder, we hypothesize that spinal cord neurons may also be affected in PD.

There are many different circuits in the brain that influence motor function, most obviously via the spinal cord. Various descending and ascending nerve projections intimately connect the brain, midbrain, and spinal cord. The brain manipulates the intrinsic reflex circuits in the spinal cord to produce volitional movement. Any detrimental factors released from degenerated neurons and axons in the brain may affect interneurons, motor neurons, and their tracts in spinal cord, which may ultimately interfere with movement. Thus, spinal cord dopaminergic neurons and catecholaminergic neurons are subjected to degeneration in MPTP-induced PD. Involvement of spinal cord in PD-associated pain has been shown. Other clinical studies have indicated degeneration of noradrenergic and serotonergic neurons, but not dopaminergic neurons in lumbar spinal cord of PD patients.[29,30] 5HT and NA projections to the spinal cord are dense and modulate pain and movement, respectively. However, in some clinical studies, involvement of spinal cord in PD remains controversial although Lewy body inclusions in spinal cord were similar to those seen in SN of PD patients.[31–33]

Because of Ca^{2+} influx in MPTP-induced PD mice and PD patients, we investigated the involvement of calpain in the pathogenesis of PD in the animal model and subsequently determined cell death in SN and spinal cord. We have found increased calpain expression in glial cells and neurons in spinal cord and correlated this with neuronal death using *in situ* TUNEL and immunofluorescence labeling. Elevated calpain activity has been previously reported in SN of patients with PD which implicated an important role for calpain in pathophysiology of PD.[34] Also, we have recently demonstrated such an increased calpain activity and transcriptional expression of calpain in the spinal cord of MPTP-induced PD mice.[34,35] The current investigation examines whether the cell types expressing increased calpain are dying of apoptosis or necrosis in spinal cord. The study was carried out in MPTP-induced C57BL/6N mouse model of parkinsonism.

MPTP-INDUCED PARKINSON'S DISEASE MODEL

Male C57BL/6N mice were used for induction of PD with intraperitoneal (i.p.) injection of MPTP.[10] A 10 mg/kg/10 mL solution of MPTP in normal saline was given i.p., and control animals received saline only. Animals were sacrificed at 24 h and 7 days following MPTP administration. The spinal cord and brain areas were removed fixed in tissue-freezing medium,[36] and frozen at −70°C. Cryostat sections from these samples were then analyzed by TUNEL and double immunofluorescent studies.[36]

CALPAIN AND CALPASTATIN SYSTEM IN CNS

Calpains, Ca^{2+}-activated neutral proteinases, are classified as ubiquitous or tissue-specific forms.[37] The present work is designed to examine the role of ubiquitous calpain, which has been implicated in the pathophysiology of neurodegenerative diseases such as Alzheimer's, demyelinating diseases such as multiple sclerosis (MS), and Parkinson's disease, as well as CNS injuries.[25,37] Ubiquitous calpain exists in two forms, micro (μ)- and milli (m)-calpain, activated by μM and mM calcium concentrations, respectively.[38] It is also regulated by a specific endogenous inhibitor, calpastatin. In the pathogenesis of diseases, the regulatory role of calpastatin is diminished or destroyed due to an increase in the calpain-calpastatin ratio, the condition in which calpastatin becomes a suicide substrate of calpain.[39] Calpain has many substrates, including myelin basic protein (MBP), cytoskeletal proteins, neurofilament protein (NFP), microtubule-associated protein (MAP), spectrin, and protein kinase C.[25] The degradation of cytoskeletal proteins has implicated calpain involvement in cell death (neurons and glial cells) related to stress and diseases.[40,41]

CALPAIN ACTIVITY AND EXPRESSION IN MPTP-INDUCED PD

An increase in the level of m-calpain has been demonstrated in mesencephalon of patients with PD and implicated in the mechanism of neuronal death.[34] This study, however, did not examine calpain activity and expression in other areas of CNS, including spinal cord. Since PD is a movement disorder and spinal cord normally coordinates movements, we have postulated that spinal motor and interneurons may be degenerated in MPTP-induced PD mice. In considering this hypothesis, we previously showed increased calpain activity and transcriptional expression in spinal cord of MPTP-induced PD mice.[35] This finding suggested a participating role for calpain in neuron death in the spinal cord of PD mice. We extended this finding to examine the demise of those cells that were expressing elevated calpain, by application of TUNEL and double immunofluorescent techniques.[36] Identification of calpain expression in TUNEL-positive cells in spinal cord were compared with those in SN. Cells were identified by specific marker antibodies to OX-42 for microglia and mononuclear phagocytes, GFAP for astrocytes, and NeuN for neurons. Calpain expression was detected by antibody raised in our laboratory.

OX-42–positive microglia or mononuclear phagocytes were activated in spinal cord both at 24 h and 1 week following treatment with MPTP. Many of these cells also showed increased calpain immunoreactivity compared to controls. Astrocytes are also reactive with substantially increased calpain staining at that time period. Spinal cord neurons were identified with NeuN antibody. Some were swollen and demonstrated increased calpain immunoreactivity compared to controls. Neurons from SN also showed greatly increased calpain immunostaining. Neurons were TUNEL-positive compared to controls. At the morphological level these neurons in both spinal cord and SN were necrotic with a granular cytoplasmic NeuN content at 1 week following treatment with MPTP. Our data indicate that increased calpain may have a crucial role in cell death in MPTP-induced parkinsonism. We and others have demonstrated such a role for calpain in neural cell death mechanism *in vitro* as well as in the pathophysiology of SCI and demyelinating diseases such as EAE and MS.[25,42] These findings also support our previous notion that not only SN, but spinal cord neurons as well as neurons in other areas of the brain may be affected in Parkinson's disease. Such an effect on the energy metabolism has been recently demonstrated in cerebelli of patients with PD.[43]

In conclusion, our study supports a crucial role for calpain, among others, in cell death in PD and suggests that in addition to SN, other CNS areas including spinal cord and cerebellum may also be affected in this devastating disorder. Our results suggest that use of calpain inhibitors as therapeutic agents may preserve or protect cells in the MPTP-induced parkinsonism.

ACKNOWLEDGMENTS

This work was supported in part by grants from NIH-NINDS (NS-31622, NS-38146, and NS-41088) and an SCE&G Summer Student Research Scholarship to Bhisham Chera. We thank Gloria Wilford and Denise Matzelle for their invaluable assistance.

REFERENCES

1. WICHMANN, T. & M.R. DELONG. 1993. Pathophysiology of parkinsonian motor abnormalities. Adv. Neurol. **60:** 53–61.
2. OLANOW, C.W. & W.G. TATTON. 1999. Etiology and pathogenesis of Parkinson's disease. Annu. Rev. Neurosci. **22:** 123–144.
3. RAJPUT, A.H. *et al.* 1987. Geography, drinking water chemistry, pesticides and herbicides and the etiology of Parkinson's disease. Can. J. Neurol. Sci. **14:** 414–418.
4. GOEDERT, M. 1997. Familial Parkinson's diseases. The awakening of alpha-synuclein [news]. Nature **388:** 232.
5. FIGUEIREDO-PEREIRA, M. & P. ROCKWELL. 2001. The ubiquitin/proteosome pathway in neurological disorders. *In* Role of Proteases in the Pathophysiology of Neurodegenerative Diseases. A. Lajtha & N.L. Banik, Eds.: 137–153. Kluwer Academic/Plenum Publishers. New York.
6. LINCOLN, S. *et al.* 1999. Low frequency of pathogenic mutations in the ubiquitin carboxy-terminal hydroxylase gene in familial Parkinson's disease. Neuroreport **10:** 427–429.
7. DAMIER, P. *et al.* 1999. The substantia nigra of the human brain. I. Nigrosomes and the nigral matrix, a compartmental organization based on calbindin D(28K) immunohistochemistry. Brain **122:** 1421–1436.
8. DAMIER, P. *et al.* 1999. The substantia nigra of the human brain. II. Patterns of loss of dopamine-containing neurons in Parkinson's disease. Brain **122:** 1437–1448.
9. DELISLE, M.B. *et al.* 1987. Motor neuron disease, parkinsonism and dementia. Report of a case with diffuse Lewy body-like intracytoplasmic inclusions. Acta Neuropathol. **75:** 104–108.
10. FREYALDENHOVEN, T.E. *et al.* 1997. Systemic administration of MPTP induces thalamic neuronal degeneration in mice. Brain Res. **759:** 9–17.
11. HEIKKILA, R.E. *et al.* 1984. Dopaminergic neurotoxicity of 1-methyl-4-phenyl-1,2,5,6-tetrahydropyridine in mice. Science **224:** 1451–1453.
12. HEIKKILA, R.E. *et al.* 1984. Protection against the dopaminergic neurotoxicity of 1-methyl-4-phenyl-1,2,5,6-tetrahydropyridine by monoamine oxidase inhibitors. Nature **311:** 467–469.
13. BURNS, R.S. *et al.* 1983. A primate model of parkinsonism: selective destruction of dopaminergic neurons in the pars compacta of the substantia nigra by *N*-methyl-4-phenyl-1,2,3,6-tetrahydropyridine. Proc. Natl. Acad. Sci. USA **80:** 4546–4550.
14. CHIBA, K. *et al.* 1984. Metabolism of the neurotoxic tertiary amine, MPTP, by brain monoamine oxidase. Biochem. Biophys. Res. Commun. **120:** 574–578.
15. JAVITCH, J.A. & S.H. SNYDER. 1984. Uptake of MPP(+) by dopamine neurons explains selectivity of parkinsonism-inducing neurotoxin, MPTP. Eur. J. Pharmacol. **106:** 455–456.
16. NIKLAS, W.J. *et al.* 1985. Inhibition of NADH-linked oxidation in brain mitochondria by 1-methyl-4-phenyl-1,2,3,6-tetrahydropyridine. Life Sci. **36:** 2505–2508.
17. RIACHI, N.J. *et al.* 1989. Entry of 1-methyl-4-phenyl-1,2,3,6-tetrahydropyridine into the rat brain. J. Pharmacol. Exp. Ther. **249:** 744–748.
18. TATTON, N.A. & S.J. KISH. 1997. *In situ* detection of apoptotic nuclei in the substantia nigra compacta of 1-methyl-4-phenyl-1,2,3,6-tetrahydropyridine-treated mice using terminal deoxynucleotidyl transferase labelling and acridine orange staining. Neuroscience **77:** 1037–1048.

19. SCHAPIRA, A.H. *et al.* 1989. Mitochondrial complex 1 deficiency in Parkinson's disease. Lancet **1:** 1269.
20. OLANOW, C.W. 1990. Oxidation reactions in Parkinson's disease. Neurology **40** (Suppl.)**:** 32–37; discussion 37–39.
21. KOSEL, S. *et al.* 1999. Role of mitochondria in Parkinson disease. Biol. Chem. **380:** 865–870.
22. PERRY, T.L. *et al.* 1982. Parkinson's disease: a disorder due to nigral glutathione deficiency? Neurosci. Lett. **33:** 305–310.
23. HARTMANN, A. *et al.* 2000. Caspase-3: a vulnerability factor and final effector in apoptotic death of dopaminergic neurons in Parkinson's disease. Proc. Natl. Acad. Sci. USA **97:** 2875–2780.
24. TURMEL, H. *et al.* 2001. Caspase-3 activation in 1-methyl-4-phenyl-1,2,3,6-tetrahydropyridine (MPTP)-treated mice. Move. Disord. **16:** 185–189.
25. RAY, S.K. & N.L. BANIK. 2001. Calpain. *In* Wiley Encyclopedia of Molecular Medicine. G. Collins, Ed.: 435–440. John Wiley & Sons, Inc. New York.
26. MITCHELL, I.J. *et al.* 1985. Sites of the neurotoxic action of 1-methyl-4-phenyl-1,2,3,6-tetrahydropyridine in the macaque monkey include the ventral tegmental area and the locus coeruleus. Neurosci. Lett. **61:** 195–200.
27. SENIUK, N.A. *et al.* 1990. Dose-dependent destruction of the coeruleus-cortical and nigral-striatal projections by MPTP. Brain Res. **527:** 7–20.
28. GOTO, S. & A. HIRANO. 1991. Catecholaminergic neurons in the parabrachial nucleus of normal individuals and patients with idiopathic Parkinson's disease. Ann. Neurol. **30:** 192–196.
29. SCATTON, B. *et al.* 1986. Degeneration of noradrenergic and serotonergic but not dopaminergic neurones in the lumbar spinal cord of parkinsonian patients. Brain Res. **380:** 181–185.
30. SAGE, J.I. *et al.* 1990. Evidence for the role of spinal cord systems in Parkinson's disease-associated pain. Clin. Neuropharmacol. **13:** 171–174.
31. LELLI, S. *et al.* 1991. Spinal cord inhibitory mechanisms in Parkinson's disease. Neurology **41:** 553–556.
32. SANDYK, R. & R. P. IACONO. 1987. Spinal dopamine mechanisms and primary sensory symptoms in Parkinson's disease. Int. J. Neurosci. **32:** 927–931.
33. SICA, R. E. & O. P. SANZ. 1976. An electrophysiological study of the functional changes in the spinal motoneurones in Parkinson's disease. Electromyogr. Clin. Neurophysiol. **16:** 409–417.
34. MOUATT-PRIGENT, A. *et al.* 1996. Increased M-calpain expression in the mesencephalon of patients with Parkinson's disease but not in other neurodegenerative disorders involving the mesencephalon: a role in nerve cell death? Neuroscience **73:** 979–987.
35. RAY, S.K. *et al.* 2000. Calpain upregulation in spinal cords of mice with 1-methyl-4-phenyl-1,2,3,6-tetrahydropyridine (MPTP)-induced Parkinson's disease. *In* Neurological Mechanisms of Drugs of Abuse: Cocaine, Ibogaine, and Substituted Amphetamines. S.F. Ali, Ed. Ann. N.Y. Acad. Sci. **914:** 275–283.
36. RAY, S.K. *et al.* 2000. Combined TUNEL and double immunofluorescence labeling for detecting apoptotic mononuclear phagocytes in autoimmune demyelinating disease. Brain Res. Protocol **5:** 305–311.
37. SHIELDS, D.C. & N.L. BANIK. 2001. Calcium-activated neutral proteinase in demyelinating diseases. *In* The Role of Proteolytic Enzymes in the Pathophysiology of Neurodegenerative Diseases. A. Lajtha & N.L. Banik, Eds.: 25–45. Plenum Press. New York.
38. CROALL, D.E. & G.N. DEMARTINO. 1991. Calcium-activated neutral protease (calpain) system: structure, function, and regulation. Physiol. Rev. **71:** 813–847.
39. SUZUKI, K. *et al.* 1987. Calcium-activated neutral protease and its endogenous inhibitor. Activation at the cell membrane and biological function. FEBS Lett. **220:** 271–277.
40. RAY, S.K. *et al.* 1999. Diverse stimuli induce calpain overexpression and apoptosis in C6 glioma cells. Brain Res. **829:** 18–27.
41. RAY, S.K. *et al.* 2000. Oxidative stress and Ca^{2+} influx upregulate calpain and induce apoptosis in PC12 cells. Brain Res. **852:** 326–334.

42. SHIELDS, D.C. *et al.* 1999. A putative mechanism of demyelination in multiple sclerosis by a proteolytic enzyme, calpain. Proc. Natl. Acad. Sci. USA **96:** 11486–11491.
43. GIBSON, G.E. *et al.* 2001. Deficit in a Krebs cycle mitochondrial enzyme in brains from patients with Parkinson's disease. J. Neurochem. **78**(Suppl.): 132(BP02-18).

Abused Inhalants and Central Reward Pathways

Electrophysiological and Behavioral Studies in the Rat

ARTHUR C. RIEGEL AND EDWARD D. FRENCH

Department of Pharmacology, University of Arizona, College of Medicine, Tucson, Arizona 85724, USA

ABSTRACT: Inhalant abuse remains a significant health problem among the younger segment of society. In fact, the use of inhalants in this population trails only that of nicotine, alcohol, and marijuana. Toluene is a common ingredient in many of the substances sought out for inhalation abuse, apparently for its euphorigenic and hallucinogenic effects. Because drugs of abuse share the common property of altering the activity of mesolimbic dopamine neurons, it is reasonable to suspect that toluene-induced changes in this CNS pathway may underlie its abuse potential. Here we will provide *in vivo* and *in vitro* electrophysiological data and behavioral evidence linking toluene exposure in rats to activation of mesolimbic dopamine neurons. Exposure of rats to 11,000 ppm of inhaled toluene produced time-dependent activation of dopamine neurons within the midbrain ventral tegmental area (VTA). In the rat brain slice preparation, perfusion with toluene (23–822 µM) also evoked an increase in activity of both dopamine and nondopamine neurons within the VTA. These excitatory effects could not be found in adjacent non-VTA nuclei, nor were they sensitive to the glutamate antagonists CGS19755 or CNQX. In behavioral studies, systemic administration of toluene produced a dose-dependent locomotor hyperactivity that was attenuated by either pretreatment with the D2 dopamine receptor antagonist remoxipride or by 6-hydroxydopamine lesions of the nucleus accumbens. These findings show that toluene can activate dopamine neurons within the mesolimbic reward pathway, an effect that may underlie the abuse potential of inhaled substances containing toluene.

KEYWORDS: toluene; inhalants; dopamine; ventral tegmental area; reward

INTRODUCTION

The widespread abuse of inhalants (i.e., spray paints, glues, and lacquers) is a significant and potentially lethal problem among youth. An epidemiological study showed that in 1995, 23% of the adolescents in the United States were experimenting with inhalants.[1] Although the overall incidence of inhalant abuse is extensive, there is little experimental data implicating the abuse liability of solvents such as toluene with a specific CNS site or mechanism of action.

Address for correspondence: Edward D. French, Department of Pharmacology, University of Arizona, College of Medicine, Tucson, AZ 85724. Voice: 520-626-4359; fax: 520-626-2204.
efrench@u.arizona.edu

Ann. N.Y. Acad. Sci. 965: 281–291 (2002). © 2002 New York Academy of Sciences.

The acute consumption of inhalants produces a variety of psychotropic effects, including an initial euphoria, intoxication, slurred speech, ataxia, numbness of the extremities, amnesia, hostile behavior, and hallucinations. As inhalation continues, seizures, tinnitus, diffuse somatic pain, tremor, and death can occur.[2] Several reports also link chronic "huffing" to permanent liver, kidney, heart, and cranial nerve damage; cerebral, cerebellar, and brainstem atrophy neuropathies; dependence; and psychosis (see Arlien-Soborg[3] and references therein). Many consider the organic solvent toluene the essential psychotropic component found in many commonly abused inhalants. Even nonhuman primates lever-press for bursts of toluene vapor.[4] Human abusers are known to consume volatiles by chewing on solvent-soaked rags or breathing vapors from paper bags or other containers (toluene concentration ~10,000 ppm).[5]

When inhaled, toluene is rapidly absorbed by the lungs and with continued exposure saturates the blood and brain in about 60 minutes, with the concentration in brain being directly proportional to the air concentration.[6,7] Toluene preferentially accumulates in lipid-rich areas such as the midbrain and, to a lesser extent, the cerebral cortex and olfactory bulbs.[8–10]

Presumably, the repeated use of inhalants would imply a positively reinforcing mechanism. To date, however, no one has associated the reinforcing effects of inhalants to a specific CNS site or mechanism of action. One possible rationale for the prevalence of abused inhalants may be that one of their components may modulate the mesolimbic dopamine system whose fibers originate in cell bodies located in the ventral tegmental area (VTA).[11] Furthermore, experiments conducted in animals have shown that other commonly abused drugs (i.e., ethanol, phencyclidine, Δ^9-tetrahydrocannabinol, opiates) can increase the firing frequency of dopamine neurons in the VTA and dopamine release within the nucleus accumbens.[12–17] Thus, enhanced dopamine neurotransmission within this circuit has been proposed to underlie the rewarding effects of drugs of abuse.[18,19]

The goal of this study was to determine whether toluene inhalation could alter dopamine neuronal activity and, if so, whether this effect resulted from a site of action within the VTA. In addition, behavioral experiments were conducted to also ascertain whether toluene-induced locomotor hyperactivity was mediated through activation of dopamine neurotransmission through the VTA–nucleus accumbens pathway. The data presented here may provide some insight into possible mechanisms underlying the reinforcing properties of this solvent.

MATERIALS AND METHODS

Adult male Sprague-Dawley rats (Harlan, Indianapolis, IN) weighing 250–350 g were used in all experiments. Toluene (analytical grade), benzene, and carbon disulfide (reagent grade) were purchased from Fisher Scientific. The preparation of the drug solutions used for the *in vivo* electrophysiological and behavioral experiments are described elsewhere.[20,21]

Presumptive dopamine neurons in the ketamine-anesthetized rat were identified according to the following well-characterized criteria: (1) biphasic or triphasic positive–negative waveform action potentials; (2) action potential duration >2 ms; (3) firing rates <10 spikes/s and regular to bursting patterns of firing.[22,23] Once a neuron with these characteristics was found, its activity was monitored for approximately 4 minutes to establish a basal firing rate before toluene challenges were begun. Toluene exposure was accomplished by placing a 5-ml glass vial containing 4 ml of toluene 5 mm from the tip of the tracheal breathing tube for various periods of time. Neuronal activity was recorded during toluene challenge, and qualitative changes in firing rates were visually displayed as ratemeter records. Subsequent quantitative analyses of the electrophysiological responses were performed off-line using periods of 10 bins of 10 s per bin (i.e., 100 s or 1.7 min). Firing rate changes (spikes/s) in each of these 1.7-min periods were calculated by measuring the number of action potentials between the time of onset of toluene exposure and point of maximum change in rate and divided by the elapsed time to yield spikes/s. Changes in firing rate and percent bursts during toluene were compared to pretoluene firing rate and percent bursts and calculated as percent change over baseline. A total of 64 cells was recorded from 42 rats. Because exposure times were not held constant, the percent changes in firing rate for the various exposure times were then assigned to a single exposure period (1.7, 3.4, 5.1 min, etc.) using a mid-range calculation as follows: exposures of 0–2.6 min to the 1.7-min timepoint, 2.6–4.3 min to 3.4 timepoint, 4.3–6.0 to 5.1, 6.0–7.7 to 6.8, 7.7–9.4 to 8.5, 9.4–11.1 to 10.2, 11.1–12.8 to 11.9, 12.8–14.2 to 13.6, and 14.2–15.9 to the 15.3-min timepoint. Neurons were classified as bursting when, within an epoch of >500 action potentials, there were at least two episodes containing two action potentials and at least one episode containing three or more action potentials. The criteria used for computer recognition of bursts included (1) an interspike interval of 80 ms or less for the first pair of spikes in a train and (2) termination when the interval between two spikes exceeded 160 ms.[23] Records were excluded from the burst analysis if fewer than 500 action potentials were recorded or the activity contained no bursts that would, with any subsequent bursting, result in an infinite change in percent bursts.

In vitro experiments were conducted in brain slices cut at 400 μm through the midbrain containing the VTA. Slices were superfused in a recording chamber with ACSF maintained at 35°C.

Samples of jugular vein blood were taken and analyzed as previously described.[21] Samples of bath perfusate containing toluene were also taken and analyzed for solvent concentration.

RESULTS

Exposure Concentration and Blood Toluene Levels

GC/FID analysis ($n = 3$) indicated that the concentration of toluene present inside the tracheal breathing tube of a rat breathing vapor generated from 4 ml toluene was 11,500 ppm. Additional blood concentration analysis further indicates that rats ($n = 24$) exposed to this concentration of toluene developed blood levels from 4 to 80 μg/ml during exposures ranging from 1.7 to 15.3 minutes. The blood toluene concentrations were proportional, rising in a linear fashion, and highly correlated with the length of inhalation of the toluene vapor ($R^2 = 0.97$). Moreover, we found that the blood toluene concentrations were not predictive of the pattern of the electrophysiological response of ventral tegmental area dopamine neurons. For example,

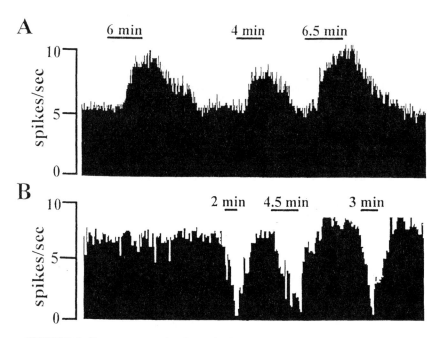

FIGURE 1. Ratemeter records of two single ventral tegmental area dopamine neurons during toluene exposure (11,500 ppm). Note that both the excitatory (**A**) and the inhibitory (**B**) effects of toluene appear to be proportional to exposure time.

over the range of 1.7 to 15.3 minutes of exposure, 12 neurons were inhibited and 12 were stimulated.

In Vivo *Electrophysiology of A10 Dopamine Cells*

Each ventral tegmental area dopamine neuron that was tested showed either an increase or decrease in firing rate during toluene exposure (FIG. 1A and 1B). When the ratemeter records (totaling $n = 64$ cells comprising 113 challenges) were ultimately grouped according to their response (excitation or inhibition) during toluene (11,500 ppm), half of the neurons ($n = 32$ cells comprising 52 challenges) responded with an increase in firing rate. With prolonged exposure to the solvent, however, this increased rate eventually progressed to an attenuation of firing (FIG. 2A and 2B). The maximum change in firing in this group averaged +221% ± 72% (mean ± SEM) during the first 8.5 minutes of inhalation in the presence of toluene blood levels ranging from 4 to 45 µg/ml. Exposure times >8.5 minutes, however, often led to a progressively diminished cell firing (+58.7% ± 6.3% over baseline activity), even with increasing toluene blood concentrations (45–80 µg/ml). In contrast, in a population of neurons showing the inhibitory response ($n = 32$ cells comprising 61 challenges), the firing rates were reduced—96% ± 6.8% below baseline with 4–80 µg/ml blood concentrations of toluene. The mean blood levels occurring with a 50% change in activity in either the excitation or inhibition groups were found to be 23 and 43 µg/ml, respectively.

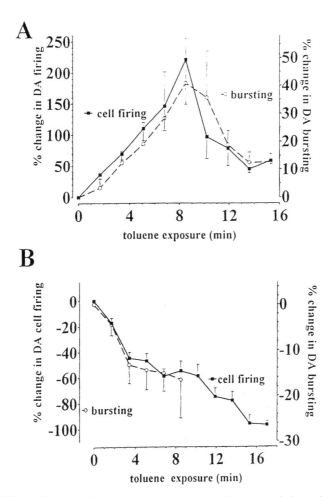

FIGURE 2. Electrophysiological response of ventral tegmental dopamine neurons stimulated (**A**) or inhibited (**B**) during periods of increasing length of inhalation exposure to toluene (11,500 ppm). The percent change in firing rate and action potentials contained in bursts were averaged from neurons that were stimulated (n = 32 cells and 52 challenges) or inhibited (n = 32 cells and 61 challenges) during exposure to toluene vapor.

Exposure to toluene vapor also altered the number of action potentials contained in bursts and the number of bursting events (FIG. 2A and 2B). In five neurons (n = 7 challenges) the firing rate changed, but the pattern of firing remained in a nonbursting state throughout the exposure to toluene. The pattern of firing of another eight neurons (n = 16 challenges) was converted from nonbursting to bursting following toluene. Generally, the toluene-induced increase in the percent of burst firing paralleled the effects of the solvent on the firing rate. Dopamine neurons responding in an excitatory manner to toluene showed a maximum change in percent bursts of

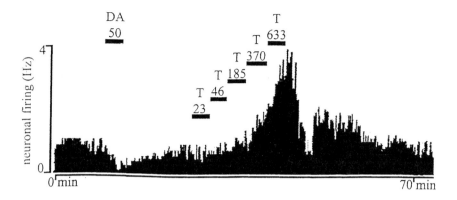

FIGURE 3. Dose-dependent activation of a VTA dopamine neuron during perfusion with sequentially increased concentrations (µM) of toluene (T). Note that at the highest concentration the activity of the neuron went into a period of reduced firing, reminiscent of a state of depolarization inactivation. The neuron from which this recording was made is a presumptive dopamine neuron, given the fact that its activity is inhibited upon application of 50 µM dopamine (DA).

+40.8 + 16% (n = 19 cells comprising 24 challenges) at <8.5 min followed by an attenuation of burst activity to only +12.6 + 3.0% at >8.5 minutes. In contrast, the percentage of action potentials contained in bursts in those neurons inhibited by toluene inhalation decreased 16.5 + 8.3% (n = 24 cells comprising 34 challenges) at <8.5 minutes. An insufficient number of cells were tested to ascertain whether the magnitude of the decrease would have continued at >8.5 minutes of exposure.

In Vitro *Electrophysiology of VTA Dopamine Neurons*

Extracellular single-unit activity of both dopamine and nondopamine neurons within the VTA was increased upon perfusion with ACSF containing toluene in concentrations ranging from 23 to 822 µM (FIG. 3). These toluene-induced excitations were concentration dependent and reversible, although at higher concentrations firing rates were observed to go into a period of decline for both the dopamine and nondopamine neurons. These toluene-induced periods of diminished firing were accompanied by a combined increase in action potential duration and amplitude, changes that have been associated with the condition of depolarization inactivation. Preliminary results comparing dopamine and nondopamine neurons, as delineated by their response or nonresponse to dopamine and serotonin, suggest that the nondopamine neuronal population is more sensitive to induction of a depolarization block induced by toluene.

Because VTA dopamine and nondopamine neurons have been shown to possess excitatory amino acid receptors and there is some evidence in an expression system to suggest an interaction between toluene and the NMDA receptor ion-channel complex, we next examined the possibility that toluene's excitatory effects in these neurons is mediated through a glutamatergic mechanism. This hypothesis was tested using the selective NMDA and AMPA receptor antagonists, CGS19755 and CNQX,

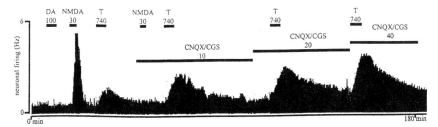

FIGURE 4. Ratemeter histogram of a nondopamine neuron within the VTA that is activated by toluene in the presence of a combination of the NMDA antagonist, CGS 19755, and the AMPA antagonist, CNQX. The concentration of the glutamate antagonist cocktail was sufficient to block the excitatory effects of NMDA itself. CGS19755 alone, but not CNQX, effectively blocks NMDA-induced excitations (data not shown).

respectively. In concentrations in which both CGS19755 and CNQX effectively eliminated the excitatory effects of NMDA and AMPA, respectively, the toluene-induced stimulations of both VTA neuronal types were not attenuated (FIG. 4). Although still quite preliminary, some of our data suggest that in the presence of AMPA the excitatory actions of toluene in the VTA are actually augmented. Further studies will be conducted to confirm this observation.

Locomotor Stimulatory Effects of Toluene

As reported previously, the systemic administration of toluene evoked an increase in forward locomotor behavior with an inverted-U dose–response relationship, the locomotor response to the highest dose (1200 mg/kg) being attenuated by an interfering ataxia.[20] In animals pretreated with the D2 dopamine receptor antagonist remoxipride, the stimulatory effects of 900 mg/kg toluene were reduced by 58%. This altered response in the presence of remoxipride appears to be specific to the blockade of dopamine receptors, since the locomotor hyperactivity produced by 1.5 mg/kg scopolamine, a muscarinic acetylcholine antagonist, was not affected. In more recent experiments, this apparent dopamine-dependent action of toluene was tested in animals that received intra-accumbens injections of 6-hydroxydopamine and were challenged with toluene 14 days later. Here, toluene-induced locomotor hyperactivity was significantly reduced by 55% in the lesioned animals compared to sham-lesioned controls. Again, the stimulatory effects of scopolamine were not affected by the lesion. At the time of this writing, the extent of dopamine depletion has yet to be measured. Earlier studies using a similar lesioning protocol found dopamine levels in the accumbens reduced by greater than 80%, however.

DISCUSSION

These results clearly demonstrate that the inhalant abuse paradigm used in a whole-animal preparation substantially alters the activity of ventral tegmental area dopamine neurons. Moreover, inhalants appear to produce electrophysiological effects similar to other drugs of abuse (e.g., ethanol, phencyclidine, Δ9-tetrahydrocannabinol, opiates).[13–16] Therefore, it is possible that in humans comparable concentrations of toluene may alter dopaminergic neurotransmission in those pathways described as playing a role in the rewarding/reinforcing effects and abuse potential of most drugs of abuse.[18,19]

The solvent for these initial studies was chosen on the basis of the finding that humans reportedly abuse pure toluene when possible.[24] Also, neurobehavioral evidence obtained in rats indicates that toluene has greater narcotic potency and a faster onset of action than other common solvents, such as acetone, xylene, and hexane.[25–27] Although the solvent benzene may exert an equipotent narcotic effect to that produced by toluene, it is not commonly found in products subject to abuse.

The exposure paradigm employed in the present study also appeared optimal, given its shared similarities with voluntary human inhalant abuse, namely brief exposure (minutes) to extremely high but sublethal concentrations (10,000–30,000 ppm) of the volatile agent followed by a period of recovery via exhalation of solvent and inhalation of clean air.[28] In terms of glue sniffing, Press and Done[5] approximated the concentration of toluene in a paper bag at 10,000 ppm, but data from our laboratory indicates that spray abusers likely ingest higher concentrations. Chromatagraphic headspace analysis of the same volume (125 ml) of the same spray paint commonly abused by "huffers" in the same receptacle (a 355-ml plastic soda bottle) measured >20,000 ppm (unpublished observations). Other protocols that use low-concentration exposures (<10,000 ppm) for long periods of time (>3 h) may be more applicable to issues related to occupational exposure, since the rate of induction and degree of narcosis are known to be dependent on the concentration of solvent inhaled.[25]

The exact mechanism of action of toluene remains unknown, but neurobehavioral studies associate toluene with biphasic (initial stimulation followed by depression) changes in CNS function.[20,29,30] Although a comparison of the temporal relationship between our measured electrophysiological responses with blood toluene concentrations and behavioral data from other groups shows some similarities,[31] caution must be used when attempting to extrapolate any of these findings to humans. Nevertheless, the first 8 minutes of our time course with <40 μg/ml blood toluene could conceivably reflect the stimulatory and euphoric effects reported by human abusers. In support of this supposition, Garriott et al.[32] reported that self-administering human inhalant abusers, demonstrating symptoms of moderate intoxication including signs of euphoria, ataxia, and inability to concentrate, had blood toluene levels of ~30 μg/ml. In contrast, the dysphoric effects also noted under some conditions of toluene use might occur with the higher blood toluene concentrations (40–80 μg/ml). This could possibly explain why abusers prefer to use repeated but short "huffs." Nevertheless, any direct correlation of global behavioral effects in humans to the electrophysiological changes observed here in rats is far from being established.

Acute exposure to our paradigm of using a high concentration of toluene produced two opposing effects on firing rates of dopamine neurons in ketamine-anesthetized rats. Because the short exposures (min) and the reproducibility of the electrophysiological response do not suggest a gross degenerative process, other mechanisms may be at work.[33] Two speculative possibilities, namely dopamine and NMDA receptor interactions, appear particularly relevant.

(1) Toluene is linked to decreased D2 autoreceptor affinity and biphasic changes in dopamine-dependent locomotor activity, the later being blocked by D2 receptor antagonists.[20,34] D2 dopamine receptors are present in high density throughout the

ventral tegmental area, and, when activated by somatodendritically released dopamine, dopamine neuronal firing is reduced.[35,36] Thus, if toluene rendered the D2 dopamine receptors of VTA dopamine neurons subsensitive to the somatodendritically released dopamine, then action potential generation would be expected to increase—at least initially. Increased dopamine neuronal activity enhances dopamine release in the nucleus accumbens, which in turn would activate inhibitory (i.e. GABA) feedback pathways to dampen dopamine neuronal excitability.[17] The attenuation of the stimulation that occurred with long exposures to toluene is particularly interesting in light of the toluene-evoked elevations in striatal dopamine release observed by Stengård et al.[37] Further electrophysiological experiments will be needed to test this hypothesis, though such a mechanism appears unlikely to explain the inhibition seen in some dopamine cells during toluene exposure.

Another clue to explain the toluene-induced stimulations and inhibitions of dopamine cell firing may lie with the observation that the changes in firing rate (for both patterns of response) were also mirrored by parallel changes in bursting activity. Intracellular recordings in tissue slices reveal that dopamine neurons display an inherent nonbursting pacemaker-like activity.[38] However, bursting can be elicited by the local administration of glutamic acid into the ventral tegmental area. In the intact organism, bursting may arise from activation of excitatory amino acid efferents to the VTA.[38] Thus, the augmentation of bursting during toluene exposure may reflect modulation of glutamatergic neurotransmission on dopamine neurons. This notion is particularly attractive in light of recent evidence showing a toluene blockade of NMDA receptors expressed in frog oocytes.[39] The blockade of NMDA receptors residing on the VTA dopamine soma and the subsequent removal of their tonic excitatory input might be expected to decrease cell firing. The blockade of NMDA receptors on local GABA interneurons, however, and the subsequent removal of this inhibitory input could lead to enhanced dopamine cell firing through disinhibition.[40] Interestingly, data from our laboratory suggest that the same exposure paradigm used in this study also inhibits VTA neurons characterized electrophysiologically as nondopamine.[41] It is also intriguing that the effects of toluene on dopamine cell activity are similar in several respects to the actions of the NMDA antagonist phencyclidine, which also appears to stimulate mesolimbic dopamine neurotransmission through indirect mechanisms.[42] Although the use of ketamine (an NMDA antagonist) as the anesthetic of choice in this study may make this hypothesis less tenable, additional studies employing an in vitro preparation will be able to assess the potential role of NMDA receptors in the actions of toluene.

In conclusion, there appears to be clear evidence that toluene inhalation can activate neurons within the rat midbrain ventral tegmental area. This effect can also be mimicked by the application of toluene directly on ventral tegmental neurons maintained in the brain slice preparation, strongly suggesting that toluene-induced activation of mesolimbic dopamine neurons likely occurs within the VTA itself. Although the preliminary data presented here do not implicate a toluene–NMDA ion-channel interaction in this effect, more experiments will be needed to definitively assess possible roles for glutamate in toluene's excitatory effects. Thus, although the mechanism by which toluene activates mesolimbic dopamine neurons remains unresolved, there is little argument that toluene produces neuronal activity changes within the brain's reward pathways that are potentially compatible with the known abuse potential of compounds containing this solvent.

ACKNOWLEDGMENTS

This work was supported in part by Grant DA 09025 from the National Institue of Drug Abuse.

REFERENCES

1. MATHIAS, R. 1996. Students' use of marijuana, other illicit drugs and cigarettes continued to rise in 1995. NIDA Notes **11:** 8–9.
2. FLANAGAN, R. & R. IVES. 1994. Volatile substance abuse. Bull. Narc. **XLVI**(No. 2): 49–78.
3. ARLIEN-SOBØRG, P. 1992. Toluene. *In* Solvent Neurotoxicity. CRC Press. Boca Raton, FL. pp. 61–125.
4. WEISS, B., R. WOOD & D. MACYS. 1979. Behavioral toxicology of carbon disulfide and toluene. Environ. Health Perspect. **30:** 39–45.
5. PRESS, E. & A. DONE. 1967. Solvent sniffing. Physiological effects and community control measures for intoxication from the intentional inhalation of organic solvents. I. Pediatrics **39:** 451–461.
6. BENIGNUS, V., K. MULLER, C. BARTON & J. BITTIKOFER. 1981. Toluene levels in blood and brain of rats during and after respiratory exposure. Toxicol. Appl. Pharmacol. **61:** 326–334.
7. BENIGNUS, V., J. MULLER, J. GRAHAM & C. BARTON. 1984. Toluene levels in blood and brain of rats as a function of toluene levels in inspired air. Environ. Res. **33:** 39–46.
8. GOSPE, S. & M. CALABAN. 1988. Central nervous system distribution of inhaled toluene. Fund. Appl. Toxicol. **11:** 540–545.
9. AMENO, K. *et al.* 1992. Regional brain distribution of toluene in rats and in a human autopsy. Arch. Toxicol. **66:** 153–156.
10. KIRIU, T. *et al.* 1990. The distribution of toluene in the brain and its effects on the brain catecholamine in acute toluene poisoning. Jpn. J. Legal Med. **44:** 25–33.
11. KALIVAS, P. 1993. Neurotransmitter regulation of dopamine neurons in the ventral tegmental area. Brain Res. Rev. **18:** 75–113.
12. DICHIARA, G. & A. IMPERATO. 1988. Drugs abused by humans preferentially increase synaptic dopamine concentrations in the mesolimbic system of freely moving rats. Proc. Natl. Acad. Sci. USA **85:** 5274–5278.
13. DICHIARA, G. & R.A. NORTH. 1992. Neurobiology of opiate abuse. Trends Pharmacol. Sci. **13:** 185–192.
14. FRENCH, E.D. 1986. Effects of phencyclidine on ventral tegmental A10 dopamine neurons in the rat. Neuropharmacology **25:** 241–248.
15. FRENCH, E., K. DILLON & W. WU. 1997. Cannabinoids excite dopamine neurons in the ventral tegmentum and substantia nigra. NeuroReport **8:** 649–652.
16. GESSA, G. *et al.* 1985. Low doses of ethanol activate dopaminergic neurons in the ventral tegmental area. Brain Res. **348:** 201–203.
17. WESTERINK, B., H. KWINT & J. DEVRIES. 1996. The pharmacology of mesolimbic dopamine neurons: a dual-probe microdialysis study in the ventral tegmental area and nucleus accumbens of the rat brain. J. Neurosci. **16:** 2605–2611.
18. KOOB, G. 1992. Drugs of abuse: anatomy, pharmacology and function of reward pathways. Trends Pharmacol. Sci. **13:** 177–184.
19. WISE, R. & M.A. BOZARTH. 1984. Brain reward circuitry: four circuit elements wired in apparent series. Brain Res. Bull. **12:** 203–208.
20. RIEGEL, A. & E.D. FRENCH. 1999. Acute toluene induces biphasic changes in rat spontaneous locomotor activity which are blocked by remoxipride. Pharmacol. Biochem. Behav. **62:** 399–402.
21. RIEGEL, A. & E.D. FRENCH. 1999. An electrophysiological analysis of rat ventral tegmental dopamine neuronal activity during acute exposure to toluene. Pharmacol. Toxicol. **85:** 37–43.

22. BUNNEY, B., J. WALTERS, R. ROTH & G. AGHAJANIAN. 1973. Dopaminergic neurons: Effects of antipsychotic drugs and amphetamine on single cell activity. J. Pharmacol. Exp. Ther. **185:** 560–571.
23. GRACE, A.A. & B.S. BUNNEY. 1984. The control of firing pattern in nigral dopamine neurons: burst firing. J. Neurosci. **4:** 2877–2890.
24. YAMANOUCHI, N. *et al.* 1995. White matter changes caused by chronic solvent abuse. Am. J. Neuroradiol. **16:** 1643–1649.
25. BRUCKNER, J. & R. PETERSON. 1981. Evaluation of toluene and acetone inhalant abuse. I. Pharmacology and pharmacodynamics. Toxicol. Appl. Pharmacol. **61:** 27–38.
26. TEGERIS, J. & R. BALSTER. 1994. A comparison of the acute behavioral effects of alkylbenzenes using a functional observational battery in mice. Fund. Appl. Toxicol. **22:** 240–250.
27. SILVA-FILHO, A., M. PIRES & N. SHIOTSUKI. 1991. Anticonvulsant and convulsant effects of organic solvents. Pharmacol. Biochem. Behav. **41:** 79–82.
28. LONGLEY, E., A. JONES, R. WELCH & O. LOMAEV. 1967. Two acute toluene episodes in merchant ships. Arch. Environ. Health **14:** 481–487.
29. HINMAN, D. 1987. Biphasic relationship for the effects of toluene inhalation on locomotor activity. Pharmacol. Biochem. Behav. **26:** 65–69.
30. KONDO, H. *et al.* 1995. Toluene induces behavioral activation without affecting striatal dopamine metabolism in the rat: behavioral and microdialysis studies. Pharmacol. Biochem. Behav. **51:** 97–101.
31. KISHI, R. *et al.* 1988. Neurobehavioral effects and pharmacokinetics of toluene in rats and their relevance to man. Br. J. Indust. Med. **45:** 396–408.
32. GARRIOTT, J.C. *et al.* 1981. Measurement of toluene in blood and breath in cases of solvent abuse. Clin. Toxicol. **18:** 471–479.
33. LADEFOGED, O. *et al.* 1991. Irreversible effects in rats of toluene (inhalation) exposure for six months: Pharmacol. Toxicol. **68:** 384–390.
34. VON EULER, G. *et al.* 1991. Subacute exposure to low concentrations of toluene affects dopamine mediated locomotor activity in the rat. Toxicology **67:** 333–349.
35. MANSOUR, A. *et al.* 1990. Localization of dopamine D2 receptors for mRNA and D1 and D2 receptor binding in the rat brain and pituitary: an in situ hybridization-receptor autoradiographic analysis. J. Neurosci. **10:** 2587–2600.
36. WHITE, F.J. & R.Y. WANG. 1984. A10 dopamine neurons: role of autoreceptors in determining firing rate and sensitivity to dopamine agonists. Life Sci. **34:** 1161–1170.
37. STENGÅRD, K., G. HOGLUND & U. UNGERSTEDT. 1994. Extracellular DA levels within the striatum increase during inhalation exposure to toluene: a microdialysis study in awake, freely moving rats. **71:** 245–255.
38. GRACE, A.A. & S. ONN. 1989. Morphology and electrophysiological properties of immunocytochemically identified rat dopamine neurons recorded in vitro. J. Neurosci. **9:** 3463–3481.
39. CRUZ, S. *et al.* 1998. Effects of the abused solvent toluene on recombinant *N*-methyl-D-aspartate receptors expressed in *Xenopus* oocytes. J. Pharm. Exp. Ther. **286:** 334–340.
40. WANG, T. & E.D. FRENCH. 1995. NMDA, kainate, and AMPA depolarize non-dopamine neurons in the rat ventral tegmentum. Brain Res. Bull. **36:** 39–43.
41. RIEGEL, A. & E.D. FRENCH. 1999. The susceptibility of rat non-dopamine ventral tegmental neurones to inhibition during toluene exposure. Pharmacol. Toxicol. **85:** 44–46.
42. WANG, T. & E.D. FRENCH. 1993. Effects on phencyclidine on spontaneous and excitatory amino acid-induced activity of ventral tegmental dopamine neurons: an extracellular in vitro study. Life Sci. **53:** 49–56.

Factors for Susceptibility to Episode Recurrence in Spontaneous Recurrence of Methamphetamine Psychosis

KUNIO YUI,[a,b] SHIGENORI IKEMOTO,[c,d] AND KIMIHIKO GOTO[c]

[a]Department of Psychiatry, Jichi Medical School, Tochigi 329-0498, Japan

[b]V.A. Honolulu, National Center for PTSD, Honolulu, Hawaii 96813, USA

[c]Nippon Veterinary and Animal Science University, Tokyo 180-8602, Japan

[d]Department of Legal Medicine and Human Genetics, Jichi Medical School, Tochigi 329-0498, Japan

ABSTRACT: The relation between increased sensitivity to stress associated with noradrenergic hyperactivity and dopaminergic changes, and susceptibility to subsequent spontaneous recurrences of methamphetamine (MAP) psychosis (flashbacks) was examined. Plasma monoamine metabolite levels were assayed in 19 flashbackers, of whom 10 experienced a single flashback and 9 exhibited subsequent flashbacks, 18 nonflashbackers with a history of MAP psychosis, 9 subjects with persistent MAP psychosis, and 22 MAP user and 10 nonuser controls. All flashbackers had undergone frightening stressful experiences during previous MAP use. They exhibited flashbacks in response to mild psychosocial stressors. There was no significant difference in the number of stressful experiences and having mild psychosocial stressors between the two flashbacker subgroups. Plasma norepinephrine (NE) levels increased with a small increase in plasma levels of 3-methoxytyramine (3-MT), an index of dopamine release, during flashbacks in the 19 flashbackers. Of the 19 flashbackers, the 9 with subsequent episodes had markedly increased NE levels and slightly increased 3-MT levels during flashbacks, while the 10 with a single episode displayed small increases in NE and 3-MT levels during flashbacks. The 9 flashbackers with subsequent episodes had a longer duration of imprisonment than the 10 flashbackers with a single episode. Thus, robust noradrenergic hyperactivity with slightly increased DA release in response to mild stress may predict subsequent flashbacks. Long-term exposure to distressing situations appears to contribute to susceptibility to subsequent flashbacks.

KEYWORDS: amphetamine; methamphetamine; flashback; methamphetamine psychosis; dopamine; noradrenergic hyperactivity

Address for correspondence: Kunio Yui, M.D., Department of Psychiatry, Jichi Medical School, Minamikawachi 3311-1, Tochigi 329-0498, Japan. Voice: +81 (48) 862-7520; fax: +81 (48) 836-1372.
    User356886177@AOL.COM

Ann. N.Y. Acad. Sci. 965: 292–304 (2002). © 2002 New York Academy of Sciences.

INTRODUCTION

It is well known that amphetamine (AMP)- or methamphetamine (MAP)-induced paranoid–hallucinatory states occasionally recur on exposure to stress (referred to as "flashbacks") in individuals with a history of MAP psychosis.[1] We have previously reported that frightening stressful experiences, together with MAP use, increases sensitivity to stress associated with noradrenergic hyperactivity[2,3] and increased dopamine release.[3,4] This increased sensitivity may be critical for the development of flashbacks.[2–4] About 50% of our subjects with flashbacks had subsequent flashbacks. In this regard, more psychosocial stressors may be involved in the first episode of major affective disorders than in subsequent episodes, so that the later episodes imply an increasing susceptibility to recurrence.[5,6] A previous study that used a prospective design to assess stress and symptom levels found a close similarity in the frequency or type of stress experienced by patients who remained well and those who relapsed in bipolar disorder.[7] Here, we examine the possibility that stress reactivity associated with noradrenergic hyperactivity and dopaminergic changes in an initial episode and in any subsequent episodes may differ in the first flashback episode.

Ruminations associated with aversive events may induce a further series of adaptive neurochemical changes.[8] It is therefore possible that some impact of stress contributes to the susceptibility to episodic recurrence of flashbacks.

Based on these possibilities, we investigated the difference in the nature of stress reactivity associated with noradrenergic hyperactivity and dopaminergic changes during the first flashback episode between subjects with a single flashback episode and those with subsequent flashback episodes. The focus of this study was to examine stress factors related to episode recurrences.

METHODS

Subject Selection

The subjects were 78 physically healthy females, recruited from inmates in a women's prison. This group was made up of 37 with a history of MAP psychosis, of whom 19 experienced flashbacks during their 15–20 months of incarceration (referred to as "flashbackers"), while the other 18 did not (referred to as "nonflashbackers"), 9 with persistent MAP psychosis, and 32 age-matched controls. The control group consisted of 22 MAP users and and 10 nonusers, none of whom had ever become psychotic. The 19 flashbackers were selected on the basis that their plasma monoamine metabolite levels were assayed during the first flashback episode, and again within 30 days of the first episode passing. Of these, 10 experienced a single flashback episode without further recurrence, and the other 9 experienced subsequent episodes (two flashbacks per subject).

All subjects were deemed physically healthy based on physical and neurological examinations and biochemical screening. None had abused other substances or experienced any psychiatric disorder in the absence of MAP use. Subjects had been tested for other substances by the police and all results were negative. The 18 nonflashbackers were selected for having broadly similar times at which MAP psychosis disappeared to when those of the 19 flashbackers ceased (within 730 days of blood sampling: the 19 flashbackers, mean ± SD = 235.1 ± 229.0 days; the 18 nonflashbackers, mean ± SD = 237.8 ± 202.5 days). The 9 subjects with persistent MAP psychosis, persisting for at least 6 months before blood collection (mean ± SD = 16.2 ± 10.7 months), were included for comparison with the 19 flashbackers (spontaneous vs. persistent recurrence) to study the relation between prior exposure to stressful experiences and plasma monoamine metabolite levels. All subjects freely gave written informed consent prior to the study, which was approved by the Medical Care and Classification Division of the Ministry of Justice of Japan. Using the DSM-IV criteria for AMP-induced psychotic disorders, the 37 subjects with a history of MAP psychosis were diagnosed as previously having had MAP psychosis, based on a structured interview and inmate record review. Subjects with schizophrenia, brief psychotic disorders, delusional disorder, anxiety disorders, and PTSD were excluded. Flashbacks due to previous MAP psychosis are defined with reference to a general definition of psychedelic drug flashbacks[9] and the DSM-IV criteria for hallucinogen-persisting perception disorder (flashbacks), as a spontaneous recurrence of MAP-induced paranoid–hallucinatory states following a period of normalcy during which the pharmacological effects of MAP had worn off.

Monitoring Secret Use of MAP

All prisoners, including our subjects, in detention houses and prisons are prevented from taking MAP or other substances. For example, all prisoners undergo repeated searches in accordance with the Cannabis Control Law, the Narcotic Control Law, and the Stimulant Drug Control Law of Japan. They are prevented from meeting any visitors apart from family members, and do not receive any sealed correspondence. Our subjects expected to be searched by methods authorized under the Prison Law, and thus they were not frightened by the searches. Moreover, venous plasma was tested for MAP in a randomly selected subsample of 9 of the 19 flashbackers at the time the flashbacks occurred, using gas chromatography/mass spectrometry, as previously described.[2] All analyses were negative for MAP.

Neuroleptic Treatment

Among the 19 flashbackers, 6 were treated with haloperidol (1–2 mg/day), chlorpromazine (25–75 mg/day), or thioridazine (25–75 mg/day) for at least 4 weeks before and during the study because of their paranoid–hallucinatory flashback states (medicated flashbackers). The other 13 flashbackers were unmedicated for at least 3 months before blood collection. They received the neuroleptic treatment specified above following blood collection during flashbacks, in response to flashback aggravation (later-medicated flashbackers). The 9 subjects with persistent MAP psychosis were maintained on haloperidol (1–9 mg/day) or chlorpromazine (25–125 mg/day) for at least one month (mean ± SD = 2.1 ± 2.0 months) before blood collection. The 18 nonflashbackers were unmedicated for at least 3 months before and during the study because of no psychiatric symptoms. All subjects were free of other medications.

Stress Factors

Details of the pattern of MAP use, stressful experiences, and symptoms of MAP psychosis during previous MAP use were obtained from structured interviews and inmate record reviews. The questions concerned details of stressful events and threatening paranoid–hallucinatory states during previous MAP use. With reference to the general definition of stress,[10] the criteria for stressful events during previous MAP use were based on whether the subjects had been overwhelmingly distressed, whether the events met the DSM-111-R criteria for a severe to catastrophic type of psychosocial stressor (axis IV scores of 4 to 6), and whether the subjects had escaped from the situations. The criteria for MAP-induced fear-related paranoid–hallucinatory states (perception of threat) during previous MAP use were based on whether the subjects had been overwhelmingly threatened and whether they had taken refuge near or in their houses out of fear. Data on the factors triggering flashbacks were obtained from structured interviews and reports made by prison staff.

Imprisonment involves confinement in a restricted area, daily penal servitude, no visitors or incoming sealed correspondence, restriction of free action and diet (low monoamine, alcohol-free, and caffeine-restricted), and disciplinary punishment, all of which distress the prisoners. To examine the effect of the duration of confinement in the prison before blood collection on stress reactivity in the flashbacker subgroups, this duration was compared across the two flashbacker subgroups.

Anxiety Levels

The State-Trait Anxiety Inventory (STAI) was used to assess anxiety levels related to stress.[11] The scale consisted of two separate 20-question scales intended to measure both levels of transitory anxiety at the time of testing (state anxiety) and longer-lasting anxiety (trait anxiety). STAI data were available for 13 of the 19 flashbackers at the times when the flashbacks occurred and at remission, and upon admission to the prison for 12 of the 18 nonflashbackers, 10 of the 22 user controls, and 9 of the 10 nonuser controls. These subsamples were random. Pulse rate was measured at the time of blood sampling.

Plasma Monoamine Metabolite Levels

All subjects were given a low-monoamine, alcohol-free, and caffeine-restricted diet for at least 3 months before and during the study while confined in detention houses and in the prison. Blood was obtained from the 19 flashbackers during the prominent paranoid–hallucinatory flashback state of the first flashback episode, as specified by subscores of 3 or more on the Brief Psychiatric Rating Scale (BPRS)[12] Hallucinatory Behavior and Suspiciousness, occurring within 14 days of the occurrence of flashbacks. Further samples were obtained 14 to 30 days after cessation of the flashback. The other subjects had a single blood sample assayed when they were transferred to the prison. Blood was obtained at random using venipuncture between 10:30 A.M. and 12:00 P.M. after a 20-min rest. Plasma was stored at −80°C until it was assayed for: norepinephrine (NE) and its metabolite normetanephrine (NM), epinephrine (E), and dopamine (DA) and its metabolites [3-methoxytyramine (3-MT) and dihydroxyphenylacetic acid (DOPAC)] using high-performance liquid chromatography with an electrochemical detector, as previously described.[2] Sensitivity was 0.01 pmol/mL, except for NM, which was 0.05 pmol/mL.

Statistical Analysis

The distributions of plasma monoamine metabolite levels were often extremely skewed. Thus, all monoaminergic values were square-root transformed to reduce the skewness and then analyzed using one-way analysis of variance (ANOVA), followed by *post hoc* test.[13] To confirm significant differences in monoamine metabolite levels between flashbacks and remission, and the absence of any significant effect of our neuroleptic treatment on monoaminergic values, the transformed data from the 19 flashbackers were analyzed using repeated ANOVA measures. The presence or absence of neuroleptic treatment was the between-subject factor, and the presence or absence of flashbacks was the within-subject repeated factor.[14] Comparison between subject subgroups was performed using the Kruskal–Wallis test followed by the Mann–Whitney U test, and the X^2 test.

RESULTS

All subjects had averaged 1–5 intravenous injections of MAP (30–60 mg per injection) per day during periods of abuse, except for the 10 nonuser controls, who had been imprisoned for theft ($n = 7$), arson ($n = 1$), and involuntary manslaughter ($n = 2$). Most subjects were reinjecting themselves before the effects of the previous MAP injection had lessened, resulting in multiple daily injections. There was no significant difference in the mean cumulative duration of MAP use before the onset of MAP psychosis among the 19 flashbackers (mean ± SD = 15.0 ± 21.1 months), the 18 nonflashbackers (mean ± SD = 23.7 ± 33.4 months), and the 9 subjects with persistent MAP psychosis (mean ± SD = 7.9 ± 15.3 months).

The 19 flashbackers exhibited reactivated MAP psychosis (a total of 28 flashbacks) without reexperiencing either the original stressful events or the symptoms of PTSD or acute stress disorder listed in the DSM-IV criteria. The incidence of psychotic symptoms during flashbacks was not significantly different from that of the previous MAP psychosis ($X^2 = 14.54$, $df = 12$, $p = 0.28$). During flashbacks, subjects continued to experience paranoid delusions, in which they developed transient auditory and visual hallucinations. Paranoid delusions abated after 3–229 days. The total duration of flashbacks, including one or more hallucinatory flashbacks and persistent paranoid delusions, was therefore 3 to 229 days (mean ± SD = 63.7 ± 58.4 days).

As shown in TABLE 1, the number of medicated subjects did not differ significantly between the 10 flashbackers with a single episode and the 9 flashbackers with subsequent episodes ($p = 0.13$). There were no significant differences in the BPRS suspiciousness ($p = 0.63$) and hallucinatory ($p = 0.36$) subscores, and the duration of flashbacks ($p = 0.20$) between the the two flashbacker subgroups.

Stressful Experiences

As shown in TABLE 2, the 19 flashbackers had been exposed to significantly higher numbers of stressful events and MAP-induced fear-related paranoid–

TABLE 1. Clinical characteristics of the two flashbacker subgroups

	Flashbackers with single episode ($n = 10$)	Flashbackers with subsequent episode ($n = 10$)
Duration of confinement before the beginning of blood sampling (days)	53.5 ± 68.1	161.9 ± 122.7[a]
Number of subjects treated with neuroleptics	2	4
BPRS suspiciousness score	3.8 ± 0.6	3.0 ± 1.3
BPRS hallucinatory behavior score	4.2 ± 1.1	3.4 ± 1.5

Data represent mean ± SD.
[a] $p < 0.05$ when compared with the flashbackers with a single episode.

hallucinatory states during previous MAP use than the 18 nonflashbackers. These events had overwhelmingly threatened the subjects. The 5 flashbackers with no history of stressful events had experienced fear-related paranoid–hallucinatory states. Thus, in comparison with the 18 nonflashbackers, all flashbackers had been exposed to frightening stressful experiences during previous MAP use. All 9 subjects with persistent MAP psychosis had experienced significantly higher numbers of threatening stressful events and fear-related psychotic symptoms than had the 18 nonflashbackers.

The factors triggering the 28 flashbacks met the DSM-111-R criteria for mild types of psychosocial stressor, involving mainly mild fear of other people ($n = 27$, 96.4%); conflicts or confrontations with inmates ($n = 10$, 35.7%); fear of emitting body odor ($n = 7$, 7.1 %); fear of the prison staff ($n = 12$, 42.9%); fear of other inmates' words and actions ($n = 3$, 10.7%). Other factors, which coincided with mild fear of other people in 3 flashbackers, were worry about family ($n = 1$, 3.6%), back pain ($n = 1$, 3.6%), and general fatigue ($n = 1$, 3.6%). It is important to point out that these factors represent nonspecific psychosocial stressors that arise from general conflicts among inmates in the prison.

The STAI-state scores did not differ significantly among the subject subgroups ($p = 0.39$): the flashbackers during flashbacks, mean ± SD = 58.9 ± 9.7; the flashbackers at remission, mean ± SD = 56.2 ± 12.5; the nonflashbackers, mean ± SD = 53.3 ± 6.9; the user controls, mean ± SD = 51.1 ± 5.5; the nonuser controls, mean ± SD = 53.1 ± 9.9. The STAI-trait scores during flashbacks (mean ± SD = 61.4 ± 9.1) were significantly higher than in the 13 nonflashbackers (mean ± SD = 51.5 ± 6.9) ($p < 0.01$), the 10 user controls (mean ± SD = 45.3 ± 27.6) ($p < 0.01$), and the 9 nonuser controls (mean ± SD = 47.8 ± 13.7) ($p < 0.05$). The STAI-trait scores at remission (mean ± SD = 60.9 ± 13.3) were significantly higher than in the nonflashbackers ($p < 0.05$) and the 10 user controls ($p < 0.01$). Pulse rate did not increase during flashbacks.

As shown in TABLE 2, the numbers of stressful events and MAP-induced fear-related symptoms in each of the two flashbacker subgroups were significantly higher than for the 18 nonflashbackers. However, the number of stressful events ($p = 0.80$) or fear-related states ($p = 0.89$) were not significantly different between the two flashbacker subgroups. There was no significant difference in the numbers having

TABLE 2. Stressful experiences during previous MAP use

	Flashbackers $n = 19$ (%)	Subgroups		Subjects with persistent MAP psychosis $n = 8$ (%)	Non-flashbackers $n = 20$ (%)
		A single episode $n = 10$ (%)	Subsequent episodes $n = 9$ (%)		
Stressful events	14 (73.7)[b]	8 (80.0)[b]	6 (66.7)[a]	5 (55.6)[a]	1 (5.6)
Physical abuse	8 (42.1)[a]	4 (48.0)	4 (44.4)[a]	4 (44.4)[a]	1 (5.6)
Sexual abuse	1 (5.3)	0 (0.0)	1 (11.1)	0 (0.0)	0 (0.0)
Divorce	2 (10.5)	2 (20.0)[a]	0 (0.0)	0 (0.0)	0 (0.0)
Rejecting parents	2 (10.5)	1 (10.0)	1 (11.1)	1 (11.1)	0 (0.0)
Unwanted pregnancy	1 (5.3)	1 (10.0)	0 (0.0)	0 (0.0)	0 (0.0)
Fear-related symptoms	12 (63.2)[b]	6 (60.0)[b]	6 (66.7)[a]	5 (55.6)[a]	1 (5.6)
Threatening auditory hallucinations	6 (31.6)[b]	3 (30.6)[b]	3 (33.3)[a]	4 (44.4)[a]	0 (0.0)
Threatening visual hallucinations	6 (31.6)[a]	3 (30.0)[a]	3 (33.3)[a]	1 (11.1)	0 (0.0)
Dead body or ghost	2 (10.5)	1 (10.0)	1 (11.1)	2 (22.2)	0 (0.0)
Blood soaked face	2 (10.5)	1 (10.0)	1 (11.1)	0 (0.0)	0 (0.0)
Grave yard or blood	2 (10.5)	1 (10.0)	1 (11.1)	0 (0.0)	0 (0.0)
Delusions of being pursued	8 (47.4)[a]	4 (45.5)	4 (50.0)[a]	2 (25.0)	1 (5.0)

Percentages in fear-related psychotic symptoms do not total 100 because some subjects had more than one symptom.

[a]$p < 0.05$; [b]$p < 0.01$ when compared with the nonflashbackers.

mild fear of other people between the 10 flashbackers with a single episode ($n = 10$ per 10 flashbacks) and the 9 flashbackers with subsequent episodes ($n = 17$ per 18 flashbacks) ($p = 0.92$). The mean duration of confinement before the beginning of blood collection during flashbacks was significantly longer in the 9 flashbackers with subsequent episodes than in the 10 flashbackers with a single episode.

Plasma Monoamine Metabolite Levels

As shown in TABLE 3, repeated ANOVA measures indicate a significant difference in plasma NE levels between flashbacks and remission [$F(1,17) = 4.68$]. There was no evidence of any interaction between the testing time (during flashbacks and remission) and neuroleptic treatment, or its effect, for any monoamine metabolite levels. Plasma NE levels during flashbacks in the 19 flashbackers were significantly higher than during remission, and were significantly higher than in the 18 nonflashbackers, and the 22 user and 10 nonuser controls. Plasma NE levels in the 9 subjects with persistent MAP psychosis were significantly higher than in the 22 user and 10 nonuser controls. Plasma 3-MT levels during flashbacks were significantly higher than during remission, and significantly higher than in the 22 user controls. Plasma E levels did not differ significantly among the subject subgroups. The 10 flashbackers with a single episode had significantly higher NE levels during flashbacks than the 22 user controls, but their NE levels during flashbacks did not differ significantly

TABLE 3. Plasma monamine metabolite levels

Subject subgroups	n	Age (y)	NE	3-MT	E	DOPAC	DA
Flashbackers during flashbacks	19	28.5 ± 5.9	0.68 ± 0.66[a,b,c,f,h]	1.42 ± 2.27[b,e]	0.48 ± 0.58	0.16 ± 0.47	0.05 ± 0.09
Flashbackers with a single episode	11	28.8 ± 8.0	0.49 ± 0.66[e]	1.41 ± 2.24[e]	0.45 ± 0.57	0.24 ± 0.65	0.04 ± 0.08
Flashbackers with subsequent episodes	8	27.2 ± 4.6	0.89 ± 0.64[b,d,f,h]	1.44 ± 2.42[e]	0.51 ± 0.62	0.07 ± 0.12	0.06 ± 0.10
Medicated flashbackers	6	26.5 ± 2.0	0.76 ± 0.89[f,h]	0.31 ± 0.76	0.34 ± 0.52	0.07 ± 0.14	0.08 ± 0.05
Later-medicated flashbackers	13	28.8 ± 7.0	0.64 ± 0.57[f,h]	1.94 ± 2.55[b,c,g,i]	0.57 ± 0.62	0.20 ± 0.57	0.04 ± 0.03
Flashbackers during remission	19	28.2 ± 6.1	0.36 ± 0.41	0.33 ± 0.77	0.39 ± 0.57	0.30 ± 0.62	0.12 ± 0.18
Flashbackers with a single episode	11	29.1 ± 7.3	0.24 ± 0.26	0.06 ± 0.26	0.24 ± 0.44	0.25 ± 0.63	0.12 ± 0.17
Flashbackers with subsequent episodes	8	27.2 ± 4.6	0.50 ± 0.51	0.62 ± 1.05	0.56 ± 0.68	0.35 ± 0.64	0.12 ± 0.20
Medicated flashbackers	6	26.5 ± 2.0	0.49 ± 0.53	0.12 ± 0.30	0.47 ± 0.55	0.14 ± 0.20	0.04 ± 0.02
Later-medicated flashbackers	13	29.0 ± 7.2	0.30 ± 0.35	0.42 ± 0.91	0.35 ± 0.60	0.37 ± 0.73	0.15 ± 0.06
Subjects with persistent MAP psychosis	9	25.0 ± 2.7	0.59 ± 0.43[e,g]	0.40 ± 0.88	0.44 ± 0.82	0.03 ± 0.09	0.13 ± 0.22
Nonflashbackers	18	30.2 ± 9.2	0.39 ± 0.35	1.03 ± 2.15	0.79 ± 1.38	0.33 ± 0.66	0.14 ± 0.22
User controls	22	31.1 ± 8.0	0.15 ± 0.24	0.10 ± 0.47	0.60 ± 1.33	0.20 ± 0.59	0.13 ± 0.20
Nonuser controls	10	30.8 ± 6.4	0.17 ± 0.16	1.18 ± 1.83	0.35 ± 0.46	0.46 ± 1.17	0.29 ± 0.26

NOTE: Data are mean ± SD pmol/mL. All monoaminergic values were square-root transformed, and analyzed using repeated-measures analysis of variance (ANOVA) and one-way ANOVA followed by post hoc test. NE, norepinephrine; 3-MT, 3-methoxytyramine; E, epinephrine; DOPAC, dihydroxyphenylacetic acid; DA, dopamine.
[a]$p < 0.05$ significant difference between flashbackers and remission, repeated measures ANOVA. [b]$p < 0.05$ compared to the flashbackers during remission. [c]$p < 0.05$; [d]$p < 0.01$ compared to nonflashbackers. [e]$p < 0.05$; [f]$p < 0.01$ compared to the user control. [g]$p < 0.05$; [h]$p < 0.01$ compared to the nonuser controls. [i]$p < 0.05$ compared to medicated flashbackers.

from levels during remission. The 9 flashbackers with subsequent episodes had significantly higher NE levels during flashbacks than during remission, and significantly higher NE levels than the 18 nonflashbackers and the 22 user and 10 nonuser controls. Both flashbacker subgroups had significantly higher 3-MT levels during flashbacks than the user controls.

During flashbacks, both the 6 medicated and the 13 later-medicated flashbackers had significantly higher NE levels during flashbacks than the 22 user and 10 nonuser controls. The 13 later-medicated flashbackers had significantly higher 3-MT levels during flashbacks than the 6 medicated flashbackers, the 18 nonflashbackers, and the 9 nonuser controls.

DISCUSSION

The 19 flashbackers had experienced paranoid–hallucinatory states after taking MAP, but not after exposure to any severe stressor. They exhibited transient paranoid–hallucinatory states closely resembling their previous MAP psychosis in response to mild psychosocial stressors. They did not exhibit characteristic symptoms of schizophrenia (i.e., disorganized speech, grossly disorganized, catatonic behavior, or negative symptoms), as listed in the DSM-IV. They did not have schizophrenic thought disorder characterized by a concreteness of abstract thought and an impairment in goal-directed thought.[15,16] There was no possibility of secret use of MAP or other substances. The flashbacks are therefore best explained as a spontaneous psychosis due to previous MAP psychosis.

The 19 flashbackers had been exposed to threatening stressful events, fear-related psychotic symptoms, or both, during previous MAP use. They then exhibited flashbacks due to previous MAP psychosis when exposed to mild psychosocial stressors involving mainly mild fear of other people. It is well known that exposure to stressful stimuli resulted in sensitization of brain and peripheral noradrenergic systems to subsequent stress that is mild enough to have no measurable effect on nonexposed animals.[8,17] Thus, reexposure to similar but less severe stress can easily increase NE turnover as well as peripheral and brain NE levels.[8,17] AMP induces lasting sensitization to stress via dopaminergic changes.[18] Collectively, frightening stressful experiences, together with MAP use, can induce noradrenergic hyperreactivity to less severe psychosocial stressors (mainly mild fear of other people). In this context, noradrenargic hyperreactivity appears to be causally related to the occurrence of flashbacks. The high trait anxiety of the flashbackers may reflect such peripheral noradrenergic hyperreactivity.[19] The 9 subjects with persistent MAP psychosis had been exposed to frightening psychotic symptoms as well as threatening stressful events during previous MAP use. They were then suffering from persisting MAP psychosis. Their plasma NE levels were elevated. Thus, noradrenergic hyperreactivity to mild stressors may be related to persistent recurrences of MAP psychosis.

Preclinical studies indicate that 3-MT levels are a more sensitive index of preferential DA release than homovanillic acid (HVA) or DOPAC levels.[20] A peripheral origin of 3-MT has be postulated,[21] suggesting an important correlation between 3-MT levels in plasma and in the brain. Thus, higher 3-MT levels during flashbacks may reflect increased DA release. Repeated stressful stimuli sensitize 3-MT release under subsequent stress in the rat brain.[22] In view of these observations, frightening stressful experiences, together with MAP use, may induce sensitization of DA release in addition to noradrenergic hyperactivity in response to mild psychosocial stressors. This increased sensitivity associated with noradrenergic hyperactivity and increased DA release may predispose the subjects to flashbacks and further episodes. In this context, some degree of increased NE levels, together with slightly increased DA release in the 10 flashbackers with a single episode, can trigger flashback. These findings strengthen our previous studies, indicating that noradrenergic hyperactivity, including increased DA release, is critical in the development of flashbacks.[2–4]

During flashbacks, the 10 flashbackers with subsequent episodes showed a much greater increase in NE levels, while the 9 flashbackers with a single episode had a smaller increase. Both subgroups had slightly increased 3-MT levels during flashbacks. It has been documented that noradrenergic hyperreactivity to mild stress may be a precipitating factor in stress-related psychiatric disorders.[8,17] Noradrenergic hyperactivity is associated with psychotic relapse in schizophrenia.[23] Taking these considerations into account, noradrenergic hyperreactivity may be related to susceptibility to episode recurrence. Therefore, robust noradrenergic hyperactivity with slightly increased DA release, in response to mild psychosocial stressors in flashbackers with subsequent episodes, may be able to trigger the initial episode and further predispose to subsequent flashbacks. By contrast, less robust noradrenergic hyperactivity with slightly increased DA release in response to mild psychosocial stressors in flashbackers with a single episode may be insufficient to predispose to subsequent flashbacks.

There was no significant difference in the number of stressful events or MAP-induced fear-related psychotic symptoms between the two flashbacker subgroups. The ratio of those with a mild fear of other people to the number of flashbacks did not differ significantly between the two flashbacker subgroups. Therefore, the impact of stress may not be related to robust noradrenergic hyperactivity. The proportion of medicated subjects did not differ significantly between the two flashbacker subgroups, suggesting that the neuroleptic treatment may not be attributed to robust noradrenergic hyperactivity. The mean duration of confinement before the start of blood sampling during the first flashback was significantly longer in the 9 flashbackers with subsequent episodes than in the 10 flashbackers with a single episode. According to recent reports, ruminations associated with aversive events have substantial impact on the reservoir of adaptive energy that may induce further NE changes.[8] Therefore, long-term exposure to distressing situations (imprisonment) in the 9 flashbackers with subsequent episodes may reflect their robust noradrenergic hyperreactivity.

Plasma levels of NE[24] and 3-MT,[25] respectively, reflect at best gross changes in whole brain noradrenergic and dopaminergic metabolism. Nevertheless, measurement of plasma monoaminergic metabolites remains the least invasive method available for evaluating central monoamine metabolism. The elevated levels of NE[19] and 3-MT[26] might be due to heightened autonomic arousal related to stress or anxiety. However, plasma E levels, which reflect fluctuations in emotional stress,[27] were not affected by the flashbacks. STAI-state scores and heart rate were likewise unaffected. Noradrenergic effusion from the locus coeruleus does not play a major role in cardiovascular responses (sympathetic activation) such as heart rate and blood pressure.[28] It follows that the elevated NE and 3-MT levels may not be secondary to sympathetic arousal.

The neuroleptics used may affect plasma NE and 3-MT levels. Previous clinical study has indicated that haloperidol (5–10 mg/day or 10–20 mg/day) decreased plasma NE levels in schizophrenics over a 6-week course of treatment,[29] and that infusion of chlorpromazine (25 mg) decreased plasma NE levels.[30] However, a number of studies have found that the neuroleptics have no effect on peripheral NE levels. Haloperidol (4 mg/day) for 5 weeks,[31] or administration of haloperidol (4–8 mg/day) or thioridazine (150–400 mg/day) for at least 10 days,[32] has no significant effect on peripheral noradrenergic activity. Treatment with haloperidol (3–20 mg/day) for at least one year,[33] or with haloperidol (5–15 mg/day) for 3 weeks,[34] does not affect plasma NE levels. There are few clinical studies of the neuroleptics' effects on plasma 3-MT levels. A preclinical study has reported that injection of haloperidol (0.5 mg/kg) or chlorpromazine (20 mg/kg) has no significant effect on brain 3-MT levels.[22] However, brain 3-MT levels increase after injections of haloperidol (0.5–1.0 mg/kg), chlorpromazine (2.3 or 14.0 mg/kg), or thioridazine (5 or 30 mg/kg).[20] Chronic haloperidol treatment reduces brain 3-MT levels in rats.[35] Therefore, neuroleptic effects on plasma NE and brain 3-MT levels may change with subject selection criteria or design of study. In our study, repeated ANOVA measures revealed no significant effect of neuroleptic treatment on plasma NE or 3-MT levels. Plasma NE levels during flashbacks in both medicated and later-medicated flashbackers were significantly higher than in user and nonuser controls. Plasma 3-MT levels during flashbacks in the later-medicated flashbackers, before they had received the neuroleptics, were significantly higher than in the medicated flashbackers and the nonuser controls. Overall, the elevated NE and 3-MT levels cannot be attributed to our neuroleptic treatment. However, since our analysis of the differences between the subject subgroups included subjects with and without neuroleptics, influence of neuroleptics on plasma NE and 3-MT levels cannot be finally ruled out.

REFERENCES

1. Sato, M., C.-C. Chen, K. Akiyama & S. Otsuki. 1983. Acute exacerbation of paranoid psychotic state after long-term abstinence in patients with previous methamphetamine psychosis. Biol. Psychiatry 18: 429–440.
2. Yui, K., K. Goto, S. Ikemoto & T. Ishiguro. 1997. Methamphetamine psychosis: spontaneous recurrence of paranoid-hallucinatory states and monoamine neurotransmitter function. J. Clin. Psychopharmacol. 17: 34–43.
3. Yui, K. et al. 1999. Neurobiological basis of relapse prediction in stimulant-induced psychosis and schizophrenia: the role of sensitization. Mol. Psychiatry 4: 512–523.
4. Yui, K., K. Goto, S. Ikemoto & T. Ishiguro. 2000. Increased sensitivity to stress in spontaneous recurrence of methamphetamine psychosis: noradrenergic hyperactivity with contribution from dopaminergic hyperactivity. J. Clin. Psychopharmacol. 20: 165–174.
5. Ellicott, A. et al. 1990. Life events and the course of bipolar disorder. Am. J. Psychiatry 147: 1194–1198.
6. Post, R.M. 1992. Transduction of psychosocial stress into the neurobiology of recurrent affective disorder. Am. J. Psychiatry 149: 999–1010.
7. Hall, K.S, D.L. Runner, G. Zeller & R.R. Fieve. 1997. Bipolar illness: a prospective study of life events. Comp. Psychiatry 18: 497–502.
8. Anisman, H. & R.M. Zacharko. 1995. Behavioral and neurochemical consequences associated with stressors. Ann. N.Y. Acad. Sci. 771: 205–225.
9. Matefy, R.E., C. Hayes & J. Hirsh. 1978. Psychedelic drug flashbacks: subjective reports and biographical data. Addict. Behav. 3: 165–178.

10. LANDAU, S.L. 1986. International Dictionary of Medicine and Biology, Vol. III. Wiley. New York.
11. SPIELBERGER, C.D. 1983. Manual for the State-Trait Anxiety. Inventory. Psychologist Press. Palo Alto, CA.
12. OVERALL, J.F. & D.R. GRAHAM. 1962. The brief psychiatric rating scale. Psychol. Rep. **10:** 799–812.
13. MILLNS, H., M. WOODWARD & C. BOITON-SMITH. 1995. Is it necessary to transform nutrient variables prior to statistical analyses? Am. J. Epidemiol. **141:** 251–262.
14. HAVILCEK, L.L. & R.D. CRAW. 1988. Practical Statistics for Physical Sciences. American Chemical Society. Washington, DC.
15. BELL, D.S. 1965. Comparison of amphetamine psychosis and schizophrenia. Br. J. Psychiatry **111:** 701–707.
16. SEGAL, D.S. & D.S. JANOUSKY. 1978. Psychostimulant-induced behavioral effects: possible models of schizophrenia. *In* Psychopharmacology: A Generation of Progress, M. A. Lipton, A. DiMascio, and K. F. Killam, Eds.: 1113–1123. Raven Press. New York.
17. IRWIN, J., P. AHILUWALIA & H. ANISMAN. 1986. Sensitization of norepinephrine activity following acute and chronic footshock. Brain Res. **379:** 98–103.
18. ROBINSON, T.E. *et al.* 1987. The effects of footshock stress on regional brain dopamine metabolism and pituitary β-endorphin release in rats previously sensitized to amphetamine. Neuropharmacology **26:** 679–691.
19. PÉRONET, F. *et al.* 1986. Plasma catecholamines at rest and exercise in subjects with high- and low-trait anxiety. Psychosom. Med. **48:** 52–58.
20. WOOD, P.L. & C.A. ALTAR. 1988. Dopamine release in vivo from nigrostriatal, mesolimbic, and mesocortical neurons utility of 3-methoxytyramine measurements. Pharmacol. Rev. **40:** 163–167.
21. DALMAZ, Y. & L. PEYRIN. 1978. Relations entre la 3-méthoxytyramine urinaire et le metabolisme périphérique de la dopamine chez l'homme et chez l'enfant. Arch. Int. Physiol. Biochim. **86:** 257–270.
22. WESTARINK, B.H.C. & S.J. SPAAN. 1982. On the significance of endogenous 3-methoxytyramine for the effects of centrally acting drugs on dopamine release in the rat brain. J. Neurochem. **38:** 680–686.
23. VAN KAMMEN, D.P. *et al.* 1994. Noradrenergic activity and prediction of psychotic relapse following haloperidol withdrawal in schizophrenia. Am. J. Psychiatry **51:** 379–384.
24. ROY, A. *et al.* 1988. Norepinephrine and its metabolites in cerebrospinal fluid, plasma, and urine. Arch. Gen. Psychiatry **45:** 849–857.
25. KENT, A.P., G.M. STERN & R.A. WEBSTER. 1990. The effect of benserazide on the peripheral and central distribution and metabolism of lovodopa after acute and chronic administration in the rat. Br. J. Pharmacol. **100:** 743–748.
26. CHARPUSTA, S.J., R.J. WYATT & J.M. MASSERANO. 1997. Effects of single and repeated footshock on dopamine release and metabolism in the brains of fisher rats. J. Neurochem. **68:** 2024–2031.
27. DIMSDALE, J.E. & J. MOSS. 1980. Plasma catecholamines in stress and exercise. JAMA **243:** 340–342.
28. VAN DEN BUUSE, M., G. LAMBERT, M. FLUTTERT & N. EIKELIS. 2001. Cardiovascular and behavioural responses to psychological stress in spontaneously hypertensive rats: effects of treatment with DSP-4. Behav. Brain Res. **119:** 131–142.
29. GREEN, A.I. *et al.* 1993. Haloperidol response and plasma catecholamines and their metabolites. Schizophr. Res. **10:** 33–37.
30. RISBO, A., K. JESSEN & J.O. HAGELSTEN. 1983. Catecholamine response to the clinical use of alpha adrenergic receptor blocking agents. Acta Anaesthesiol. Scand. **27:** 72–74.
31. BREIER, A. *et al.* 1994. The effect of clozapine on plasma norepinephrine: relationship to clinical efficacy. Neuropsychopharmacology **10:** 1–7.
32. TUCK, J.R. 1973. Effects of chlorpromazine, thioridazine and haloperidol on adrenergic transmitter mechanisms in man. Eur. J. Clin. Pharmacol. **6:** 81–87.
33. NAGAOKA, S., N. IWAMOTO & H. ARAI. 1997. First-episode neuroleptic-free schizophrenics: concentrations of monoamines and their metabolites in plasma and their

correlations with clinical response to haloperidol treatment. Biol. Psychiatry **41:** 857–864.
34. BROWN, A.S. *et al.* 1987. Effects of clozapine on plasma catecholamines and relation to treatment response in schizophrenia: a within-subject comparison with haloperidol. Neuropsychopharmacology **17:** 317–325.
35. VONVOIGTLANDER, P.F., M.A. BURIAN, T.S. ALTHAUS & L.R. WILLIAMS. 1990. Effects of chronic haloperidol on vitamin E levels and monoamine metabolism in rats fed normal and vitamin E deficient diets. Res. Commun. Chem. Pathol. Pharmacol. **68:** 343–352.

Environmental Chemical Compounds Could Induce Sensitization to Drugs of Abuse

RICARDO DUFFARD AND ANA MARÍA EVANGELISTA DE DUFFARD

Experimental Toxicology Laboratory, Faculty of Biochemistry and Pharmaceutical Sciences, UNR, Suipacha 531, Rosario, Argentina

ABSTRACT: Chemical environment should be considered as an additional factor that influences drugs of abuse. Besides, maternal exposure to environmental chemicals has increased, and fetuses as well as neonates may be at greater risk than adults. Studies from our laboratory have described a permanent effect of the worldwide use of the herbicide 2,4-dichlorophenoxyacetic acid (2,4-D) on serotonin and dopamine content in total brain and specific brain areas of adult rats born of mothers treated during lactation and fed with 2,4-D–treated diet after weaning. These animals show a modified neurotransmitter-related behavioral pattern in their developmental young and in adult age. Drugs that could be used to challenge the dopaminergic or serotoninergic systems include amphetamine or haloperidol, a postsynaptic dopamine receptor blocker. 2,4-D–exposed animals showed exacerbated response to challenges. Postnatal alterations in central dopaminergic and serotoninergic systems due to environmental chemical exposure may contribute to the enhanced/reduced behavioral sensitization to drugs of abuse.

KEYWORDS: 2,4-dichlorophenoxyacetic acid; amphetamine; environmental compounds; sensitization

INTRODUCTION

Drugs of Abuse and Addiction

The various pharmacological substances classified as drugs of abuse differ in molecular structure, specific neural substrate, or target system and have quite different, and sometimes opposite, unconditioned behavioral effects. However, these agents share the ability to act as positive reinforcers and, more importantly, to induce addiction. Drug addiction or drug abuse defines a particular consuming attitude which results in a compulsive and uncontrollable drug intake that becomes the principal goal-directed behavior of the individual. The fact that only certain compounds are able to induce addiction suggests that this process depends on intrinsic properties of these molecules.[1]

Address for correspondence: Dr. Ricardo Duffard, Laboratorio de Toxicología Experimental, Facultad de Ciencias Bioquímicas y Farmacéuticas, Universidad Nacional de Rosario, Suipacha 531, 2000 Rosario, Argentina. Fax: +54-341-4804598.
rduffard@fbioyf.unr.edu.ar

Ann. N.Y. Acad. Sci. 965: 305–313 (2002). © 2002 New York Academy of Sciences.

Many people have tried taking drugs at least once, but only a few persist in taking them and develop a true addiction. For others, drug intake remains just a recreational activity. These observations indicate that drugs require a special vulnerability substrate to develop their abuse potential. Comprehension of the "how" of this vulnerability substrate represents a key to understanding the "why" of addiction.

From the standpoint of a drug-centered vision of addiction, vulnerable individuals are the ones whose environment provides them with a greater opportunity of exposure to the drug. Peer and/or social pressure are often the most cited causes. Repeated exposure to the drug—via the development of tolerance, sensitization, and conditioning—induces drug dependence, which, in a drug-centered vision of addiction, represents the real cause of abuse.

However, from the point of view of an individual-centered vision of addiction, certain individuals, because of a particular functional state of the biological substances that interact with the drug, experience singular effects of the drug that promote a shift from use to abuse. Such individual vulnerability might be considered a drug-specific phenomenon or the behavioral expression of an addictive personality.[1]

Pre- and Postnatal Exposure to Environmental Compounds

Insecticides and herbicides used in agriculture are the classic example of anthropogenic chemicals that enter the earth's environment in large amounts via no specific sources. These compounds can adversely affect no target organisms and may be detrimental to human health if people are exposed either to direct contact, or to residues of the molecules in food, water, or agricultural products. In this paper, we try to demonstrate that these environmental compounds might also modify the chemistry and biochemistry of the brain and make those individuals sensitized to drugs of abuse. The aim of the present work is to define whether individuals that have been perinatally exposed to environmental chemical compounds such as a herbicide like 2,4-dichlorophenoxy acetic acid (2,4-D) show differential reactivity to drugs of abuse.

Our laboratory has described changes in biogenic amine levels in different brain areas in pups and in adult rats exposed to 2,4-D during different developmental periods through mother's milk,[2,3] as well as to increased immunoreactive astrocytes, detected by immunostaining with antibodies to GFAP and S-100 protein. This increase took place in all layers of the cerebellar cortex, mainly in its granular layer, in the alveus and stratum radiato of the hippocampus and in the dorsal nucleus of the mesencephalon.[4] Changes in SER-IR neurons of the dorsal raphe nucleus (DRN) and medial raphe nucleus (MRN) in 2,4-D–exposed pups during early life were also observed.[5]

Consequently, if these animals were exposed to drugs of abuse or other compounds that act via those systems, their dopaminergic and serotoninergic systems would respond differently than would those that were not exposed to chemical compounds which modify these neurotransmitter systems; the behavioral answers would be different.

Taking into account these paradigms as well as the fact that certain lesions of the central nervous system (CNS) have obvious manifestations, while other CNS lesions may remain undetected for long periods because they do not have such manifestations evident under ordinary conditions and because behavioral functions served by the involved brain areas may be subtle and difficult to test and measure, our previous studies have suggested that this could be caused by some 2,4-D–derived CNS lesions that remain undetected.[6]

One strategy for detecting subclinical damage to dopaminergic and serotoninergic systems is the specific pharmacological challenge to a compromised neurotransmitter system. This method would take into account the fact that the neurotransmitter system in question has limited reserves or increased quantities of neurotransmitters. In essence, under normal conditions, a compromised neurotransmitter system might be able to function, but if it is stressed abnormalities might become apparent.

It has been proposed that a pharmacological neuronal stress test might be useful in the evaluation of patients with suspected subclinical neurotoxicity. In an individual with a history of significant methamphetamine use, diminished dopaminergic neurotransmission might be expected but, under ordinary conditions, it might be clinically inapparent because it was not sufficiently severe. If that individual were given a drug that specifically interfered with dopaminergic neurotransmission, it might be anticipated that the subject would demonstrate exquisite sensitivity to its effects.[7]

Differential Effects of Challenges to Neurochemical and Neurobehavioral Outcomes

Drugs that could be used to challenge the serotonergic or dopaminergic systems include amphetamine (AMPH) or haloperidol (HAL), a postsynaptic dopamine-receptor blocker. Amphetamine and other psychomotor stimulants produce substantial behavioral effects through activation of the mesolimbic and mesocortical dopaminergic system. Part of that evidence is derived from pharmacological studies: drugs that either directly or indirectly stimulate DA receptors have a characteristic profile of behavioral effects. Amphetamine is an indirect DA agonist. At low-to-moderate doses, AMPH increases locomotion, apparently involving DA in the limbic forebrain, decreases food and water intake, has rate-dependent effects on schedule-controlled behavior, and functions as a positive reinforcer. At higher doses, AMPH induces species-specific stereotypic behaviors involving striatal DA. In humans, AMPH increases positive mood, has a high abuse liability, and when used in high doses can induce stereotypic and maladaptive behaviors. When AMPH is used repeatedly, paranoid psychosis develops which may also be related to a hyperdopaminergic state.

THE 2,4-D MODEL AND BEHAVIORAL RESPONSES

Our experimental model of study consisted of offsprings of dams treated with a daily oral dose by diet of about 50 or 70 mg/kg/day of 2,4-D from gestational day (GD) 16 to postnatal day (PND) 23. 2,4-D (Sigma Chemical Co., St. Louis, MO) was dissolved in alcohol solution, mixed with food, and dried before starting to feed the diet, according to Evangelista de Duffard *et al*.[2,8,9] Dietary levels were adjusted based on the most recent body weight and food consumption determinations in order to deliver a constant average dietary intake (mg/kg body weight/day). The dose of herbicide (about one-tenth of the reported LD_{50}—639 and 764 mg/kg/day for male and female, respectively)[10] was selected based on a previous study that demonstrated behavioral changes in adult rats exposed to 2,4-D butyl ester.[8]

Control dams were fed the same diet as untreated rodents, based on consumption by a weight-matched 2,4-D–fed dam. As parturition approached, dams were checked for birth twice daily. Twenty-four hours following parturitions (parturition was PND 0), litters were examined and culled to eight pups, with equal representation of sex within litter whenever possible. Pups were weaned at PND 23 and housed separately by sex per cage until termination of the experiment (PND 90). After weaning, the pups from the 2,4-D–treated group were randomly assigned to one of the following experimental subgroups:

T1 group. This group consisted of offspring of dams exposed to 2,4-D in their diet from GD 16 to PND 23; after weaning, these pups were fed with untreated diet until PND 90.

T2 group. This group consisted of offspring of dams exposed to 2,4-D in their diet from GD 16 to PND 23, as described above, but after weaning these pups were maintained with diet treated with 2,4-D until PND 90.

In all these adult rats, behaviors were observed and measured before and at

- 30, 300, or 1440 min following a single injection of 5 or 10 mg/kg i.p. injection of (+)-amphetamine sulfate dissolved in 0.9% saline solution. The dose of AMPH had been selected in a previous work,[6] which demonstrated that the rotation at low doses was masked by the rat's hyperactivity.
- 30, 60, or 90 min after a single injection of 0.05 or 1.0 mg/kg HAL, which was dissolved in warm lactic acid to prepare a stock solution of 1 mg/mL in 1 mg/mL acid. This stock was diluted with distilled water to yield 0.1 mg/mL at pH 3.6. These doses of HAL were chosen because, in a pilot study, neither akinesia nor catalepsy was produced in adult rats.[6]

Testing procedures were conducted between 0900 and 1700 h. During all behavioral studies, the experimenter was blinded to the experimental design. The testing was conducted only once in each rat, and on only one day of the whole experiment.

Interpretation of 2,4-D Effects

When T1 and T2 animals were injected with amphetamine (AMPH), they showed an exacerbated serotoninergic and dopaminergic behavioral response and when they were injected with HAL, at noncataleptic doses (0.05 or 0.1 mg/kg), they displayed significant catalepsy.

In that manner, following i.p. injection of amphetamine, 5 or 10 mg/kg, all 2,4-D–exposed animals (from T1 or T2 groups) showed the "serotonin syndromc" (SS) involving altered behaviors and postures (TABLE 1). These included forepaw movements (forepaw treading, excessive placement or tapping), hunching (back arching), sprawling of limbs, backing, hindlimb abduction, mobility (ability of rat for locomotion despite gait abnormalities, including padding), abnormal head movements (vertical or lateral side-to-side respective movements), wet-dog shakes (including head shakes), lying on side, limb extension, dystonic and flat-body posture. The observers also registered the presence of piloerection, moist fur, and stiff tail (defined as the raising of the tail to a level higher than that of the body axis). In addition,

TABLE 1. 5-HT syndrome behaviors in male and female rats exposed to 2,4-D

			5-HT syndrome behaviors					
Treatment	Age (days)	Sex	Flat body posture	Hunching	Stiff tail	Forepaw treading	Hindlimb abduction	Head movement
Control	30	M	0	0.50 ± 0.12	0.32 ± 0.10	0.31 ± 0.09	0	1.25 ± 0.38
		F	0	0.58 ± 0.18	0.29 ± 0.05	0.28 ± 0.10	0	0.95 ± 0.15
T1		M	0	0.46 ± 0.10	0.39 ± 0.08	0.35 ± 0.05	0	1.38 ± 0.58
		F	0	0.54 ± 0.11	0.41 ± 0.19	0.32 ± 0.01	0	$1.52 \pm 0.60*$
T2		M	0	$1.12 \pm 0.33*$	$2.32 \pm 0.65*$	0.52 ± 0.10	0	$2.00 \pm 0.32*$
		F	0	$0.98 \pm 0.25*$	$1.98 \pm 0.33*$	0.58 ± 0.07	0	$1.89 \pm 0.25*$
Control	60	M	0	0	0.29 ± 0.02	0	0	0
		F	0	0	0.33 ± 0.01	0	0	0
T1		M	0	0	0.55 ± 0.03	0	0	0
		F	0	0.75 ± 0.19	0.45 ± 0.12	0	0	0
T2		M	$1.10 \pm 0.25*$	$0.91 \pm 0.33*$	$1.95 \pm 0.23*$	0	0	0
		F	$0.82 \pm 0.20*$	$1.57 \pm 0.22*$	$2.06 \pm 0.42*$	0	0	0
Control	90	M	0.25 ± 0.08	0	0.30 ± 0.09	0	0	0
		F	0.15 ± 0.09	0	0.28 ± 0.05	0	0	0
T1		M	0.22 ± 0.13	0	0.41 ± 0.15	0	0	0
		F	0.12 ± 0.09	0	0.55 ± 0.10	0	0	0
T2		M	$2.60 \pm 0.28*$	$1.15 \pm 0.54*$	$2.10 \pm 0.25*$	0	0	0
		F	$1.58 \pm 0.58*$	$2.19 \pm 0.39*$	$2.22 \pm 0.39*$	0	0	0

Each animal was observed for several seconds at 5-min intervals of the 60-min test period. Behaviors were scored as described in the text with a maximum score of 4. The results are presented as mean ± SEM. * Significantly different from respective control group $p < 0.05$. (Data from Bortolozzi et al.[9])

dopaminergic behaviors like rearing and rotation were also shown, and all behaviors and postures were sex dependent.

Several lines of evidence suggest that the development of central serotonergic neurons may be affected by the prenatal or neonatal environment and that the intensity of the 5-HT syndrome is related to their functional and differential activities.[12,13]

We have just described high immunoreactivity to S-100, GFAP proteins, and 5-HT-IR neurons—especially in dorsal and medial raphe nucleus—in T1 2,4-D–exposed rats; these processes are not reversible, at least not in these brain areas.[14]

On the other hand, it is known that blockade of either D_1 or D_2 receptors leads to a suppression of spontaneous exploratory and motor behavior and the elicitation of a state known as catalepsy. Catalepsy refers to a marked difficulty in initiating voluntary motor activity, usually experimentally demonstrated by showing that the subject does not change position when placed in an awkward or uncomfortable posture. Cataleptic effects in adult rats were assessed by reference to three criteria according to Waldmeier and Delini-Stula:[11] (a) the forepaws of the animals were placed alter-

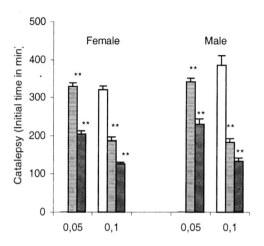

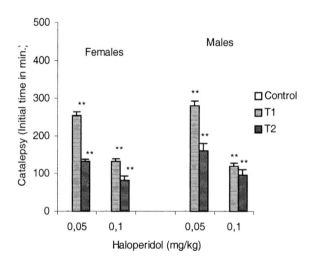

FIGURE 1. Effects of 0.05 and 0.10 mg/kg haloperidol on cataleptic response in PND 60 and PND 90 rats of both sexes exposed to 2,4-D. Data are presented as means ± SEM of initial time of catalepsy (in min). **Significant differences from haloperidol-treated control rats ($p < 0.01$). (Data from Bortolozzi et al.[9])

natively on a cork 3 cm high. Failure to remove the paw within 10 s scored as a positive response of stage 1 of catalepsy; (b) the same procedure and ratings were used as above, but with a cork 8 cm high, and for each paw held in place for 10 s stage 2 of catalepsy was given; (c) homolateral fore- and hindpaws were crossed and, similarly, if held for 60 s, it was considered as stage 3 of catalepsy. An average score for the group was calculated and expressed as the time in minutes in which catalepsy was unchained after HAL. For this study, two rats/sex/dose from each of four litters were tested at 30-min intervals for several hours postinjection. The testing was conducted only once in each rat and on one day only of the whole experiment.

Our behavioral data also indicated that HAL in noncataleptic doses induced catalepsy in the T1 and T2 groups. Again, T1 rats of 60 and 90 days of age (apparently "normal" rats) were capable of producing catalepsy induced by HAL (FIG. 1). This response in 90-day-old rats of the T2 group with both doses of HAL, and in T1 group rats with the higher HAL dose only (0.1 mg/kg), maintained the catalepsy even 24 h after HAL (data not shown). There was no significant noticeable effect in catalepsy on sex at both doses of HAL, and 2,4-D alone did not cause any obvious cataleptic response. The degree of catalepsy produced by HAL differed according to dose level, rat age, and duration of 2,4-D exposure.

We have also shown that there was an increase of DA D_2-like receptors in the T1 and T2 groups, but to elicit the increase of DA D_2-like receptors in the T1 group the rats had to be challenged with AMPH.[15] In this manner, 2,4-D exposure at a dose producing no overt signs of toxicity may cause long-term alterations in the functional state of the rat CNS, detected through a neurobehavioral test battery. The exposure to the herbicide during pre- and postnatal development induces behavioral abnormalities that seem to disappear in adulthood after cessation of 2,4-D. However, exposure to 2,4-D during early postnatal development prevents the normal behavior of a rat in its adult life, and this may be unmasked after additional chemical stress.

The enhancement of the behavioral effects by both AMPH and HAL, in the 2,4-D–exposed animals would resemble that of the repeated intermittent administration of psychostimulants, like amphetamine or cocaine. This phenomenon—referred to as sensitization—can persist for weeks or months after cessation of drug use; our results confirm that statement.

Studies have shown that the repeated intermittent administration of cocaine and other psychostimulants can result in enhancement of their behavioral effects[16]—that is, the efficacy and/or potency of these agents in producing a given effect are increased. Sensitization has been implicated in drug craving and the reinstatement of drug addiction. The results from the T1 group (withdrawal group) confirm the persistence of the sensitization-derived effect of 2,4-D.

VULNERABILITY TO DRUG ABUSE

Although current advances in research on drugs of abuse have resulted in many exciting developments, we do not know yet about the factors that determine the use of, dependence on, and adaptations in the CNS by drugs of abuse.

The development of addiction does not seem to be the simple consequence of the intrinsic effects of drugs of abuse, but rather the result of their interaction with specific individual substrates. Consequently, comprehension of the biological mechanisms of individual vulnerability to drugs seems an essential step to the development of new therapies of addiction.

Briefly, with our these results we have demonstrated that:

(a) a xenobiotic neonatal exposure such as that to 2,4-D produces neurochemical, but functionally hidden, alterations that may be elicited in the presence of the challenge treatment.

(b) the 2,4-D–exposed animals would be more vulnerable or sensitized to serotoninergic and dopaminergic drugs, like drugs of abuse.

(c) vulnerability to drugs of abuse can be innate as it was demonstrated by genetic studies, or acquired by exposure to environmental compounds like 2,4-D, a member of the chemical family of chlorophenoxy alkanoic compounds.

ACKNOWLEDGMENT

This research was supported by grants from the Consejo Nacional de Investigaciones Científicas y Técnicas (CONICET), Argentina to Ricardo Duffard and Ana María Evangelista de Duffard.

REFERENCES

1. PIAZZA, P.V. & M. LE MOAL. 1996. Pathophysiological basis of vulnerability to drug abuse: role of an interaction between stress, glucocorticoids, and dopaminergic neurons. In Annual Review of Pharmacology and Toxicology, Vol. 36. A.K. Cho, T.F. Blaschke, I.K. Ho, and H.H. Loh, Eds.: 359–378. Annual Reviews Inc. Palo Alto, CA.

2. EVANGELISTA DE DUFFARD, A.M., M. NICOLA DE ALDERETE & R. DUFFARD. 1990. Changes in brain serotonin and 5-hydroxyindolacetic acid levels induced by 2,4-dichlorophenoxyacetic butyl ester. Toxicology 64: 265–270.

3. FERRI, A., A. BORTOLOZZI, R. DUFFARD & A.M. EVANGELISTA DE DUFFARD. 2000. Monoamine levels in neonate rats lactationally exposed to 2,4-dichlorophenoxyacetic acid. Biog. Amines 16: 73–100.

4. BRUSCO, A. et al. 1997. 2,4-Dichlorophenoxyacetic acid through lactation induces astrogliosis in rat brain. Mol. Chem. Neuropathol. 30: 175–185.

5. EVANGELISTA DE DUFFARD, A.M. et al. 1995. Changes in serotonin-immunoreactivity in the dorsal and median raphe nuclei of rats exposed to 2,4-dichlorophenoxyacetic acid through lactation. Mol. Chem. Neuropathol. 26: 187–193.

6. EVANGELISTA DE DUFFARD, A.M., A. BORTOLOZZI & R. DUFFARD. 1995. Altered behavioral responses in 2,4-dichlorophenoxyacetic acid treated and amphetamine challenged rats. Neurotoxicology 16: 479–488.

7. MCCANN, U.D. & G.A. RICAURTE. 1993. Strategies for detecting subclinical monoamine depletions in human. In Assessing Neurotoxicity of Drug Abuse. National Institute on Drug Abuse Research Monograph Series, Vol. 136. L. Erinoff, Ed.: 53–62. U.S. Department of Health and Human Services. Rockville, MD.

8. EVANGELISTA DE DUFFARD, A.M., C. ORTA & R. DUFFARD. 1990. Behavioral changes in rats fed a diet containing 2,4-dichlorophenoxyacetic butyl ester. Neurotoxicology 11: 563–572.

9. BORTOLOZZI, A., R. DUFFARD & A.M. EVANGELISTA DE DUFFARD. 1999. Behavioral alterations induced in rats by a pre- and postnatal exposure to 2,4-dichlorophenoxyacetic acid. Neurotoxicol. Teratol. 21: 451–465.

10. MUNRO, I.C., G.L. CARLO, J.C. ORR, et al. 1992. A comprehensive, integrated review and evaluation of the scientific evidence relating to the safety of the herbicide 2,4-D. J. Am. Coll. Toxicol. 11: 662–664.

11. WALDMEIER, P. & A. DELINI-STULA. 1979. Serotonin-dopamine interactions in the nigrostriatal system. Eur. J. Pharmacol. **55:** 363–373.
12. PETERS, D.A. 1988. Both prenatal and postnatal factors contribute to the effects of maternal stress on offspring behavior and central 5-hydroxytryptamine receptors in the rat. Pharmacol. Biochem. Behav. **30:** 669–673.
13. PRANZATELLI, M.R. 1992. Serotonin receptors ontogeny: effects of agonists in 1-day-old rats. Pharmacol. Biochem. Behav. **43:** 1273–1277.
14. GARCIA, G. *et al.* 2002. Morphological study of 5-HT neurons and astroglial cells on brain of adult rats perinatal or chronically exposed to 2,4-dichlorophenoxyacetic acid. Neurotoxicol. In press.
15. BORTOLOZZI, A., R. DUFFARD, M.C. ANTONELLI & A. M. EVANGELISTA DE DUFFARD. 2002. Increased sensitivity in dopamine D2-type brain receptors from 2,4-dichlorophenoxyacetic (2,4-D) exposed and amphetamine challenged. Ann. N.Y. Acad. Sci. This volume.
16. STRAKOWSKI, S.M. & K.W. SAX.1998. Progressive behavioral response to repeated d-amphetamine challenge: further evidence for sensitisation in humans. Biol. Psychol. **44:** 1171–1177.

Increased Sensitivity in Dopamine D_2-like Brain Receptors from 2,4-Dichlorophenoxyacetic Acid (2,4-D)-Exposed and Amphetamine-Challenged Rats

ANALÍA BORTOLOZZI,[a] RICARDO DUFFARD,[a] MARTA ANTONELLI,[b] AND ANA MARÍA EVANGELISTA DE DUFFARD[a]

[a]Experimental Toxicology Laboratory, Faculty of Biochemistry and Pharmaceutical Sciences, UNR, Suipacha 531, Rosario, Argentina

[b]Chemistry and Biological Physical-Chemistry Institute (UBA-CONICET), Faculty of Pharmacy and Biochemistry, UBA, Buenos Aires, Argentina

ABSTRACT: To determine whether the dopamine D_2 receptor plays a crucial role in chemically acquired sensitivity to drugs of abuse like amphetamine (AMPH) after an exposure to aryloxoalkanoic compounds, we examined in the present work the impact of AMPH (10 mg/kg, i.p.) on the dopaminergic D_2-like receptors. Rats were exposed to 2,4-D 70 mg/kg/day from gestation day (GD) 16 to postnatal day (PND) 23. After weaning, the pups were assigned to one of the two subgroups: T1 (fed with untreated diet until PND 90) and T2 (maintained with 2,4-D diet until PND 90). After that, an acute challenge with AMPH was administered to each animal. Rats were sacrificed at 0, 5, 24, 72, and 168 h after AMPH, and membranes of striatum (CPu), prefrontal cortex (PfC), hippocampus (H), and cerebellum (Ce) were obtained. Binding studies employing [^{3}H]nemonapride showed that AMPH caused an increase in DA D_2-like receptors of all brain areas between 5 and 24 h after the treatment, with a reduction to the basal levels one week later. The AMPH challenge to (T1 and T2) 2,4-D–exposed rats showed an alteration on receptor density depending on brain area and on sex, more than on the 2,4-D exposure time. This D_2-like receptor density increase could explain the exacerbated behaviors of the 2,4-D–exposed and amphetamine-challenged animals, as previously observed by us. The withdrawal of 2,4-D did not produce a real reversion to basal levels of D_2-like receptors, indicating that herbicide exposure during the preweaning period caused a sensitization and a stable DA D_2-like receptor increase that was elicited when the system was challenged with this dopaminergic drug.

KEYWORDS: 2,4-dichlorophenoxyacetic acid; amphetamine; dopaminergic D_2-like receptors; binding studies; rat brain areas

Address for correspondence: Dr. Ana María Evangelista de Duffard, Laboratorio de Toxicología Experimental, Facultad de Ciencias Bioquímicas y Farmacéuticas, Universidad Nacional de Rosario, Suipacha 531, 2000 Rosario, Argentina. Fax: +54-341-4804598.
aevangel@fbioyf.unr.edu.ar

Ann. N.Y. Acad. Sci. 965: 314–323 (2002). © 2002 New York Academy of Sciences.

INTRODUCTION

Chlorophenoxyalkanoic compounds—particularly 2,4-dichlorophenoxyacetic acid (2,4-D)—are being extensively used as effective broad-leaf herbicide in agriculture and forestry.[1] The use of herbicides has generated a series of toxicological and environmental problems in developing countries.[2,3] It has been reported that the central nervous system (CNS) is one of the targets for the toxic effects of phenoxyherbicides.[3–5] A variety of neurotoxic effects of 2,4-D have been reported in experimental animals, among them neurobehavioral changes in rats associated with alterations in both serotoninergic and dopaminergic systems.[6–12]

Normal expression and maturation of DA receptors in the forebrain region are of particular interest because disturbances in their development have been involved in psychotic disorders.[13] In a previous work we also reported a vulnerability of D$_2$-like receptors to 2,4-D exposure. Subchronic exposure to 2,4-D elicited a regional increase of D$_2$ receptor density at different ages during development, with the caudate-putamen the most affected brain area. However, no changes were observed in the dopamine D$_2$-like receptors in brain areas of 90-day-old rats with a subacute exposure to 2,4-D and the withdrawal of the drug.[14]

It is accepted that the administration of challenges to an organism previously exposed to xenobiotics may unmask possible subtle behavioral abnormalities. We have previously reported behavioral alterations in rats induced by an acute or a pre- and postnatal exposure to 2,4-D and amphetamine challenge.[8,15]

Amphetamine (AMPH) induces short-term and long-term behavioral changes when it is administered to humans or rodents. Acute administration of AMPH produces locomotor hyperactivity and stereotypy behaviors in rodents. The major target for this psychostimulant is thought to be the brain monoamine (DA, NE, and 5-HT) systems. Repeated dosing can lead to long-lasting behavioral changes, such as sensitization and tolerance. AMPH induces dopamine (DA) release, resulting in increased occupancy of dopamine receptors, and blocks DA reuptake by binding to the DA transporter.[16–18]

Humans could be either occupationally or environmentally exposed to herbicides and may also be exposed to an occasional amphetamine experience. The goal of the present study was to examine the impact of AMPH on the sensitivities of dopaminergic D$_2$-like receptors in specific brain areas of adult rats exposed to 2,4-D, either through their mothers' milk since the last gestation days and nursing period (with 2,4-D withdrawal) or until pups were 90 days old.

MATERIAL AND METHODS

2,4-D Exposure

Pregnant female Wistar rats were individually housed in plastic breeding cages in a temperature-controlled nursery (22–24°C) and maintained on a 12-h light/dark cycle. Food and water were available *ad libitum*. In gestational day (GD) 16, the pregnant females were randomly divided into two groups.

2,4-D-Treated Group: Dams were treated with a daily oral dose by diet of about 70 mg/kg of 2,4-D from GD 16 to postnatal day 23 (PND 23). 2,4-D (Sigma Chemical Co., USA) was dissolved in an alcohol solution, according to Duffard et al.[5]

Control Group: Dams were fed with untreated rodent diet, with the same amount consumed by a weight-matched 2,4-D–fed dam.

The day after the dam delivered, postnatal day (PND) 1, litters were examined and culled to 8 pups, 4 of each sex, if possible. At PND 23, rats from 2,4-D–treated group were randomly assigned to one of the following experimental subgroups. The T1 group consisted of offspring of dams exposed to 2,4-D in their diet from GD 16 to PND 23. But after weaning, these pups were fed untreated diet until PND 90 (withdrawn 2,4-D rats). The T2 group consisted of offspring of dams exposed to 2,4-D in their diet from GD 16 to PND 23, as just described, but after weaning these pups were maintained on the 2,4-D diet until PND 90.

On PND 90, all rats were challenged with 10 mg/kg of (+)-amphetamine sulfate dissolved in 0.9% saline solution, i.p., and 3 h later sacrificed. Brain tissue was rapidly removed and prefrontal cortex (PFc), caudate-putamen (CPu), hippocampus (H), and cerebellum (Cer) were isolated by free-hand dissection.

Dopamine Receptor Binding Procedure

For the binding assays of the dopamine receptors, membranes were obtained according to Borodinsky et al.[19] Briefly, a crude membrane fraction was prepared from each brain area by homogenization of the tissue in 10 volumes of chilled solution of 0.32 M sucrose, and then centrifuged at $1000 \times g$ for 10 min. The supernatant was centrifuged at $12,000 \times g$ for 20 min. The pellet was suspended in bi-distilled water, centrifuged at $20,000 \times g$ for 30 min, and resuspended in binding buffer (see below) to a final protein concentration of 3 mg/mL. Protein content was determined by the method of Bradford,[21] using bovine serum albumin as the standard.

D_2-like receptor binding assay followed a standard method described in Defagot and Antonelli,[20] using [^{3}H]nemonapride for DA receptor specific binding. Nonspecific binding was determined using flupexintol. Ligand-binding assays were performed by incubating the membrane preparations for 100 min at 22°C in a final volume of 500 mL binding buffer (50 mM Tris-HCl, pH 7.8, 120 mM NaCl, 5 mM KCl, 5 mM $MgCl_2$, 1.5 mM $CaCl_2$, and 1 mM EDTA).

The reaction was started by adding 2 mL cold binding buffer and stopped by rapid filtration through Whatman GF/B glass fiber filters. Then, filters were washed twice with 2 mL of the same buffer and assayed for radioactivity on a liquid scintillation counter (45–50% efficiency). Binding assays were determined by triplicate. Specific binding was calculated by subtracting the binding observed in the presence of 50 mM flupentixol (nonspecific binding: 30–35%).

DRUGS AND CHEMICALS

R,S-(±)-[N-metyl-H]-nemonapride (85 Ci/mmol) was purchased from New England Nuclear Co. (Boston, MA). 2,4-D, amphetamine, flupentixol, and other chemicals were from Sigma/RBI (St. Louis, MO).

STATISTICAL ANALYSES

The results of binding experiments were analyzed for the effect of sex, 2,4-D exposure, and acute amphetamine injection using ANOVA. Significant main effects and interactions were further analyzed employing Student's *t* test (two-tailed) or Student-Newman-Keuls.

RESULTS

In control rats, a single dose of amphetamine increased the DA D$_2$-like receptor density 70–80% in hippocampus and cerebellum, but only 40% in striatum, a week after amphetamine injection (FIGS. 3 and 4). A diminution of DA D$_2$-like receptors in prefrontal cortex was registered at 72 h after AMPH injection (FIG.1 and 2). No sex difference was registered. However, the alteration in D$_2$-like receptors produced by the 2,4-D and manifested with one single injection of AMPH—in both experimental subgroups—depended on sex more than on the 2,4-D exposure time.

When AMPH was administered to T2 animals, AMPH enhanced the amount of dopamine D$_2$-like receptors more than in control and 2,4-D rats, in all four brain areas studied (FIGS. 2 and 4). Although during the first hours after AMPH, the basal receptor amount—different in each area—was similar for females and males, an onward sex difference by amphetamine was registered.

Unexpectedly, amphetamine-enhanced D$_2$-like receptors in T1 rats (FIGS. 1 and 3). D$_2$-like receptor density in T1 rats was similar to 90-day-old control animals at 0 time. When an amphetamine challenge was administered, a dopamine D$_2$-like receptor increase was registered in all the brain areas studied with regard to that of corresponding ones of controls, and in females it was different from that found in males.

Compared to the controls, PFc was the most affected area and AMPH did not affect receptor density of T1 rats' hippocampus. Similar to what occurred with PFc, in CPu and Cer, males increased these receptors to 70% sooner after AMPH, then normalized to control values, and a week later DA D$_2$-like receptors were reduced to basal values.

DISCUSSION

Dopamine mediates neurochemical and physiological effects by interacting with at least five different receptors, among them the D$_2$-like (D$_2$, D$_3$, and D$_4$) receptors. Anatomically, D$_2$-like receptors occur in the brain areas (caudate-putamen, frontal cortex, hippocampus, and cerebellum[22]) that we studied.

In previous work we have demonstrated an increase in the DA D$_2$-like receptors in offspring's brain exposed to 2,4-D *in utero* and until PND 90 (T2 group). When the herbicide was removed at the end of their lactation period and apparently recovered and stabilized to control level (T1 group), no variation in DA D$_2$-like binding was observed.[14] Thus, we showed that DA D$_2$ binding induced in adult rats by a subacute or chronic 2,4-D exposure has different levels from DA D$_2$-like receptors.

Our present data indicate that an amphetamine challenge to 90-day-old rats—in both treated groups of rats—produce enhanced dopamine D$_2$-like receptor binding.

A

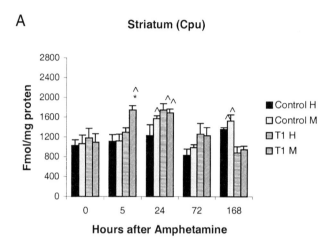

B

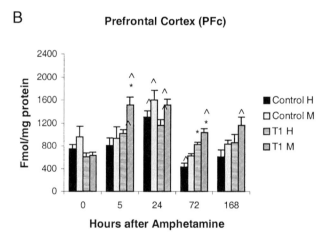

FIGURE 1. (A) Amphetamine effect on [³H]nemonapride binding in striatum (CPu) and **(B)** prefrontal cortex (PFc) brain membranes of control and T1 rats. Results are expressed as the average ± SEM. $^*p < 0.05$, $^{**}p < 0.01$ compared to the corresponding controls. $^\wedge p < 0.05$, $^{\wedge\wedge}p < 0.01$ compared to 0 time.

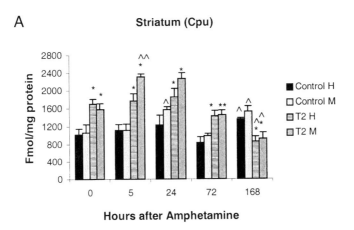

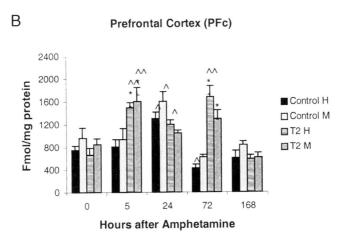

FIGURE 2. (A) Amphetamine effect on [³H]nemonapride binding in striatum (CPu) and **(B)** prefrontal cortex (PFc) brain membranes of control and T2 rats. Results are expressed as the average ± SEM. $^*p < 0.05$, $^{**}p < 0.01$ compared to the corresponding controls. $^\wedge p < 0.05$, $^{\wedge\wedge}p < 0.01$ compared to 0 time.

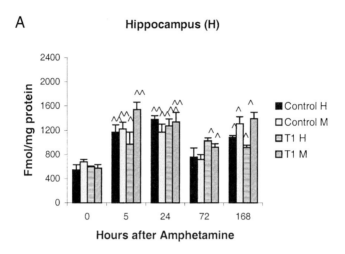

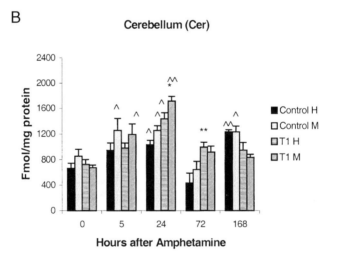

FIGURE 3. (**A**) Amphetamine effect on [³H]nemonapride binding in hippocampus (H) and (**B**) cerebellum (Cer) brain membranes of control and T1 rats. Results are expressed as the average ± SEM. $^*p < 0.05$, $^{**}p < 0.01$ compared to the corresponding controls. $^\wedge p < 0.05$, $^{\wedge\wedge}p < 0.01$ compared to 0 time.

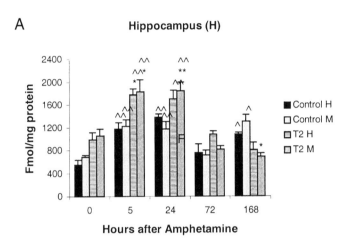

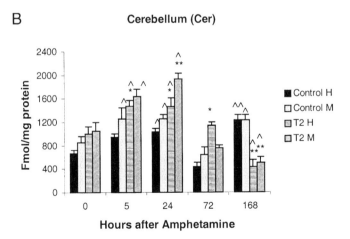

FIGURE 4. (**A**) Amphetamine effect on [^{3}H]nemonapride binding in hippocampus (H) and (**B**) cerebellum (Cer) brain membranes of control and T2 rats. Results are expressed as the average ± SEM. $^*p < 0.05$, $^{**}p < 0.01$ compared to the corresponding controls. $^\wedge p < 0.05$, $^{\wedge\wedge}p < 0.01$ compared to 0 time.

In this way an acute administration of amphetamine can potently induce binding activity in dopamine-innervated brain areas of rats exposed early in their life to 2,4-D. These results suggest a strong modulator role for the 2,4-D in the brain areas studied. Adult offspring exposed only to 2,4-D *in utero* and lactation did not exhibit any changes in DA D_2-like receptors, but after an amphetamine challenge a remarkable increase of these receptors was observed. It is evident that the withdrawal of 2,4-D produces a reversion to basal levels of D_2-like receptors. However, after an amphetamine challenge, an increase of receptors was observed in certain brain areas, particularly PFc. These results suggest the ability of the system to induce an internalization of DA D_2 receptors subsequent to the withdrawal of 2,4-D. This fact also indicates that herbicide exposure during the preweaning period causes a sensitization of D_2-like receptors and, in consequence, a DA D_2-like receptors increase elicited when the system was challenged with other dopaminergic drugs. Besides, it is possible that the increase in DA receptors obtained by AMPH in rats with a long-term 2,4-D pretreatment was produced by a synergic response on the 2,4-D effect.

Neurons and their projections in the brain areas studied provide an important excitatory drive necessary for the development of sensitization. When given alone, 2,4-D might sensitize the rats to subsequent stimulant challenges. Behavioral sensitization in rat, typically associated with augmented levels of cerebral DA and 5-HT, was observed when 2,4-D rats were co-administered with an acute injection of AMPH.[15] Dopamine D_2 receptors are implicated in stimulant-induced behavioral sensitization.[23,16] These D_2-like receptors' density increases could explain the appearance of abnormal behaviors (motor alterations, serotonin syndrome, facilitation of circling, and catalepsy), previously reported by us,[15] in 2,4-D–exposed rats. Such behaviors have been associated with sensitization and are involved in the pathological mechanisms of the drug.

ACKNOWLEDGMENTS

This research was supported by a grant from the Consejo Nacional de Investigaciones Científicas y Técnicas (CONICET), Argentina, to Ana María Evangelista de Duffard and by a grant from ANPCYT (PICT 0287) to Marta Antonelli.

REFERENCES

1. BAGE, G., E. CEKANOVA & K. LARSSON. 1973. Teratogenic and embryotoxic effects of the herbicides di- and trichlorophenoxycetic acids (2,4-D and 2,4,5-T). Acta Pharmacol. Toxicol. **32:** 408–416.
2. ROWE, V.K. & T.A. HYMAS. 1954. Summary of toxicological information on 2,4-D and 2,4,5-T type herbicides and an evaluation of the hazards to livestock associated with their use. Am. J. Vet. Res. **15:** 622–629.
3. DUFFARD, R., L. TRAINI & A.M. EVANGELISTA DE DUFFARD. 1981. Embryotoxic and teratogenic effects of phenoxyherbicides. Acta Physiol. Latinoam. **35:** 39–41.
4. DUFFARD R., G. MORI DE MORO & A.M. EVANGELISTA DE DUFFARD.1987. Vulnerability of the myelin development of the chicks to the herbicide 2,4-dichlorophenoxyacetic butyl ester. Neurochem. Res. **12:** 1077–1080.
5. DUFFARD, R. *et al.* 1996. Central nervous system myelin deficit in rats exposed to 2,4-dichlorophenoxyacetic acid through lactation. Neurotoxicol. Teratol. **18:** 691–696.

6. EVANGELISTA DE DUFFARD, A.M., C. ORTA & R. DUFFARD. 1990. Behavioral changes in rats fed a diet containing 2,4-dichlorophenoxyacetic butyl ester. Neurotoxicology **11:** 563–572.
7. EVANGELISTA DE DUFFARD, A.M., M. NICOLA DE ALDERETE & R. DUFFARD.1990. Changes in brain serotonin and 5-hydroxyindolacetic acid levels induced by 2,4-dichlorophenoxyacetic butyl ester. Toxicology **64:** 265–270.
8. EVANGELISTA DE DUFFARD, A.M., A. BORTOLOZZI & R. DUFFARD. 1995. Altered behavioral responses in 2,4-dichlorophenoxyacetic acid treated and amphetamine challenged rats. Neurotoxicology **16:** 479–488.
9. BRUSCO, A. *et al.* 1997. 2,4-dichlorophenoxyacetic acid through lactation induces astrogliosis in rat brain. Mol. Chem. Neuropathol. **30:** 175–185.
10. BORTOLOZZI, A. *et al.* 1998. Regionally specific changes in central brain monoamine levels by 2,4-dichlorophenoxyacetic acid in acute treated rats. Neurotoxicology **19:** 839–852.
11. BORTOLOZZI, A., C. SARTORIO, R. DUFFARD & A.M. EVANGELISTA DE DUFFARD. 1998. Peripheral serotoninergic system alterations in rats exposed during different periods of their life to neurotoxic 2,4-dichlorophenoxyacetic acid. Biog. Amines **14:** 667–689.
12. BORTOLOZZI, A. *et al.* 2001. Intracerebral administration of 2,4-diclorophenoxyacetic acid induces behavioral and neurochemical alterations in the rat brain. Neurotoxicology **23:** 221–232.
13. BENES, F.M. 1995. Is there a neuroanatomic basis for schizophrenia? An old question revisited. J. Neuroscientist **1:** 104–115.
14. BORTOLOZZI, A., A.M. EVANGELISTA DE DUFFARD, R. DUFFARD & M. ANTONELLI. 2000. Effects of 2,4-dichlorophenoxyacetic acid exposure on dopamine D2-like receptors in rat brain. Society for Neuroscience 30th Annual Meeting (Abstr.), New Orleans, LA.
15. BORTOLOZZI, A., R. DUFFARD & A.M. EVANGELISTA DE DUFFARD. 1999. Behavioral alterations induced in rats by a pre- and postnatal exposure to 2,4-dichlorophenoxyacetic acid. Neurotoxicol. Teratol. **21:** 451–465.
16. PIERCE, R.C. & P.W. KALIVAS. 1997. A circuitry model of the expression of behavioral sensitization to amphetamine-like psychostimulants. Brain Res. Rev. **25:** 192–216.
17. SEGAL, D.S. & R. KUCZENSKI. 1997. A circuitry model of the expression of behavioral sensitization to amphetamine-like stimulants. Brain Res. Rev. **25:** 192–216.
18. JONES, S.R., R.R. GAINETDINOV, R.M. WIGHTMAN & M.G. CARON. 1998. Mechanism of amphetamine action revealed in mice lacking the dopamine transporter. J. Neurosci. **18:** 1979–1986.
19. BORODINSKY, L.N., G. PESCE, P. POMATA & M.L. FISZMAN. 1997. Neurosteroid modulation of GABA_A receptors in the developing rat brain cortex. Neurochem. Int. **31:** 313–317.
20. DEFAGOT, M.C.& M.C. ANTONELLI. 1997. Autoradiographic localization of the putative D4 dopamine receptor in rat brain. Neurochem. Res. **22:** 401–407.
21. BRADFORD, M.M. 1976. A rapid and sensitive method for the quantification of microgram quantities of proteins utilising the principle of protein dye binding. Anal. Biochem. **72:** 243–254.
22. BALDESSARINI, R.J. & F.I. TARAZI. 1996. Brain dopamine receptors: a primer on their current status, basic and clinic. Harv. Rev. Psychiatry **3:** 301–325.
23. KALIVAS, P.W. & J. STEWART. 1991. Dopamine transmission in the initiation and expression of drug- and stress-induced sensitization of motor activity. Brain Res. **16:** 223–244.

Developmental Expression of the β-Amyloid Precursor Protein and Heat-Shock Protein 70 in the Cerebral Hemisphere Region of the Rat Brain

D.K. LAHIRI, C. NALL, D. CHEN, M. ZAPHIRIOU, C. MORGAN, AND J.I. NURNBERGER, SR.[a]

Laboratory of Molecular Neurogenetics, Institute of Psychiatric Research, Department of Psychiatry, Indiana University School of Medicine, Indianapolis, Indiana 46202, USA

ABSTRACT: Alzheimer's disease (AD) is characterized by depositions of the amyloid β protein (Aβ) in the brain in the form of extracellular plaques and cerebrovascular amyloid. Aβ (~4 kDa) is derived from a family of large (~110 kDa) β-amyloid precursor proteins (APP), which are integral membrane glycoproteins. Although a connection between AD and alcoholism has recently been suggested, this relationship has not been explored at the molecular level. Our hypothesis is that APP has a role in brain development and that abnormal APP levels may be involved in dementia associated with AD and alcoholism. We compared the profile of total APP levels between ethanol naïve alcohol-preferring (P) and alcohol-nonpreferring (NP) rats. We also investigated the possibility that APP levels can be regulated in an age-dependent manner in young rats. We studied the distribution of two proteins in the cerebral hemisphere region of the rat brain at various developmental periods. Six groups composed of the following different ages of rats were used: 7, 14, 21, 36, 43, and 78 (postnatal) days. Cell extracts from different regions of the brain were subjected to Western immunoblotting using mAb22C11. Our results suggest that levels of high-molecular-weight APP bands were greater in brain extracts from 7-day-old P rats than in other samples tested, and that the distribution of APP levels was more uneven in brain extracts from different ages of P than from NP rats. These initial results suggest that APP may play an important role in the early development of the rat brain and the alcohol-preferring trait may influence APP processing in the developing brain.

INTRODUCTION

Alzheimer's disease (AD) is a progressive, degenerative disease of the brain and is the most common form of dementia, with unique neuropathological and biochemical characteristics.[1] In addition, there are recent reports of possible interactions of

Address for correspondence: Dr. D.K. Lahiri, Institute of Psychiatric Research, Indiana University School of Medicine, Room No. PR-313, 791 Union Drive, Indianapolis, IN 46202-4887. Voice: 317-274-2706; fax: 317-274-1365.
dlahiri@iupui.edu
[a]Deceased June 14, 2001.

Ann. N.Y. Acad. Sci. 965: 324–333 (2002). © 2002 New York Academy of Sciences.

AD and alcoholism.[2,3] Notably, the effects of a history of heavy alcohol consumption on AD have also been studied.[4] Nevertheless, the relationship between alcohol and AD has not been explored at the molecular level. This is partly due to the lack of appropriate cellular and *in vivo* models. Our hypothesis is that β-amyloid precursor protein (APP) has a role in brain development and that abnormal APP levels may be involved in dementia associated with AD and alcoholism. We also investigated the possibility that APP levels can be regulated in an age-dependent manner in young rats. Our objective here is to study the function of Alzheimer's APP in brain development using alcohol-preferring (P) and alcohol-nonpreferring (NP) strains of rats.[5,6]

Neuropathologically, AD is characterized by depositions of the amyloid β–protein (Aβ) in the brain in the form of extracellular plaques and cerebrovascular amyloid.[1] Aβ is derived from a family of large β-amyloid precursor proteins that are highly conserved, integral membrane glycoproteins.[1] The function of APP and its role in the pathogenesis of AD are still unclear despite the extensive efforts to determine both. However, the finding of mutations in Aβ that are tightly linked to AD makes APP an important target for understanding the etiology of this disease.[7] Currently, we are engaged in studying the effects of various cholinergic drugs on the processing of APP.[8,9] In order to understand the biological function of APP, we are investigating the expression and processing of these proteins during the early stages of rat development. We have also extended this study to include the effects of genetic predisposition to alcoholism on the levels of APP. In the study presented here, we have used ethanol-naïve P and NP strains of rats that were selectively bred for voluntary alcohol drinking under two-bottle choice conditions, one containing alcohol and the other water.[5] The P rats also show higher operant responding for ethanol than do the NP rats, indicating a genetically mediated difference in the reward value of alcohol. Our aim in this study is to compare the levels of APP and heat-shock protein 70/72 (HSP-70) between P and NP rats as a function of the age of the animal. Our initial results suggest a differential expression of APP in early rat development.

EXPERIMENTAL PROCEDURES

Animals and Brain Regions

Rats (Sprague-Dawley) of different ages, 7 to 76 days (postnatal), were obtained from the Indiana University Alcohol Research Center. A representative set of animals from each age group was used for the tissue preparation. The weight of the animals varied depending on the age of the animal (~10–250 g), and brains from 2–4 animals were pooled for each experiment. At each time point studied, brains of appropriate ethanol-naïve animals were perfused first with volumes of 0.5% sodium nitrite and then with 4% paraformaldehyde (PFA) in sodium phosphate buffer. Following perfusion, tissues were placed in cold PFA overnight and transferred to 30% buffered sucrose at 4°C. Brains from P and NP rats at various age groups were dissected into the following four sections: brain stem, cerebellum, cerebral hemispheres, and olfactory bulb. Extracts from each region were subjected to Western immunoblot analysis as described in the following sections.

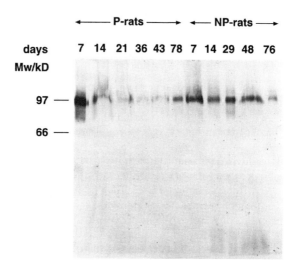

FIGURE 1. Detection of APP levels in brain extracts from different ages of P and NP rats. Western immunoblot of brain extracts from the cerebral hemisphere is shown. The brain region was obtained from the various age groups (days) of either P or NP rats as indicated. Briefly, the rat brain tissue was homogenized, and cell extracts (lysates) were obtained in IP buffer as described in the EXPERIMENTAL PROCEDURES section. Thirty micrograms of protein from the total cell lysate were separated on a 12% polyacrylamide gel containing SDS. Western immunoblot analysis was performed in the Mini-PROTEAN II system, and immunodetection of specific bands was performed using the 22C11 antibody as described previously. Brains from two to four animals were pooled, cell extracts prepared, and the Western blot analysis was performed. The experiment was performed in duplicate, and the blot was run three times; a typical result is shown here. The protein molecular mass markers in kilodaltons are shown to the left of the blot. The specific APP signal is seen as ~100-kDa bands.

Preparation of Rat Brain Extracts

Briefly, the brain tissue from each rat brain was homogenized in a Brinkman PT 10/35 homogenizer for 10 s in IP buffer containing Tris-Cl, pH 7.4; NaCl; NP-40; sodium deoxycholate; and a cocktail of protease inhibitors.[9] They were centrifuged at $11,000 \times g$ for 20 min at 4°C, and the proteins of the supernatant solution (cell lysate) were measured. Brains from 2–4 animals were pooled, cell extracts prepared, and Western blot analysis was performed. The experiment was done in duplicate, and the blot was run three times; typical results are shown in FIGURES 1 and 2.

SDS-PAGE and Western Immunoblot Analysis

Thirty micrograms of proteins from the total cell lysate were separated on a 12% polyacrylamide gel containing sodium dodecyl sulfate (SDS-PAGE). Western immunoblot analysis was performed in the Mini-PROTEAN II system of Bio-Rad (Hercules, CA), and immunodetection of specific bands was performed as described previously.[8] Immunoreactive bands were compared densitometrically with the use of a UVP-GDS5000 Gel Documentation System (San Gabriel, CA). The analysis was performed using the NIH Image 1.49 software.

Detection of the Levels of Different Intracellular Proteins

Each blot was sequentially probed with two antibodies: (i) mouse monoclonal antibody, 22C11 (Boehringer Mannheim), against the amino-terminus of APP and (ii) mouse monoclonal antibody against the carboxy-terminus of the 70-kDa heat-shock protein (Sigma, St. Louis, MO).[9] The epitope region of 22C11 antibody was mapped to APP_{66-81} in the ectoplasmic cysteine-containing domain.[10] The 22C11 clone recognizes all mature forms of APP found in cell membranes as well as the APP-like proteins (APLPs).[11] The biotinylated secondary antibodies, horse anti-mouse (Boehringer Mannheim), were also used. The blot of FIGURE 1 was probed with one antibody only (22C11). The blot of FIGURE 2 was first probed with 22C11, the specific APP band was observed, and then the blot was reprobed with anti-HSP-70 IgG without removing the signal from the first antibody. This way, signals from both the proteins could be detected and compared in the same blot at the same time.

RESULTS

A typical Western blot from brain extracts could detect APP as 95- to 120-kDa immunoreactive protein bands that represent different isoforms of APP as well as their posttranslationally modified derivatives.[8] These represent the glycosyslated and sulfated full-length mature forms as well as the alternatively spliced forms of the protein in cell lysates as detected by SDS-PAGE. Here, we compared the profile of total protein levels of APP and HSP-70 between ethanol-naïve P and NP rats as described below.

Detection of APP in Brain Regions from Different Ages of P and NP Rats

When relative levels of APP in the cerebral hemisphere region were compared among the different age groups, it was found to be at the maximum on day 7 in both strains of rats under the conditions studied here (FIG. 1). However, this early accumulation of APP on day 7 was more pronounced in P than in NP rats. For instance, while there was a sharp drop of APP levels over time in P rats up to day 43, there was a uniform level of APP during the postnatal development period from day 14 to 76 in NP rats. In general, levels of APP were constant in NP rats throughout the time points studied. There is a similar trend for APP levels in the cerebellum and brain stem regions of the brain (data not shown). In the olfactory bulb, however, APP levels were not at their highest on day 7, and no specific trend like that of other brain regions was observed in P and NP rats (data not shown). These results suggest that in the cerebral hemisphere levels of high-molecular-weight APP bands were maximal in brain extracts from 7-day-old P rats, higher than in other samples tested, and that there was an uneven distribution of APP levels in brain extracts from different ages of P rats.

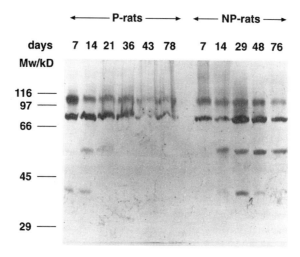

FIGURE 2. Comparative analysis of APP and HSP-70 levels in brain extracts of P and NP rats. Western immunoblot of brain extracts from the cerebral hemisphere is shown. The brain region was obtained from either P or NP rats of various ages (days) as indicated. A Western immunoblot similar to that shown in FIGURE 1 was reprobed with antibody against HSP-70 without stripping off the signal from the APP bands. The rest of the procedure is the same as in FIGURE 1 and as described in the text. The specific signal from APP and HSP-70 is seen as ~100- and 70-kDa bands, respectively.

Detection of APP and HSP-70 in Brain Regions from Different Ages of P and NP Rats

In the cerebral hemisphere, levels of HSP-70 were not found to be at the maximum on day 7, unlike the levels of APP. The general trend of the protein was not as sharp as with APP in either P or NP rats. Levels of HSP-70 were higher, however, in the younger P rats than in the younger NP rats. In NP rats, the levels were higher at later ages. It is apparent from the intensity of the immunoreactive signal that the overall expression of HSP-70 is greater than APP during development. HSP-70 was not at its highest in the olfactory bulb on day 7 (data not shown).

Densitometric analysis revealed that the trend of the APP signal was very similar in two independent experiments (FIGS. 1 and 2). Moreover, the trend of the signal in different experiments was similar when relative levels of APP were compared by plotting the APP signal either alone (FIG. 1) or with that of HSP-70 (FIG. 2).

DISCUSSION

One of the major hallmarks of AD is the brain deposition of Aβ, which is derived from a large β-amyloid precursor protein. Although the role of APP metabolism in Aβ generation is being thoroughly studied, the physiological function of APP is not completely understood. One of our objectives was to investigate the role of APP in rat brain development. We have also considered whether there is a connection between AD and alcohol at the molecular level. This approach is based on the reports of a possible interaction between AD and alcoholism.[2,3] The interaction of chronic alcohol consumption and aging on brain structure and function has also been investigated.[12] However, only a few studies have been published about APP, Aβ, and alcohol. For example, one of the cellular cofactors for Aβ-induced cellular perturbation is reported to be ABAD (Aβ-binding alcohol dehydrogenase).[13] The lack of studies in this area is most probably due to the absence of proper *in vivo* models. Our aim here is to investigate the function of APP in developing rat brains. We have used selectively bred alcohol-preferring and alcohol-nonpreferring lines of rats, which were used to study the biology of alcohol-seeking behavior.[14] The ethanol-preferring line of rats has been reported to be a suitable animal model of alcoholism.[5] In our set of experiments, the purpose was to compare protein levels at different ages between alcohol-naive, alcohol-preferring and alcohol-nonpreferring rats. Because P and NP rats are genetically bred for high and low alcohol drinking behavior, respectively, our results suggest the possibility that increased levels of APP in the cerebral hemisphere may be associated with the high alcohol drinking behavior of P rats.

The mechanisms underlying neuronal adaptation to ethanol are poorly understood but appear to involve alterations in cellular membrane structure and/or function. A recent report characterizes the gene for heat-shock protein 70 as an ethanol-responsive gene.[15] HSP-70 is a constitutive member of the 70-kDa stress protein family, which plays an important role in protein trafficking and coated vesicle processing. There is evidence for a protective role for the stress protein response in cultured neurons in excitotoxicity.[16] Thus, modulation of HSP-70 by ethanol could produce widespread changes in cellular membrane functioning. In this report we have studied the level of this protein in parallel with APP. In addition to stress proteins, there is also a recent report of differential gene expression in human alcoholism using microarray analysis of the frontal cortex.[17] We are also examining the levels of other proteins such as synatophysin (SNAP-25) in the same samples; that report will be published elsewhere.

In this study, we have analyzed the levels of two important proteins at different ages of the brain under two conditions. These two proteins are APP and HSP-70. In the typical Western blot of brain lysates, APP could be detected as 95- to 120-kDa protein bands that represent different isoforms of APP (695 to 770) and/or their post-translationally modified derivatives. In our blots, we did not detect any specific immunoreactive protein bands other than these high-molecular-weight bands when immunoblots from brain extract samples were probed against the mAb 22C11. Some of these bands could also represent an APP-related homologue such as APLP2.[1] We could predominantly detect APP and not APLP2.[9]

Our results suggest that there is a differential level of expression between these proteins as far as development of the brain is concerned. For example, APP levels were found to be higher at earlier ages, the maximum being at day 7 among the age groups studied here. In contrast, levels of HSP were maximal at later ages. In our hands, the APP antibody detected proteins in the molecular mass range of 95–120 kDa normally observed for APP but did not detect proteins in the 160- to 200-kDa range nor smaller proteins of 25, 40, and 50 kDa previously described in a developmental study of APP expression.[18] Levels of APP-immunoreactive proteins in the regions of brain stem, cerebellum, and cerebral hemisphere were significantly higher in 7-day-old animals than in other age groups studied (data not shown). Levels of APP bands in the region of the olfactory bulb were significantly lower than in the three other regions studied, and the level in the olfactory bulb remained constant throughout development. A significant difference was observed between the levels of APP in extracts prepared from P rats versus those of NP rats. About three- to five-fold more APP bands were detected in extracts from P rats than NP rats at day 7. Our initial results suggest that APP expression is high during early development in rats and may therefore play a significant role during this period. Our present results are supported by other important published studies.

Recently, developmental changes in the APP levels in growth cones and synaptosomes were studied from embryonic day 14 up to postnatal day (PD) 400. Kirazov and colleagues[19] observed that the APP level in growth cones was low during prenatal stages, that it continuously increased from PD 3 up to PD 10, and the highest APP level in synaptosomes was found between PD 7 and 10, followed by a considerable decrease up to PD 30. The increase in APP level during synaptogenesis suggests a "functional role of APP in the processes of neurite outgrowth and cell targeting."[19] Another study detected a gradual increase in the soluble APP level in the archicerebellum during the first three weeks, whereas in the neo- and paleocerebellum the levels reach a plateau as early as the first week.[20] A comparative analysis of different proteins indicates that the postnatal expressions of the soluble and membrane-bound forms of APP, synaptophysin and presenilin-1, are regulated differently during the ontogenetical development of the archi-, paleo-, and neocerebellum of rat.[20] However, we have not studied the levels of synaptophysin and presenilin proteins in our present study. Another study showed that the expression of APP mRNA isoforms in rat brain is differentially regulated during postnatal maturation and by cholinergic activity.[21] The immunohistochemical identification of APP in various developmental stages revealed APP to be widely distributed through the nervous system, existing mainly in the cytoplasm, dendrites, and axons of the neurons.[22] They observed dramatic changes in APP expression in the cerebellum from the embryonic stage. These findings suggested that APP played an important role in neuronal maturation and synaptogenesis.

The expression of the APP gene has been examined in the basal forebrain of rats from birth to adulthood. Levels of total APP mRNA are highest at birth and at postnatal day 15 (PD 15), when APP-695 message levels are over sixfold higher than KPI-containing APP mRNA (APP-751, APP-770).[23] This large difference in the APP-695/KPI-APP ratio observed during postnatal development coincided with the period of maximal neurotrophic responsiveness in the basal forebrain. Another study examined various APP isoforms in different rat brain regions and during brain development and found that the highest level of most APP forms was reached in the second postnatal week, which is the time of brain maturation and completion of synaptic connections.[24] Sandbrink and colleagues[25] studied the expression of the APP gene family and observed a differential expression of various alternatively spliced APP transcripts in brain cells during brain development and aging. We have not, however, examined different isoforms of APP in this study.

The results given here should be discussed from the following perspective of known APP functions. Although the role of APP in the biogenesis of Aβ, which is involved in the neuropathology of AD, is well recognized, the function of APP is poorly understood. The work presented here was initiated in order to understand the physiological functions of APP. Three known functions have been reported. First, a role has been attributed for APP in the inhibition of certain blood coagulation factors and thrombin.[26] Second, APP may be involved in the modulation of cell adhesion, as APP contains heparin-binding and integrin-binding sites.[27–29] A third potential function of APP is as cell surface receptors that bind unknown ligands to transmit signals into the cell. This report suggests a role for APP in brain development.

APP is a physiologically important protein, and it is a part of a family of at least three proteins in mammals, which includes APLP1, APLP2, and APP.[30] The importance of APP in biological function can be deduced from recent knockout animal studies. Notably, a knockout mouse model lacking APLP2 and either APLP1 or APP is lethal soon after birth, suggesting that these proteins play a critical role in the postnatal mouse.[30,31] The finding that the APLP2–APP double mutant is lethal indicates that APLP1 cannot compensate for the function of these two proteins.

APP and its homologues are physiologically important, because similar proteins are detected throughout evolution. In this regard, the following studies of APP-like proteins in other species and in systems deficient in the protein are noteworthy. For example, APP homologues are known in lower invertebrates, such as the apl-1 of *Caenorhabditis elegans*[32] and APPL of *Drosophila melanogaster*.[33] Loss of the apl-1 protein is lethal in *C. elegans* but can be restored by neuronal expression, suggesting that its major function is in neurons. In *Drosophila*, the APPL protein is expressed exclusively in neurons and is processed to secreted derivatives like APP.[33,34] *Drosophilas* deficient in the APP protein are viable but show subtle behavioral deficits that can be ameliorated by expression of human APP.

The interpretation of the study presented here should, however, be examined in the light of several caveats. First, a limited number of animal samples are used in the present work. This is due to the strict time points of the development and the inclusion of several ages of animals. However, it should be mentioned here that the two proteins analyzed were from the same sample under the same blotting conditions, so the level of HSP may act as a control for other proteins, such as APP. In other words, the change in relative levels of APP with HSP may reduce other experimental variations. Second, the choice of the selected time point in development is rather arbitrary. This is due to our poor understanding of the developmental process. Other time points that are earlier than day 7 have been considered. However, at this early time point it is difficult to get enough protein material from the different brain regions to work with. But future work should address this issue of including other equally important time points in the context of development. Third, this work is limited to only two proteins. We are currently studying the changes in levels of other proteins, such as synaptic and vesicular proteins, to determine their role in the development process. The work presented here is meant to include only representative protein markers and provide a model to study the molecular mechanism of development. Fourth, we have not studied other isoforms of APP such as the Kunitz protease inhibitor, which contains APP (APP-751). We have mainly focused on examining the levels of total cellular APP, and the study can be extended to other isoforms of APP as well in the same samples. Finally, the very choice to use the NP and P rats can be questioned. It should be mentioned here that these animals were ethanol naïve and have not previously been given ethanol for this kind of experiment. However, the lack of studies on AD and alcohol at the molecular level has prompted us to utilize these unique P and NP rat lines. Our present study will, in turn, encourage future investigators to study the molecular connection between these two disorders using these novel and other appropriate animals.

ACKNOWLEDGMENTS

These studies were supported by grants from the National Institutes of Health and from the Indiana Division of Mental Health to the Institute of Psychiatric Research (IPR). We also sincerely thank Dr. John I. Nurnberger, Jr., Director of IPR, and Dr. Kumar Sambamurti (Mayo Clinic, Jacksonville) for their help.

This paper is dedicated to the late Prof. (Dr.) John I. Nurnberger, Sr. for his scientific vision and his contribution to and constant support for neuroscience research.

REFERENCES

1. SELKOE, D.J. 1997. Alzheimer's disease: genotypes, phenotypes, and treatments. Science **75:** 630–631.
2. FREUND, G. & W.E. BALLINGER, JR. 1992. Alzheimer's disease and alcoholism: possible interactions. Alcohol **9:** 233–240.
3. SAXTON, J. *et al.* 2000. Alcohol, dementia, and Alzheimer's disease: comparison of neuropsychological profiles. J. Geriatr. Psychiatr. Neurol. **13:** 14114–14119.
4. ROSEN, J. *et al.* 1993. Effects of a history of heavy alcohol consumption on Alzheimer's disease. Br. J. Psychiatry **163:** 358–363.
5. WALLER, M.B. *et al.* 1984. Intragastric self-infusion of ethanol by ethanol-preferring and -nonpreferring lines of rats. Science **225:** 78–80.
6. CRABBE, J.C., *et al.* 1994. Genetic animal models of alcohol and drug abuse. Science **264:** 1715–1723.
7. HARDY, K.J. & K. GWINN-HARDY. 1998. Genetic classification of primary neurodegenerative disease. Science **282:** 1075–1079.
8. LAHIRI, D.K. *et al.* 1998. The secretion of amyloid beta-peptides is inhibited in the tacrine-treated human neuroblastoma cells. Mol. Brain Res. **62:** 131–140.
9. LAHIRI, D.K. *et al.* 1994. Tacrine alters the processing of beta-amyloid precursor protein in different cell lines. J. Neurosci. Res. **37:** 777–787.
10. HILBICH, C. *et al.* 1993. Amyloid-like properties of peptides flanking the epitope of amyloid precursor protein-specific monoclonal antibody 22C11. J. Biol. Chem. **268:** 26571–26577.
11. SLUNT, H.H. *et al.* 1993. Expression of a ubiquitous, cross-reactive homologue of the mouse β-amyloid precursor protein (APP). J. Biol. Chem. **269:** 2637–2644.
12. FREUND, G. 1982. The interaction of chronic alcohol consumption and aging on brain structure and function. Alcohol. Clin. Exp. Res. **6:** 13–21.
13. YAN, S.D. *et al.* 2000. Cellular cofactors potentiating induction of stress and cytotoxicity by amyloid beta-peptide. Biochim. Biophys. Acta **1502:** 145–157.
14. LI, T.K. *et al.* 1987. Rodent lines selected for factors affecting alcohol consumption. Alcohol Alcohol. Suppl. **1:** 91–96.
15. MILES, M.F. *et al.* 1991. Mechanisms of neuronal adaptation to ethanol. Ethanol induces Hsc70 gene transcription in NG108-15 neuroblastoma × glioma cells. J. Biol. Chem. **266:** 2409–2414.
16. LOWENSTEIN, D.H. *et al.* 1991. The stress protein response in cultured neurons: characterization and evidence for a protective role in excitotoxicity. Neuron **7:** 1053–1060.
17. LEWOHL, J.M. *et al.* 2000. Gene expression in human alcoholism: microarray analysis of frontal cortex. Alcohol. Clin. Exp. Res. **24:** 1873–1882.

18. ANDERSON, J.P. *et al.* 1989. Cellular forms of the rat and human beta-amyloid precursor protein (BAPP). Brain Res. **478:** 391–398.
19. KIRAZOV, E. *et al.* 2001. Ontogenetic changes in protein level of amyloid precursor protein (APP) in growth cones and synaptosomes from rat brain and prenatal expression pattern of APP mRNA isoforms in developing rat embryo. Int. J. Dev. Neurosci. **19:** 287–296.
20. FAKLA, I. *et al.* 2000. Expressions of amyloid precursor protein, synaptophysin and presenilin-1 in the different areas of the developing cerebellum of rat. Neurochem. Int. **36:** 143–151.
21. APELT, J. *et al.* 1997. Expression of amyloid precursor protein mRNA isoforms in rat brain is differentially regulated during postnatal maturation and by cholinergic activity. Int. J. Dev. Neurosci. **15:** 95–112.
22. OHTA, M. *et al.* 1993. Immunohistochemical distribution of amyloid precursor protein during normal rat development. Dev. Brain Res. **75:** 151–161.
23. SHERMAN, C.A. & G.A. HIGGINS. 1992. Regulated splicing of the amyloid precursor protein gene during postnatal development of the rat basal forebrain. Dev. Brain Res. **66:** 63–69.
24. LOFFLER, J. 1992. Beta-amyloid precursor protein isoforms in various rat brain regions and during brain development. J. Neurochem. **59:** 1316–1324.
25. SANDBRINK, R. *et al.* 1997. Expression of the APP gene family in brain cells, brain development and aging. Gerontology **43:** 119–131.
26. SMITH, R.P. *et al.* 1990. Platelet coagulation factor XIa-inhibitor, a form of Alzheimer amyloid precursor protein. Science **248:** 1126–1128.
27. CLARRIS, H.J. *et al.* 1997. Identification of heparin-binding domains in the amyloid precursor protein of Alzheimer's disease by deletion mutagenesis and peptide mapping. J. Neurochem. **68:** 1164–1172.
28. GHISO, J. *et al.* 1992. A 109-amino-acid C-terminal fragment of Alzheimer's-disease amyloid precursor protein contains a sequence, -RHDS-, that promotes cell adhesion. Biochem. J. **288:** 1053–1059.
29. YAMAZAKI, T. *et al.* 1997. Cell surface amyloid beta-protein precursor colocalizes with beta 1 integrins at substrate contact sites in neural cells. J. Neurosci. **17:** 1004–1010.
30. VON KOCH, C.S. *et al.* 1997. Generation of APLP2 KO mice and early postnatal lethality in APLP2/APP double KO mice. Neurobiol. Aging **18:** 661–669.
31. HEBER, S. *et al.* 2000. Mice with combined gene knock-outs reveal essential and partially redundant functions of amyloid precursor protein family members. J. Neurosci. **20:** 7951–7963.
32. DAIGLE, I. & C. LI. 1993. apl-1, a *Caenorhabditis elegans* gene encoding a protein related to the human beta-amyloid protein precursor. Proc. Natl. Acad. Sci. USA **90:** 12045–12049.
33. LUO, L. *et al.* 1992. Human amyloid precursor protein ameliorates behavioral deficit of flies deleted for *Appl* gene. Neuron **9:** 595–605.
34. FOSSGREEN, A. *et al.* 1998. Transgenic *Drosophila* expressing human amyloid precursor protein show gamma-secretase activity and a blistered-wing phenotype. Proc. Natl. Acad. Sci. USA **95:** 13703–13708.

Alcohol Exposure During Adulthood Induces Neuronal and Astroglial Alterations in the Hippocampal CA-1 Area

PATRICIA TAGLIAFERRO, MAITE DUHALDE VEGA, SERGIO GUSTAVO EVRARD, ALBERTO JAVIER RAMOS,[a] AND ALICIA BRUSCO

Instituto de Biología Celular y Neurociencias "Prof. Eduardo De Robertis," Facultad de Medicina, Universidad de Buenos Aires, Paraguay 2155 (1121), Buenos Aires, Argentina

ABSTRACT: Ethanol (ETOH) exposure can result in neuronal damage. Astrocytes are morphologic and functionally related to neurons, and astrocyte-neuron interactions provide strategic sites for the actions of many chemical compounds. The aim of the present work was to study the morphologic alterations of glial cells and neurons on the hippocampus after long-term ETOH exposure using GFAP and S-100β protein, neurofilaments of 200 kDa (Nf200), MAP2, and serotonin transporter (5HT-T) immunocytochemical staining. Adult Wistar male rats (200–250 g) were orally exposed to ETOH (6.6% v/v ad libitum) for 6 weeks. Control rats received water ad libitum. Brain sections from control and exposed rats were processed by immunocytochemistry. After ETOH exposure we observed in the CA1 area of the hippocampus: (1) an important astroglial reaction evidenced by the presence of GFAP+ reactive astrocytes; (2) an increase in S-100β immunostaining in astroglial cells; and (3) a decrease in Nf200, 5HT-T, and MAP2 immunoreactivity. The current study provides evidence that long-term ETOH exposure induces alterations in the neuronal cytoskeleton and an astroglial reaction, which is a common response to brain injury and may promote functional recovery of the nervous system, as by the release of glial-derived trophic factors (such as S-100β) that promote cell survival and neurite growth.

KEYWORDS: ethanol; astrocytes; serotonin transporter; S100β; neurofilaments; GFAP; MAP2

INTRODUCTION

Alcohol abuse and dependence are serious health problems throughout the world. It is well known that ethanol (ETOH) administration alters several brain functions and behaviors in humans[1–3] as well as in laboratory animals.[1] There are several mechanisms by which ETOH can exert its damaging effects on the central nervous

Address for correspondence: Dra. Alicia Brusco, Rivera Indarte 132 1ro. A, (1406) Ciudad de Buenos Aires, Argentina. Voice: 54-11-5950-9626; fax: 54-11-4566-1901.
hbrusco@fmed.uba.ar
[a]Current address: Universidad Austral, B1629 AHJ Derqui, Pilar, Buenos Aires, Argentina.

Ann. N.Y. Acad. Sci. 965: 334–342 (2002). © 2002 New York Academy of Sciences.

system (CNS) during development[4] and adulthood, including the possibility that ETOH may alter the levels of essential neurotrophic factors.[5] Some of these neurotrophic factors have an important role in the maintenance of neuronal function.

ETOH exposure induces an important response from astroglial cells, and because astrocytes are morphologic and functionally related to neurons, astrocyte-neuron interactions provide strategic sites for actions of many chemical compounds. The neurotoxic effects of ETOH may also include disruption of several neurotransmitter systems, the serotoninergic system being one of them.

Serotonin (5HT) is a classic neurotransmitter that also plays an important role during CNS development. In the adult CNS, 5HT-astrocyte interactions are involved in neuronal and glial plasticity. The 5HT actions in these events appear to be mediated by S100β, a glial-derived growth factor. This protein belongs to a family of diverse Ca^{2+} binding proteins and is released by astrocytes after astroglial $5HT_{1A}$ receptor stimulation.[6,7] Once outside the astrocyte, S-100β participates in neurite extension,[8] stabilizes the neuronal cytoskeleton,[9] and regulates GAP-43 phosphorylation.[10]

ETOH exposure is reported to induce depletion of 5HT level during CNS development.[11] Other investigators indicate that serotoninergic system plays a role in alcohol intake reinforcement.[12] 5HT depletion induces significant changes in the CNS, such as astroglial reaction[13,14] and alterations in the neuronal cytoskeleton.[15,16]

The aim of the present work was to study the morphologic alterations of astroglial cells and neurons in the hippocampus after long-term ETOH exposure. Studies focused on the serotoninergic system because of its actions during the CNS plasticity phenomenon and its close relation to astrocytes.

MATERIAL AND METHODS

Animal Treatment. Adult Wistar male rats weighing 250–300 g were exposed orally to ethanol (6.6% v/v) in drinking water ad libitum for 6 weeks. The control group received water ad libitum. Control and treated animals were kept in the same environment (12-hour light/dark cycle, free access to standard rat food and water or water + ethanol). All procedures were consistent with the principles established by the Society for Neuroscience in their guidelines for the humane treatment of animals.

Tissue Processing. After 6 weeks of ethanol exposure, control and exposed rats were anesthetized with 300 mg/kg of chloral hydrate (Mallinckrodt). Their left ventricle was perfused with a cold fixative solution containing 4% (w/v) paraformaldehyde and 0.25% (v/v) glutaraldehyde in 0.1 M phosphate buffer, pH 7.4. A brief wash with 30 ml of saline solution containing 0.05% (w/v) $NaNO_2$ plus 50 IU of heparin was passed through their circulatory system prior to fixation. Brains were kept in cold fixative solution for 2–4 hours, washed three times in the same buffer plus 5% (w/v) sucrose, and then left in this washing solution for 18 hours at 4°C. Sagittal brain sections (thickness 40 μm) were obtained in an Oxford vibratome. Sections were stored at −20°C in 0.1 M phosphate buffer, pH 7.4, plus 25% (w/v) sucrose.

Immunocytochemistry. Free-floating sections of control and exposed animals were processed by immunocytochemistry. To inhibit endogenous peroxidase activity, sections were previously dehydrated, treated with 0.5% (v/v) H_2O_2 in methanol for 30 minutes at room temperature and rehydrated. Sections were then incubated with 3% (v/v) normal bovine serum (NBS) in phosphate-buffered saline (PBS) for 1 hour. After two rinses in PBS plus 0.025% (v/v) Triton X-100 (PBS-X), sections were incubated for 48 hours at 4°C with one of the after primary antibodies against: 5HT-T (serotonin transporter), neurofilaments of 200 kDa (Nf200), microtubular associated protein (MAP2), S-100β protein, and gliofibrillar acidic protein (GFAP) diluted 1:1000, 1:2000, 1:700, 1:500, and 1:3000, respectively. Thereafter, sections were washed three times in PBS-X and incubated for 1 hour with biotinylated secondary antibodies diluted 1:100 at room temperature. Sections were then washed three times in PBS-X and incubated with streptavidin-peroxidase complex solution diluted 1:200 for 1 hour. In all cases, antibodies were dissolved in PBS solution containing 1% (v/v) NBS and 0.3% (v/v) Triton X-100, pH 7.4.

After washing three times in PBS-X and twice in 0.1 M acetate buffer (AcB), pH 6, development of peroxidase activity was carried out with 0.035% (w/v) 3,3' diaminobencidine plus 2.5% (w/v) nickel ammonium sulfate and 0.1% (v/v) H_2O_2 dissolved in AcB. Finally, after two washes in AcB and one in distilled water, sections were mounted on gelatin-coated slides, dehydrated, and cover-slipped using Permount for light microscopic observations. Sections were observed and photographed by light microscopy in an Axiophot Zeiss light microscope. Brain sections of both exposed and control animals were simultaneously processed for both immunocytochemical and morphometric studies.

Image Analysis and Statistics. Mean gray of immunolabeled astrocytes and morphometric parameters, such as cell area and total area of fibers, and cellular processes were measured in an Axiophot Zeiss light microscope equipped with a video camera on line with a Zeiss-Kontron VIDAS image analyzer. Observations and measurements obtained in the light microscope were transferred to an attached video camera connected to an interactive image analysis system on line. The images were digitized into an array of 512×512 pixels corresponding to field of 140×140 μm (40× primary magnification). Each pixel resolution was of 256 gray levels. Relative optical density (ROD) was obtained after a transformation of mean gray values into ROD using the formula: $ROD = \log (256/mean\ gray)$. The ROD value was chosen to evaluate the intensity of S-100β immunoreactivity. A background parameter was obtained from each section out of the immunolabelled structures and subtracted from each cell ROD before statistically processing values. To evaluate 5HT-T, Nf-200, and MAP2 positive neuronal processes, the total area of immunolabeled fibers was related to the total area of the evaluated field, giving a fiber density parameter. Cellular area of astrocytes immunolabeled for GFAP was directly measured on the cell body. These analyses were performed in five different staining experiments, and for each experiment, more than seven sections from both control and treated groups were measured The statistical study was performed by applying a two-tailed *t* test to the results of the quantitative analysis and by assuming that data were normally distributed. The equality of variance for control and treated values was analyzed by an F test. For the same group interanimal differences as well as interexperimental differences were not significant.

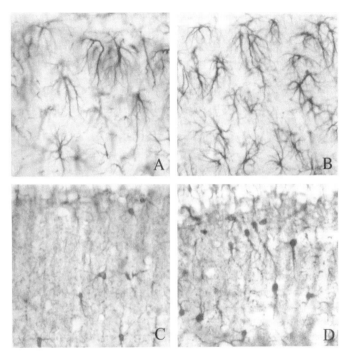

FIGURE 1. Astrocytes immunostained for GFAP (*upper row*) and S-100β protein (*lower row*) from control (**A** and **C**) and treated (**B** and **D**) rats. Note the presence of hypertrophied astrocytes (**B**) and the increase in S100β immunostaining (D) in treated rats. Primary magnification 400×.

RESULTS

All studies were performed on the stratum radiatum of the hippocampal CA1 area.

Glial Markers. In control rats, GFAP-immunolabeled astrocytes presented a classic appearance with large and thin cellular processes (FIG. 1A). In exposed rats, an important astroglial reaction was observed as an increase in the cellular area (control: 80.96 μm^2 ± 21.12; exposed: 155.66 μm^2 ± 6.77) (FIG. 2). Reactive astrocytes present not only larger cellular bodies but also thicker and more abundant cellular processes (FIG. 1B).

In normal astrocytes, S-100β protein has a cytosolic distribution limited to the cellular body and the astrocytic processes appear hardly immunolabeled (FIG. 1C). In exposed rats, the distribution pattern of S-100β immunoreactivity was the same, but the intensity of the intracellular immunostaining was significantly increased (control: 0.92 ± 0.17; exposed: 1.45 ± 0.16) (FIGS. 1D and 3).

Neuronal Markers. 5HT-T is expressed in the serotoninergic fibers, not only at the synaptic terminal but also all along the fiber. 5HT-T–immunolabeled fibers were

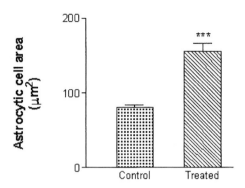

FIGURE 2. Cell area of GFAP-immunolabeled astrocytes. Values are expressed in μm^2 as mean and $\pm$ SD. Values were analyzed by two-tailed t test. ***$p < 0.001$.

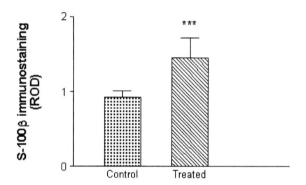

FIGURE 3. Image analysis of S-100β protein-immunolabeled astrocytes. Values are expressed as relative optical density (ROD), mean $\pm$ SD. Values were analyzed by two-tailed t test. ***$p < 0.001$.

present in every analyzed section from control and exposed animals, although in exposed rats there was an important reduction in 5HT-T fibers in the stratum radiatum (compare FIG. 4A and 4B). These observations were confirmed by image analysis when fibers were measured as total area of immunolabeled fibers related to total area of the evaluated field. Statistical analysis determined that reduction in serotoninergic innervation was very significant (control: 0.170 ± 0.002; exposed: 0.120 ± 0.020) (FIG. 5).

Nf-200 are very important cytoskeletal components in neuronal processes. Nf-200 immunoreactivity was also reduced after ETOH exposure (compare FIG. 4C and 4D). In sections from exposed rats, the relative area covered by Nf-200–immunolabeled neuronal processes was significantly minor compared to that in control ones (control: 0.30 ± 0.02; exposed: 0.15 ± 0.02) (FIG. 6).

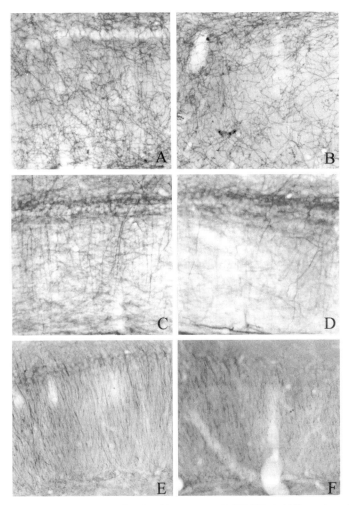

FIGURE 4. Immunostaining for 5HT-T (*upper row*), Nf-200 (*middle row*), and MAP2 (*lower row*) in control (**A, C,** and **E**) and treated (**B, D,** and **F**) rats. Note the important reduction in expression of the three markers in the treated sections. Primary magnification 200×.

MAP2 is a microtubule-associated protein present in dendrites. Stratum radiatum contains apical dendrites of pyramidal neurons, MAP2 being a useful marker for demonstrating morphologic alterations in those neuronal processes. After ETOH exposure, we observed in exposed sections a decrease in MAP2-immunolabeled processes (compare FIG. 4E and 4F). On the other hand, dendrites showed an irregular and fragmented structure. Image analysis demonstrated a significant reduction in MAP2-immunoreactive dendrites in exposed rats (control: 0.12 ± 0.02; exposed: 0.07 ± 0.01) (FIG. 7).

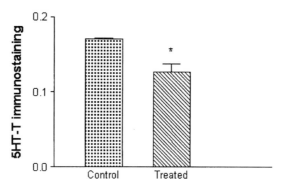

FIGURE 5. Area of 5HT-T–immunolabeled fibers. Data are expressed as area of 5HT-T–immunolabeled fibers per μm^2 of tissue, mean ± SD. Values were analyzed by two-tailed *t* test. *$p < 0.05$.

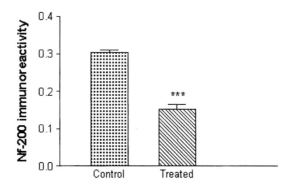

FIGURE 6. Area of Nf-200–immunolabeled neuronal processes. Data are expressed as area of immunolabeled processes per μm^2 of tissue, mean ± SD. Values were analyzed by two-tailed *t* test. ***$p < 0.001$.

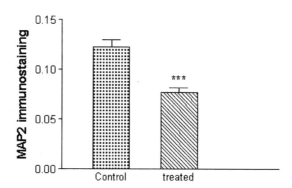

FIGURE 7. Area of MAP2-immunoreactive neuronal processes. Data are expressed as the area of immunolabeled processes per μm^2 of tissue. Values were analyzed by two-tailed *t* test. ***$p < 0.001$.

DISCUSSION

The current work shows the adverse effects of long-term ETOH exposure on neuronal and astroglial cells in adults. Glial cells are very important cell types in vertebrate CNS; they provide the structural and nutritive support for neurons.[17] One of the most remarkable characteristics of astrocytes is their response to diverse neurologic insults.[14,18,19] After long-term ETOH exposure we found an important astroglial reaction evidenced by the hypertrophy of GFAP+ astrocytes. These kind of modified astrocytes are termed reactive astrocytes. Cellular components of those glial cells can synthesize neurotrophic factors and thus affect the fate of the neuronal population in injured tissue.[20]

A substantial reduction in hippocampal serotoninergic innervation was demonstrated by a decrease in 5HT-T–immunolabeled fibers. The mechanism by which ETOH induces this serotoninergic dennervation is unknown, but some reports indicate that ETOH or its metabolite has a deleterious effect on raphe neurons.[11] Over adult life, 5HT is a classic neurotransmitter that also plays a role in the maintenance of some neuronal populations. It has been proposed that this serotoninergic effect is mediated by S-100β, an astroglial-derived growth factor.[6] This protein is released by astroglial cells when their $5HT_{1A}$ receptors are stimulated. Once outside the cytoplasm, S-100β has important effects on neuronal differentiation.[8–10] Interestingly, after ETOH exposure we found an increase in S-100β intracellular immunoreactivity. We believe that the increased immunoreactivity might indicate decreased S-100β release. If the hippocampal 5HT level is reduced after ETOH exposure (as indicated by the serotoninergic dennervation), the astroglial $5HT_{1A}$ receptors may be less stimulated, resulting in a decrease in S-100β release.

On the other hand, we observed an important reduction in Nf-200- and MAP2-immunolabeled processes. Specially, MAP2+ neuronal processes showed a fragmented and abnormal structure. Considering that MAP2 is associated with dendrites, we think that the altered neuronal processes would be mainly dendrites, probably proceeding from the pyramidal neurons. We may speculate that the decrease in the available S-100β in the extracellular surroundings could result in alterations in dendrites. We have already demonstrated, in a model of 5HT depletion, that S-100β accumulation in astroglial cells leads to neuronal cytoskeletal alterations in adult rats.[16] Moreover, the involvement of S-100β and $5HT_{1A}$ receptors on ETOH-induced alterations has recently been recognized.[21,22]

In conclusion, morphometric analysis shows that ETOH exposure induces morphologic alterations in both neuronal and astroglial populations probably related to a lower release of trophic factors, such as S-100β, which are necessary for CNS maintenance. However, we cannot rule out the possibility that other molecules or neurotransmitters could be involved in these complex neural-glial interactions. Further studies are necessary to confirm our suggestion.

ACKNOWLEDGMENTS

We would like to thank Alejandro Ferrari for his collaboration. This work was supported by grants from Beca Carrillo-Oñativia 2000 Ministerio de Salud, Rep. Argentina; UBACYT B-033, Universidad de Buenos Aires, Argentina. A.J. Ramos is a postdoctoral fellow of CONICET.

REFERENCES

1. CREWS, F.T. 1999. Alcohol and neurodegeneration. CNS Drug Rev. **5:** 397–394.
2. SCHUCKIT, M.A. 1995. Alcohol-related disorders. *In* Comprehensive Textbook of Psychiatry. 6th ed. H.I. Kaplan and B.J. Sadock, Eds.: 2207–2241. Williams & Wilkins. Baltimore.
3. REINBERG, A. 1992. Circadian changes in psychologic effects of ethanol. Neuropsychopharmacology **7:** 149–156.
4. DRUSE, M.J. 1992. Effects of *in utero* ethanol exposure on the development of CNS neurotransmitter system. *In* Effects of Alcohol and Opiates. M.W. Miller, Ed.: 139–167. Wiley-Liss. New York.
5. KIM, J. & M.J. DRUSE. 1996. Deficiency of essential neurotrophic factor in conditioned media produced by ethanol-exposed cortical astrocytes. Dev. Brain Res. **96:** 1–10.
6. AZMITIA, E.C., P.M. DOLAN & P.M. WHITAKER-AZMITIA. 1990. S-100β but not NGF, EGF, insulin, or calmodulin is a CNS serotoninergic growth factor. Brain Res. **516:** 354–356.
7. WHITAKER-AZMITIA, P.M. & E.C. AZMITIA. 1994. Astroglial 5-HT$_{1A}$ receptors S-100 beta in development and plasticity. Perspect. Dev. Neurobiol. **2:** 2333–2338.
8. MULLER, C.M., A.C. AKHAVAN & M. BETTE. 1993. Possible role of S100 in glia-neuronal signalling involved in activity-dependent plasticity in developing mammalian cortex. J. Chem. Neuroanat. **6:** 215–227.
9. HESKETH, J. & J. BAUDIER. 1986. Evidence that S100 proteins regulate microtubule assembly and stability in rat brain extract. Int. J. Biochem. **18:** 691–695.
10. LIN, L.H., L.J. VAN ELDIK, N. OSHEROFF & N.J. NORDEN. 1994. Inhibition of protein kinase C- and casein kinase II-mediated phosphorylation of GAP-43 by S100ß. Mol. Brain Res. **25:** 297–304.
11. SARI, Y., T. POWROZEK & F.C. ZHOU. 2001. Alcohol deters the outgrowth of serotoninergic neurons at midgestation. J. Biomed. Sci. **8:** 119–125.
12. O'BRIEN, C.P, M.J. ECKARDT & M.I. LINNOILA. 1995. Pharmacotherapy of alcoholism. *In* Psycopharmacology: The Fourth Generation of Progress. F.E. Bloom and D.J. Kupfer, Eds.: 1745–1755. Raven Press. New York.
13. FAGES, C. *et al.* 1994. Long term astroglial reaction to serotoninergic fiber degeneration. Brain Res. **639:** 161–166.
14. TAGLIAFERRO, P. *et al.* 1997. Neural and astroglial effects of chronic parachlorophenylalanine-induced serotonin synthesis inhibition. Mol. Chem. Neuropathol. **32:** 195–211.
15. AZMITIA, E.C. *et al.* 1995. 5HT$_{1A}$ agonist and dexomethasone reversal of *p*-chloroamphetamine induced loss of MAP-2 and synaptophysin immunoreactivity in adult rat brain. Brain Res. **677:** 181–192.
16. RAMOS, J.A. *et al.* 2000. Neuroglial interaction in a model of *para*-chlorophenylalanine-induced serotonin depletion. Brain Res. **883:** 1–14.
17. VALLES, S. *et al.* 1997. Ethanol exposure affects glial fibrillary acidic protein gene expresión and transcription during rat brain development. J. Neurochem. **69:** 2484–2492.
18. ZHOU, F.C., E.C. AZMITIA & S. BLEDSOE. 1995. Rapid serotoninergic fiber sprouting in response to ibotenic acid lesion in the striatum and hippocampus. Dev. Brain Res. **84:** 89–98.
19. BRUSCO, A. *et al.* 1997. 2,4-Dichlorophenoxyacetic acid through lactation induces astrogliosis in rat brain. Mol. Chem. Neuropathol. **30:** 175–185.
20. JUNIER, M.P. *et al.* 1994. Target-deprived CNS neurons express the NGF gene while reactive glia around their axonal terminals contain low and high affinity NGF receptors. Mol. Brain Res. **24:** 247–260.
21. ZHOU, F.C. *et al.* 2001. Prenatal alcohol exposure retards the migration and development of serotonin neurons in fetal C57BL mice. Dev. Brain Res. **126:** 147–155.
22. ERIKSEN, J.L. & M.J. DRUSE. 2001. Potential involvement of S100β in the protective effects of a serotonin-1a agonist on ethanol-treated astrocytes. Dev. Brain Res. **128:** 157–164.

Effects of Chronic Maternal Ethanol Exposure on Hippocampal and Striatal Morphology in Offspring

ALBERTO JAVIER RAMOS, SERGIO GUSTAVO EVRARD,
PATRICIA TAGLIAFERRO, MARÍA VICTORIA TRICÁRICO,
AND ALICIA BRUSCO

Instituto de Biología Celular y Neurociencias "Prof. Eduardo De Robertis,"
Facultad de Medicina, Universidad de Buenos Aires, Paraguay 2155 (1121),
Buenos Aires, Argentina

ABSTRACT: Astrocytes and serotoninergic neurons play a role in central nervous system (CNS) development, probably through serotonin (5HT) stimulation of the glial $5HT_{1A}$ receptor. Activation of $5HT_{1A}$ receptors causes the release of S-100β, a glial derived growth factor. *In vitro*, astrocytes are profoundly altered by chronic maternal ethanol exposure (CMEE). CMEE is also associated with reduced 5HT brain levels and abnormal development of the serotoninergic system. In the present study we analyzed the hippocampal and striatal serotoninergic innervation and astroglial cells in the offspring of CMEE mothers. Female Wistar rats were orally exposed to ethanol 6.6% (v/v) ad libitum for 6 weeks before breeding and during gestation. After parturition, rat mothers continued receiving ethanol until pups reached 21 days old. The control group received water ad libitum. Rat offspring brains were processed by immunocytochemistry using antibodies directed to GFAP, serotonin transporter (5HTT), or S-100β protein. Hippocampus and striatum were studied by computer-assisted image analysis. Cell area of GFAP⁺ astrocytes, surface of 5HTT⁺ fibers per area unit, and relative optical density (ROD) of S-100β⁺ astrocytes were measured and statistically processed. Our results show that astroglial GFAP was increased (astrocytes were hypertrophied) and 5HTT⁺ fibers were increased in both the hippocampal CA-1 area and the striatum. On the other hand, S-100β ROD was increased only in the hippocampal CA-1 area but not in the striatum. The different response of the studied regions is an interesting result considering evidence of a close 5HT/astroglial relation during CNS development. These differences could be due to different gradients of development in the studied areas and/or different responses of those areas to the effect of maternal ethanol exposure since the first stages of embryonic development.

KEYWORDS: ethanol; pregnancy; maternal ethanol exposure; serotonin; S-100β; serotonin transporter; astroglia

Address for correspondence: Dra. Alicia Brusco, Rivera Indarte 132 1° A, (1406) Buenos Aires, Argentina. Voice: 54-11-5950-9626; fax: 54-11-4556-1901.
hbrusco@fmed.uba.ar

Ann. N.Y. Acad. Sci. 965: 343–353 (2002). © 2002 New York Academy of Sciences.

INTRODUCTION

Chronic maternal ethanol exposure (CMEE) during pregnancy is one of the greatest health problems world-wide. It is probably the most prevalent teratogenic cause of mental retardation.[1] CMEE during pregnancy is believed to be the cause of fetal alcohol syndrome (FAS),[2–4] a clinical condition characterized by a variety of brain and physical malformations. Children affected by FAS exhibit a typical physical phenotype and varying degrees of central nervous system (CNS) dysfunction, ranging from mild cognitive disorders to profound mental retardation, including reduced intelligence, different learning and linguistic disorders, psychomotor and mental dysfunction, and, finally, epilepsy.[5–8] It has been well established that CMEE alters neuroblast generation and migration during cortical development in offspring[9–11] and can induce different histopathologic types of cortical dysplasia, which ultimately gives rise to neuropsychiatric handicapped infants and adults.

CMEE has been associated with alterations in the development of several neurotransmitter systems including the serotoninergic system. Offspring of CMEE mothers have marked deficiency of brain serotonin (5HT) and 5-hydroxyindoleacetic acid (5-HIAA) in cerebral cortices, cerebellum, and brain stem; a decreased number of $5HT_{1A}$ receptors in brain stem and cerebral cortical regions;[12–14] a significant reduction in 5HT reuptake sites in cortical regions;[15,16] and a decreased number of 5HT neurons in the developing mesencephalic raphe nuclei in early postnatal rats.[17]

5HT is a classic neurotransmitter and one of the earliest to be expressed in the CNS. 5HT fibers are among the first to reach the cortical plate in the developing cortex and have widespread distribution in the adult brain.[18] The early expression of 5HT in brain development[19,20] was initial evidence for the hypothesis of the role of 5HT as a differentiation signal in CNS development. The role of 5HT in the development and plasticity of the CNS seems to be mediated by the glial $5HT_{1A}$ receptor stimulation that causes S-100β release.[21] S-100β is a glial cell-derived growth factor with multiple functions such as neurite outgrowth promotion, interaction with cytoskeletal proteins, regulation of enzymatic activities, promotion of neuronal survival and plasticity, and inducible nitric oxide synthase (iNOS) induction.[22–25]

Ethanol-exposed rat offspring are reported to show decreased 5HT and 5-HIAA concentrations in the brain stem and cortical regions.[12] Astroglial cells are also affected by CMEE during pregnancy.[26,27] Our laboratory has previously reported neuronal and glial alterations after sustained 5HT depletion in neonatal[28] and adult rats.[29] In the current work we studied the 5HT/astroglial relationship in a model of CMEE during pregnancy. To determine the response of glial cells in this model, glial fibrillary acidic protein (GFAP) and S-100β protein were evaluated. Because it was reported that 5HT concentrations are reduced in several brain areas, we evaluated 5HT transporter (5HTT) immunoreactive fibers to study serotoninergic projections.

MATERIAL AND METHODS

Animal Treatment

Nulliparous female Wistar rats from the same litter, initially weighing 180–200 g, were divided into two groups: control and treated. The treated group was orally exposed to ethanol 6.6% (v/v) in drinking water ad libitum for 6 weeks before breeding and during gestation. After delivery, rat mothers continued receiving ethanol 6.6% v/v in drinking water until pups reached 21 days old. The control group received water ad libitum. Both groups were fed a standard rat food.

Fixation

At postnatal day 21, rat offspring were deeply anesthetized with 300 mg/kg of chloral hydrate. The left ventricle was perfused, initially with 15 ml of a cold saline solution containing 0.05% (w/v) $NaNO_2$ plus 50 IU of heparin and subsequently with 150 ml of a cold fixative solution containing 4% (w/v) paraformaldehyde and 0.25% (v/v) glutaraldehyde in 0.1 M phosphate buffer, pH 7.4. Brains were removed and kept in the same cold fixative solution for 4 hours. After that, brains were washed three times in cold 0.1 M phosphate buffer, pH 7.4, containing 5% (w/v) sucrose and left in this washing solution for 18 hours at 4°C. Sagittal 40-μm thick brain sections were cut with a vibratome and stored at −20°C in 0.1 M phosphate buffer, pH 7.4, with 25% (w/v) sucrose added as cryoprotector.

Immunocytochemistry

To inhibit endogenous peroxidase activity, tissue sections were previously dehydrated, treated with 0.5% (v/v) H_2O_2 in methanol for 30 minutes at room temperature, and rehydrated. Brain sections were treated for 1 hour with 3% (v/v) normal goat serum (NGS) in phosphate-buffered saline (PBS) solution to block unspecific immunogen sites. After two rinses in PBS plus 0.025% (v/v) Triton X-100 (PBS-X), sections were incubated for 48 hours at 4°C with antibodies against 5HTT, GFAP, or S-100β protein. After five rinses in PBS-X, sections were incubated 1 hour at room temperature with biotinylated secondary antibodies diluted 1:100. After further washing in PBS-X, sections were incubated 1 hour with a streptavidin-peroxidase complex solution diluted 1:200. Sections were washed again, five times in PBS-X and two times in 0.1 M acetate buffer, pH 6 (AcB), and development of peroxidase activity was performed with 0.035% (w/v) 3,3′-diaminobenzidine plus 2.5% (w/v) nickel ammonium sulfate and 0.1% (v/v) H_2O_2 dissolved in AcB. Following the enzymatic incubation step, sections were washed three times in AcB and once in distilled water. Sections were mounted, dehydrated, and cover-slipped using Permount for light microscopic observation.

All the antibodies as well as the streptavidin-peroxidase complex were dissolved in PBS containing 1% (v/v) NGS and 0.3% (v/v) Triton X-100, pH 7.4.

Morphometric Analysis

All measurements were performed on coded slides to ensure objectivity. Tissue images were obtained through an Axiophot Zeiss light microscope equipped with a video camera on line with a Zeiss-Kontron VIDAS image analyzer. Video images were digitized into an array of 512×512 pixels corresponding to a tissue area of 140 μm × 140 μm (40× primary magnification). Each pixel resolution was of 256 gray levels. To evaluate the 5HTT immunoreactive (5HTT-IR) fibers, the total area of immunolabeled fibers was related to the total area of the evaluated field, rendering a relative fiber density parameter. In GFAP-immunoreactive (GFAP-IR) astrocytes, the cell area was measured by interactively determining each cell's limits. The intensity of S-100β immunoreactivity (S-100β-IR) was evaluated by means of a relative optical density (ROD) value. ROD was obtained after transformation of mean gray values into ROD using the formula: ROD = log (256/mean gray). A background parameter was obtained from each section out of the immunolabeled structures and subtracted from each cell ROD before statistically processing the obtained values.

Statistical Analysis

Seven to fifteen separate immunocytochemical experiments were run for each primary antibody. Individual experiments were composed of 6–10 tissue sections of each animal from each group. Seven to ten fields were measured for each brain area in each section of each animal. Interanimal differences in each group were not statistically significant. Values represent the means of experiments performed for each marker and each brain area. Differences among the means were statistically analyzed by means of Student's two-tailed t test. Statistical significance was set to $p < 0.05$.

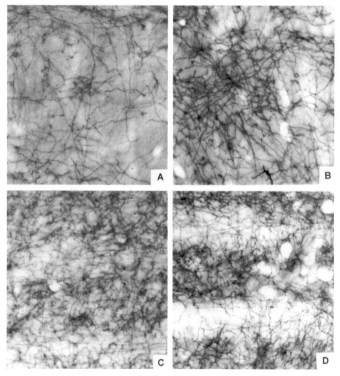

FIGURE 1. 5HTT immunostaining. (*Above*) 5HTT immunostaining in the stratum radiatum of the hippocampal CA-1 area. (**A**) Control group; (**B**) ethanol-exposed offspring. (*Below*) 5HTT immunostaining in the striatum; (**C**) control group; (**D**) ethanol-exposed offspring. Note that 5HTT+ fibers are increased in both hippocampus and striatum. Primary magnification 400×.

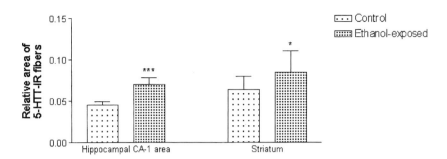

FIGURE 2. Area of 5HTT immunostained fibers in hippocampal CA1 area (*left*) and striatum (*right*). Data are expressed as area of 5HTT+ fibers per μm^2 of tissue. Note the increased area of 5HTT immunoreactive fibers in the ethanol-exposed offspring. ***p <0.001; *p < 0.05; after two-tailed Student's t test. Bars represent mean ± SD.

RESULTS

5HTT Immunostaining

5HTT is expressed in every 5HT fiber. This marker is useful to follow 5HT fibers when they are depleted of neurotransmitter, because the 5HTT-IR is not affected by the 5HT level inside the fiber. 5HTT expression was observed in all studied areas as thin fibers with dense branching. Quantitative studies allowed the evaluation of fiber density and were expressed as the area of 5HTT-IR fibers per unit area of tissue. In the stratum radiatum of the hippocampal CA-1 area of ethanol-exposed rat offspring, there was an extremely significant increase in the relative area of 5HTT-IR fibers, reaching 155% of controls (p < 0.001) (FIG. 1A and 1B and FIG. 2). In control and treated animals, striatal 5HTT-IR fibers were observed in the matrix, sparing the striatosomes. Image analysis was focused on the matrix, where dense 5HT innervation is present. In the striatum of ethanol-exposed rat offspring, there was a significant increase in the relative area of 5HTT-IR fibers reaching 132.9% of controls (p < 0.05) (FIG. 1C and 1D and FIG. 2).

GFAP Immunostaining

Because GFAP-IR specifically labels the intermediate filaments of the astroglial cytoskeleton, allowing the study of astrocyte morphology, its morphometric analysis is a sensitive parameter for evaluating astroglial reaction. In the stratum radiatum of the hippocampal CA-1 area of ethanol-exposed rat offspring, astrocytes presented enlarged, tortuous cytoplasmic processes and increased soma size. Morphometric analysis showed a very significant increase in astroglial cell area, reaching 194.9% of controls (p < 0.01) (FIG. 3A and 3B and FIG. 4). In the striatum of ethanol-exposed rat offspring, astroglial hypertrophy was also observed, and morphometric analysis showed a significant increase in the astroglial cell area, reaching 139.1% of controls (p < 0.05) (FIG. 3C and 3D and FIG. 4). This characteristic hypertrophy is typical of

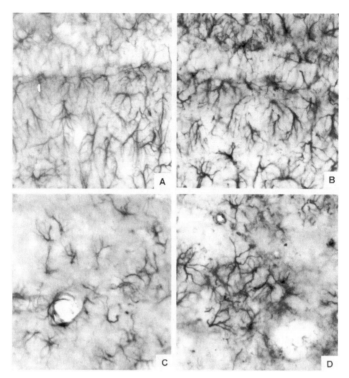

FIGURE 3. GFAP immunostaining. (*Above*) GFAP immunostaining in the stratum radiatum of the hippocampal CA-1 area. (**A**) Control group; (**B**) ethanol-exposed offspring. (*Below*) GFAP immunostaining in the striatum. (**C**) Control group; (**D**) ethanol-exposed offspring. Note that GFAP-immunolabeled astrocytes increased their size and extended the processes in both hippocampus and striatum. Primary magnification 400×.

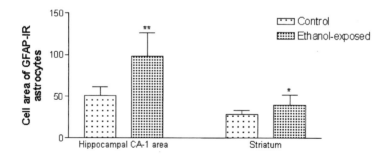

FIGURE 4. Area of GFAP-immunostained astrocytes in hippocampal CA1 area (*left*) and striatum (*right*). Data are expressed as area of GFAP-immunolabeled astrocytes in μm^2. Note the increased area of GFAP-immunoreactive astrocytes in ethanol-exposed offspring. **$p < 0.01$; *$p < 0.05$; after two-tailed Student's t test. Bars represent mean ± SD.

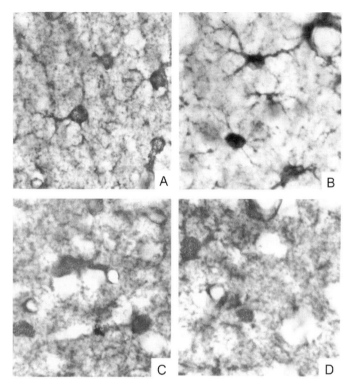

FIGURE 5. S-100β immunostaining. (*Above*) S-100β immunostaining in the stratum radiatum of the hippocampal CA-1 area. (**A**) Control group; (**B**) ethanol-exposed offspring. (*Below*) S-100β immunostaining in the striatum. (**C**) Control group; (**D**) ethanol-exposed offspring. Note that S-100β immunostaining increased only in the hippocampus. Primary magnification 1,000×.

an astroglial reaction. Interestingly, astroglial hypertrophy was more important in the hippocampus than in the striatum of ethanol-exposed rat offspring.

S-100β Immunostaining

Intracellular S-100β-IR was observed in the astroglial cells of every analyzed brain region in control and treated groups. S-100β immunostaining labeled the astrocyte cell body and some cytoplasmic projections. The intensity of S-100β-IR was evaluated by digital image analysis. In the stratum radiatum of the hippocampal CA-1 area of ethanol-exposed rat offspring, a very significant increase was noted in the intensity of intracellular S-100β-IR, evaluated as ROD units, reaching 157.1% of control ($p < 0.01$) (FIG. 5A and 5B and FIG. 6). In the striatum, anti-S-100β antibodies labeled astrocytes in the matrix, presenting intense staining in the astrocyte soma. In the striatum of ethanol-exposed rat offspring, S-100β-IR was not significantly different from that of the control group, reaching 115.3% of control (FIG. 5C and 5D and FIG. 6).

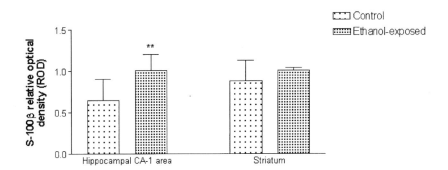

FIGURE 6. Relative optical density (ROD) of S-100β-immunostained glial cells in hippocampal CA1 area (*left*) and striatum (*right*). Data are expressed as ROD units. Note the increased ROD of S-100β-immunostained glial cells only in the hippocampus of ethanol-exposed offsprings. **$p < 0.01$ after two-tailed Student's t test. Bars represent mean ± SD.

DISCUSSION

In 21-day-old offspring of CMEE Wistar rats we studied the expression of 5HTT, GFAP and S-100β in two CNS areas receiving a dense serotoninergic innervation: hippocampus and striatum. It was previously described that 5HT brain content is reduced after ethanol exposure,[12,14] using anti-5HTT antibodies we could describe the 5HT innervation in spite of the reduced 5HT levels. 5HTT-IR is not affected by the 5HT content in each fiber. Our results showed that in the pups of CMEE mothers, 5HTT-IR fibers present normal morphology but there was an increase in the surface covered by 5HTT-IR fibers. In fact, this is an interesting result because it could be indicating a phenomena of neuronal sprouting. To our knowledge, this is the first morphologic description showing an increase in the 5HT innervation in the pups of CMEE mothers. Our observation raises the question on the hypothetical adaptive mechanisms triggered by the early ethanol exposure during CNS development.

It is well known that S-100β stimulates neurite outgrowth specially on 5HT fibers.[24,29] Interestingly, our results showed increased S-100β-IR in the hippocampus, where 5HTT-IR fibers are also augmented. However, S-100β-IR is not significantly increased in the striatum, where 5HTT-IR fibers are slightly increased. These evidences show that 5HTT-IR fibers sprouting after CMEE could also be related to other substances besides S-100β. Probably different brain regions elicit a different profile of neuronal and glial response to early ethanol exposure during CNS development. In fact, we have already demonstrated that S-100β-IR is increased in a model of 5HT depletion, presenting very different profiles accordingly with the studied brain areas.[29]

GFAP, a classical marker of astroglial cytoskeleton, was used to follow the astroglial response after CMEE. Our results showed increased astrocytic cell area, indicating an astroglial hypertrophy and an astroglial reaction. Astroglial reaction is a well characterized glial response showed after many different kinds of CNS injuries.[30–33] Controversial reports on astroglial response to ethanol exposure have been published with different paradigms of ethanol exposure and methodologic procedures, showing both increased[34–37] and decreased GFAP expression.[26,27] Clearly, in our studies both analyzed areas have presented an important glial reaction which is in accordance with other previous morphologic studies.[36]

In summary, we reported here that early ethanol exposure during pre and postnatal CNS development altered significantly the 5HT/astroglial relation in two brain areas (hippocampus and striatum) which are critical in the development of FAS symptoms in children of alcoholic mothers. In the last years the role of 5HT/astroglial relationship have been proposed as a pharmacologic target possible to develop successful strategies to reach neuroprotection as well as to prevent ethanol effects during development.[38–40] The complete description of ethanol effects in early development is essential to complete those pharmacologic studies.

ACKNOWLEDGMENTS

This work was supported by grants Beca Carrillo-Oñativia 2000 Ministerio de Salud, Rep. Argentina, and UBACYT B-033, Universidad de Buenos Aires, Argentina. We would like to thank Alejandro Ferrari and Maite Duhalde Vega for their collaboration. A.J. Ramos is a postdoctoral fellow of CONICET; his present address is Universidad Austral, B1629AHJ Derqui, Pilar, Buenos Aires, Argentina.

REFERENCES

1. BREGMAN, J.D. & J.C. HARRIS. 1995. Mental retardation. *In* Comprehensive Textbook of Psychiatry. 6th ed. H.I. Kaplan and B.J. Sadock, Eds.: 2207–2241. Williams & Wilkins. Baltimore.
2. ADAMS, R.D. & M. VICTOR. 1995. Principles of Neurology. 5th ed.: 903–921. McGraw-Hill. New York.
3. KINSELLA, L.J. & D.E. RILEY. 1999. Nutritional deficiencies and syndromes associated with alcoholism. *In* Textbook of Clinical Neurology. C.G. Goetz and E.J. Pappert, Eds.: 798–818. W.B. Saunders. Philadelphia.
4. SCHUCKIT, M.A. 1995. Alcohol-related disorders. *In* Comprehensive Textbook of Psychiatry. 6th ed. H.I. Kaplan and B.J. Sadock, Eds.: 2207–2241. Williams & Wilkins. Baltimore.
5. CONRY, J. 1990. Neuropsychological deficits in fetal alcohol syndrome and fetal alcohol effects. Alcohol. Clin. Exp. Res. **14**: 650–655.
6. FAMY, C., A.P. STREISSGUTH & A.S. UNIS. 1998. Mental illness in adults with fetal alcohol syndrome or fetal alcohol effects. Am. J. Psychiatry **155**: 552–554.
7. MATTSON, S.N., E.P. RILEY, D.C. DELIS, *et al.* 1996. Verbal learning and memory in children with fetal alcohol syndrome. Alcohol. Clin. Exp. Res. **20**: 810–816.
8. MATTSON, S.N. *et al.* 1997. Heavy prenatal alcohol exposure with or without physical features of fetal alcohol syndrome leads to IQ deficits. J. Pediatr. **131**: 718–721.
9. MILLER, M.W. 1986. Effects of alcohol on the generation and migration of cerebral cortical neurons. Science **233**: 1308–1311.
10. MILLER, M.W. 1987. Effect of prenatal exposure to alcohol on the distribution and time of origin of corticospinal neurons in the rat. J. Comp. Neurol. **257**: 372–382.
11. MILLER, M.W. 1997. Effects of prenatal exposure to ethanol on callosal projection neurons in rat somatosensory cortex. Brain Res. **766**: 121–128.
12. RATHBUN, W.E. & M.J. DRUSE. 1985. Dopamine, serotonin and acid metabolites in brain regions from the developing offspring of ethanol-treated rats. J. Neurochem. **44**: 57–62.

13. TAJUDDIN, N.F. & M.J. DRUSE. 1989. Chronic maternal ethanol consumption results in decreased serotonergic $5HT_1$ sites in cerebral cortical regions from offspring. Alcohol **5:** 465–470.
14. DRUSE, M.J., A. KUO & N. TAJUDDIN. 1991. Effects of *in utero* ethanol exposure on the developing serotonergic system. Alcohol. Clin. Exp. Res. **15:** 678–684.
15. DRUSE, M.J. & L.H. PAUL. 1989. Effects of *in utero* ethanol exposure on serotonin uptake in cortical regions. Alcohol **5:** 455–459.
16. KIM, J.-A. & M.J. DRUSE. 1996. Protective effects of maternal buspirone treatment on serotonin reuptake sites in ethanol-exposed offspring. Dev. Brain Res. **92:** 190–198.
17. TAJUDDIN, N.F. & M.J. DRUSE. 1999. *In utero* ethanol exposure decreased the density of serotonin neurons. Maternal ipsapirone treatment exerted a protective effect. Dev. Brain Res. **117:** 91–97.
18. LAUDER, J.M. *et al.* 1982. *In vivo* and *in vitro* development of serotonergic neurons. Brain Res. Bull. **9:** 605–625.
19. LAUDER, J.M. & H. KREBS. 1978. Serotonin as a differentiation signal in early neurogenesis. Dev. Neurosci. **1:** 15–30.
20. LAUDER, J.M. 1990. Ontogeny of the serotonergic system in the rat: serotonin as a developmental signal. Ann. N.Y. Acad. Sci. **600:** 297–314.
21. WHITAKER-AZMITIA, P.M., R. MURPHY & E.C. AZMITIA. 1990. Stimulation of astroglial 5HT1A receptors releases the serotoninergic growth factor, protein S-100, and alters astroglial morphology. Brain Res. **528:** 155–158.
22. FANO, G. *et al.* 1995. The S-100: a protein family in search of a function. Prog. Neurobiol. **46:** 71–82.
23. LIU, J.P. & J.M. LAUDER. 1992. S-100β and insulin-like growth factor–II differentially regulate growth of developing serotonin and dopamine neurons *in vitro*. J. Neurosci. Res. **33:** 248–256.
24. AZMITIA, E.C., D.R. MARSHAK & P.M. WHITAKER-AZMITIA. 1990. Functional interactions between glial S-100β protein and CNS 5HT neurons. J. Cell. Biochem. **14F:** 8.
25. HU, J., F. CASTETS, J.L. GUEVARA & L.J. VAN ELDIK. 1996. S-100β stimulates inducible nitric oxide synthase activity and mRNA levels in rat cortical astrocytes. J. Biol. Chem. **271:** 2543–2547.
26. VALLÉS, S. *et al.* 1996. Glial fibrillary acidic protein expression in rat brain and in radial glia culture is delayed by prenatal ethanol exposure. J. Neurochem. **67:** 2425–2433.
27. VALLÉS, S., J. PITARCH, J. RENAU-PIQUERAS & C. GUERRI. 1997. Ethanol exposure affects glial fibrillary acidic protein gene expression and transcription during rat brain development. J. Neurochem. **69:** 2484–2493.
28. BRUSCO, A. *et al.* 2000. Morphological effects of neonatal parachloroamphetamine treatment on the hippocampus. J. Neurochem. **74** (Suppl): S61D.
29. RAMOS, A.J. *et al.* 2000. Neuroglial interactions in a model of parachlorophenylalanine-induced serotonin depletion. Brain Res. **883:** 1–14.
30. TAGLIAFERRO, P. *et al.* 1997. Neural and astroglial effects of a chronic parachlorophenylalanine-induced serotonin síntesis inhibition. Mol. Chem. Neuropathol. **32:** 195–211.
31. MATHEWSON, A.J. & M. BERRY. 1985. Observations on the astrocyte response to a cerebral stab wound in adult rats. Brain Res. **327:** 61–69.
32. SELVIN-TESTA, A., J.J. LÒPEZ-COSTA, A.C. NESSI DE AVIÑON & J. PECCI SAAVEDRA. 1991. Astroglial alterations in rat hippocampus during chronic lead exposure. Glia **4:** 384–392.
33. BRUSCO, A. *et al.* 1997. 2,4-Dichlorophenoxyacetic acid through lactation induces astrogliosis in rat brain. Mol. Chem. Neuropathol. **30:** 175–185.
34. FLETCHER, T.L. & W. SHAIN. 1992. Ethanol exposure increases GFAP mRNA in developing rat cortex and cultured cortical astrocytes. Soc. Neurosci. Abstr. **18:** 1115.
35. FLETCHER, T.L. & W. SHAIN. 1993. Ethanol-induced changes in astrocyte gene expression during rat central nervous system development. Alcohol. Clin. Exp. Res. **17:** 993–1001.
36. MILLER, M.W. & S. ROBERTSON. 1993. Prenatal exposure to ethanol alters the postnatal development and transformation of radial glia to astrocytes in the cortex. J. Comp. Neurol. **337:** 253–266.

37. GOODLETT, C.R. *et al.* 1993. Transient cortical astrogliosis induced by alcohol exposure during the neonatal brain growth spurt in rats. Dev. Brain Res. **72:** 85–97.
38. AHLEMEYER, B. *et al.* 2000. S–100β protects cultured neurons against glutamate- and staurosporine-induced damage and is involved in the antiapoptotic action of the 5HT$_{1A}$ agonist, Bay X 3702. Brain Res. **858:** 121–128.
39. ERIKSEN, J.L. & M.J. DRUSE. 2001. Potential involvement of S-100β in the protective effects of a serotonin-1a agonist on ethanol-treated astrocytes. Dev. Brain Res. **128:** 157–164.
40. ZHOU, F.C. *et al.* 2001. Prenatal alcohol exposure retards the migration and development of serotonin neurons in fetal C57BL mice. Dev. Brain Res. **126:** 147–155.

Brain Regions Mediating the Discriminative Stimulus Effects of Nicotine in Rats

HISATSUGU MIYATA,[a] KIYOSHI ANDO,[b] AND TOMOJI YANAGITA[c]

[a]Department of Psychiatry, [c]Department of Pharmacology I, Jikei University School of Medicine, Tokyo 105-8461, Japan

[b]Central Institute for Experimental Animals, Kawasaki 216-0001, Japan

ABSTRACT: The involvement of cerebral regions in the discriminative stimulus (DS) effects of nicotine was studied using rats. Substitution tests with nicotine administered into the medial prefrontal cortex, nucleus accumbens, and ventral tegmental area, all of which are located on the mesolimbocortical dopaminergic neurons, and into the dorsal hippocampus and medial habenular nucleus, which possess high densities of nicotinic cholinergic receptors, were conducted in rats trained to discriminate nicotine (0.5 mg/kg sc) from saline solution in a two-lever, food-reinforced, operant task. Nicotine administered into the medial prefrontal cortex substituted for nicotine (0.5 mg/kg sc), whereas nicotine administered into the nucleus accumbens and ventral tegmental area partially substituted for sc injected nicotine. However, nicotine administered into the dorsal hippocampus and medial habenular nucleus did not substitute for sc injected nicotine. These results suggest that the medial prefrontal cortex is primarily involved in the DS effects of nicotine, whereas the nucleus accumbens and ventral tegmental area are partially involved.

KEYWORDS: nicotine; discriminative stimulus effect; medial prefrontal cortex; nucleus accumbens; ventral tegmental area; dorsal hippocampus

INTRODUCTION

Nicotine is reported to play a major role in the establishment and maintenance of tobacco smoking behavior.[1–3] The ability of nicotine to serve as the discriminative stimulus (DS) effects is obviously a necessary condition for nicotine self-administration.[4] Much work has been done to investigate central mechanisms underlying the DS effects of nicotine using experimental animals. Firstly, it has been reported that the DS effects of nicotine are blocked by mecamylamine, a centrally and peripherally acting nicotinic antagonist,[4–6] but not by hexamethonium, a peripherally acting nicotinic antagonist.[7] Secondly, intraventricularly administered nicotine substituted for subcutaneously (sc) injected nicotine,[8,9] but peripherally administered nicotine isomethonium, at a dose that did not penetrate the blood-brain barrier, did not substitute for sc injected nicotine.[10] These results indicate that the DS effects of nicotine

Address for correspondence: Hisatsugu Miyata, Department of Psychiatry, Jikei University School of Medicine, 3-25-8 Nishi-shimbashi, Minato-ku, Tokyo 105-8461, Japan. Voice: +81-3-3433-1111; fax: +81-3-3437-0228.
miyata@jikei.ac.jp

Ann. N.Y. Acad. Sci. 965: 354–363 (2002). © 2002 New York Academy of Sciences.

are mediated by a central nicotinic mechanism. Furthermore, the drugs that produce nicotine-like DS effects are known to inhibit the binding of [^{3}H] nicotine in *in vitro assays*. In addition, the potency of the drugs in producing nicotine-like DS effects was correlated with their potency as inhibitors of [^{3}H] nicotine binding with the exception of cytisine. Thus, these results also indicate that the DS effects of nicotine are mainly mediated through the high affinity binding site for [^{3}H] nicotine.[11]

On the other hand, central dopaminergic neurons are considered to be involved in the DS effects of nicotine. Part of the evidence for this comes from the demonstration that α-methyl-*p*-tyrosine[12] and 6-hydroxydopamine[13] attenuate the DS effects of nicotine and that partial substitution of amphetamine for nicotine is observed in rats trained to discriminate nicotine from saline.[6,14] More direct proof derives from the demonstration that the presynaptic dopamine release inhibitor CGS 10746B as well as the centrally active calcium blocker isradipine blocks nicotine discrimination, suggesting that dopamine release and calcium influx in the brain are necessary conditions for nicotine discrimination.[15]

Among various types of central dopaminergic neurons, mesolimbocortical dopaminergic neurons were demonstrated to be involved in the DS effects of nicotine in recent studies from our laboratory.[16–18] These behavioral data are supported by various lines of neurochemical studies. Autoradiographic and immunohistochemical studies have revealed that the mesolimbocortical dopaminergic neurons possess nicotinic receptors at the level of cell bodies and/or dentrites within the ventral tegmental area and in their terminal fields such as the nucleus accumbens and the prefrontal cortex in rat brain.[19–21] Functional studies have also indicated that the stimulation of these receptors leads to activation of the mesolimbocortical dopaminergic neurons.[22–24]

In addition, among the central regions that possess high densities of [^{3}H] nicotine binding located on the cholinergic neurons, the dorsal hippocampus has been reported to be partially involved in the DS effects of nicotine.[25] Therefore, we investigated the involvement of the medial habenular nucleus in the DS effects of nicotine,[18] because the region has been reported to possess high densities of [^{3}H] nicotine binding and to be implicated in the transmission of neuronal information from hippocampus to the raphe nuclei.[26]

The purpose of this article is to summarize the results of our studies[16–18] on the investigation of cerebral regions mediating the DS effects of nicotine and to discuss the neural mechanisms underlying them.

MATERIAL AND METHODS

Animals. Male Sprague-Dawley rats (234–290 g) were obtained from Clea Japan Inc. (Tokyo). Rats were individually housed in an animal room at a regulated temperature (22 ± 2°C) with a light/dark cycle of 12/12 hours (light on at 8:00 A.M.). Each rat was fed 15 g of food per day (water freely available) throughout the experiment, except for a period of 3 days before and 7 days after cannulation surgery. This experiment was performed in accordance with the Principles of Laboratory Animal Care (NIH publication No. 85-23, revised 1985).

Drugs. (-)-Nicotine (Tokyo Kasei Co., Tokyo) was diluted in physiologic saline solution. The concentration of nicotine administered into one side of each cerebral

region was adjusted to result in an injection volume of 0.4 μl. The concentration of
sc injected nicotine was 0.5 mg/ml.

Apparatus. Operant chambers, each containing two response levers, were contained in sound-insulated, ventilated enclosures. On one wall of the chamber, a light
was mounted centrally above a food cup, which was located between the levers. A
food pellet (50 mg) was delivered by a pellet dispenser. White noise was present at
all times to mask external sounds. The operant schedule and recording of data were
controlled by an LSI-11 microcomputer (Digital Equipment Co., Maynard, MA), using software developed at this laboratory.

Nicotine Discrimination Training. The procedure for establishing nicotine discrimination has been described in detail.[16] In summary, after acquisition of lever-
pressing behavior under a fixed ratio 10 schedule (FR-10), nicotine discrimination
training was instituted: pressing one of two levers (randomly assigned) was reinforced with food pellets (50 mg) following nicotine (0.5 mg/kg sc) on certain days,
whereas pressing the other lever was reinforced following saline solution (1 ml/kg
sc) on other days. Rats were given injections of either nicotine or saline 10 minutes
prior to daily training sessions (4 days a week) in a double alternation sequence (i.e.,
nicotine, nicotine, saline, saline, nicotine, ...). Sessions were terminated after 30
minutes or 100 reinforcements, whichever occurred first. The discrimination criterion to determine establishment and maintenance of drug discrimination behavior was
that the appropriate lever was chosen for (a) at least 80% of the responses for the first
food pellet in a session, and also for (b) at least 80% of the responses in a session
overall, for at least five consecutive training sessions.

Cannulation. After the discrimination between nicotine (0.5 mg/kg sc) and saline
was successfully established, guide cannulas were bilaterally implanted into the lateral ventricle ($n = 10$), medial prefrontal cortex ($n = 7$), nucleus accumbens ($n = 11$),
ventral tegmental area ($n = 7$), dorsal hippocampus ($n = 9$), and medial habenular nucleus ($n = 5$) under sodium pentobarbital (Nembutal, 40 mg/kg iv) anesthesia. The
tips of the guides were located 1 mm above the final injection sites. The coordinates
for each region were as follows: lateral ventricle: 1.3 mm posterior (P), 1.9 mm lateral (L), and 3.6 mm ventral (V) to bregma; medial prefrontal cortex: 3.4 mm anterior (A), 0.8 mm (L), and 4.0 mm (V); nucleus accumbens: 1.7 mm (A), 1.4 mm (L),
and 7.1 mm (V); ventral tegmental area: 5.3 mm (P), 0.9 mm (L), and 8.1 mm (V);
dorsal hippocampus: 4.8 mm (P), 2.4 mm (L), and 3.0 mm (V); medial habenular nucleus: 3.5 mm (P), 0.25 mm (L), and 4.5 mm (V) according to the atlas of Paxinos
and Watson.[27] The guide cannula assemblies were made from No. 26 gauge stainless
steel hypodermic tubing. The injection unit consisted of a No. 33 gauge needle
attached to a 10-μl Hamilton microsyringe via a piece of polyethylene tubing. A volume of 0.4 μl solution per side for each region was injected into hand-held conscious
rats over a 30-second period. After termination of the injection, the cannula was left
in place for another 30 seconds.

Substitution Tests. After cannulation surgery, the substitution of nicotine administered directly into each cerebral region for nicotine (0.5 mg/kg sc) was tested. In
each substitution test, nicotine was tested in doses ranging from 40–140 μg (20–70
μg per side) for the lateral ventricle, 10–40 μg (5–20 μg per side) for the medial prefrontal cortex, 20–140 μg (10–70 μg per side) for the nucleus accumbens, 10–80 μg
(5–40 μg per side) for the ventral tegmental area, 5–20 μg (2.5–10 μg per side) for

the dorsal hippocampus, or 5–40 μg (2.5–20 μg per side) for the medial habenular nucleus. Saline in a volume of 0.4 μl per side was also administered into each region as control. The substitution tests were interspersed with daily discrimination training sessions and were only performed again after the discrimination criterion just described had been satisfied for at least three consecutive daily discrimination training sessions. In the substitution test sessions, the procedure was identical with that in the discrimination training sessions except for the duration of a test session (2 minutes) and the fact that every tenth consecutive response on either lever elicited reinforcement. Following the experiment, the rats were killed under deep pentobarbital anesthesia, and the injection sites were identified histologically. Data were discarded from rats in which the injection sites were not found to be clearly within the expected regions.

Data Analysis. The percentage of nicotine-appropriate response data and the response rate data were analyzed with a one-way repeated measures analysis of variance (ANOVA) followed by post-hoc Dunnett's tests ($p < 0.05$) where appropriate.

RESULTS

Rats attained the training criterion for the establishment of nicotine discrimination within 64 sessions (about 4 months) from the beginning of the experiment. Once the discrimination behavior was established, it was stable throughout the experiment.

The results of the substitution tests are presented in TABLES 1 and 2. With saline administered into each cerebral region, the mean percentage of nicotine-appropriate responses ranged between 0.6 and 3.4%, and the mean total response rate per minute ranged between 27.1 and 50.9 across groups.

Substitution Tests with Nicotine Administered into the Lateral Ventricle

Nicotine administered into the lateral ventricle increased the mean percentage of nicotine-appropriate responses in a dose-dependent manner [$F(6, 54) = 15.656, p < 0.001$]. The maximum percentage of nicotine-appropriate responses was 85.3% at 100 μg ($p < 0.01$), and eight of ten rats showed 80% or more nicotine-appropriate responses at this dose. Nicotine administered into the lateral ventricle decreased the mean total response rate per minute [$F(6, 54) = 3.841, p < 0.01$], and a significant decrease was observed at 140 μg ($p < 0.05$).

Substitution Tests with Nicotine Administered into the Medial Prefrontal Cortex

Nicotine administered into the medial prefrontal cortex increased the mean percentage of nicotine-appropriate responses in a dose-dependent manner [$F(3, 18) = 24.481, p < 0.001$]. The maximum percentage of nicotine-appropriate responses was 88.2% at 40 μg ($p < 0.05$), and four of seven rats showed 80% or more nicotine-appropriate responses at this dose. Nicotine administered into the medial prefrontal cortex did not change the mean total response rate per minute [$F(3, 18) = 0.793, p > 0.05$].

TABLE 1. Results of substitution tests with nicotine administered into each brain region in rats discriminating nicotine (0.5 mg/kg, sc) from saline

Brain region and drugs	Doses (μg/rat)	Nicotine-appropriate responses (%)[a]	Response rate per min[a]	n/N[b]
Lateral ventricle				
Saline	1 μl	0.7 ± 0.3	48.6 ± 5.6	0/10
Nicotine	40	22.0 ± 14.5	57.5 ± 8.9	2/10
Nicotine	60	50.8 ± 16.3	61.0 ± 3.9	5/10
Nicotine	80	59.8 ± 14.0	47.4 ± 8.2	5/10
Nicotine	100	85.3 ± 10.1	54.7 ± 6.3	8/10
Nicotine	120	83.0 ± 12.5	50.9 ± 9.7	6/10
Nicotine	140	62.8 ± 19.0	20.3 ± 7.9*	3/10
Medial prefrontal cortex				
Saline	0.4 μl	1.0 ± 1.0	27.1 ± 2.3	0/7
Nicotine	10	1.0 ± 1.0	33.6 ± 3.3	0/7
Nicotine	20	37.1 ± 17.8	26.4 ± 5.7	2/7
Nicotine	40	88.2 ± 7.0	26.6 ± 5.2	4/7
Nucleus accumbens				
Saline	0.4 μl	0.6 ± 0.4	50.9 ± 4.9	0/11
Nicotine	20	19.3 ± 12.1	53.7 ± 1.8	2/11
Nicotine	40	46.2 ± 15.5	50.6 ± 7.5	5/11
Nicotine	60	46.3 ± 15.2	50.1 ± 5.8	5/11
Nicotine	80	51.2 ± 14.4	51.7 ± 4.3	4/11
Nicotine	100	77.6 ± 12.1	45.5 ± 8.1	8/11
Nicotine	120	66.2 ± 16.4	38.6 ± 6.6	6/11
Nicotine	140	75.0 ± 25.0	14.1 ± 7.5**	3/11
Ventral tegmental area				
Saline	0.4 μl	3.4 ± 1.6	38.9 ± 5.4	0/7
Nicotine	10	24.0 ± 16.2	44.3 ± 2.4	1/7
Nicotine	20	55.4 ± 14.7	40.2 ± 7.5	3/7
Nicotine	40	58.7 ± 16.2	28.6 ± 8.1	3/7
Nicotine	60	60.6 ± 17.4	24.4 ± 6.7	3/7
Nicotine	80	47.5 ± 20.5	10.1 ± 7.2	2/7

[a]Mean and SE during each 2-min test session.

[b]n/N indicates the number of rats showing 80% or more nicotine-appropriate responses (n) out of the total number of rats tested (N).

*$p < 0.05$; **$p < 0.01$ compared to saline control (Dunnett's test).

TABLE 2. Results of substitution tests with nicotine administered into each brain region in rats discriminating nicotine (0.5 mg/kg, sc) from saline

Brain region and drugs	Doses (μg/rat)	Nicotine-appropriate responses (%)[a]	Response rate per min[a]	n/N[b]
Dorsal hippocampus				
Saline	0.4 μl	1.6 ± 0.9	30.9 ± 3.1	0/9
Nicotine	5	3.0 ± 2.5	31.1 ± 7.3	0/9
Nicotine	10	44.1 ± 17.2	25.0 ± 7.6	3/9
Nicotine	20	30.5 ± 16.8	16.3 ± 5.1	2/9
Medial habenular nucleus				
Saline	0.4 μl	2.3 ± 2.3	29.5 ± 1.9	0/5
Nicotine	5	2.2 ± 2.0	32.7 ± 1.6	0/5
Nicotine	10	3.2 ± 2.1	35.5 ± 3.0	0/5
Nicotine	40	2.2 ± 1.2	10.1 ± 4.5***	0/5

[a]Mean and SE during each 2-min test session.
[b]n/N indicates the number of rats showing 80% or more nicotine-appropriate responses (n) out of the total number of rats tested (N).
***$p < 0.001$ compared to saline control (Dunnett's test).

Substitution Tests with Nicotine Administered into the Nucleus Accumbens

Nicotine administered into the nucleus accumbens increased the mean percentage of nicotine-appropriate responses in a dose-dependent manner [$F(7, 70) = 18.358$, $p < 0.001$]. The maximum percentage of nicotine-appropriate responses was 77.6% at 100 μg ($p < 0.05$), and 8 of 11 rats showed 80% or more nicotine-appropriate responses at this dose. Nicotine administered into the nucleus accumbens decreased the mean total response rate per minute [$F(7, 70) = 3.761, p < 0.01$], and a significant decrease was observed at 140 μg ($p < 0.01$).

Substitution Tests with Nicotine Administered into the Ventral Tegmental Area

Nicotine administered into the ventral tegmental area increased the mean percentage of nicotine-appropriate responses [$F(5, 30) = 5.033$, $p < 0.01$]. The maximum percentage of nicotine-appropriate responses was 60.6% at 60 μg ($p < 0.05$), and three of seven rats showed 80% or more nicotine-appropriate responses at this dose. Nicotine administered into the dorsal hippocampus tended to decrease the mean total response rate per minute, but the change did not reach a significant level [$F(5, 30) = 2.016, p < 0.05$].

Substitution Tests with Nicotine Administered into the Dorsal Hippocampus

Nicotine administered into the dorsal hippocampus tended, but not significantly, to increase the mean percentage of nicotine-appropriate responses [$F(3, 24) = 2.351$, $p > 0.05$]. The maximum percentage of nicotine-appropriate responses was 44.1% at 10 μg, and three of nine rats showed 80% or more nicotine-appropriate responses at this dose. Nicotine administered into the dorsal hippocampus tended to decrease the mean total response rate per minute, but the change did not reach a significant level [$F(3, 24) = 2.662, p > 0.05$].

Substitution Tests with Nicotine Administered into the Medial Habenular Nucleus

Nicotine administered into the medial habenular nucleus did not increase the mean percentage of nicotine-appropriate responses [$F(3, 12) = 0.845, p > 0.05$]. The maximum percentage of nicotine-appropriate responses was 3.2% at 10 μg, and none of five rats showed 80% or more nicotine-appropriate responses. Nicotine administered into the medial habenular nucleus decreased the mean total response rate per minute [$F(3, 12) = 19.995, p < 0.001$], and a significant decrease was observed at 40 μg ($p < 0.001$).

DISCUSSION

As Chance et al.[8] and Schechter[9] reported, our studies showed that nicotine (100 and 120 μg) administered into the lateral ventricle substituted for nicotine (0.5 mg/kg sc), which confirmed the mediation of the DS effects of nicotine by a central mechanism. The main purpose of our studies was to clarify the involvement of the mesolimbocortical dopaminergic neurons in manifesting the DS effects of nicotine. In the substitution tests with nicotine administered into each region of the mesolimbocortical dopaminergic neurons, nicotine administered into the medial prefrontal cortex and the nucleus accumbens substituted for sc injected nicotine, and the degree of substitution observed in the aforementioned two regions (88.2 and 77.6% of nicotine-appropriate responses at 40 μg in the medial prefrontal cortex and at 100 μg in the nucleus accumbens, respectively) was almost equivalent to that in the lateral ventricle (85.3% of nicotine-appropriate responses at 100 μg). However, the fact that the dose of nicotine for substitution was higher in the nucleus accumbens (100 μg) than in the medial prefrontal cortex (40 μg) and was almost equivalent to that in the lateral ventricle (100 and 120 μg) indicates that the nucleus accumbens is less sensitive to nicotine than the medial prefrontal cortex in manifesting the DS effects of nicotine. These results thus suggest that involvement of the medial prefrontal cortex is more significant than that of the nucleus accumbens. On the other hand, a lesser degree of substitution (58.7 and 60.6% of nicotine-appropriate responses at 40 μg and 60 μg, respectively) was observed in the ventral tegmental area than in the aforementioned two regions. However, the sensitivity to nicotine in the ventral tegmental area was higher than that in the nucleus accumbens and was almost equivalent to that in the medial prefrontal cortex in terms of the dose range of nicotine tested. These results suggest that the ventral tegmental area is also partially involved in the DS effects of nicotine. These findings may indicate that the medial prefrontal cortex is primarily involved in the DS effects of nicotine, whereas the nucleus accumbens and the ventral tegmental area are only partially involved. The results reported by Shoaib and Stolerman,[28] which indicate that nicotine administered into the nucleus accumbens did not substitute for the training dose of sc injected nicotine, contradict the aforementioned findings. The inconsistency in the results of the substitution tests between the two studies may depend on the methodologic differences of the experiments. For example, (1) the test doses (20–140 μg) of nicotine were quite high in our studies compared with those (2–8 μg) used in their study; (2) the training dose (0.5 mg/kg) of nicotine was also higher in our studies than that (0.2 mg/kg) used in their study; and (3) the discrimination criterion for the substitution tests was set more strictly in our studies than in their study, that is, at least 80% nicotine-appropriate responses both for the first food pellet in the session and for the session overall was required for at least three consecutive training sessions in our studies, whereas a difference of greater than 60% between the percentage of nicotine-appropriate responses after sc injection of nicotine and saline was required in their study.

As for the cerebral regions that possess high densities of nicotinic cholinergic receptors, the role of the dorsal hippocampus and the medial habenular nucleus in mediating the DS effects of nicotine was investigated. Nicotine (10 μg) administered into the dorsal hippocampus produced 44.1% of the maximum nicotine-appropriate responses, which is almost equivalent to 51.8% at 8 μg of the corresponding value reported by Meltzer and Rosecrans.[25] However, in contrast to their report indicating involvement of the dorsal hippocampus in the DS effects of nicotine, in our studies statistical analysis failed to demonstrate that significant effects of nicotine administered into the above region on nicotine-appropriate responses. The reason for the inconsistency in the results between the two studies is not clear, but the differences in the experimental procedures are considered to be related to the contradictory findings. For example, (1) the training dose (0.5 mg/kg) of nicotine was lower in our studies than that (1.14 mg/kg) used in their study; and (2) the schedule of reinforcement was FR-10 in our studies, whereas it was a variable-interval 12-second schedule in their study. As for the medial habenular nucleus, nicotine administered into that region did not substitute for nicotine (0.5 mg/kg sc). These results suggest that neither the dorsal hippocampus nor the medial habenular nucleus is involved in the DS effects of nicotine.

A problem in our studies[16–18] was that the doses of nicotine for substitution were relatively high in comparison with those in other studies.[25,28] However, the dose range of nicotine in our studies was wide enough to cover both the lower doses producing no changes in the total response rate and the higher doses producing either obvious effects on nicotine-appropriate responses or decreases in the response rate. Thus, the selection of the drug doses seemed to be appropriate. One possibility to explain the discrepancy in the doses of nicotine for substitution is that the training criterion for nicotine discrimination reached 64 sessions (about 4 months) in our studies, which is a longer period than that reported in other studies.[25,28] Therefore, tolerance to certain effects of nicotine may have developed more markedly during the training sessions in our studies than in other studies. Another more likely possibility is that cerebral regions other than those tested in our studies or complex neural networks rather than a single neural system are involved in mediating the DS effects of nicotine. In support of this possibility, Meltzer and Rosecrans[25] reported the involvement of the mesencephalic reticular formation, in which the presence or absence of cholinergic receptors is not clear. These questions await resolution.

In conclusion, our studies suggest that the mesolimbocortical dopaminergic neurons are involved in the DS effects of nicotine. The mesolimbocortical dopaminergic neurons are known to play a prominent role in the reinforcing effects of nicotine.[29,30] Therefore, it is considered that the neural mechanisms of the DS effects of nicotine may overlap with those of the reinforcing effects of nicotine, which suggests that cues of the DS effects of nicotine are associated with the reinforcing effects of nicotine to a certain degree. Furthermore, our studies also demonstrated that the involvement of each region of the mesolimbocortical dopaminergic neurons was different in degree. That is, the medial prefrontal cortex is primarily involved in the DS effects of nicotine, whereas the nucleus accumbens and the ventral tegmental area are partially involved.

ACKNOWLEDGMENTS

This work was supported by grants from the Smoking Research Foundation.

REFERENCES

1. JAFFE, J.H. 1990. Drug addiction and drug abuse. *In* The Pharmacological Basis of Therapeutics. A.G. Gilman, T.W. Rall, A.S. Nies and P. Taylor, eds.: 522–573. Pergamon Press. New York.
2. JARVIK, M.E. 1973. Further observations on nicotine as the reinforcing agent in smoking. *In* Smoking Behavior: Motives and Incentives. W.L. Dunn, ed.: 33–49. Winston. Washington, DC.
3. RUSSELL, M.A.H. 1976. Tobacco smoking and nicotine dependence. *In* Research Advances in Alcohol and Drug Problems. R.J. Gibbins, Y. Israel, H. Kalant, R.E. Popham, W. Schmidt, & R.G. Smart, Eds.: 1–47. John Wiley & Sons. New York.
4. ROMANO, C., A. GOLDSTEIN & N.P. JEWELL. 1981. Characterization of the receptor mediating the nicotine discriminative stimulus. Psychopharmacology 74: 310–315.
5. HIRSCHHORN, I.D. & J.A. ROSECRANS. 1974. Studies on the time course and the effect of cholinergic and adrenergic receptor blockers on the stimulus effects of nicotine. Psychopharmacologia 40: 109–120.
6. STOLERMAN, I.P., H.S. GARCHA, J.A. PRATT & R. KUMAR. 1984. Role of training dose in discrimination of nicotine and related compounds by rats. Psychopharmacology 84: 413–419.
7. STOLERMAN, I.P., R. KUMAR & C. REAVILL. 1988. Discriminative stimulus effects of cholinergic agonists and the actions of their antagonists. *In* Transduction Mechanisms of Drug Stimuli. F.C. Colpaert and R.L. Balster, eds.: 32–43. Springer-Verlag. Berlin.
8. CHANCE, W.T., M.D. KALLMAN, J.A. ROSECRANS & R.M. SPENCER. 1978. A comparison of nicotine and structurally related compounds as discriminative stimuli. Br. J. Pharmacol. 63: 609–616.
9. SCHECHTER, M.D. 1973. Transfer of state-dependent control of discriminative behaviour between subcutaneously and intraventricularly administered nicotine and saline. Psychopharmacologia 32: 327–335.
10. SCHECHTER, M.D & J.A. ROSECRANS. 1972. Nicotine as a discriminative cue in rats: inability of related drugs to produce a nicotine-like cueing effect. Psychopharmacologia 27: 379–387.
11. STOLERMAN, I.P. 1990. Behavioural pharmacology of nicotine: implications for multiple brain nicotinic receptors. *In* The Biology of Nicotine Dependence (Ciba Foundation Symposium 152). G. Bock and J. Marsh, eds.: 3–22. Wiley. Chichester.
12. SCHECHTER, M.D & J.A. ROSECRANS. 1972. Nicotine as a discriminative stimulus in rats depleted of norepinephrine or 5-hydroxytryptamine. Psychopharmacologia 24: 417–429.
13. ROSECRANS, J.A., W.T. CHANCE & M.D. SCHECHTER. 1976. The discriminative stimulus properties of nicotine, d-amphetamine and morphine in dopamine depleted rats. Psychopharmacol. Commun. 2: 349–356.

14. CHANCE, W.T., D. MURFIN, G.M. KRYNOCK & J.A. ROSECRANS. 1977. A description of the nicotine stimulus and tests of its generalization to amphetamine. Psychopharmacology **55:** 19–26.
15. SCHECHTER, M.D. & S.M. MEEHAN. 1992. Further evidence for the mechanisms that may mediate nicotine discrimination. Pharmacol. Biochem. Behav. **41:** 807–812.
16. ANDO, K., H. MIYATA, N. HIRONAKA, *et al.* 1993. The discriminative effects of nicotine and their central sites in rats. Jpn. J. Psychopharmacol. **13:** 129–136.
17. MIYATA, H., K. ANDO & T. YANAGITA. 1991. Studies on the involvement of the nucleus accumbens in the discriminative effects of nicotine in rats. (Abstr.) Nippon Yakurigaku Zasshi **98:** 389–397.
18. MIYATA, H., K. ANDO & T. YANAGITA. 1999. Medial prefrontal cortex is involved in the discriminative stimulus effects of nicotine in rats. Psychopharmacology **145:** 234–236.
19. CLARKE, P.B.S. & A. PERT. 1985. Autoradiographic evidence for nicotine receptors on nigrostriatal and mesolimbic dopaminergic neurons. Brain Res. **348:** 355–358.
20. SWANSON, L.W., D.M. SIMMONS, P.J. WHITING & J. LINDSTROM. 1987. Immunohistochemical localization of neuronal nicotinic receptors in the rodent central nervous system. J. Neurosci. **7:** 3334–3342.
21. WADA, E. *et al.* 1989. Distribution of alpha2, alpha3, alpha4, and beta2 neuronal nicotinic receptor subunit m-RNAs in the central nervous system: a hybridization histochemical study in the rat. J. Comp. Neurol. **284:** 314–335.
22. CALABRESI, P., M.G. LACEY & R.A. NORTH. Nicotinic excitation of rat ventral tegmental neurones *in vitro* studies by intracellular recording. Br. J. Pharmacol. **98:** 135–140.
23. IMPERATO, A., A. MULUS & G. DI CHIARA. 1986. Nicotine preferentially stimulates dopamine released in the limbic system of freely moving rats. Eur. J. Pharmacol. **132:** 337–338.
24. LAPIN, E.P., H.S. MAKER, H. SERSHEN & A. LAJTHA. Action of nicotine on accumbens dopamine and attenuation with repeated administration. Eur. J. Pharmacol. **160:** 53–59.
25. MELTZER, L.T. & J.A. ROSECRANS. 1981. Investigations on the CNS sites of action of the discriminative stimulus effects of arecoline and nicotine. Pharmacol. Biochem. Behav. **15:** 21–26.
26. NIEUWENHUYS, R., J. VOOGD & VAN C. HUIJZEN. 1988. The Human Central Nervous System: A Synopsis and Atlas. Springer-Verlag. Berlin.
27. PAXINOS, G. & C. WATSON. 1986. The Rat Brain in Stereotaxic Coordinates. Academic Press. San Diego.
28. SHOAIB, M. & I.P. STOLERMAN. 1996. Brain sites mediating the discriminative stimulus effects of nicotine in rats. Behav. Brain Res. **78:** 183–188.
29. CORRIGALL, W.A., K.B.J. FRANKLIN, K.M. COEN & B.S. CLARKE. 1992. The mesolimbic dopaminergic system is implicated in the reinforcing effects of nicotine. Psychopharmacology **107:** 285–289.
30. CORRIGALL, W.A. 1991. Understanding brain mechanisms in nicotine reinforcement. Br. J. Addiction **86:** 507–510.

Nicotine Reduces the Secretion of Alzheimer's β-Amyloid Precursor Protein Containing β-Amyloid Peptide in the Rat without Altering Synaptic Proteins

D.K. LAHIRI,[a] T. UTSUKI,[b] D. CHEN,[a] M.R. FARLOW,[a] M. SHOAIB,[b]
D.K. INGRAM,[b] AND N.H. GREIG[b]

[a]Laboratory of Molecular Neurogenetics, Department of Psychiatry
and Neurology, Institute of Psychiatric Research, Indiana University
School of Medicine, Indianapolis, Indiana 46202, USA

[b]Laboratory of Neurosciences, Intramural Research Program,
National Institute on Aging, Baltimore, Maryland 21224, USA

ABSTRACT: Alzheimer's disease (AD) is characterized by cerebrovascular deposition of the amyloid β-peptide (Aβ), which is derived from a larger β-amyloid precursor protein (βAPP). Altered metabolism of βAPP, resulting in increased Aβ production, appears central in the neuropathology of AD. The processing of the holoprotein βAPP by different "secretase" enzymes results in three major carboxyl-truncated species. One species, which results from the cleavage of βAPP by γ-secretase, is secreted into the cerebrospinal fluid (CSF) and is called sAPPγ as it contains an intact Aβ domain. Moreover, AD is characterized by cholinergic dysfunction and the loss of synaptic proteins. Reports of an inverse relation between nicotine intake, due to cigarette smoking, and the incidence of AD prompted us to investigate the effects of nicotine on βAPP processing and synaptic proteins in rats and in cell culture. Nicotine, 1 and 8 mg/kg/day, doses commensurate with cigarette smoking, and a higher but well tolerated dose, respectively, was administered over 14 days to rats. Levels of sAPP in the CSF sample were evaluated by Western blot analysis. The higher dose significantly increased levels of total sAPP; however, both doses significantly reduced sAPPγ, which contains the amyloidogenic portion of Aβ. These actions were blocked by nicotinic receptor antagonism. Nicotinic antagonists alone had no effect on either total sAPP or sAPPγ levels in CSF. Nicotine did not significantly change the intracellular levels of total βAPP in rat brain extracts, which is consistent with neuronal cell culture data. Similarly, levels of vesicular protein, such as synaptophysin, and presynaptic terminal protein SNAP-25 were unaffected by nicotine treatment both *in vivo* and in cell culture experiments. Taken together, these results suggest that nicotine modifies βAPP

Address for correspondence: Dr. D.K. Lahiri, Institute of Psychiatric Research, Indiana University School of Medicine, Room No. PR-313, 791 Union Drive, Indianapolis, IN 46202-4887. Voice: 317-274-2706; fax: 317-274-1365.
  dlahiri@iupui.edu

Ann. N.Y. Acad. Sci. 965: 364–372 (2002). © 2002 New York Academy of Sciences.

processing away from the formation of potentially amyloidogenic products, without altering the levels of synaptic proteins, and that this can potentially offer therapeutic potential for Alzheimer's disease.

KEYWORDS: nicotine; Alzheimer's disease; β-amyloid precursor protein; β-amyloid peptide; cholinergic system; synaptic proteins

INTRODUCTION

Alzheimer's disease (AD) is characterized by a severe loss of presynaptic cholinergic neurons and decreased levels of acetylcholine and choline acetyl transferase in the cortex.[1] Inhibition of cholinergic activity in the central nervous system (CNS) of patients with AD correlates with deterioration in scores on dementia rating scales.[2] Several lines of investigation suggest that the nicotinic cholinergic system, like the muscarinic system, is involved in memory processing and in AD.[3,4] First, epidemiologic studies have reported a consistent inverse relation between nicotine intake, as a consequence of cigarette smoking, and the incidence of AD.[5] These findings suggest that nicotine reduces the risk of AD through some protective mechanism. Second, a marked loss occurs in the total number of nicotinic cholinergic receptors (nAChR) in the AD brain.[6] This loss is generally more substantial than the reduction found in muscarinic cholinergic receptors (mAChR) in AD[1] and contrasts with the higher density of nAChRs reported present in the brain of normal smokers.[7,8] Third, the degree of cognitive impairment found in AD correlates well with the central cholinergic deficiency.[2] Fourth, acute and chronic nicotine administration has improved the cognitive performance of both animals and healthy humans, and studies have demonstrated small improvements in patients with AD.[3,9] By contrast, deficits in cognitive performance can be produced by selective nicotinic antagonism induced by mecamylamine administration.[10,11]

Chronic nicotine administration is known to upregulate its own receptor number,[12] possibly attenuating the deficit found in AD. Whether these receptors are functional remains to be elucidated. Nicotine additionally affects the release of several neurotransmitters depleted in AD. Recent results suggest that cholinergic activity regulates the synthesis, processing, and secretion of βAPP,[13] which is the source of the putative AD toxic peptide amyloid beta-peptide (Aβ) that contains 40–42 amino acids.[14] Neuronal cells constitutively secrete Aβ, which can be detected in CSF. In AD, a major neurochemical change is the cortical extracellular and vascular deposition of the 4-kDa peptide Aβ, which is derived from a larger (110–130 kDa) glycosylated membrane-bound beta-amyloid precursor protein (βAPP).[14] The holoprotein βAPP is processed by alternative proteolytic pathways to generate different breakdown products.[14] In a secretory pathway, three different secretases have been implicated. First, a constitutively expressed putative α-secretase enzyme bisects the Aβ domain within βAPP to release carboxyl-truncated soluble derivatives (sAPPα) in the CSF and in the conditioned media of cells. A majority of βAPP is processed by α-secretase to generate nonamyloidogenic sAPPα. Second, beta-secretase cleaves βAPP on the amino side of Aβ to produce a large secreted derivative (sAPPβ), which does not contain intact Aβ. Third, gamma-secretase cleaves βAPP on the carboxyl side of Aβ, producing another secreted derivative (sAPPγ), which contains intact Aβ. The synthesis, processing, and secretion of βAPP and its derivatives occur *in vivo* in the brain[14,15] and also in cell cultures.[16,17] Identification of factors regulating these processes could be central to both understanding and preventing the pathogenesis of AD. In the present study, we report that nicotinic stimulation alters the secretion of total sAPP *in vivo* and reduces levels of potentially amyloidogenic sAPPγ. To understand possible mechanisms, we performed pharmacologic manipulations to alter levels of both total sAPP and sAPPγ in the CSF of rats. In addition to the amyloid pathway, there is a severe loss of (1) presynaptic protein markers, such as SNAP-25, and (2) vesicular proteins, such as synaptophysin, in AD. Synaptophysin (SYPH), which is a 38-kDa phosphoprotein, is a synaptic vesicle-associated integral membrane protein.[19] SNAP-25, a synaptosomal associated protein, is located at the presynaptic terminal, and these proteins are involved in neuronal transmission. From the reported beneficial effect of nicotine on cognition and memory, based on epidemiologic and initial clinical studies, it is reasonable to hypothesize that nicotine may synergistically regulate the processing of βAPP and of presynaptic terminal proteins in a way that can lead to lowered levels of Aβ without compromising neuronal transmission. We therefore, additionally, investigated the levels of synaptophysin and SNAP-25 in nicotine-treated rat brain tissue samples.

MATERIAL AND METHODS

Material and Preparation. Nicotine, chlorisondamine, and mecamylamine hydrochloride were purchased from Research Biochemicals International (Natick, MA). Osmotic minipumps (Alzet, Palo Alta, CA, 2ML2, 4.84 ml/h) were used for the administration of nicotine, mecamylamine, and scopolamine and were implanted sc to provide steady-state levels of these normally only short-acting agents. Osmotic pumps for control groups administered buffered saline solution alone. All pumps were incubated at 37°C (5 hours) to attain equilibration prior to subcutaneous implantation, which was undertaken under aseptic conditions. Chlorisondamine was dissolved into buffered artificial CSF and administered by lateral ventricle injection (5 μg in 5 μl). Appropriate control animals received similar injections of buffered artificial CSF.

In Vivo Pharmacologic Treatment. Male Fischer-344 rats, weighing between 300 and 350 g (22–24 months old) and obtained from the NIA colony maintained by Harlan Sprague-Dawley (Indianapolis, IN), were separated into groups of 8–12 animals and treated for 14 days as described (Utsuki *et al.*, manuscript in preparation). Thereafter, rats were killed, and total brain and CSF were immediately obtained from the cisterna magna, frozen, and kept at −80°C until assay.

Detection of Secreted Forms of sAPP. Levels of total sAPP in CSF samples (5 μl) were assayed by immunoblot analysis using 10% tris-glycine gels (Novex, San Diego, CA). Proteins were blotted onto polyvinylidene difluoride (PVDF) paper (Novex) and probed with affinity-purified anti-βAPP antibody 22C11 (Roche Molecular Biochemicals, Indianapolis, IN). The 22C11 clone recognizes all mature forms of βAPP as well as the APP-like proteins (APLP). The latter, however, migrate at a slightly different rate, to ~70 kDa, and were not quantitated. CSF samples (20 μl) were assayed for levels of sAPPγ, specifically sAPP with at least the 1–28 sequence of Aβ attached, by using 266 antibody (courtesy of Elan Corporation, San

Francisco, CA) directed to residues 13–28 of Aβ. Immunoluminescence, ECL (Amersham Life Science Inc., Arlington Heights, IL), was used for visualizing total βAPP, sAPPγ, and sAPPβ, and densitometric quantification was undertaken using a CCD camera and NIH-IMAGE (version 4.1).

Detection of the Levels of Different Intracellular Proteins. Briefly, cortical tissue sections from each rat brain were homogenized with a Brinkman PT 10/35 homogenizer for 10 seconds in IP buffer containing Tris-Cl, pH 7.4, NaCl, NP-40, sodium, and a cocktail of protease inhibitors.[17] They were centrifuged at $11,000 \times g$ for 20 minutes at 4°C, and the proteins of the supernatant solution (cell lysate) were measured. Thirty micrograms of protein from the total cell lysate were separated on a 12% polyacrylamide gel containing sodium dodecyl sulfate (SDS-PAGE), and immunoblot analysis was performed as described previously. Each blot was sequentially probed with four different antibodies: (1) mouse monoclonal IgG (22C11) against the N-termnius of βAPP, (2) goat polyclonal IgG against the carboxyl terminus of SNAP-25, (3) goat polyclonal IgG against the amino terminus of synaptophysin, and (4) goat polyclonal IgG against the carboxyl terminus of β-actin. The preceding three antibodies were obtained from Santa Cruz Biotechnology, Santa Cruz, CA.

Statistics. A two-tailed Student's t test was carried out to compare two means. When more than two means were compared, one-way analysis of variance together with a Bartlett's test for homogeneity of variance and a Dunnett's multiple comparison test was used. The level of significance was defined as $p < 0.05$.

RESULTS

To investigate the effect of nicotine *in vivo* in rats, we measured (1) the secreted levels of sAPP species in the extracellular fluid and (2) the intracellular levels of βAPP holoprotein, SYPH, SNAP-25, and β–actin in the rat brain extracts, as described below.

Nicotine Treatment Reduced the Release of Total sAPPγ in Rat CSF. The presence of secreted total sAPP and sAPPγ was detected in rat CSF samples by Western blot analysis at ~90–110 kDa (based on molecular mass markers; data not shown). In contrast to controls, nicotine administration dramatically reduced levels of secreted sAPPγ. For instance, nicotine (1 and 8 mg/kg/day) significantly reduced CSF levels of sAPPγ to $36.3 \pm 4.7\%$ and $52.0 \pm 4.1\%$ of control values, respectively (as measured by mAb 266). By contrast, neither the long-acting nicotinic antagonist chlorisondamine nor the noncompetitive antagonist mecamylamine significantly altered CSF levels of sAPPγ ($90.5 \pm 9.7\%$ and $105.2 \pm 10.2\%$ of controls, respectively).

Coadministration of Chlorisondamine Blocked the Nicotine-Mediated Reduction of sAPPγ. Notably, coadministration of chlorisondamine to rats administered nicotine (8 mg/kg/day) prevented nicotine's ability to reduce CSF sAPPγ, and resulting levels were no different from those of controls (nicotine $59.3 \pm 6.5\%$ versus nicotine + chlorisondamine $83.7 \pm 7.6\%$ of controls). The action of nicotine on levels of total sAPP in CSF was different from that on sAPPγ (see below and TABLE 1).

Nicotine Treatment at Low Doses Had No Effect on the Release of Total sAPP in Rats CSF. The action of nicotine on levels of total sAPP in CSF was measured using mAb 22C11 antibody that recognizes all forms of the amyloid precursor protein. Nicotine (1 mg/kg/day) did not significantly alter the level of total sAPP in CSF

TABLE 1. Summary of the Western immunoblot results with different proteins

Treatments	Dose	sAPPγ	Total sAPP	Total βAPP (β-actin adjusted)	SYPH (β-actin adjust.)	SNAP-25 (β-actin adjust.)
		90–110 kDa	95–115 kDa	110–130 kDa	38 kDa	25 kDa
		mAb 266	mAb 22C11	mAb 22C11	C-terminus Ab	C-terminus Ab
Control	—	—	—	—	—	—
Nicotine	1 mg/kg/day	Decreased	Unchanged	Unchanged	Unchanged	Unchanged
Nicotine	8 mg/kg/day	Decreased	Increased	Unchanged	Unchanged	Unchanged
Chlorisondamine	5 μg in 5 μL icv	Unchanged	Unchanged	Unchanged	Unchanged	Unchanged
Mecamylamine	9 mg/kg/day	Unchanged	Unchanged	Unchanged	Unchanged	Unchanged
Nicotine + chlorisondamine	8 mg/kg/day 5 μg in 5 μL icv	Unchanged	Unchanged	Not done	Not done	Not done

NOTE: The effects of nicotine and other treatment on levels of sAPPγ, total sAPP, total βAPP, synaptophysin (SYPH), and synaptosomal associated protein (SNAP-25) were compared with respect to the control as described in the text.

(105.1 ± 4.9% of controls), whereas nicotine (8 mg/kg/day) significantly elevated total sAPP levels (146 ± 10.5% of controls). Similar to that found for sAPPγ measurement, the nicotinic antagonists chlorisondamine and mecamylamine did not significantly alter levels of total sAPP in CSF (107.6 ± 8.7% and 94.2 ± 3.5% of their respective controls), and coadministration of chlorisondamine to rats administered nicotine (8 mg/kg/day) likewise blocked the ability of nicotine to increase total sAPP in CSF.

Nicotine Treatment Had No Effect on Levels of Total βAPP and Synaptic Proteins. At the intracellular level, we examined the profile of βAPP bands in brain extracts from either vehicle-treated or nicotine (2 doses)-treated rats by Western blotting analysis. Using 22C11 antibody, we detected full-length βAPP as 110–130 kDa protein bands of 695–770 amino acids in different samples. There was no significant change in its level with nicotine treatment (data not shown). As expected, the βAPP holoprotein was found to be a slower migrating band (larger) than either sAPP or sAPPγ. When the immunoblot was probed with anti-SYPH antibody, we observed synaptophysin as a 38-kDa protein band, but no change occurred in SYPH levels with nicotine treatment under our conditions. A similar result with nicotine was obtained with SNAP-25 protein, which migrates as a 25-kDa band. For comparative purposes, all these proteins were adjusted against levels of a constitutive protein, β-actin, that yielded a characteristic 43-kDa band in our Western blot (TABLE 1).

DISCUSSION

The present study illustrates that nicotine at both a low dose (1 mg/kg/day), consistent with that achieved by smoking,[3–5] and a high but well tolerated dose (8 mg/kg/day) significantly lowered the level of sAPPγ (sAPP containing the amyloidogenic sequence) in the CSF of rats *in vivo*. As compared to that in controls, levels of total sAPP in the CSF of the same animals were unchanged by the lower nicotine dose and were significantly elevated by the higher dose. This indicates that nicotine modifies the normal processing of βAPP, away from βAPPγ, to favor a nonamyloidogenic route and, additionally, that a high dose elevates the secretion of sAPP, which does not contain the amyloidogenic sequence. This interpretation should be discussed in the light of the following perspective. First, to ensure steady-state conditions between brain and CSF, this study was undertaken over a protracted period of 14 days. Our prior studies demonstrated that cortical tissue total βAPP levels, which would include both cellular and secreted protein, mirror those determined in CSF.[15,18] Secondly, we view CSF and, hence, brain levels of sAPPγ in rat as a potential source of Aβ, as beta-secretase, which is minimally present in rat, has a potential to cleave sAPPγ to release Aβ. In both naive adult and elderly rats, secreted sAPP within the CSF was predominantly in the form of sAPPγ, the form first described by Anderson *et al.*,[20] with minimal amounts of Aβ.[15] Likewise in the present study, readily detectable amounts of secreted total sAPP and sAPPγ were present in CSF as determined by probing with mAbs 22C11 and 266, respectively. The latter is directed to a portion of Aβ beyond the cleavage point of α-secretase, Aβ$_{17}$, and it thus contains at least the Aβ$_{1-28}$ portion, which has been shown to be sufficient to cause neurotoxicity. Third, in contrast, levels of sAPPβ in CSF, as detected by mAb 92, were minimal in all groups and were unaltered by nicotine. Fourth, the present study did not differentiate between the various forms of CSF sAPP (695, 751, and 770). It is therefore possible that in addition to the described changes in the levels of total sAPP or sAPPγ, the ratio of the sAPP isoforms may also have changed to a lesser or greater degree. Fifth, the present study did not include the measurements of Aβ species, such as Aβ40 and Aβ42, as well as different carboxyl-terminal fragments (CTFs). The physiologic consequences of changes in these, however, remain yet to be fully elucidated.

Our demonstration of altered processing of total sAPP, away from sAPPγ, to favor a nonamyloidogenic route by nicotine 1 mg/kg/day is significant. It reduced sAPPγ levels by 63.7% without significantly affecting the total soluble sAPP and intracellular βAPP levels. Studies by Monteggia et al.[21] demonstrated that continuous administration of a comparable dose of nicotine (approximately 1.5 mg/kg/day) does not alter either total βAPP mRNA or the relative percentage of βAPP isoforms associated with it. Together with our study, this suggests that such doses of nicotine act to modify the processing and not the synthesis or relative abundance of βAPP isoforms.

In our experience, a higher but nevertheless well tolerated dose of nicotine (8 mg/kg/day), which is known to induce dependence in rodents,[21] significantly increased CSF levels of total sAPP, and, similar to the lower nicotine dose, significantly decreased sAPPγ levels. The reduction of sAPPγ levels, coupled with an increase in the CSF levels of total sAPP and no change in the minimal level sAPPβ, leads, by subtraction, to an increase in the levels of carboxyl-terminally truncated forms of sAPP in CSF which do not contain an amyloidogenic sequence, that is, sAPPα. Indeed, in vitro studies by Kim et al.[23] reported that nicotine, in both a time- and concentration-dependent (1-100 μM) manner, increased the secretion of carboxyl-terminally truncated forms of βAPP, termed βAPP^s and equivalent to sAPPα, from PC12 cells without affecting the ratio of the isoforms. Several studies have demonstrated that sAPP possesses both potent trophic and protective activities in a variety of cell culture models, promoting neurite outgrowth and cellular proliferation as well as cell survival.[24] In addition, in vivo studies have reported that i.c.v. administration of a peptide sequence representing a trophic domain of βAPP^s increased both memory retention and synaptic density in cortical tissue[25] and reduced neurologic damage in an animal model of ischemia.[6]

Inhibition of the effects of nicotine on both sAPPγ and total sAPP by selective nicotinic antagonism (chlorisondamine) indicates that the observed actions occur via a specific interaction with the neuronal nAChR, as chlorisondamine blocks the nAChR ion channel. The neuronal nAChR is a ligand-gated ion channel that exists as various subtypes in a temporally and regionally specific pattern and that is formed from a combination of at least eight α-like, $α_2$–$α_9$, and three β-like, $β_2$–$β_4$, subunit isoforms.[26] Nicotinic receptor subtypes have been studied in human brain aging, Alzheimer and Lewy body diseases.[8] Additionally, decreased uptake and binding of [^{11}C]-nicotine in brain of AD patients were visualized by positron emission tomography. Studies strongly implicate Ca^{2+} cellular entry via nAChR voltage-sensitive Ca^{2+} channels, with corresponding activation of assorted Ca^{2+}-dependent cellular processes.[27,28] This is critical not only for neurotransmitter release but likely also for βAPP regulation. The nicotinic antagonists chlorisondamine and mecamylamine alone did not alter CSF levels of either sAPPγ or total sAPP. These nicotinic antagonists were administered in concentrations known to produce substantial nAChR inhibition.[10,11] The demonstration that nicotine administration in the rat, in levels readily achieved in man, alters the processing of ßAPP *in vivo* away from an amyloidogenic route has a number of potential physiologic consequences in man. The expected elevated levels of carboxyl-terminally truncated forms of sAPP that are known to have trophic actions could account for the widely described neuroprotective role of nicotine.[24] Nicotine also has been reported to inhibit Aβ aggregation *in vitro*.[29] Recently, the roles of nicotine and its receptor on sAPP secretion and Aβ or CT(105)-induced toxicity were studied.[30–32] Clearly, cerebral nAChR stimulation has favorable actions on cognitive performance, which may prove beneficial in the treatment of AD dementia. In conclusion, the early use of safe and well tolerated agents that beneficially modulate the processing of βAPP towards trophic rather than toxic products to potentially delay the onset of AD represents perhaps the best therapeutic strategy for future AD treatment.

ACKNOWLEDGMENTS

We would like to acknowledge the support of grants from Axonyx, the Alzheimer's Association (IIRG), and the National Institutes of Health.

REFERENCES

1. GUELA, C. & M.M. MESULUM. 1994. The cholinergic system. *In* Alzheimer's Disease. R.D. Terry, R. Katzman, and K.L. Blick, Eds.: 263–303. Raven. New York.
2. PERRY, E.K. *et al.* 1978. Correlation of cholinergic abnormalities with senile plaques and mental test scores in senile dementia. Br. Med. J. **2:** 1457–1459.
3. NEWHOUSE, P.A. *et al.* 2001. Nicotinic treatment of Alzheimer's disease. Biol. Psychiatry **49:** 268–278.
4. REZVANI, A.H. & E.D. LEVIN. 2001. Cognitive effects of nicotine. Biol. Psychiatry **49:** 258–267.
5. LEE, P.N. 1994. Smoking and Alzheimer's disease: a review of the epidemiological evidence. Neuroepidemiology **13:** 131–144.
6. KELLAR, K.J. *et al.* 1987. Muscarinic and nicotinic binding sites in Alzheimer's disease cerebral cortex. Brain Res. **436:** 62–68.
7. BENWELL, M.E.M. *et al.* 1988. Evidence that tobacco smoke increased the density of [^{3}H]-nicotine binding sites in human brain. J. Neurochem. **50:** 1243–1247.
8. PERRY, E. *et al.* 2000. Nicotinic receptor subtypes in human brain ageing, Alzheimer and Lewy body diseases. Eur. J. Pharmacol. **393:** 215–222.
9. SAHAKIAN, B.J. *et al.* 1989. The effect of nicotine on attention, information processing and short-term memory in patients with dementia of the Alzheimer's type Br. J. Psychiatry **154:** 797–800.
10. CLARKE, P.B.S. & R. KUMAR. 1983. Characterization of the locomotor stimulant action of nicotine in tolerant rats. Br. J. Pharmacol. **80:** 587–594.
11. EL-BIZRI, H. *et al.* 1995. Intraneuronal accumulation and persistence of radiolabel in rat-brain following *in vivo* administration of [H^3]-chlorisondamine. Br. J. Pharmacol. **116:** 2503–2509.
12. MARKS, M.J. *et al.* 1983. Effects of chronic nicotine infusion on tolerance development and nicotinic receptors. J. Pharmacol. Exp. Ther. **226:** 817–826.
13. NITSCH, R.M. *et al.* 1992. Release of Alzheimer amyloid precursor derivatives stimulated by activation of muscarinic acetylcholine receptors. Science **258:** 304–307.

14. SELKOE, D.J. 1997. Alzheimer's disease: genotypes, phenotype, and treatment. Science
    275: 630–631.
15. WALLACE, W.C. *et al.* 1995. Chronic elevation of secreted amyloid precursor protein in
    subcortically lesioned rats, and its exacerbation in aged rats. J. Neurosci. **15:** 4896–
    4905.
16. LAHIRI, D.K. *et al.* 1994. Tacrine alters the secretion of beta-amyloid precursor protein
    in cell lines. J. Neurosci. Res. **37:** 777–787.
17. LAHIRI, D.K. *et al.* 1998. The secretion of amyloid beta-peptides is inhibited in the
    tacrine-treated human neuroblastoma cells. Mol. Brain Res. **62:** 131–140.
18. HAROUTUNIAN, V. *et al.* 1997. Pharmacological modulation of Alzheimer's β-amyloid
    precursor protein levels in the CSF of rats with forebrain cholinergic system lesions.
    Mol. Brain Res. **46:** 161–168.
19. SCHELLER, R.H. 1995. Membrane trafficking in the presynaptic nerve terminal. Neuron
    14: 893–897.
20. ANDERSON, J.P. *et al.* 1992. An alternative secretase cleavage produces soluble Alzhe-
    imer amyloid precursor protein containing a potentially amyloidogenic sequence. J.
    Neurochem. **59:** 2328–2331.
21. MONTEGGIA, L.M. *et al.* 1994. Nicotine effects on the regulation of amyloid precursor
    protein splicing, neurotrophin and glucose transporter RNA levels in aged rats. Int. J.
    Dev. Neurosci. **12:** 133–142.
22. MALIN, D.H. *et al.* 1992. Rodent model of nicotine abstinence syndrome. Pharmacol.
    Biochem. Behav. **43:** 779–784.
23. KIM, S.H. *et al.* 1997. Enhanced release of secreted form of Alzheimer's amyloid pre-
    cursor protein from PC12 cells by nicotine. Mol. Pharm. **52:** 430–436.
24. ROBERSON, M.R. & L.E. Harrell. 1997. Cholinergic activity and amyloid precursor pro-
    tein metabolism. Brain Res. Rev. **25:** 50–69.
25. ROCH, J.M. *et al.* 1994. Increase of synaptic density and memory retention by a peptide
    representing the trophic domain of the amyloid β/A4 protein precursor. Proc. Natl.
    Acad. Sci. USA. **91:** 7450–7454.
26. LEUTJE, C. & J. PATRICK. 1991. Both α and β subunits contribute to the agonist sensi-
    tivity of neuronal nicotinic receptors. J. Neurosci. **7:** 2153–2162.
27. MULLE, C. *et al.* 1992. Calcium influx through nicotinic receptor in rat central neu-
    rons: its relevance to cellular regulation. Neuron **8:** 135–143.
28. VERNINO, S. *et al.* 1992. Calcium modulation and high calcium permeability of neu-
    ronal nicotinic acetylcholine receptors. Neuron **8:** 127–134.
29. SALOMON, A.R. *et al.* 1996. Nicotine inhibits amyloid formation by the beta-peptide.
    Biochemistry **35:** 13568–13578.
30. SEO, J. *et al.* 2001. Effects of nicotine on APP secretion and Abeta- or CT(105)-
    induced toxicity. Biol. Psychiatry **49:** 240–247.
31. SHIMOHAMA, S. & T. KIHARA. 2001. Nicotinic receptor-mediated protection against
    beta-amyloid neurotoxicity. Biol. Psychiatry **49:** 233–239.
32. ZENG, H. *et al.* 2001. Nicotine and amyloid formation. Biol. Psychiatry **49:** 248–257.

Serotonergic Neurotoxicity of MDMA (Ecstasy) in the Developing Rat Brain

JERROLD S. MEYER[a] AND SYED F. ALI[b]

[a]Department of Psychology, Neuroscience and Behavior Program,
University of Massachusetts, Amherst, Massachusetts 01003, USA

[b]Neurochemistry Laboratory, Division of Neurotoxicology,
National Center for Toxicological Research, Jefferson, Arkansas 72079, USA

ABSTRACT: The abused drug 3,4-methylenedioxymethamphetamine (MDMA) damages fine serotonergic fibers and nerve terminals in adult organisms; however, developing animals seem less susceptible to this effect. One proposed hypothesis is that neonates are less sensitive to MDMA neurotoxicity because they fail to show drug-induced hyperthermia. We tested this hypothesis by producing hyperthermia in neonatal rats for 2 hours after each of twice-daily MDMA (10 mg/kg sc) or saline injections given over the period from postnatal day (PD) 1 to 4. Other drug-treated and control litters were maintained at normothermic temperatures after injection. Differential core body temperatures were achieved by placing pups (without the dam) in humidified, thermostatically controlled incubators. Temperatures were monitored with a thermocouple probe at 30-minute intervals. Pups subsequently remained undisturbed until sacrifice at PD 25 and PD 60 for assessment of serotonergic damage by measuring 5-HT transporter (SERT) binding in the hippocampus and neocortex as well as 5-HT and 5-HIAA concentrations (PD 25 only). Neonatal MDMA exposure led to significant reductions in both SERT binding and 5-HT levels in the hippocampus at PD 25, independent of body temperature during treatment. Hippocampal SERT binding increased between PD 25 and PD 60 in both the MDMA and saline groups, but the MDMA-related deficit remained unchanged. Interestingly, the neocortex showed no effect of MDMA at PD 25, but SERT binding was significantly reduced at PD 60. Thus, MDMA can exert serotonergic neurotoxicity in developing animals in the absence of elevated body temperature. Hippocampal serotonergic innervation is damaged early, whereas neocortical effects emerge at a later time. Furthermore, the tendency for serotonergic recovery may be less after neonatal MDMA exposure than exposure of adult animals.

KEYWORDS: neurotoxicity; 3,4-methylenedioxymethamphetamine; MDMA; ecstasy; brain

Address for correspondence: Jerrold S. Meyer, Ph.D., Department of Psychology, Tobin Hall, University of Massachusetts, Amherst, MA 01003. Voice: 413-545-2168; fax: 413-545-0996. jmeyer@psych.umass.edu

Ann. N.Y. Acad. Sci. 965: 373–380 (2002). © 2002 New York Academy of Sciences.

INTRODUCTION

The use of 3,4-methylenedioxymethamphetamine (MDMA, or Ecstasy) among adolescents and young adults has been rising.[1] Within this group are many women of child-bearing age, and there are now at least three published reports of MDMA use during pregnancy.[2–4] Nevertheless, epidemiologic data on the overall prevalence of MDMA use by pregnant women are unavailable, nor is it known whether developmental MDMA exposure causes neurologic or behavioral deficits in human offspring.

In adult animals and possibly humans as well, MDMA exerts a neurotoxic action on the serotonin (5-HT) system by pruning serotonergic fibers and terminals from forebrain target areas such as the neocortex and hippocampus.[5,6] This effect can be produced by a single moderate dose of MDMA, although even greater deficits are observed with multiple dose regimens. Studies examining the effects of prenatal or neonatal MDMA exposure have indicated that immature animals are less susceptible than adults to the drug's serotonergic effects. For example, offspring of pregnant rats given MDMA either twice-daily or once every other day showed no changes in brain 5-HT or 5-hydroxyindoleacetic acid (5-HIAA), despite the fact that levels of these compounds were significantly reduced in the brains of the dams.[7,8] Rat pups given a single dose of as much as 40 mg/kg MDMA on postnatal day (PD) 10 displayed a temporary decline in frontal cortical 5-HT concentration that returned to normal within 72 hours postinjection.[9] Multiple doses of MDMA given to pups over a period of either 4 days or 10 days do cause later reductions in 5-HT levels or 5-HT transporter (SERT) binding; however, the effect sizes are smaller than would be expected from the same treatments given to adult rats.[10,11]

The fact that repeated exposure to MDMA can produce serotonergic deficits in developing animals raises obvious concerns for human infants born of MDMA-using women. On the other hand, it is not yet clear why the neurotoxic effects are less severe during development. One hypothesis to explain this disparity stems from the finding that MDMA treatment leads to significant hyperthermia in adult animals but not in infants.[11,12] Because the hyperthermic response to MDMA contributes to its effects on the 5-HT system in adults, Broening and coworkers[12] proposed that the lack of hyperthermia in infants is an important factor in their relative resistance to MDMA neurotoxicity.

The current study was designed to test the hyperthermia hypothesis more thoroughly than in previous work. This was accomplished by treating rat pups with MDMA twice daily from PD 1 through PD 4 and by subjecting half of the litters to a 2-hour period of severe hyperthermia after each of the eight treatments. Control pups received saline vehicle injections, and half of those litters were subjected to the same hyperthermic challenge. Serotonergic projections to the neocortex and hippocampus were assessed neurochemically at approximately PD 25 and PD 60 to determine the long-term effects of neonatal treatment and to ascertain whether such effects were exacerbated by inducing hyperthermia during periods of MDMA exposure.

METHODS

Sprague-Dawley rats (Charles River CD strain) were bred in our laboratory. On the day after birth (PD 1), litters were culled to eight (usually four males and four females) and were randomly assigned to one of four treatment groups: MDMA-treated low-temperature, MDMA-treated high-temperature, saline-treated low-temperature, and saline-treated high-temperature ($n = 6$–7 litters per group). MDMA pups received s.c. injections of 10 mg/kg (±)-MDMA HCl (Sigma Chemical Co., St. Louis) in saline b.i.d. The first injection was given in the morning between 0900 and 1100 hours; the second injection was given in the afternoon between 1300 and 1500 hours. Saline pups received s.c. injections of physiological saline at the same times.

After each litter was injected, the pups were placed together in a $13 \times 13 \times 5$ cm polypropylene container with a shallow bedding of wood shavings. Each container was covered but was ventilated by means of holes drilled in the sides and top. The containers and their pups were then placed for a 2-hour period inside a thermostatically controlled incubator (Boekel model 133000) with a water trough at the bottom to provide humidification. The incubator for the low-temperature groups was set to a temperature of 31°C, which we determined in preliminary studies would maintain the core body temperature (35–36°C) that is normal for this age.[13] The high-temperature groups were placed in an incubator set to 37°C, which was designed to raise core body temperature to 39–40°C, which is maximum amount of hyperthermia typically produced in adult rats given a relatively high dose of MDMA.[14] For each 2-hour period in the incubators, one pup per litter was chosen in a pseudorandom manner (balanced across gender) to have its core temperature monitored at 30-minute intervals using a Physitemp model IT-18 thermocouple probe (0.625 mm diameter) attached to a Physitemp TH-5 digital thermometer.

Two (one male and one female) pups from each litter were removed on PD 5 for determination of apoptotic activity in the brain (results to be presented elsewhere). All litters otherwise remained undisturbed until PD 24–26, at which time two additional pups (either one male and one female, or two females) per litter were lightly anesthetized by CO_2 inhalation and were then killed by decapitation. The hippocampus and parietal cortex were rapidly dissected, frozen on dry ice, and stored at −70°C for subsequent neurochemical analyses. The remaining animals were weaned and group-housed by litter and gender. At PD 5–61, another male was killed and brain samples were obtained as before. For the sake of convenience, subsequent references to the PD 24–26 and PD 59–61 time points will be shortened to PD 25 and PD 60, respectively.

PD 25 hippocampal and cortical samples from one animal per litter were analyzed for 5-HT, dopamine (DA), and their respective metabolites by high-performance liquid chromatography with electrochemical detection.[15] Tissue samples from littermates killed at PD 25 and PD 60 were homogenized in ice-cold buffer consisting of 10 mM sodium phosphate, 120 mM sodium chloride, and 5 mM potassium chloride, pH 7.4. Washed membrane fractions prepared from these homogenates were assayed in triplicate for 5-HT transporter (SERT) binding using a fixed 1.0 nM concentration of [³H]paroxetine (21.5 Ci/mmol; New England Nuclear) with or without 10 µM unlabeled imipramine to define nonspecific binding.[16] Membrane protein concentrations were measured by means of the Bradford dye-binding method with bovine gamma globulin as the standard.[17]

All data were analyzed statistically by analyses of variance (ANOVA) with drug treatment and incubator condition as independent variables. For core temperature and body weight measurements during the 4-day treatment period, we also included day as a repeated measures factor.

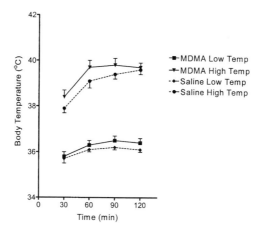

FIGURE 1. Time course of core body temperature of rat pups as a function of treatment and incubator condition (high or low temperature). Values are shown as the mean ± SEM averaged across gender and across the 4 treatment days (PD 1–4). There was a highly significant effect of incubator condition ($p < 0.001$) but no significant effect of MDMA treatment.

RESULTS

Temperature measurements verified that the incubator conditions produced the desired hyperthermic and normothermic core body temperatures in the pups (FIG. 1). There was a slight trend for the MDMA-treated pups to have higher body temperatures than the controls, although this difference failed to reach statistical significance. MDMA administration led to significantly slower weight body gain during the treatment period (data not shown). By PD 25, however, there was no significant difference between MDMA-treated and control animals.

Production of hyperthermia had no effect on any of the neurotransmitter or metabolite concentrations measured at PD 25 except that hippocampal levels of homovanillic acid (HVA) were significantly increased in both saline and MDMA groups that had been placed in the high-temperature incubator (not shown). Consequently, the neurotransmitter and metabolite data were pooled across incubator condition for the purpose of presentation. Serotonin concentrations in the hippocampus were significantly reduced in the MDMA group compared to the saline controls (TABLE 1). There was a trend for 5-HIAA levels to be lower as well; however, this difference did not reach statistical significance. Surprisingly, 5-HT and 5-HIAA concentrations in the neocortex were unaffected by MDMA at PD 25. There were no group differences in either the hippocampus or cortex in the levels of DA or its metabolites dihydroxyphenylacetic acid (DOPAC) or HVA.

Results of the SERT binding assays are shown in FIGURE 2. Importantly, the data from PD 25 are completely consistent with the 5-HT measurements. That is, MDMA pretreatment was associated with a significant 20% reduction in SERT binding in the hippocampus, but there was no change at all in the neocortex. Comparing the PD 60 binding data with those obtained at PD 25 shows that there was an expected age-

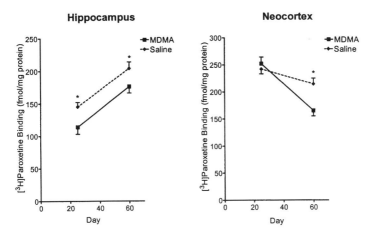

FIGURE 2. [³H]Paroxetine binding to SERT in the hippocampus and neocortex of rats at PD 25 and PD 60 as a function of neonatal treatment. *MDMA-treated animals showed a significant reduction in hippocampal SERT binding across both time points, whereas SERT binding in the neocortex was reduced only at PD 60 (all $p < 0.05$).

TABLE 1. Regional neurotransmitter and metabolite concentrations at PD 25

Neurotransmitter/metabolite	Saline	MDMA
	(ng/100 mg wet tissue weight)	
Neocortex		
5-HT	12.14 ± 0.54	12.56 ± 1.02
5-HIAA	8.51 ± 0.31	8.80 ± 0.40
DA	45.40 ± 3.64	46.85 ± 8.34
DOPAC	22.45 ± 0.74	22.47 ± 1.52
HVA	12.28 ± 0.60	12.55 ± 0.88
Hippocampus		
5-HT	17.97 ± 1.00	$14.02 \pm 1.17^*$
5-HIAA	8.20 ± 0.46	6.99 ± 0.63
DA	ND	ND
DOPAC	ND	ND
HVA	3.73 ± 0.37	3.43 ± 0.71

*Significantly different ($p < 0.025$) from the saline group. Note that all data have been collapsed across incubator condition because body temperature generally had no effect on neurotransmitter and metabolite concentrations (see text). ND, not detected.

related increase in SERT density in the hippocampus. However, the difference between the MDMA and control groups remained the same at both ages, with no evidence for convergence over time. Even more strikingly, at PD 60 there was now a significant MDMA-related decrease in SERT binding in the cortex. Consequently, an effect of MDMA emerged at PD 60 that was not present at PD 25.

DISCUSSION

There are several important findings from the present study. First, we found no evidence that changes in body temperature contribute to the differences in serotonergic neurotoxicity produced by MDMA in neonatal compared to adult rats. Second, the results show that the present dosing regimen leads to long-lasting (i.e., at least until PD 60) serotonergic deficits in both hippocampus and neocortex, but that the effect in the cortex emerges some time after PD 25. Third, the differences between MDMA and control groups in hippocampal SERT binding were similar at PD 25 and PD 60, suggesting a lack of "catch-up" growth following the initial neurotoxic insult.

In adult rats, MDMA-induced hyperthermia persists for a number of hours after the treatment.[14] For purposes of the present study, however, we did not wish to subject either the MDMA-treated or control pups to an excessive period of maternal deprivation. Consequently, we chose a period of 2 hours for exposure of litters to their respective incubators while being separated from the dam. It could be argued that only 2 hours of hyperthermia following each MDMA dose was insufficient to reveal an effect of elevated body temperature. However, we emphasize that there were eight such periods (twice-daily dosing for 4 days), which should have been ample to demonstrate a role for hyperthermia if such a role was important. Therefore, we conclude that there must be some other factor responsible for the difference between neonatal and adult rats in their sensitivity to MDMA-induced serotonergic neurotoxicity. Aguirre and colleagues[18] have suggested that an immaturity of the DA system is the key variable that causes pups to be more resistant to the effects of MDMA. Further studies are necessary to confirm this hypothesis.

The neocortex unexpectedly showed no effect of MDMA at PD 25 but a significant serotonergic deficit at PD 60. There are at least two possible explanations for this result. First, it is possible that in this brain area, the neonatal treatment produced an immediate insult to the ingrowing serotonergic fibers that did not manifest itself until much later in development. Various developmental studies with serotonergic drugs other than MDMA have found complex, time-related changes in 5-HT uptake sites.[19,20] Such findings indicate that the effects of early serotonergic perturbations depend on how these perturbations interact with the normal developmental trajectory of the serotonergic system. Second, the delayed loss of SERT binding could be partly related to the fact that our sample of neocortical tissue included the barrel field of primary somatosensory cortex (S-1). In this area of cortex, which receives input from the rat's vibrissae, the thalamocortical afferents transiently express SERT during postnatal development. Boylan and coworkers[21] recently demonstrated the presence of thalamocortical-associated SERT binding in S-1 as late as PD 30. If these SERT-expressing but nonserotonergic fibers are not damaged by MDMA, then their presence at PD 25 but not at PD 60 might contribute to the lack of a treatment effect at the earlier time point.

Based on both neurochemical studies of SERT binding and immunostaining for serotonergic axons, adult rats treated with MDMA exhibit a gradual recovery of their forebrain 5-HT innervation. Although maximal recovery may take up to a full year, partial regrowth can be seen much earlier. For example, in one study by Battaglia and colleagues[22] in which rats were given twice-daily injections of 20 mg/kg MDMA for 4 days, 5 weeks post-treatment was sufficient for a noticeable increase of [³H]paroxetine-labeled binding sites. In contrast, there was no evidence in the present study for recovery of SERT binding over the 5-week period between PD 25 and PD 60. With respect to the hippocampus, the amount of [³H]paroxetine binding in the MDMA group was reduced to the same extent at PD 60 as it was at PD 25. And as discussed earlier, there emerged in the neocortex an MDMA-related deficit in binding that was not apparent at PD 25. It will be important to determine whether MDMA exposure during the neonatal period potentially causes permanent damage to the serotonergic system. To address this question, we are currently performing SERT immunohistochemistry on brain sections from littermates of the present subjects that were killed at approximately 9 months of age. The density of SERT-immunoreactive fibers in various forebrain areas will be assessed to determine whether there are long-lasting decreases in serotonergic innervation associated with neonatal MDMA treatment.

In conclusion, a typical multidose regimen of MDMA given to newborn rat pups led to subsequent reductions in SERT binding in the hippocampus and neocortex. These effects, which can be interpreted as a pruning of serotonergic fibers, emerged with a different temporal pattern in the two brain areas. Furthermore, MDMA-related serotonergic deficits were independent of experimentally induced changes in core body temperature, which argues against the hyperthermia hypothesis of differential MDMA sensitivity in neonatal vs. adult rats.

ACKNOWLEDGMENTS

The authors would like to thank Laura Marks and Bonnie Robinson for technical assistance. This research was supported by NIH grants DA 00499 and RR 11122, and a Faculty Research Grant from the University of Massachusetts.

REFERENCES

1. POPE, H.G., JR., M. IONESCU-PIOGGIA & K.W. POPE. 2001. Drug use and life style among college undergraduates: a 30-year longitudinal study. Am. J. Psychiatry 158: 1519–1521.
2. HO, E., L. KARIMI-TABESH & G. KOREN. 2001. Characteristics of pregnant women who use Ecstasy (3,4-methylenedioxymethamphetamine). Neurotoxicol. Teratol. 23: 561–567.
3. MCELHATTON, P.R. et al. 1999. Congenital anomalies after prenatal ecstasy exposure. Lancet 354: 1441–1442.
4. VAN TONNINGEN-VAN DRIEL, M.M., J.M. GARBIS-BERKVENS & W.E. REUVERS-LODEWIJKS. 1999. Pregnancy outcome after ecstasy use; 43 cases followed by the Teratology Information Service of the National Institute for Public Health and Environment. Ned. Tijdschr. Geneeskd. 143: 27–31.

5. BOOT, B.P., I.S. MCGREGOR & W. HALL. 2000. MDMA (Ecstasy) neurotoxicity: assessing and communicating the risks. Lancet **355:** 1818-1821.
6. RICAURTE, G.A., J. YUAN & U.D. MCCANN. 2000. (±)3,4-Methylenedioxymethamphetamine ('Ecstasy')-induced serotonin neurotoxicity: Studies in animals. Neuropsychobiology **42:** 5–10.
7. COLADO, M.I. *et al.* 1997. A study of the neurotoxic effect of MDMA ('ecstasy') on 5-HT neurones in the brains of mothers and neonates following administration of the drug during pregnancy. Br. J. Pharmacol. **121:** 827–833.
8. ST. OMER, V.E.V. *et al.* 1991. Behavioral and neurochemical effects of prenatal methylenedioxymethamphetamine (MDMA) exposure in rats. Neurotoxicol. Teratol. **13:** 13–20.
9. BROENING, H.W., L. BACON & W. SLIKKER, JR. 1994. Age modulates the long-term but not the acute effects of the serotonergic neurotoxicant 3,4-methylenedioxymethamphetamine. J. Pharmacol. Exp. Ther. **271:** 285–293.
10. BROENING, H.W. *et al.* 2001. 3,4-Methylenedioxymethamphetamine (Ecstasy)-induced learning and memory impairments depend on the age of exposure during early development. J. Neurosci. **21:** 3228–3235.
11. WINSLOW, J.T. & T.R. INSEL. 1990. Serotonergic modulation of rat pup ultrasonic vocal development: studies with 3,4-methylenedioxymethamphetamine. J. Pharmacol. Exp. Ther. **254:** 212–220.
12. BROENING, H.W., J.F. BOWYER & W. SLIKKER, JR. Age-dependent sensitivity of rats to the long-term effects of the serotonergic neurotoxicant (±)-3,4-methylenedioxymethamphetamine (MDMA) correlates with the magnitude of the MDMA-induced thermal response. J. Pharmacol. Exp. Ther. **275:** 325–333.
13. SULLIVAN, R.M., N. SHOKRAI & M. LEON. 1988. Physical stimulation reduces the body temperature of infant rats. Dev. Psychobiol. **20:** 225–235.
14. O'SHEA, E.R. *et al.* 1998. The relationship between the degree of neurodegeneration of rat brain 5-HT nerve terminals and the dose and frequency of administration of MDMA ('ecstasy'). Neuropharmacology **37:** 919–926.
15. ALI, S.F. *et al.* 1994. Low environmental temperatures or pharmacologic agents which produce hypothermia decrease methamphetamine neurotoxicity in mice. Brain Res. **658:** 33–38.
16. DEWAR, K.M., T.A. READER, L. GRONDIN & L. DESCARRIES. 1991. [^{3}H]Paroxetine binding and serotonin content of rat and rabbit cortical areas, hippocampus, neostriatum, ventral mesencephalic tegmentum, and midbrain raphe nuclei region. Synapse **9:** 14–26.
17. BRADFORD, M.M. 1976. A rapid and sensitive method for the quantification of microgram quantities of protein utilizing the principle of protein-dye binding. Anal. Biochem. **72:** 248–254.
18. AGUIRRE, N., M. BARRIONUEVO, B. LASHERAS & J. DEL RIO. 1998. The role of dopaminergic systems in the perinatal sensitivity to 3,4-methylenedioxymethamphetamine-induced neurotoxicity in rats. J. Pharmacol. Exp. Ther. **286:** 1159–1165.
19. SHEMER, A.V., E.C. AZMITIA & P.M. WHITAKER-AZMITIA. 1991. Dose-related effects of prenatal 5-methyoxytryptamine (5-MT) on development of serotonin terminal density and behavior. Dev. Brain Res. **59:** 59–63.
20. WHITAKER-AZMITIA, P.M., X. ZHANG & C. CLARKE. 1994. Effects of gestational exposure to monoamine oxidase inhibitors in rats: preliminary behavioral and neurochemical studies. Neuropsychopharmacology **11:** 125–132.
21. BOYLAN, C.B., C.A. BENNETT-CLARKE, N.L. CHIAIA & R.W. RHOADES. 2000. Time course of expression and function of the serotonin transporter in the neonatal rat's primary somatosensory cortex. Somatosen. Motor Res. **17:** 52–60.
22. BATTAGLIA, G., S.Y. YEH & E.B. DE SOUZA. 1988. MDMA-induced neurotoxicity: parameters of degeneration and recovery of brain serotonin neurons. Pharmacol. Biochem. Behav. **29:** 269–274.

Striatal Postsynaptic Ultrastructural Alterations Following Methylenedioxymethamphetamine Administration

F. FORNAI,[a,b] M. GESI,[a] P. LENZI,[a] M. FERRUCCI,[a] A. PELLEGRINI,[a] S. RUGGIERI,[b] A. CASINI,[c] AND A. PAPARELLI[a]

[a]Department of Human Morphology and Applied Biology, University of Pisa, Pisa, Italy

[b]I.R.C.C.S. I.N.M. Neuromed, Pozzilli, Italy

[c]Department of Experimental Pathology, University of Pisa, Pisa, Italy

ABSTRACT: Amphetamine derivatives, such as methamphetamine (METH) and 3,4-methylenedioxymethamphetamine (MDMA), act as monoaminergic neurotoxins in the central nervous system. Although there are slight differences in their mechanism of action, these compounds share a final common pathway, which involves dopamine release and oxidative stress. Apart from striatal toxicity involving monoamine axons, no previous report evidenced any alteration at the striatal level concerning postsynaptic sites. Given the potential toxicity for extracellular dopamine at the striatal level, and the hypothesis for neurotoxic effects of dopamine on striatal medium-sized neurons in Huntington's disease, we evaluated at an ultrastructural level the effects of MDMA on intrinsic striatal neurons of the mouse. In this study, administering MDMA, we noted ultrastructural alterations of striatal postsynaptic GABAergic cells consisting of neuronal inclusions shaped as whorls of concentric membranes. These whorls stained for ubiquitin but not for synuclein and represent the first morphologic correlate of striatal postsynaptic effects induced by MDMA.

KEYWORDS: dopamine; ecstasy; MDMA; whorls; ubiquitin

INTRODUCTION

Amphetamine derivatives, such as methamphetamine (METH) and 3,4-methylenedioxymethamphetamine (MDMA), act as monoaminergic neurotoxins in the central nervous system (CNS).[1] Although there are slight differences in their mechanism of action, these compounds share a final common neurotoxic mechanism, which involves oxidative stress.[2]

Address for correspondence: Francesco Fornai, Department of Human Morphology and Applied Biology, University of Pisa 56100, Pisa, Italy. Voice: +39-050-835927; fax: +39-050-835925.

f.fornai@med.unipi.it

Ann. N.Y. Acad. Sci. 965: 381–398 (2002). © 2002 New York Academy of Sciences.

In particular, METH and MDMA administration, apart from releasing serotonin (5HT), produces a marked release of dopamine (DA) in several brain areas, the striatum[3] being the main target region. Such DA release represents the triggering mechanism that induces oxidative stress.

In fact, although there are species differences in the neuronal system selectively involved in amphetamine-induced neurotoxicity,[4] DA plays a major role in the pathogenesis of the lesions.[5,6] In keeping with this, enhancement of DA metabolism, by producing toxic quinones and cysteinyl derivatives, is thought to be responsible for the rapid increase in cerebral content of free radicals and reactive oxygen species (ROS),[2,7] leading to damage of striatal DA terminals arising from the substantia nigra pars compacta (SNpc) and 5HT striatal terminals arising from the dorsal raphe nucleus. Potential neurotoxicity of cerebral DA extends not only to DA neurons, but also to the surrounding 5HT axons[8] and nonmonoaminergic neurons.[9] Recent studies lend substance to these effects, showing that endogenous DA might trigger the degeneration of striatal medium-sized γ-aminobutyric acid (GABA) neurons in Huntington's disease.[10]

The main mechanism responsible for DA-mediated neurotoxicity consists of the high production of free radicals and ROS. Indeed, neurons are particularly susceptible to the toxic effects of ROS, as compared with other cell types;[11] on the other hand, brain metabolism requires great amounts of molecular oxygen, resulting in the generation of high levels of oxygen-free radicals, also in basal conditions.[11] Therefore, the role of antioxidant systems in the CNS is critical to preventing cell death during both acute injuries and chronic degenerative disorders.[11]

Therefore, it is likely that oxidative stress might arise not only from the enhancement of free radical production, but also from the depletion of physiologic antioxidant mechanisms.

In line with this, it has been shown that MDMA produces a significant reduction in the concentrations of antioxidant molecules, such as vitamin E and ascorbic acid (AA) in the brain. This latter effect, in addition to MDMA-induced oxidative stress, can contribute to enhancing the toxicity of this neurotoxin.[12] Ascorbic acid has great importance in the CNS, where it has different effects. Recently, the key role of AA as a brain antioxidant was pointed out as consisting of scavenging aqueous free radicals and ROS and decreasing quinone formation.[13]

Accordingly, pretreatment with AA can prevent MDMA-induced hydroxyl radical formation.[12] A new enzyme, a glutathione (GSH)-dependent dehydroascorbate (DHA) reductase, plays a pivotal role in regenerating AA from its oxidation product, DHA.[14] In previous studies we localized DHA reductase within the CNS, where it was found to be particularly abundant in certain brain areas (i.e., cerebellum, striatum, rhinencephalon, brain stem, and substantia nigra). At subcellular levels, DHA reductase was found in the cytosol, in the nucleus, associated with the chromatin filaments, and spared in the axoplasm.[15] In the present study we evaluated at ultrastructural levels the occurrence of this enzyme in those subcellular compartments that appear to be affected by the administration of amphetamine derivatives.

Another system that appears crucial to counteract degenerative processes selectively involving the SNpc DA neurons is the locus coeruleus (LC), the most rostral noradrenaline (NA) complex, representing the major source of NA in the CNS. In fact, recent studies suggest that impairment of LC can increase the nigrostriatal DA toxicity produced in various experimental models.[16,17]

In the present study, therefore, we evaluated at an ultrastructural level the modulation of the NA system on subcellular alterations induced by amphetamines. Besides oxidative stress, the striatum is extremely sensitive to different types of injury such as cerebral ischemia, virus infections, and specific neuronal genetic alterations, which provoke cell suffering or degeneration.[18–20] The latter conditions involve striatal intrinsic neurons. By contrast, amphetamine derivatives have been extensively studied for their effects on striatal nerve endings arising from brain stem monoaminergic nuclei.

Therefore, apart from the well characterized methamphetamine-induced striatal toxicity involving monoamine axons, no previous report evidenced any alteration at the striatal level concerning postsynaptic sites. This refers mainly to biochemical and immunohistochemical studies. Therefore, given the potential toxicity for extracellular DA at the striatal level, as just reviewed, and the hypothesis for neurotoxic effects of DA on striatal medium-sized neurons in Huntington's disease,[10] we decided to evaluate at an ultrastructural level the effects of amphetamines on the striatal neurons of the mouse.

In addition, since, as reported above, previous studies indicated a crucial role for the endogenous NA system in conditioning the toxicity of amphetamines on DA neurons, we investigated the importance of LC integrity on amphetamine-induced ultrastructural changes in striatal neurons. For this purpose, we administered the neurotoxin N-(-2-chloroethyl)-N-ethyl-2-bromobenzylamine (DSP-4), which selectively destroys NA axons arising from LC neurons and spares extra-coeruleus NA terminals.[21]

MATERIAL AND METHODS

Animals

Male C57 Black mice (C57BL/6J) 9–10 weeks old were obtained from Harlan Industries (San Pietro al Natisone, Italy). Mice were kept under controlled conditions (12-hour light/dark cycle with lights on between 07:00 and 19:00) and were fed and allowed to drink water *ad libitum*. As the toxicity of amphetamine derivatives is highly variable, critically depending on room temperature and number of animals per cage,[8] we carefully kept a constant room temperature (21°C); 24 hours before treatment, we housed animals one per cage (size of the cage: 11 × 10 cm wide and 15 cm high), allowing the mouse to move freely inside. Animals were handled in accordance with the Guidelines for Animal Care and Use developed by the National Institutes of Health. All appropriate efforts were made to minimize animal suffering and to reduce the number of animals used.

Drug Administration

Intraperitoneal injection of neurotoxin DSP-4 hydrochloride (RBI, Natick, MA) was carried out at a dose of 50 mg/kg, which produces the maximal NA lesions in different brain areas.[8] DSP-4 solution was freshly prepared in 0.9% NaCl.

Two days after DSP-4 injection, MDMA hydrochloride (Sigma Chemical Co., St. Louis, MO) was administered at a dose of 30 mg/kg × 3, 2 hours apart, which has been shown to produce depletion of striatal DA in mice.[8] MDMA solutions were freshly prepared in distilled water. Each treatment group was composed of 10 animals.

Biochemical Procedures and HPLC Analysis

One week after treatment, the animals were killed by decapitation, and their brains were removed and dissected in order to obtain the striatum. Tissue samples were homogenized in ice-cold 0.6 mL of perchloric acid (0.1 M), and an aliquot of homogenate (50 µL) was assayed for protein content.[8] After centrifugation at 8,000 g for 10 minutes, 20 µL of the clear supernatant was injected into an HPLC system to measure levels of NA, DA, 5HT, and metabolites, as previously described.[8]

Morphological Procedures

Light Microscopy and Immunohistochemistry

Under i.p. chloral hydrate anesthesia, mice were sacrificed, and the brain was removed and frozen at −80°C until sectioning. Twenty-micrometer thick cryostate sections were mounted on slides and maintained at 37°C for 15 minutes. Slices processed for tyrosine hydroxylase (TH) were fixed in cold methanol, whereas slices for DA transporter (DAT) and glial fibrillar acidic protein (GFAP) immunohistochemistry were first fixed in 4% paraformaldehyde and then permeabilized in phosphate-buffered saline (PBS) solution with 0.1% Triton 100 SX; after washing, endogenous peroxidase activity was removed by a 30-minute wash in methanol with 0.3% hydrogen peroxide and pre-blocked with normal goat serum (Vector Laboratories, Burlingame, CA) for 2 hours. They were then incubated for 24 hours with primary antibodies (Ab-I) IgG in PBS solution containing normal goat serum. We used mouse Ab-I anti-TH IgG (Sigma Chemical Co., St. Louis, MO) diluted 1:2000; rat Ab-I anti-DAT IgG (Chemicon International, Temecula, CA) diluted 1:1000; and rabbit Ab-I anti-GFAP IgG (Chemicon International, Temecula, CA) diluted 1:400.

After careful washing, sections incubated with anti-TH and anti-DAT Ab-I were incubated with byotinylated secondary antibodies (Vector Laboratories, Burlingame, CA), washed and revealed by using the ABC kit (Vector Laboratories, Burlingame, CA), followed by diaminobenzidine as chromogen (Vector Laboratories, Burlingame, CA). Sections incubated with anti-GFAP Ab-I were then processed with a secondary fluorescein-conjugated antibody (Vector Laboratories, Burlingame, CA).

Electron Microscopy

Perfusion-Fixation. Mice were anesthetized with chloral hydrate (4 mL/kg), thoracotomized, and perfused transcardially. In a pilot series of experiments, we empirically established the optimal fixing solution: 2.0% paraformaldehyde/0.1% glutaraldehyde in 0.1 M PBS, pH 7.4.

After perfusion, brains were maintained *in situ* overnight at 4°C. They were then removed from the skull, and the caudate-putamen was dissected from a thick coronal section of brain by a clean cut, removing the surrounding white matter and cortex.

Immunocytochemical Methods. Dihydroxynonenal, α/β-synuclein, and DHA reductase immunocytochemistry were carried out using post-embedding immunogold;

ubiquitin immunocytochemistry was carried out by both immunoperoxidase pre-embedding and immunogold post-embedding.

For pre-embedding experiments, after perfusion, thin slices (approximately 200 μm) were washed in PBS, and endogenous peroxidase activity was blocked using 0.3% hydrogen peroxide. Specimens were preblocked using 10% normal goat serum and 0.2% saponine (Sigma Chemical Co., St. Louis, MO) in PBS for 20 minutes and then incubated with rabbit primary antibodies against ubiquitin (Chemicon International, Temecula, CA) in PBS containing 0.2% saponine and 1% normal goat serum for 24 hours at 4°C. Samples were further rinsed in PBS and incubated with secondary anti-rabbit peroxidase-labeled IgG (Sigma Chemical Co., St. Louis, MO) for 60 minutes at room temperature, washed carefully, and revealed with diaminobenzidine (Vector Laboratories, Burlingame, CA) for 10 minutes as a chromogen. After immunocytochemistry, samples were post-fixed in 1% OsO_4, dehydrated in ethanol, and embedded in an epon-araldite mixture.

For post-embedding experiments, we used only immunogold staining. Briefly, specimens were post-fixed in 1% OsO_4 in buffered solution, dehydrated in ethanol, and embedded in epon-araldite mixture. Thin sections, collected on nickel grids, were deosmicated in Na-metaperiodate solutions for 30 minutes at room temperature, washed in PBS (15 minutes), incubated for 24 hours with primary antibodies against ubiquitin (Chemicon International, Temecula, CA), dihydroxynonenal (kind gift from Prof. Alfonso Pompella, University of Pisa), α/β-synuclein (kind gift from Oliver Schlueter, Max Planck Institute, Goettingen), and DHA reductase, obtained as described in a previous report,[14] and finally processed as described for pre-embedding, using secondary gold conjugate antibodies (diameter 10 nm) (Sigma Chemical Co., St. Louis, MO). Control sections were incubated only with secondary antibody, and they never showed any detectable levels of immunostaining. All thin sections were contrasted with uranyl acetate and lead citrate and examined in a Jeol JEM SX 100 transmission electron microscope (TEM).

Statistical Analysis of Striatal Whorls

Striatal whorls were measured by counting the number of either cytosolic or nuclear whorls out of the total number of neurons under observation. In particular, for each animal from each different group we randomly chose two tissue blocks dissected from the dorsolateral striatum. From each block we got 10 grids, every grid containing several nonserial slices to observe 10 different neurons and count a final number of 2,000 cells.

Data concerning the percentage of whorls in the cytosol or the nucleus of striatal cells were compared using ANOVA with Sheffè post hoc analysis. Null hypothesis (H_0) was rejected when $p < 0.05$.

RESULTS

Striatal Monoamine Levels

In line with previous reports,[8] administration of MDMA to intact mice caused a significant decrease in both striatal DA and DOPAC levels as compared with controls. By contrast, striatal DA and DOPAC levels were not affected by DSP-4 treat-

TABLE 1. Effect of DSP-4 on MDMA-induced striatal DA and DOPAC loss

	CONTROL	DSP-4	MDMA	DSP-4 + MDMA
DA	120.48 ± 7.15	128.07 ± 5.14	78.34 ± 7.06*	31.11 ± 4.89**
DOPAC	8.61 ± 0.22	6.07 ± 0.36	5.41 ± 0.17*	3.10 ± 0.11**

NOTE: Striatal dopamine (DA) and DOPAC levels are expressed as ng/mg protein. Mice were sacrificed after saline (controls) or after various treatments (DSP-4, MDMA, and combined DSP-4 + MDMA administration). MDMA produces a significant striatal DA loss that is exacerbated in mice carrying a previous lesion of LC neurons induced by DSP-4. DSP-4 (50 mg/kg) administration is carried out 3 days before MDMA (30 mg/kg × 3, 2 hours apart). Values are expressed as the percentage of the means ± SEM of 10 animals per group.
*$p < 0.05$ compared with controls; **$p < 0.05$ compared with MDMA.

ment. Administration of MDMA to mice that had undergone a previous NA loss induced by the neurotoxin DSP-4 showed enhancement of MDMA-induced striatal DA and DOPAC loss (TABLE 1), but no decrease in 5HT levels (data not shown).

Striatal Immunohistochemistry

Control mice had marked immunostaining for TH, and a similar positivity was present in the striatum after DSP-4 administration (FIG. 1A and 1B). Following MDMA administration, the striatum exhibited less intense TH immunostaining (FIG. 1C), which was further reduced in NA-depleted mice receiving MDMA (FIG. 1D). Similar results were obtained with striatal DAT immunohistochemistry (data not shown). In line with that, GFAP immunohistochemistry was more intense after combined treatment (data not shown).

Normal Ultrastructural Features of Striatal Neurons

The neuronal population of the striatum consists of different pharmacological and anatomical types; correspondingly, striatal neurons exhibit a certain degree of morphological variability. Nonetheless, the most frequent cell type (>90%) is represented by medium-sized neurons, which possess a large and round nucleus, with an evident nucleolus and abundant cytosol containing cisterns of rough endoplasmic reticulum (RER) and Golgi apparatus, mitochondria, and particles of glycogen (FIG. 2A).

Striatal Ultrastructural Features after MDMA Treatment

Methylenedioxymethamphetamine administration produced morphological changes within the striatal neurons. These alterations consisted of various slight alterations in the striatal ultrastructure, which were evident in some cells as enlarged cistern clusters in the Golgi apparatus (FIG. 2B). Nonetheless, typical features appearing as intracellular concentric and multilamellar bodies known as whorls were present both in the cytosol and within the nucleus of the striatal cells, mainly in the typical medium-sized neurons (FIG. 2C and 2D). The whorls, with a diameter ranging from 0.1–2.4 μm, exhibited concentric single membranes surrounding an amor-

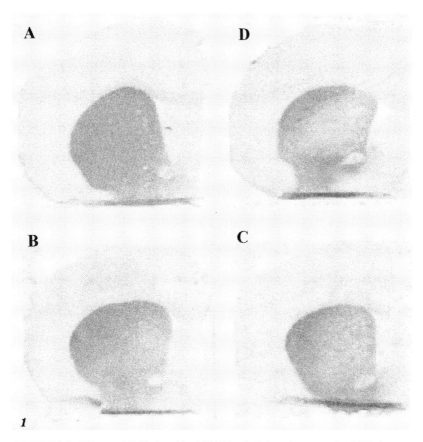

FIGURE 1. Effects of DSP-4 and/or MDMA administration on striatal TH immuno-hystochemistry. (**A**) Section from control mouse in which intense TH immunoreactivity is specifically located in the striatum. (**B**) A similar pattern occurs in section from DSP-4–treated mice. (**C**) After MDMA administration TH immunostaining is attenuated. (**D**) The immunostaining appears further reduced following DSP-4 and MDMA treatment. (X 2,9).

phous material (FIG. 2E and 2F). Apart from the different localization, no structural differences were detected between cytosolic and nuclear whorls (FIG. 2E and 2G). After MDMA administration 12.13 ± 1.69% of striatal cells showed cytosolic whorls that were often associated with smooth endoplasmic reticulum and/or the outer nuclear membrane (FIG. 2H); on the other hand, 29.02 ± 2.04% of striatal cells possessed nuclear whorls (FIG. 2G). Both cytoplasmic and nuclear whorls were absent in striatal cells of control mice.

Striatal Ultrastructural Features after DSP-4 Treatment

DSP-4 treatment induced ultrastructural modifications in striatal neurons similar to those observed after MDMA administration. Indeed, membranous whorls were observed at both cytosolic (15.8 ± 1.3%) and nuclear (25.38 ± 1.7%) levels.

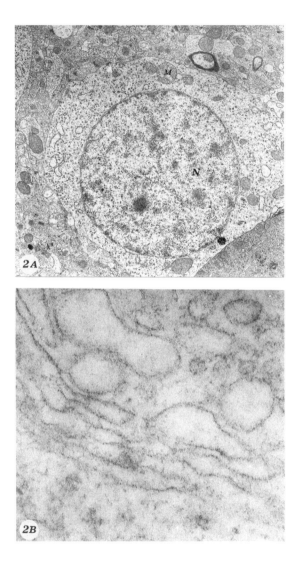

FIGURE 2. Effects of MDMA administration on the ultrastructure of striatal medium-sized neurons. (**A**) Medium-sized striatal neuron from control mouse shows round nucleus and cytoplasm rich of ribosomes and glycogen particles; cisterns of rough endoplasmic reticulum (*arrow*) and mitochondria are evident (× 7000). (**B**) After MDMA administration, Golgi apparatus shows enlargement of cisterns (× 110,000).

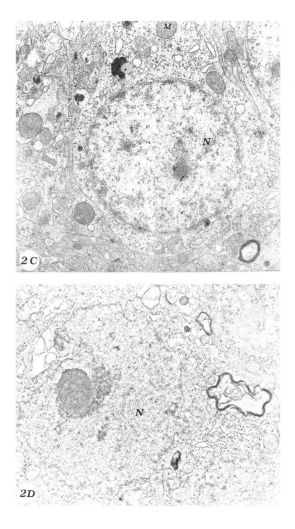

FIGURE 2—*continued*. **(C and D)** MDMA-induced membranous bodies in the nucleus and cytoplasm (*arrows*). (× 7000; × 10,000).

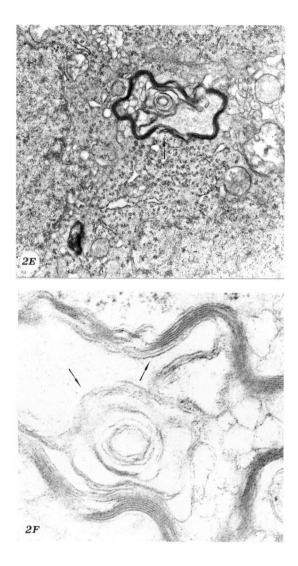

FIGURE 2—*continued*. At higher magnifications (**E and F**), a cytoplasmic membranous body shows electron-dense single membranes whorled around an amorphous material (*arrows*) (× 20,000; × 33,000).

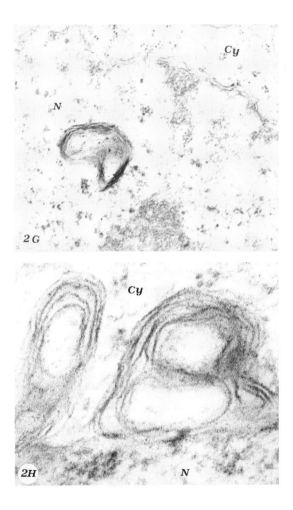

FIGURE 2—*continued.* In the nucleus (**G**), a membranous whorl appears in the neighbor of the nucleolus (Nu) (× 40,000) or (**H**) at the level of the outer nuclear envelope, where membranes are blebbing into the cytoplasm (× 130,000). Cy, cytoplasm; M, mitochondria; N, nucleus.

DSP-4 Enhances MDMA-Induced Morphological Alterations in the Striatum

Similar ultrastructural alterations, such as membranous cytosolic and nuclear whorls, were observed in the striatal cells after combined treatment (not shown). A comparable number of striatal cells (15.03 ± 1.2%) exhibited cytoplasmic membranous whorls, whereas a significant enhancement in the number of nuclear whorls (41.22 ± 2.45%) was counted, in comparison with what occurred after DSP-4 or MDMA treatment.

Immunocytochemical Characterization of the Striatal Whorls

Immunocytochemical investigation revealed that whorls were positive for ubiquitin and that the immunogold reaction was specifically located on the membrane of whorls (FIG. 3A), whereas it was not detected in the surrounding cytosol. Similar findings were obtained using immunoperoxidase (FIG. 3B). Membranous whorls also showed immunopositivity for DHA reductase (FIG. 3C), whereas they were not stained by antibodies directed against dihydroxynonenal (FIG. 3D) even when dihydroxynonenal positivity was found scattered in the nucleoplasm (FIG. 3E). Negative immunolabeling was also found for the presynaptic protein α- and β-synuclein (not shown).

DISCUSSION

Even though several hypotheses suggest a potential striatal toxicity of substituted amphetamines, to our knowledge this is the first work showing the occurrence of constant ultrastructural alterations of striatal postsynaptic GABAergic neurons. Although we did not report these data, medium-sized neurons, which have been studied here, positively stain for GAD 67 and GAD 65.

These inclusions appear as whorls of concentric membranes. Although these membranous whorls have been generally described in the brain and periphery for decades,[22,23] they remain undefined. At first, they were considered an artifact due to fixation procedures; however, it has been established that this may occur only when specimens are stored for months in glutaraldehyde.[24] In our experimental conditions storage time was limited to a few hours, and we found that these alterations occurred rarely (up to 1 in 100 cells) in control mice. In the brain, due to the abundance of phospholipids and free fatty acids, these artifacts might occur more frequently; however, it is necessary to wait for 1 month to observe an increase in whorls as a consequence of tissue storage in glutaraldehyde. The other variable, which might interfere with the formation of whorls, consists in fixation temperature. In particular, whorls increase in size as the temperature of fixation rises from 4° to 37°C.[24] In our experimental procedures we stored the tissue at 0°–4°C, ruling out even this variable.

Positive staining for ubiquitin is accompanied by positive staining for the antioxidant enzyme DHA reductase, which strongly suggests that these formations represent a functional appendix of the ubiquitin-proteasome pathway in conditions of oxidative stress. This is confirmed by the localization of whorls in association with the smooth endoplasmic reticulum and the nuclear membrane. Ascorbic acid, which is regenerated by the enzyme DHA reductase, plays an important role in preventing brain damage induced by lipid peroxidation;[25] this might explain why membranous

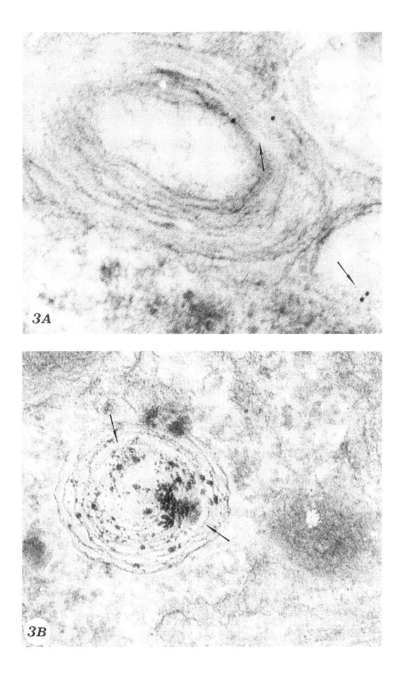

FIGURE 3. Immunocytochemistry of striatal whorls. High magnifications of whorls. (**A** and **B**) Anti-ubiquitin immunogold and immunoperoxidase staining (*arrows*) are placed on the surface of the concentric membranes (× 100,000; × 70,000).

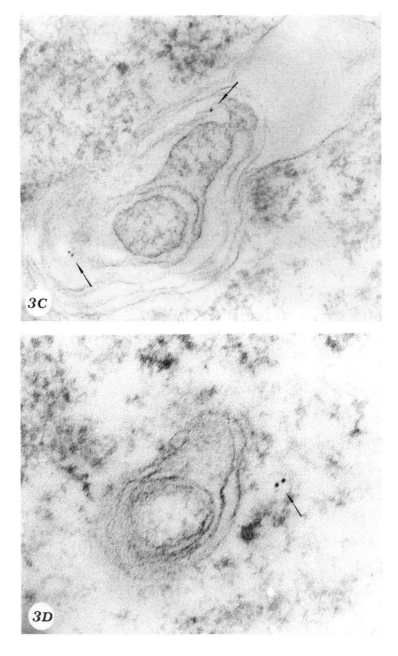

FIGURE 3—*continued*. (C) Anti-DHA reductase immunogold particles (*arrows*) are similarly placed on a whorl (× 50,000), whereas (**D**) dihydroxynonenal immunostaining (*arrow*) is located out of the external membrane of the whorl (× 100,000) and (**E**) widespread in the nucleoplasm (*arrows*) (× 80,000).

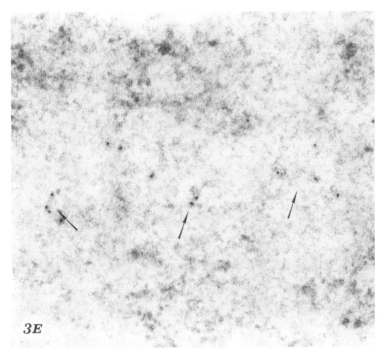

FIGURE 3—*continued.*

whorls, which possess a phospholipid structure,[26] are formed in conditions of lipid peroxidation.

Recently, membranous whorls were described in cell cultures transfected with the gene for the mutant torsinA; these inclusions positively stain for mutated torsinA, which belongs to the wide class of heat-shock proteins, which are believed to provide a protective effect against oxidative stress.[27]

Previous studies in which these ultrastructural membranous bodies were described may help again to understand their significance. They are structurally arranged similar to multivesicular bodies contained in type II pneumocytes as precursors of the lung surfactant. Interestingly, after exposure to high oxygen concentrations up to pure oxygen, there is a marked increase in these multivesicular bodies.[23] Also, following cerebral ischemia in the dorsolateral striatum, some cells show structural abnormalities consisting of cytoplasmic membranous whorls.[18]

Membranous whorls are found in several different conditions characterized by functional alterations in neurons of specific brain areas associated with hormonal deficits[28] or genetic diseases.[29] Whorls were described as a characteristic feature of a few viral infections[19] and resulted from unusual proliferation of the inner mesaxon of innumerable myelinated fibers in an experimental model of Creutzfeldt-Jacob disease.[30] Ultrastructural alterations consisting in whorls of membrane were found in axonal profiles from experimental models of Alzheimer's disease.[20] Moreover, intramitochondrial membranous whorls were observed in liver cells, after chloroform-induced hepatotoxicity,[31] and after pharmacological therapy.[32]

Ubiquitin represents a selective signal for intracytosolic protein degradation, which occurs in the proteasome. The ubiquitin-proteasome pathway has a central role in catalyzing proteolysis, and it is involved in the selective elimination of abnormal proteins.[33] Intracellular multiubiquitinated aggregates were found in some diseases such as inclusion body myositis[34] and cystic fibrosis.[35] Within the CNS, ubiquitin specifically marks intracytoplasmic inclusions such as Loewy bodies within SNpc DA neurons, LC, and other brain areas in Parkinson's disease.[36]

Ubiquitin-positive whorls, which we have observed after amphetamine treatment, might represent the morphological profile of the ubiquitin-proteasome pathway, enhanced by the neurotoxic activity of these compounds. In particular, MDMA produces hydroxyl radicals and peroxynitrite.[2] These highly reactive species can oxidase a large amount of intracellular proteins, altering their normal structures and making them ideal substrates for ubiquitin linkage and their entry into the ubiquitin-proteasome pathway.

The significance of these inclusions is still unknown. In the presence of an intact cellular machinery to recognize and degrade misfolded proteins, it is likely that these aggregation bodies could occur when the capacity of the proteasome is exceeded or their activity is inhibited.

The presence of ubiquitin in MDMA-induced whorls suggests that these formations contain misfolded proteins produced by neurotoxic treatment. For instance, it is established that both MDMA and METH produce marked striatal DA release[6] which is enhanced in mice bearing an NA lesion.[17] Interestingly, a recent study demonstrated that DA inhibits the proteasome pathway,[37] and there is evidence for such inhibition in Huntington's disease[38] in which DA release is supposed to play a causative role.[10] This might be crucial in light of new evidence showing that huntingtin inhibits the proteasome,[38] thereby making more critical the oxidative effects of DA on "proteasome-impaired" GABAergic cells.

We hypothesize that the observed membranous whorls might be the ultrastructural evidence of a functional alteration in membranes consisting of impairment of molecular trafficking.

REFERENCES

1. SEIDEN, L.S. & G.A. RICAURTE. 1987. Neurotoxicity of methamphetamine and related drugs. In Psychopharmacology: The Third Generation of Progress. H.Y. Meltzer, Ed.: 359–366. Raven Press. New York.
2. CADET, J.L. et al. 1995. Superoxide radicals mediate the biochemical effects of methylenedioxymethamphetamine (MDMA): evidence from using CuZn-superoxide dismutase transgenic mice. Synapse 21: 169–176.
3. SCHMIDT, C.J. & V.L. TAYLOR. 1987. Depression of rat brain tryptophan hydroxylase activity following the acute administration of methylenedioxymethamphetamine. Biochem. Pharmacol. 36: 747–755.
4. LOGAN, B.J. et al. 1988. Differences between rats and mice in MDMA (methylenedioxymethamphetamine) neurotoxicity. Eur. J. Pharmacol. 152: 227–234.
5. STONE, D.M. et al. 1988. Role of endogenous dopamine in the central serotonergic deficits induced by 3,4-methylenedioxymethamphetamine. J. Pharmacol. Exp. Ther. 247: 79–87.

6. O'DELL, S.J., F.B. WEIHNMULLER & J.F. MARSHALL. 1991. Multiple methamphetamine injections induced marked increases in extracellular striatal dopamine which correlate with subsequent neurotoxicity. Brain Res. **564:** 256–260.
7. FERRUCCI, M. *et al.* 2000. Recent advances in dopamine metabolism in relation to neuropsychiatric disorders. *In* Recent Research Developments in NeuroChemistry. S.G. Pandalai, ed. Vol. 3. :105–124. Research Signpost. Trivandrum, India.
8. FORNAI, F. *et al.* 2001. Biochemical effects of the monoamine neurotoxins DSP-4 and MDMA in specific brain regions of MAO-B-deficient mice. Synapse **39:** 213–221.
9. FILLOUX, F. & J.J. TOWNSEND. 1993. Pre- and postsynaptic neurotoxic effects of dopamine demonstrated by intrastriatal injection. Exp. Neurol. **119:** 79–88.
10. JAKEL, R.J. & W.F. MARAGOS. 2000. Neuronal cell death in Huntington's disease: a potential role for dopamine. Trends Neurosci. **23:** 239–245.
11. SIMONIAN, N.A. & J.T. COYLE. 1996. Oxidative stress in neurodegenerative diseases. Ann. Rev. Pharmacol. Toxicol. **36:** 83–106.
12. SHANKARAN, M., B.K. YAMAMOTO & G.A. GUDELSKY. 2000. Ascorbic acid prevents MDMA-induced hydroxyl radical formation and the behavioral and neurochemical consequences of the depletion of brain 5-HT. Soc. Neurosci. Abstr. 2321,16.
13. PARDO, B. *et al.* 1993. Ascorbic acid protects against levodopa-induced neurotoxicity on a catecholamine-rich neuroblastoma cell line. J. Neurochem. **8:** 278–284.
14. MAELLARO, E. *et al.* 1994. Purification and characterization of glutathione-dependent dehydroascorbate-reductase from the rat liver. Biochem. J. **301:** 471–476.
15. FORNAI, F. *et al.* 2001. Subcellular localization of a glutathione-dependent dehydroascorbate reductase within specific rat brain regions. Neuroscience **104:** 15–31.
16. MARIEN, M., M. BRILEY & F. COLPAERT. 1993. Noradrenaline depletion exacerbates MPTP-induced striatal dopamine loss in mice. Eur. J. Pharmacol. **236:** 487–489.
17. GESI, M. *et al.* 2000. The role of the locus coeruleus in the development of Parkinson's disease. Neurosci. Biobehav. Rev. **24:** 655–668.
18. PETITO, C.K. & W.A. PULSINELLI. 1984. Sequential development of reversible and irreversible neuronal damage following cerebral ischemia. J. Neuropathol. Exp. Neurol. **43:** 141–153.
19. LIBERSKI, P.P. *et al.* 1989. Serial ultrastructural studies in hamster. J. Comp. Pathol. **101:** 429–442.
20. OSRE-GRANITE, M.L. *et al.* 1996. Age-dependent neuronal and synaptic degeneration in mice transgenic for the C terminus of the amyloid precursor protein. J. Neurosci. **16:** 6732–6741.
21. FRITSCHY, J.M. & R. GRZANNA. 1989. Immunohistochemical analysis of the neurotoxic effects of DSP-4 identifies two populations of noradrenergic axon terminals. Neuroscience **30:** 181–197.
22. STOECKENIUS, W. 1962. The molecular structure of lipid-water systems and cell membrane models studied with the electron microscope. *In* The Interpretation of Ultrastructure. R.J.C. Harris, Ed.: 349–360. Academic Press. New York.
23. ROSENBAUM, R.M., M. WITTNER & M. LENGER. 1969. Mitochondrial and other ultrastructural changes in great alveolar cells of oxygen-adapted and poisoned rats. Lab. Invest. **20:** 516–528.
24. ROBARDS, A.W. & A.J. WILSON. 1994. Fixatives and fixation. *In* Procedures in Electron Microscopy. A.W. Robards and A.J. Wilson, Eds.: 5:1.1–48. Wiley. York, UK.
25. BANO, S. & M.S. PARIHAR. 1997. Reduction of lipid peroxidation in different brain regions by a combination of alpha-tocopherol and ascorbic acid. J. Neural Transm. **104:** 1277–1286.
26. GHADIALLY, F.N. 1988. Lysosomes. *In* Ultrastructural Pathology of the Cell and Matrix, 3rd ed.: 240–244. Butterworths. London.
27. HEWETT, J. *et al.* 2000. Mutant torsinA, responsible for early-onset torsion dystonia, forms membrane inclusions in cultured neural cells. Hum. Mol. Genet. **9:** 1403–1413.
28. PRICE, M.T., J.W. OLNEY & T.J. CICERO. 1977. Proliferation of lamellar whorls in arcuate neurons of the hypothalamus of male rats treated with estradiol benzoate or cyproterone acetate. Cell Tissue Res. **182:** 537–540.

29. FOX, J. *et al.* 1999. Naturally occurring GM2 gangliosidosis in two Muntjak deer with pathological and biochemical features of human classical Tay-Sachs disease (type B GM2 gangliosidsis). Acta Neuropathol. (Berl.) **97:** 57–62.
30. WALIS, A. & P.P. LIBERSKI. 1999. Echigo-1: a panencephalopathic strain of Creutzfeld-Jacob disease: ultrastructural studies of the optic nerve. Folia Neuropathol. **37:** 281–282.
31. GUASTADISEGNI, C. *et al.* 1999. Liver mitochondria alterations in chloroform-treated Sprague-Dawley rats. J. Toxicol. Environ. Health **57:** 415–429.
32. SHAPIRO, S.H. & J.V. KLAVINS. 1993. Concentric membranous bodies and giant mitochondria in hepatocytes from a patient with AIDS. Ultrastruct. Pathol. **17:** 557–563.
33. DE MARTINO, G.N. & C.A. SLAUGHTER. 1999. The proteasome, a novel protease regulated by multiple mechanisms. J. Biol. Chem. **274:** 22123–22126.
34. GAYATHRI, N. *et al.* 2000. Inclusion body myositis (IBM). Clin. Neuropathol. **19:** 13–20.
35. JOHNSTON, J.A., C.L. WARD & R.R. KOPITO. 1998. Aggresomes: a cellular response to misfolded proteins. J. Cell Biol. **143:** 1883–1898.
36. OLANOW, C.W. & W.G. TATTON. 1999. Etiology and pathogenesis of Parkinson's disease. Annu. Rev. Neurosci. **22:** 123–144.
37. KELLER, J.N. *et al.* 2000. Dopamine induces proteasome inhibition in neural PC12 cell line. Free Radic. Biol. Med. **29:** 1037–1042.
38. BENCE, N.F., R.M. SAMPAT & R.R. KOPITO. 2001. Impairment of the ubiquitin-proteasome system by protein aggregation. Science **292:** 1552–1555.

Action of MDMA (Ecstasy) and Its Metabolites on Arginine Vasopressin Release

J.K. FALLON,[a] D. SHAH,[b] A.T. KICMAN,[a] A.J. HUTT,[a] J.A. HENRY,[c]
D.A. COWAN,[a] AND M. FORSLING[b]

[a] Drug Control Centre and Department of Pharmacy, King's College London,
Franklin-Wilkins Building, London SE1 9NN, UK

[b] Neuroendocrine Laboratories, New Hunts House, King's College London,
Guy's Hospital, London Bridge, London SE1 1UL, UK

[c] Academic Department of Accident and Emergency Medicine,
Imperial College School of Medicine, London, W2 1NY, UK

ABSTRACT: 3,4-Methylenedioxymethamphetamine (MDMA) has been reported
to cause hyponatraemia, which appears to result from inappropriate secretion
of the antidiuretic hormone arginine vasopressin (AVP). After administration
of a low dose of (R,S)-MDMA (40 mg) to eight healthy drug-free male volunteers, concentrations of AVP in plasma increased significantly at 1, 2, and 4
hours. Although no relation between plasma MDMA and AVP was found on an
examination of the entire data set over the 24-hour study period, a statistically
significant negative correlation was observed at 1 hour. As this occurred at a
time when both AVP and MDMA concentrations were rising, it was postulated
that a metabolite, or metabolites, could primarily be responsible for the increase in AVP. To test this hypothesis we examined the effect of MDMA and five
of its metabolites, in the dose range 0.1–1,000 nM, on AVP release from the isolated rat hypothalamus. All compounds tested were found to increase AVP release (using 10 nM and 1,000 nM concentrations), with 4-hydroxy-3-
methoxymethamphetamine (HMMA), the major metabolite of MDMA, being
the most potent, and 3,4-dihydroxymethamphetamine (DHMA) the least potent. Each compound (1,000 nM), with the exception of DHMA, also enhanced
the response to 40-mM potassium stimulation. Our findings confirm that metabolites of MDMA, in addition to the parent drug, contribute to AVP secretion
in vitro. Further work will demonstrate whether this is also true in vivo.

KEYWORDS: MDMA; ecstasy; arginine vasopressin

INTRODUCTION

3,4-Methylenedioxymethamphetamine (MDMA; "ecstasy," "E," "Adam") ingestion
has been associated with disturbances of body water homeostasis. In the 1980s and early
1990s the literature concentrated on hyperthermia and associated complications as the

Address for correspondence: Dr Andrew T. Kicman, Drug Control Centre, King's College
London, Franklin-Wilkins Building, 150 Stamford Street, London SE1 9NN, UK. Voice:
+44-20-78484779; fax: +44-20-78484980.
andrew.kicman@kcl.ac.uk

Ann. N.Y. Acad. Sci. 965: 399–409 (2002). © 2002 New York Academy of Sciences.

main problems of MDMA use.[1–4] As a result, users were often advised to maintain adequate hydration to help counter these effects. Subsequent reports on the effects of MDMA ingestion described cases of hyponatraemia, sometimes fatal, that were postulated to result from the syndrome of inappropriate antidiuretic hormone secretion (SIADH), especially in young women.[5–9] Despite these reports, perhaps because this adverse reaction was considered to be idiosyncratic, the effect of MDMA administration on the underlying mechanism of arginine vasopressin (AVP) release has not been investigated.

Here we describe results from a pharmacokinetic study in healthy MDMA naïve male volunteers in which the effect of a low dose of (R,S)-MDMA (40 mg) on AVP release was also examined. Following examination of the data obtained, we advanced the hypothesis that a metabolite (or metabolites) rather than, or together with, the parent drug may be responsible for the observed effects on AVP release. To test this hypothesis we examined the effect of MDMA, and five of its metabolites, on AVP release from the isolated rat hypothalamus.

Demethylenation is the most important pathway of MDMA metabolism in man,[10–14] with N-demethylation being a minor pathway. The major cytochrome P-450 (CYP) involved in demethylenation is CYP2D6, and other isoforms, such as 2B6, 3A4, and 1A2, are also believed to make a contribution.[15–18] Hence, the major product of this transformation is 3,4-dihydroxymethamphetamine (DHMA; FIG. 1), with 3,4-dihydroxyamphetamine (DHA) also being formed via demethylenation of the minor product 3,4-methylenedioxyamphetamine (MDA; the demethylated metabolite). These two products (DHMA and DHA) subsequently undergo methylation at the 3-hydroxy group on the phenyl ring by catechol-O-methyl transferase to form 4-hydroxy-3-methoxymethamphetamine (HMMA) and 4-hydroxy-3-methoxy-

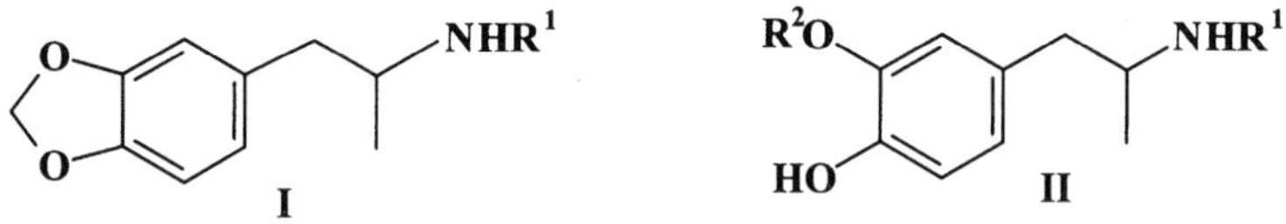

Compound	Structure	R^1	R^2
MDMA	I	CH_3	-
MDA	I	H	-
HMMA	II	CH_3	CH_3
DHMA	II	CH_3	H
HMA	II	H	CH_3
DHA	II	H	H

FIGURE 1. Structure of MDMA and its metabolites.

amphetamine (HMA), respectively. HMMA is believed to be the predominant metabolite of MDMA in humans,[11,12,14,19] and together with HMA, DHMA, and DHA it is excreted as glucuronide or sulfate conjugates in urine. The effect and relative potency of these metabolites, together with the parent drug, on the release of AVP are reported herein.

METHODS

Material. (±)-(R,S)-MDMA hydrochloride and (±)-(R,S)-MDA hydrochloride were obtained from Sigma Chemical Company Ltd, Poole, UK; (−)-(R)- and (+)-(S)-MDMA hydrochloride and (−)-(R)- and (+)-(S)-MDA hydrochloride were generously donated by the Research Technology Branch of the National Institute on Drug Abuse, Rockville, Maryland, USA. Hydrochloride salts of the racemates of HMMA, HMA, DHMA, and DHA were synthesized as described previously.[20-23]

Analytical Techniques. MDMA and MDA plasma enantiomer concentrations were measured by a validated GC-MS assay.[24] AVP concentrations in plasma[25] and in Earles balanced salt solution (EBSS, Gibco, Biocult, Paisley, UK) media[26] were determined by validated radioimmunoassay using the first International Standard for vasopressin (77/501). Intra- and interassay coefficients of variation for plasma were 7.5 and 11.6% at 2.5 pmol/L, respectively, and the corresponding values in media were 5.0 and 8.9%, respectively. Cortisol was also measured by validated radioimmunoassay (Diagnostic Products Corporation, Coat-A-Count, Gwynedd, UK) and osmolalities by freezing point depression (Microosmometer Model 3MO Plus, Advanced Instruments Inc., Vitec Scientific Ltd.). Sodium concentrations were determined using potentiometric dry slide technology.

Human Study. (±)-(R,S)-MDMA (47.6 mg HCl salt; equivalent to 40 mg free base) was administered in capsule form to eight healthy nondrug-using (MDMA naïve) male volunteers (22–32 years) at 10:00 AM on the study day with ~200 mL of water as described by Fallon *et al.*[24] Briefly, blood samples were collected from a forearm vein immediately prior to drug administration and at 0.5, 1, 2, 4, 6, 8, and 24 hours postdose. Immediately after each collection the plasma was separated and rapidly frozen using liquid nitrogen. It was stored at −20°C until required for analysis. Approval to administer the compound was obtained from the UK Home Office and the King's College London Ethics Committee, and each subject received full details prior to giving written informed consent. A control study in which three of the eight volunteers acted as untreated controls was undertaken at least 2 weeks later.

Treatment of data: Repeated measures ANOVA, with time as the within subject factor, was used to test for overall change from basal AVP and MDMA concentrations, using the SPSS software statistics package (SPSS, UK). The simple contrasts were performed to locate differences indicated, comparing mean values at each postadministration time to respective basal values. Regression analysis was applied at each sampling time to examine the relation between MDMA and AVP concentrations as well as between MDA and AVP concentrations.

In Vitro Study. The study was performed on isolated rat hypothalami using a previously validated method.[27] Specific pathogen-free male Wistar rats (Banting & Kingman Ltd., Aldeburgh, UK) weighing 225–275 g were used. Animals were given free access to food (Rat and Mouse no 1 maintenance diet; Special Diet Services

Ltd., Witham, Essex, UK) and water, and were housed under conditions of fixed lighting (12 h light: 12 h dark) and constant temperature and humidity.

Hypothalamus dissection: Decapitation of groups of rats took place between 9:00 and 10:00 AM. The brain was removed immediately and a hypothalamic block dissected within the following limits: anterior border of the optic chiasm, anterior border of the mamillary bodies, and lateral hypothalamic sulci. The dissection depth was approximately 3.0 mm. The blocks were bisected longitudinally through the midsaggital plane and the two hypothalamic halves incubated in one vial. Total dissection time was less than 2 minutes from decapitation.

Hypothalamic incubation: Each hypothalamus was incubated in polyethylene vials containing 400 µL of EBSS. The solution was supplemented with human serum albumin (0.2%), ascorbic acid (60 mg/mL), and aprotinin (concentration in EBSS; 40 kallikrein-inhibiting units [KIU]/mL). The vials were placed in a shaking water bath at 37°C and gassed with 95% O_2 and 5% CO_2. An 80-minute equilibration period was chosen as previously described.[28] After equilibration, fresh media were added for a control period of 20 minutes, after which time the media were again replaced by either fresh media (control hypothalami) or media containing MDMA or metabolites (test hypothalami) for a further 20-minute incubation period. Following each incubation period the media were analyzed for AVP. Each compound was examined at concentrations in medium of 0.1, 10, and 1000 nM ($n = 5$). The single enantiomers of MDMA and MDA were also examined at a concentration of 500 nM ($n = 5$). Additionally (±)-(R,S)-MDMA was reexamined in the presence of (±)-(R,S)-HMMA, each at a concentration of 500 nM ($n = 5$). Following these steps the hypothalami were also exposed to KCl in EBSS (40 mM) and then to KCl in EBSS also containing the compound under investigation (for the control hypothalami, no compound was added). Hypothalami were bathed in EBSS alone for a 20-minute control period prior to this. At the end of the experiment the viability of the tissue was confirmed by incubation with 56 mM KCl. Hypothalami not responding to the 56 mM KCl stimulation were excluded from the data analysis. EBSS medium from each incubation period was stored at –20°C until analyzed for vasopressin.

Treatment of data: Results were expressed as the ratio of hormone release in the test period with that in the preceding control period, being calculated for basal and stimulated release. These were compared with ratios calculated from the control hypothalami. Overall significance for each series of observations (e.g., test:control ratios, following incubation with (±)-(R,S)-MDMA at 0.1, 10, and 1000 nM concentrations, in comparison with ratios obtained for control hypothalami) was tested by one-way ANOVA. If statistical significance was found ($p < 0.05$), then sets of data were compared using Student's t test with Dunnett's correction for multiple comparisons.

RESULTS AND DISCUSSION

Human Study. A significant rise in plasma AVP concentrations was observed in all volunteers between 1 and 4 hours after administration of 40 mg (R,S)-MDMA (repeated measures ANOVA, simple contrasts, $p < 0.05$ at 1 and 4 hours, $p < 0.01$ at 2 hours) (FIG. 2).[29] Concentrations had returned to basal at 8 and 24 hours ($p > 0.05$). The rise was accompanied by a small but significant decrease in plasma sodi-

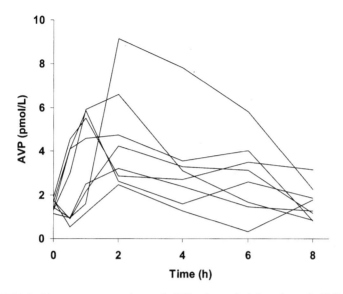

FIGURE 2. Plasma concentrations of AVP after administration of (R,S)-MDMA (40 mg) to eight drug-free healthy male volunteers. Mean increases from basal were significant at 1, 2, and 4 hours (repeated measures ANOVA, $p < 0.05$ at 1 and 4 hours, $p < 0.01$ at 2 hours).

um concentration between 0.5 and 2 hours (t test, $p < 0.05$), although plasma osmolality remained unchanged up to 8 hours after drug administration ($p > 0.05$). No marked increase in plasma cortisol concentration was seen ($p > 0.05$), the significant decreases at 6 and 8 hours ($p \leq 0.05$) being representative of a characteristic circadian rhythm. None of the measurements changed significantly in the control subjects ($p > 0.05$) up to 8 hours, with the exception of plasma cortisol, which again showed a characteristic circadian rhythm.

Although plasma total MDMA concentrations (i.e., the sum of the individual enantiomer concentrations) rose to a maximum (geometric mean) of 47.0 µg/L ± 20.9% at 4 hours (the corresponding value at 2 hours was 45.2 µg/L ± 18.5%), no correlation between (R,S)-MDMA and AVP concentrations was seen over the total sampling period (Spearman $r = 0.2$, $p = 0.1$). However, following examination of the data at each sampling time, a highly significant negative correlation was observed between total MDMA and AVP concentrations at 1 hour ($r = -0.94$, $p < 0.001$; $n = 8$) (FIG. 3).[30] This was the case whether single or total enantiomer MDMA concentrations and whether actual AVP concentrations or AVP concentration changes from basal ($r < -0.90$, $p < 0.002$) were used for data analysis. At 0.5 hour the correlation tended towards significance in the same direction (for total MDMA versus AVP, $r = 0.61$, $p = 0.11$; for total MDMA versus changes in AVP from basal, $r = 0.66$, $p = 0.11$), whereas at 2, 4, 6, and 8 hours no correlation was seen (e.g., total MDMA versus AVP or AVP concentration changes from basal at 2 hours, $r < 0.09$, $p > 0.84$).

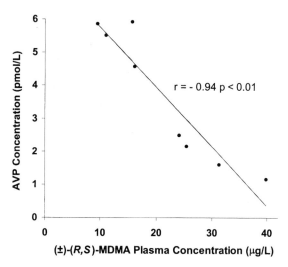

FIGURE 3. Correlation of plasma AVP concentrations with total MDMA enantiomer plasma concentrations at 1 hour after oral administration of 40 mg (R,S)-MDMA to eight drug-free healthy male volunteers. Reproduced with kind permission of the *Journal of Pharmacy and Pharmacology.*[30]

There was no significant correlation between AVP concentration and single or total enantiomer MDA concentrations at any time from 1 to 8 hours after drug administration ($p > 0.05$). The values at 0.5 hour were not examined as some of the enantiomeric concentrations of MDA were below the limit of quantification of 0.025 µg/L at this time.[24]

The rise in AVP occurred at a time of day when no change in basal AVP would be expected.[25] It did not appear to be associated with changes in water homeostasis, as plasma sodium concentrations decreased between 0.5 and 2 hours postadministration. Neither did it appear to be part of a stress response, as plasma cortisol concentrations remained relatively unchanged up to 4 hours postdose.

The lack of overall correlation between MDMA and AVP may have resulted from the short half-life of AVP, which is initially about 6 minutes,[31] whereas the half-life of MDMA is measured in hours.[19,24] The negative correlation observed at 1 hour after drug administration may have been a chance occurrence, but nonetheless the possibility that a metabolite (or metabolites) of MDMA rather than, or as well as, the parent compound may be responsible for the AVP release should be considered. Also, although a negative correlation could signify inhibition of AVP release by MDMA, the fact that the relation was seen at 1 hour, at which time AVP concentrations had increased significantly (FIG. 2), suggested that involvement of an active metabolite(s) was more likely. The lack of correlation at 2 hours could be explained by the possible diminishing responsiveness of the magnocellular neurones secreting vasopressin, even though plasma AVP concentrations were significantly greater than basal values at this time (paired t test, $p = 0.006$). Because of the lack of correlation between (R,S)-MDA and AVP shortly after (R,S)-MDMA administration, it was not

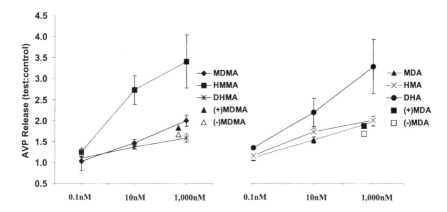

FIGURE 4. Effect of MDMA and five of its metabolites (racemates unless stated) on AVP release from isolated rat hypothalamus *in vitro*. Bars represent mean ± SEM. Response (ratio of test period:control period) to 10 nM and 1000 nM concentrations was significantly greater for each compound ($p < 0.01$) compared to data obtained from control hypothalami. At 0.1 nM concentrations, only the response to DHA was significant ($p < 0.05$). The response to 500 nM concentrations of the (+)-*S*-enantiomers of MDMA and MDA was significantly greater ($p < 0.05$) than that for their corresponding (−)-*R*-enantiomers.

thought that MDA was the metabolite causing the AVP release. MDA is known, in addition, to be a relatively minor metabolite of MDMA,[24] in comparison with catechol-derived products which are major metabolites.[10,11,14]

To examine the hypothesis that a metabolite, or metabolites, of MDMA, in addition to the parent drug, may influence the AVP release observed in humans, an *in vitro* study using isolated rat hypothalami was undertaken.

In Vitro *Study.* All compounds (MDMA and five of its metabolites) were found to increase AVP release from the isolated rat hypothalamus in a dose-related manner (FIG. 4). (*R,S*)-HMMA was the most potent compound and (*R,S*)-DHMA the least potent, compared to data from control hypothalami. Each compound, except DHMA, also enhanced the response to 40 mM potassium stimulation at a concentration of 1000 nM ($p < 0.05$). Thus, our previous observations that MDMA administration can stimulate vasopressin release in man were confirmed *in vitro*, and evidence was provided for the involvement of a metabolite or metabolite(s) in the response. The concentrations employed in the experiment covered the range of concentrations of MDMA and MDA found in plasma. They were also similar to those measured by other investigators.[14] The concentrations employed for the drug:metabolite and single enantiomer mixtures also fell within these ranges. In addition, the results confirm that MDMA can act directly on the hypothalamus. If this is also true in humans, then vasopressin release following MDMA ingestion could occur from direct action as well as other changes such as hyperthermia.[3,4]

The increase in AVP release observed was significant for each compound (parent drug and metabolites) at 10 nM and 1000 nM concentrations. For the 0.1 nM concentrations the increase was only significant for the primary amine catechol (R,S)-DHA. For the single enantiomer solutions the response to 500 nM of the (+)-S-enantiomer was significantly greater than that for the (−)-R-enantiomer, at the same concentration, for both MDMA and MDA ($p < 0.05$). This agrees with findings from other animal studies which show (+)-(S)-MDMA to have greater neurochemical activity than (−)-(R)-MDMA.[32] The response in incubates containing equal amounts of (R,S)-HMMA and (R,S)-MDMA (each 500 nM) was less than for the equivalent concentrations of (R,S)-HMMA alone (1000 nM)($p < 0.05$). This confirmed the observation that (R,S)-HMMA was more active than (R,S)-MDMA in effecting the AVP response, whether the MDMA acted as an inhibitor for the HMMA or simply reduced the total response by its lower activity.

Stimulation of AVP release could account for the sometimes fatal hyponatremia often observed following MDMA ingestion.[5,9,33] All cases of hyponatremia and SIADH reported in the literature have occurred in premenopausal women (see, for e.g., Refs. 8 and 34–36). Hyponatremia has a high incidence of morbidity and mortality in premenopausal women (Ref. 35 and references therein) as compared to young men, and some animal studies have suggested that renal responsiveness to AVP is affected by reproductive status in women.[37] Combined with any gender-dependent differences in the metabolism of MDMA, it is therefore possible that women are more susceptible than men to abnormalities of body water homeostasis following the ingestion of MDMA.

AVP release is believed to be controlled by both serotonergic and aminergic pathways.[38–40] Whereas the serotonergic effects of MDMA are well documented,[32,41,42] aminergic effects have also been reported.[43–45] Considering the similarity of the MDMA catechol and methoxy metabolite structures to common monoamine neurotransmitters, it is possible that the aminergic actions of MDMA and/or its metabolites are important for the stimulation of AVP release after the ingestion of MDMA. From animal studies it is not clear whether MDMA is metabolized inside the blood-brain barrier.[46,47] Neither is it known whether it (or its metabolites) is active at the magnocellular neurons (circumventricular organs) in vivo. Considering SIADH as a well-known side effect of neuroleptic and other psychoactive drugs,[48,49] it is perhaps not surprising that MDMA, with its catechol and catechol-like metabolites, has also been associated with SIADH.

In conclusion, we have shown an increase in plasma AVP concentration after administration of (R,S)-MDMA to healthy drug-free male volunteers. The observation of a highly significant inverse correlation between plasma drug and hormone at 1 hour postdose suggested the possible involvement of an active metabolite in hormonal release. This hypothesis was confirmed in vitro using rat hypothalamic preparations where HMMA, a major metabolite of MDMA in humans, was shown to be a more potent stimulator of AVP release than the parent drug. The significance of this observation to the adverse effects of MDMA in humans awaits further work.

NOTE ADDED IN PROOF: Since the submission of this manuscript, a paper on the effect of MDMA, and its metabolites, on neurohypophysial hormone release from the isolated rat hypothalamus has been published.[50] The response to drug and metabolite stimulation on oxytocin release was found to be dose-dependent, but less marked than that for AVP.

REFERENCES

1. BROWN, C. & J. OSTERLOH. 1987. Multiple severe complications from recreational ingestion of MDMA ('Ecstasy'). JAMA **258:** 780–781.
2. CHADWICK, I.S. *et al.* 1991. Ecstasy, 3-4 methylenedioxymethamphetamine (MDMA), a fatality associated with coagulopathy and hyperthermia. J. R. Soc. Med. **84:** 371.
3. HENRY, J.A., K.J. JEFFREYS & S. DAWLING. 1992. Toxicity and deaths from 3,4-methylenedioxymethamphetamine ("ecstasy"). Lancet **340:** 384–387.
4. SCREATON, G.R. *et al.* 1992. Hyperpyrexia and rhabdomyolysis after MDMA ("ecstasy") abuse. Lancet **339:** 677–678.
5. MAXWELL, D.L., M.I. POLKEY & J.A. HENRY. 1993. Hyponatraemia and catatonic stupor after taking "ecstasy." Br. Med. J. **307:** 1399.
6. KESSEL, B. 1994. Hyponatraemia after ingestion of ecstasy. Br. Med. J. **308:** 414.
7. HOLDEN, R. & M.A. JACKSON. 1996. Near-fatal hyponatraemic coma due to vasopressin over-secretion after "ecstasy" (3,4-MDMA). Lancet **347:** 1052.
8. MATTHAI, S.M., D.C. DAVIDSON, J.A. SILLS & D. ALEXANDROU. 1996. Cerebral oedema after ingestion of MDMA ("ecstasy") and unrestricted intake of water. Br. Med. J. **312:** 1359.
9. PARR, M.J., H.M. LOW & P. BOTTERILL. 1997. Hyponatraemia and death after "ecstasy" ingestion. Med. J. Aust. **166:** 136–137.
10. LIM, H.K. & R.L. FOLTZ. 1989. Identification of metabolites of 3,4-(methylenedioxy)methamphetamine in human urine. Chem. Res. Toxicol. **2:** 142–143.
11. HELMLIN, H.J., K. BRACHER, D. BOURQUIN, *et al.* 1996. Analysis of 3,4-methylenedioxymethamphetamine (MDMA) and its metabolites in plasma and urine by HPLC-DAD and GC-MS. J. Anal. Toxicol. **20:** 432–440.
12. LANZ, M., R. BRENNEISEN & W. THORMANN. 1997. Enantioselective determination of 3,4-methylene-dioxymethamphetamine and two of its metabolites in human urine by cyclodextrin-modified capillary zone electrophoresis. Electrophoresis **18:** 1035–1043.
13. DE LA TORRE, R., M. FARRE, P.N. ROSET, *et al.* 2000. Pharmacology of MDMA in humans. Ann. N.Y. Acad. Sci. **914:** 225–237.
14. SEGURA, M. *et al.* 2001. 3,4-Dihydroxymethamphetamine (HHMA). A major *in vivo* 3,4-methylenedioxymethamphetamine (MDMA) metabolite in humans. Chem. Res. Toxicol. **14:** 1203–1208.
15. TUCKER, G.T. *et al.* 1994. The demethylenation of methylenedioxymethamphetamine ("ecstasy") by debrisoquine hydroxylase (CYP2D6). Biochem. Pharmacol. **47:** 1151–1156.
16. LIN, L.Y. *et al.* 1997. Oxidation of methamphetamine and methylenedioxymethamphetamine by CYP2D6. Drug Metab. Dispos. **25:** 1059-1064.
17. WU, D. *et al.* 1997. Interactions of amphetamine analogs with human liver CYP2D6. Biochem. Pharmacol. **53:** 1605-1612.
18. KRETH, K., K. KOVAR, M. SCHWAB & U.M. ZANGER. 2000. Identification of the human cytochromes P450 involved in the oxidative metabolism of "Ecstasy"-related designer drugs. Biochem. Pharmacol. **59:** 1563–1571.
19. DE LA TORRE, R. *et al.* 2000. Non-linear pharmacokinetics of MDMA ('ecstasy') in humans. Br. J. Clin. Pharmacol. **49:** 104–109.
20. BECKETT, A.H., G. KIRK & A.J. SHARPEN. 1965. The configuration of α-methyldopamine. Tetrahedron **21**: 1489–1493.
21. BORGMAN, R.J., M.R. BAYLOR, J.J. McPHILLIPS & R.E. STITZEL. 1974. Alpha-methyldopamine derivatives. Synthesis and pharmacology. J. Med. Chem. **17:** 427–430.
22. GLENNON, R.A., S.M. LIEBOWITZ, D. LEMING-DOOT & J.A. ROSECRANS. 1980. Demethyl analogues of psychoactive methoxyphenalkylamines: synthesis and serotonin receptor affinities. J. Med. Chem. **23:** 990–994.
23. DE BOER, D. *et al.* 1997. Gas chromatographic/mass spectrometric assay for profiling the enantiomers of 3,4-methylenedioxymethamphetamine and its chiral metabolites using positive chemical ionization ion trap mass spectrometry. J. Mass Spectrom. **32:** 1236–1246.

24. FALLON, J.K. *et al.* 1999. Stereospecific analysis and enantiomeric disposition of 3,4-methylenedioxymethamphetamine (Ecstasy) in humans. Clin. Chem. **45**: 1058–1069.
25. FORSLING, M.L. *et al.* 1998. Daily patterns of secretion of neurohypophysial hormones in man: effect of age. Exp. Physiol. **83**: 409–418.
26. FORSLING, M.L. & K. PEYSNER. 1988. Pituitary and plasma vasopressin concentrations and fluid balance throughout the oestrous cycle of the rat. J. Endocrinol. **117**: 397–402.
27. TSAGARAKIS, S. *et al.* 1988. Acetylcholine and norepinephrine stimulate the release of corticotropin-releasing factor–41 from the rat hypothalamus *in vitro*. Endocrinology **123**: 1962–1969.
28. YASIN, S.A. *et al.* 1993. Melatonin and its analogs inhibit the basal and stimulated release of hypothalamic vasopressin and oxytocin *in vitro*. Endocrinology **132**: 1329–1336.
29. HENRY, J.A. *et al.* 1998. Low-dose MDMA ("ecstasy") induces vasopressin secretion. Lancet **351**: 1784.
30. FORSLING, M.L. *et al.* 2001. Arginine vasopressin release in response to the administration of 3,4-methylenedioxymethamphetamine ('ecstasy'); is metabolism a contributory factor? J. Pharm. Pharmacol. **53**: 1357–1363.
31. FABIAN, M., M.L. FORSLING, J.J. JONES & J.S. PRYOR. 1969. The clearance and antidiuretic potency of neurohypophysial hormones in man, and their plasma binding and stability. J. Physiol. **204**: 653–668.
32. STEELE, T.D., U.D. MCCANN & G.A. RICAURTE. 1994. 3,4-Methylenedioxymethamphetamine (MDMA, "Ecstasy"): pharmacology and toxicology in animals and humans. Addiction **89**: 539–551.
33. BALMELLI, C., H. KUPFERSCHMIDT, K. RENTSCH & M. SCHNEEMANN. 2001. Fatal brain edema after ingestion of ecstasy and benzylpiperazine. Dtsch. Med. Wochenschr. **126**: 809–811.
34. BOX, S.A., L.F. PRESCOTT & S. FREESTONE. 1997. Hyponatraemia at a rave. Postgrad. Med. J. **73**: 53–54.
35. WATSON, I.D., M. SERLIN, P. MONCUR & F. TAMES. 1997. Acute hyponatraemia. Postgrad. Med. J. **73**: 443–444.
36. MAGEE, C., H. STAUNTON, W. TORMEY & J.J. WALSHE. 1998. Hyponatraemia, seizures and stupor associated with ecstasy ingestion in a female. Ir. Med. J. **91**: 178.
37. FORSLING, M.L., Y. ZHOU & R.J. WINDLE. 1996. The natriuretic actions of vasopressin in the female rat: variations during the 4 days of the oestrous cycle. J. Endocrinol. **148**: 457–464.
38. SKLAR, A.H. & R.W. SCHRIER. 1983. Central nervous system mediators of vasopressin release. Physiol. Rev. **63**: 1243–1280.
39. IOVINO, M. & L. STEARDO. 1985. Effect of substances influencing brain serotonergic transmission on plasma vasopressin levels in the rat. Eur. J. Pharmacol. **113**: 99–103.
40. COIRO, V. *et al.* 1995. Dopaminergic and cholinergic control of arginine-vasopressin secretion in type I diabetic men. Eur. J. Clin. Invest. **25**: 412–417.
41. KANKAANPAA, A., E. MERIRINNE, P. LILLSUNDE & T. SEPPALA. 1998. The acute effects of amphetamine derivatives on extracellular serotonin and dopamine levels in rat nucleus accumbens. Pharmacol. Biochem. Behav. **59**: 1003–1009.
42. MCCANN, U.D. *et al.* 1998. Positron emission tomographic evidence of toxic effect of MDMA ("Ecstasy") on brain serotonin neurons in human beings. Lancet **352**: 1433–1437.
43. YAMAMOTO, B.K. & L.J. SPANOS. 1988. The acute effects of methylenedioxymethamphetamine on dopamine release in the awake-behaving rat. Eur. J. Pharmacol. **148**: 195–203.
44. HIRAMATSU, M. & A.K. CHO. 1990. Enantiomeric differences in the effects of 3,4-methylenedioxymethamphetamine on extracellular monoamines and metabolites in the striatum of freely-moving rats: an in vivo microdialysis study. Neuropharmacology **29**: 269–275.
45. WHITE, S.R., T. OBRADOVIC, K.M. IMEL & M.J. WHEATON. 1996. The effects of methylenedioxymethamphetamine (MDMA, "'Ecstasy") on monoaminergic neurotransmission in the central nervous system. Prog. Neurobiol. **49**: 455–479.

46. LIM, H.K. & R.L. FOLTZ. 1988. In vivo and in vitro metabolism of 3,4-(methylene-dioxy)methamphetamine in the rat: identification of metabolites using an ion trap detector. Chem. Res. Toxicol. **1:** 370–378.
47. ESTEBAN, B. *et al.* 2001. 3,4-Methylenedioxymethamphetamine induces monoamine release, but not toxicity, when administered centrally at a concentration occurring following a peripherally injected neurotoxic dose. Psychopharmacology **154:** 251–260.
48. ANANTH, J. & K.M. LIN. 1986. SIADH: a serious side effect of psychotropic drugs. Int. J. Psychiatry Med. **16:** 401–407.
49. JACKSON, E.K. 1996. Vasopressin and other agents affecting the renal conservation of water. *In* Goodman & Gilman's The Pharmacological Basis of Therapeutics. J.G. Hardman *et al.*, eds.: 715–731. McGraw-Hill. London, UK.
50. FORSLING, M.L. *et al.* 2002. The effect of 3,4-methylenedioxymethamphetamine (MDMA, "ecstasy") and its metabolites on neurohypophysial hormone release from the isolated rat hypothalamus. Br. J. Pharmacol. **135:** 649–656.

Comparative Effects of Substituted Amphetamines (PMA, MDMA, and METH) on Monoamines in Rat Caudate

A Microdialysis Study

BOBBY GOUGH,[a] SYED Z. IMAM,[a] BRUCE BLOUGH,[b] WILLIAM SLIKKER, JR.,[a] AND SYED F. ALI[a]

[a]Neurochemistry Laboratory, Division of Neurotoxicology, National Center for Toxicological Research/FDA, Jefferson, Arkansas 72079, USA

[b]Research Triangle Institute, Research Triangle Park, North Carolina 27709, USA

ABSTRACT: Paramethoxyamphetamine (PMA) is a methoxylated phenethylamine derivative that has been used illicitly in Australia since 1994. PMA is also becoming popular at rave parties in the United States. PMA raised concern when a series of fatalities resulted after its use in South Australia, where it was marketed as "ecstasy," which is the colloquial name for MDMA. In the present study, we evaluated the comparative neurotoxicity of substituted amphetamines in rats. Extracellular levels of dopamine (DA), 3,4-dihydroxyphenylacetic acid (DOPAC), homovanillic acid (HVA), serotonin (5-HT), and 5-hydroxyindoleacetic acid (5-HIAA) were assayed in the caudate of freely moving rats using microdialysis and HPLC-EC. Dialysates were assayed every 20 minutes for 4 hours after an intraperitoneal (i.p.) injection of PMA (2.5, 5, 10, 20 mg/kg), MDMA (10 and 20 mg/kg), or METH (2.5 mg/kg). METH produced a significant increase in extracellular DA (700%), and significant decreases in extracellular DOPAC and HVA (30% and 50%), with no detectable changes in either 5-HT or 5-HIAA. MDMA produced significant increases in DA (700% at 10 mg/kg and 950% at 20 mg/kg) and decreases in DOPAC (15% for both 10 and 20 mg/kg), and HVA (50% at 10 mg/kg and 35% at 20 mg/kg). MDMA also increased 5-HT (350% at 10, and 575% at 20 mg/kg), and decreased 5-HIAA to 60% for both dose levels. PMA produced no detectable increases in DA at dose levels of 2.5, 5, or 10 mg/kg, but significantly increased DA (975%) at a dose of 20 mg/kg. However, PMA significantly decreased DOPAC at all dose levels (75% at 2.5; 40% at 5; 30% at 10; 10% at 20 mg/kg), with comparable decreases in HVA at all dose levels. PMA also produced significant increases in 5-HT at 10 and 20 mg/kg (350% for both dose levels), with no detectable changes in 5-HT at 2.5 or 5 mg/kg. All dose levels of PMA significantly decreased 5-HIAA (50 to 70%). These data suggest that PMA, like MDMA and METH, is capable of producing dopaminergic and serotonergic neurotoxicity.

KEYWORDS: paramethoxyamphetamine; MDMA; monoamine; caudate nucleus; microdialysis

Address for correspondence: Syed F. Ali, Ph.D., Head, Neurochemistry Laboratory, HFT-132, Division of Neurotoxicology, National Center for Toxicological Research/US FDA, 3900 NCTR Rd., Jefferson, AR 72079. Voice: 870-543-7123; fax: 870-543-7745.

sali@nctr.fda.gov

Ann. N.Y. Acad. Sci. 965: 410–420 (2002). © 2002 New York Academy of Sciences.

INTRODUCTION

The recreational use of amphetamine derivatives among young people is common. 3,4-Methylenedioxymethamphetamine (MDMA), popularly known as "ecstasy," was first identified in street use in 1972.[1] Another amphetamine derivative, paramethoxyamphetamine (PMA), also appeared in recreational use during the 1970s. PMA, MDMA, and other amphetamine derivatives such as 3,4-methylenedioxyethylamphetamine (MDEA) and 3,4-methylenedioxyamphetamine (MDA) have all been sold on the street as ecstasy.[2,3] Within a few years, PMA was associated with several fatalities in Canada and earned the street name "death."[4] PMA has been reported to cause various fatalities in the late 1990s in various parts of Australia.[2] Recently, PMA has been reported to be used in the United States also, as a very popular drug of abuse which has been purportedly sold under the guise of MDMA. Three recent fatalities occurred in the midwestern United States in which each of the decedents ingested PMA believing that they were ingesting MDMA.[5]

Early studies with PMA have revealed that PMA administration results in myoclonic twitch activity and induces release of 5-HT in the central nervous system.[6] It has also been demonstrated that PMA induces hyperthermia and that this hyperthermia is primarily a result of influence on the 5-HT system.[7] *In vitro* studies have revealed that PMA is more than 20 times as potent as (+)-amphetamine as an inhibitor of 5-HT oxidation by monoamine oxidase in mouse brain with a K_I value of 0.22 μM.[8]

Recent studies have shown that the acute adverse effects of PMA are more likely to be associated with alterations in serotonergic rather than dopaminergic neurotransmission.[9]

We have reported that METH and MDMA produce significant change in both the dopaminergic and serotonergic system in rodents.[10,11] The present study was designed to observe the effect of PMA and to compare it with the effects of related analogues such as methamphetamine (METH) and MDMA on the onsite release of monoamines in the caudate nucleus of freely moving rats.

MATERIALS AND METHODS

Adult male Sprague-Dawley rats (three to four months old) were anesthetized with sodium pentobarbital and placed into a stereotaxic frame. The dorsal skull was exposed and a small hole was drilled to allow implantation of intracerebral guide cannula into the caudate. The cannula was fixed to the skull with dental acrylic and two anchor screws. To avoid effects of surgery and anesthesia, the dialysis experiments were started not sooner than 7 days or later than 10 days after surgery.

Animals were always tested in pairs. On the day of tests, animals were hand-held and the dialysis probe was slowly inserted through the guide cannula into the caudate. Microdialysis probes and guide cannula used in these studies were CMA-12 (Carnegie Medicine, Sweden). The membrane tip measured 2.0×0.5 mm and had an *in vitro* efficiency of between 15 and 18% at a flow rate of 1.0 μL/min using BAS Bee family pumps and controller (BAS, West Lafayette, IN). The dialysis solution used in these studies was a modified Ringers' solution of the following composition, in mM (145 Na^+, 1.2 Ca^{2+}, 2.7 K^+, 150 Cl^-, 1.0 Mg^{2+}), at a pH of 7.0.

Dialysates were analyzed alternately between the two animals under study using a dual-channel, on-line injector (BAS) with the injection time set at 10-minute intervals. Each sample was analyzed for DA, DOPAC, HVA, 5-HT, and 5-HIAA by HPLC with electrochemical detection, using a Phase-II cartridge column (BAS). The mobile phase consisted of 0.1 M monochloroacetic acid, 1.0 mM sodium octyl sulfate, 0.5 mM EDTA, and 6% methanol, degassed and filtered at a pH of 3.0. Flow through the column was 0.8 ml/min at a controlled temperature of 30°C and an applied voltage of 0.7 V.

Test compounds PMA, MDMA, and METH were dissolved in normal saline solution and injected intraperitoneally. Samples were collected for 3 hours after treatment. After each experiment, animals were sacrificed and probe placements were verified histologically.

RESULTS

FIGURE 1A represents the effect of METH and MDMA on extracellular levels of DA. METH produced a significant increase in extracellular DA (700%). MDMA also produced significant increases in DA (700% at 10 mg/kg and 950% at 20 mg/kg). The values are represented as the percentage of baseline values of control, which is 12 pg/10 µL. The significance between the control and treatments was observed at $p < 0.05$.

FIGURE 1B represents the effect of PMA on extracellular levels of DA. PMA produced no detectable increases in DA at dose levels of 2.5, 5, or 10 mg/kg, but significantly increased DA (975%) at a dose of 20 mg/kg. The values are represented as the percentage of baseline values of control, which is 12 pg/10 µL. The significance between the control and treatments was observed at $p < 0.05$.

FIGURE 2A represents the effect of METH and MDMA on extracellular levels of DOPAC. METH caused a significant decrease in DOPAC (30%). MDMA also significantly decreased DOPAC (15% for both 10 and 20 mg/kg). The values are represented as the percentage of baseline values of control, which is 650 pg/10 µL. The significance between the control and treatments was observed at $p < 0.05$.

FIGURE 2B represents the effect of PMA on extracellular levels of DOPAC. PMA significantly decreased DOPAC at all dose levels (75% at 2.5; 40% at 5; 30% at 10; 10% at 20 mg/kg). The values are represented as the percentage of baseline values of control, which is 650 pg/10 µL. The significance between the control and treatments was observed at $p < 0.05$.

The effect of METH and MDMA on extracellular levels of HVA is presented in FIGURE 3A. METH caused a significant 50% decrease in HVA levels. MDMA also resulted in a significant decrease of HVA levels (50% at 10 mg/kg and 35% at 20 mg/kg). The values are represented as the percentage of baseline values of control, which is 1650 pg/10 µL. The significance between the control and treatments was observed at $p < 0.05$.

The effect of PMA on extracellular levels of HVA is presented in FIGURE 3B. PMA resulted in siginificant decreases in the extracellular levels of HVA at all dose levels. The values are represented as the percentage of baseline values of control, which is 1650 pg/10 µL. The significance between the control and treatments was observed at $p < 0.05$.

DOPAMINE

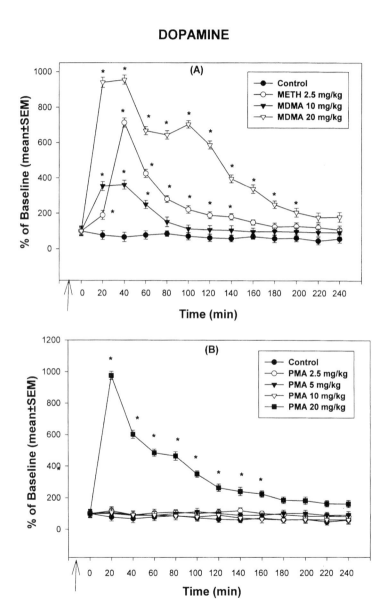

FIGURE 1. Effects of METH and MDMA (**A**) and PMA (**B**) on the extracellular levels of DA. The values are represented as the mean of percentage baseline of the values of control, which is 12 pg/10 μL. *Significant from control at $p < 0.05$.

DOPAC

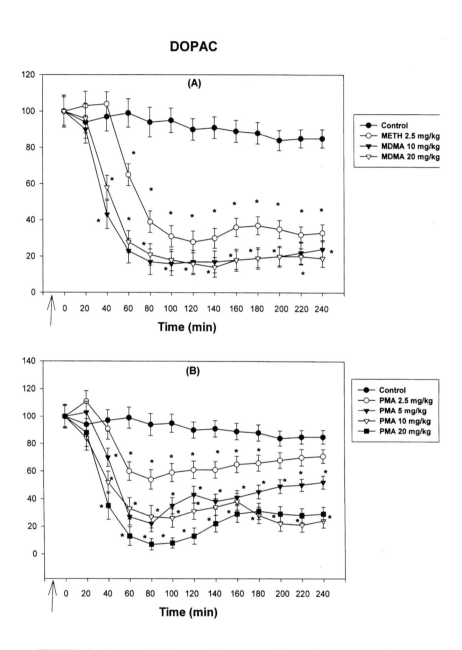

FIGURE 2. Effects of METH and MDMA (**A**) and PMA (**B**) on the extracellular levels of DOPAC. The values are represented as the mean of percentage baseline of the values of control, which is 650 pg/10 μL. *Significant from control at $p < 0.05$.

HVA

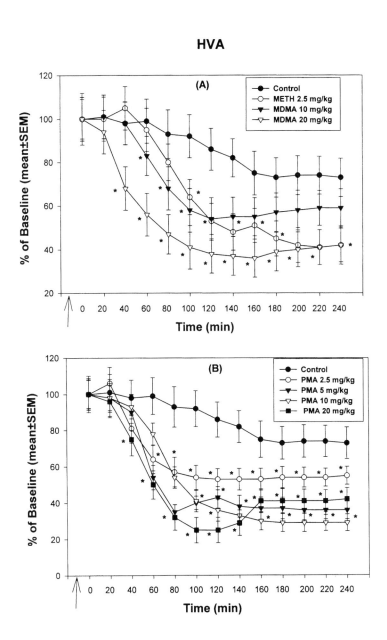

FIGURE 3. Effects of METH and MDMA (**A**) and PMA (**B**) on the extracellular levels of HVA. The values are represented as the mean of percentage baseline of the values of control, which is 1650 pg/10 µL. *Significant from control at $p < 0.05$.

SEROTONIN

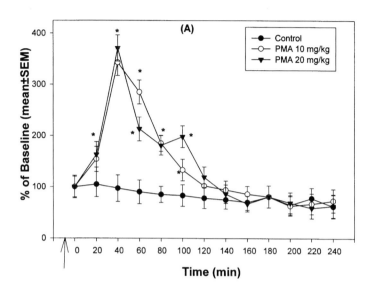

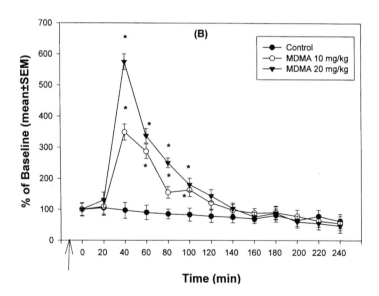

FIGURE 4. Effects of PMA (**A**) and MDMA (**B**) on the extracellular levels of 5-HT. The values are represented as the mean of percentage of baseline of the values of control, which is 4 pg/10 μL. *Significant from control at $p < 0.05$.

5-HIAA

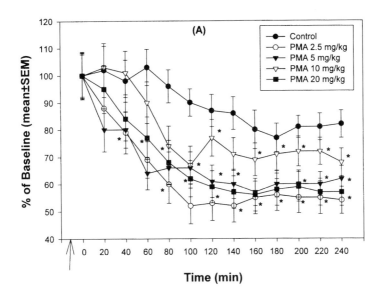

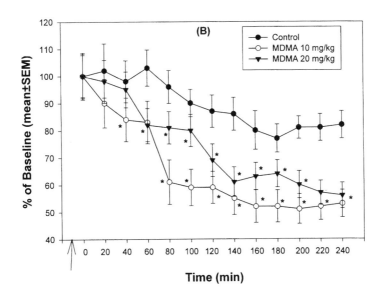

FIGURE 5. Effects of PMA (**A**) and MDMA (**B**) on the extracellular levels of 5-HT. The values are represented as the mean of percentage baseline of the values of control, which is 290 pg/10 μL. *Significant from control at $p < 0.05$.

The effect of PMA on extracellular levels of 5-HT is presented in FIGURE 4A. PMA produced significant increases in 5-HT at 10 and 20 mg/kg (350% for both dose levels), with no detectable changes in 5-HT at 2.5 or 5 mg/kg. The values are represented as the percentage of baseline values of control, which is 4 pg/10 μL. The significance between the control and treatments was observed at $p < 0.05$.

The effect of MDMA on extracellular levels of 5-HT is presented in FIGURE 4B. METH did not produce any detectable changes in 5-HT. MDMA increased 5-HT (350% at 10, and 575% at 20 mg/kg). The values are represented as the percentage of baseline values of control, which is 4 pg/10 μL. The significance between the control and treatments was observed at $p < 0.05$.

The effect of PMA on extracellular levels of 5-HIAA is presented in FIGURE 5A. All dose levels of PMA significantly decreased 5-HIAA (50 to 70%). The values are represented as the percentage of baseline values of control, which is 290 pg/10 μL. The significance between the control and treatments was observed at $p < 0.05$.

The effect of MDMA on extracellular levels of 5-HIAA is presented in FIGURE 5B. MDMA decreased 5-HIAA to 60% for both dose levels. The values are represented as the percentage of baseline values of control, which is 290 pg/10 μL. The significance between the control and treatments was observed at $p < 0.05$.

DISCUSSION

PMA and MDMA are structurally and pharmacologically similar, producing there effects through serotonergic, dopaminergic, and noradrenergic mechanisms.[12] The recent case reports of PMA-related deaths in South Australia[13,14] suggest that PMA is more toxic than MDMA, but do not provide a clinical explanation for this difference. A recent clinical study has shown that most people with PMA poisoning present with clinical features that are qualitatively similar to those of people with ecstasy poisoning such as hyperthermia, coma, and seizures, but that these symptoms occur more frequently and are more severe in those who took PMA.[12] The clinical presentation is similar to that seen in "serotonin syndrome," a potentially fatal event which is associated with increased central extracellular concentrations of serotonin (5-HT).[15,16] Early *in vitro* studies suggest that PMA stimulates release and inhibits the uptake of 5-HT and that this action is more prominent than its effects on DA and norepinephrine (NE).[17–19] Behavioral studies support these data. In rats, PMA has no effects on locomotor activity, whereas MDMA increased locomotor activity.[20,21]

To further explore the neurochemical effects of PMA *in vivo*, microdialysis was used to measure the ability of PMA to evoke the release of transmitter in the striatum of freely moving rats. We also studied the transmitter-releasing effects of MDMA and methamphetamine (METH) in freely moving rats to compare the effects of PMA with these common amphetamine derivatives. Both METH and MDMA resulted in significant release of extracellular DA, as anticipated.[10] PMA produced significant evoked release of DA at high dose. PMA has been reported to evoke the similar release of DA as MDMA in the dorsal striatum of anesthetized rats.[9] In the present study, we have also shown that PMA evoked extracellular DA release in striatum in freely moving rats. Similar effect of PMA was observed on DOPAC and HVA. PMA also caused a significant decrease in the extracellular concentrations of DOPAC and HVA as METH and MDMA.

PMA has also been reported to evoke the release of 5-HT and inhibit the uptake of 5-HT in the dorsal striatum of anesthetized rats.[9] In our present study, PMA also produced significant release of 5-HT in the striatum of freely moving rats. As anticipated, both METH and MDMA also produced significant release of 5-HT. Similar effects were observed in case of 5-HIAA with all these amphetamine derivatives.

In summary, the present data suggest that PMA, like METH and MDMA, is capable of producing dopaminergic and serotonergic neurotoxicity. Further studies are under way to understand the mechanism underlying the dopaminergic and serotonergic neurotxicity produced by PMA.

ACKNOWLEDGMENTS

This research was supported in part by an appointment (S.Z.I) to the Research Participation Program at the National Center for Toxicological Research administered by the Oak Ridge Institute of Science and Education through an interagency agreement between the U.S. Department of Energy and the U.S. Food and Drug Administration.

REFERENCES

1. BUCHANAN, J.F.& C.R. BROWN. 1988. "Designer drugs": a problem in clinical toxicology. Med. Toxicol. Adverse Drug Exp. **3**: 1–17.
2. FELGATE, H.E. *et al.* 1998. Recent paramethoxyamphetamine deaths. J. Anal. Toxicol. **22**: 169–172.
3. MILROY, C. 1999. Ten years of "ecstasy." J. R. Soc. Med. **92**: 68–71.
4. CIMBURA, G. 1974. PMA deaths in Ontario. CMAJ **110**: 1263–1267.
5. KRANER, J.C. *et al.* 2001. Fatalities caused by the MDMA-related drug paramethoxyamphetamine (PMA). J. Anal. Toxicol. **25**: 645–648.
6. TSENG, L.F. 1979. Hydroxytryptamine uptake inhibitors block para-methoxyamphetamine-induced 5-HT release. Br. J. Pharmacol. **66**: 185–190.
7. FJALLAND, B. 1979. Neuroleptic influence on hyperthermia induced 5-hydroxytryptophan and p-methoxy-amphetamine in MAOI-pretreated rabbits. Psychopharmacology **63**: 113–117.
8. GREEN, A.L. & M.A.S. EL HAIT. 1980. p-Methpxyamphetamine, a potent reversible inhibitor of type-A monoamine oxidase in vitro and in vivo. J. Pharm. Pharmacol. **32**: 262–266.
9. DAWS, E.C. *et al.* Prog. Neuropsychopharmacol. Biol. Psychiatry **24**: 955–977.
10. GOUGH, B., S.F. ALI, W. SLIKKER, JR. & R.R. HOLSON. 1991. Acute effects of 3,4-methylenedioxymethamphetamine (MDMA) on monoamines in rat caudate. Pharmacol. Biochem. Beh. **39**: 619–623.
11. IMAM, S.Z. & S.F. ALI. 2001. Aging increases the susceptibility to methamphetamine-induced dopaminergic neurotoxicity in rats: correlation with peroxynitrite production and hyperthermia. J. Neurochem. **78**: 952–959.
12. LING, L.H. *et al.* 2001. Poisoning with the recreational drug paramethoxyamphetamine ("death"). Med. J. Aust. **174**: 453–455.
13. BYARD, R.W., J. GILBERT, R. JAMES & R.J. LOKAN. 1998. Amphetamine derivative fatalities in South Australia: Is "ecstasy" the culprit? Am. J. Forensic Med. Pathol. **19**: 261–265.
14. BYARD, R.W., R.A. JAMES, J.D. GILBERT & P.D. FELGATE. 1999. Another PMA-related fatality in Adelaide. Med. J. Aust. **170**: 139–140.

15. GREEN, A.R., A.J. CROSS & G.M. GOODWIN. 1995. Review of the pharmacology and clinical pharmacology of 3,4-methylenedioxymethamphetamine (MDMA or "Ecstasy"). Psychopharmacology **119:** 247–260.
16. HEGARDOREN, K.M., G.B. BAKER & M. BOURIN. 1999. 3,4-Methylenedioxy analogues of amphetamine: defining the risks to humans. Neurosci. Biobehav. Rev. **23:** 539–553.
17. NICHOLS, D.E., D.H. LLOYD, A.J. HOFFMAN, *et al.* 1982. Effects of certain hallucinogenic amphetamine analogues on the release of ^{3}[H] serotonin from rat brain synaptosomes. J. Med. Chem. **25:** 530–535.
18. TSENG, L.F., R.J. HITZEMAN & H.H. LOH. 1974. Comparative effects of dl-p-methoxyamphetamine and d-amphetamine on catecholamine release and reuptake in vitro. J. Pharmacol. Exp. Ther. **189:** 708–715.
19. TSENG, L.F., M.K. MENON & H.H. LOH. 1976. Comparative actions of monomethoxyamphetamined on the release and reuptake of biogenic amines in brain tissues. J. Pharmacol. Exp. Ther. **197:** 263–271.
20. HEGADOREN, K.M., M.T. MARTIN-IVERSON & G.B. BAKER. 1995. Comparative behavioral and neurochemical studies with a psychomotor stimulant, a hallucinogen and 3, 4-methylenedioxy analogues of amphetamine. Psychopharmacology **118:** 295–304.
21. TSENG, L.F. & H.H. LOH. 1974. Significance of dopamine receptor activation in d,l-p-methoxyamphetamine and D-amphetamine-induced locomotor activity. J. Pharmacol. Exp. Ther. **189:** 717–723.

Cell-Mediated Immune Response in MDMA Users After Repeated Dose Administration

Studies in Controlled versus Noncontrolled Settings

R. PACIFICI,[a] P. ZUCCARO,[a] M. FARRÉ,[b] S. PICHINI,[a] S. DI CARLO,[a] P.N. ROSET,[b] I. PALMI,[a] J. ORTUÑO,[b] E. MENOYO,[b] J. SEGURA,[b] AND R. DE LA TORRE[b]

[a]*Clinical Biochemistry Department, Istituto Superiore di Sanità, Rome, Italy*

[b]*Pharmacology Unit, Institut Municipal d'Investigació Mèdica (IMIM), Universitat Autònoma de Barcelona and Universitat Pompeu Fabra, Barcelona, Spain*

ABSTRACT: Acute administration of 3,4-methylenedioxymethamphetamine (MDMA, "ecstasy") produces time-dependent immune dysfunction in humans. Recreational use of MDMA generally includes repeated drug consumption, often in association with other drugs, such as alcohol and cannabis. In the laboratory setting, repeated MDMA administration to healthy MDMA consumers produced a time-dependent immune dysfunction similar to that observed with the ingestion of a single dose, and the first of the two administrations paralleled the time-course of MDMA-induced cortisol stimulation kinetics and MDMA plasma concentrations. A significant decrease in CD4 T-helper cells with simultaneous increase in natural killer (NK) cell and a decrease in functional responsiveness of lymphocytes to mitogenic stimulation was observed. Response to the second dose was either long-lasting compared with the first dose or disproportionate and did not show any parallelism with cortisol and MDMA plasma concentrations. This circumstance extended the critical period during which immunocompetence is highly impaired as a result of MDMA use. Accumulation of MDMA in the body of a poor metabolizer induced higher immunomodulatory effects with statistically significant differences in NK cell function compared with extensive metabolizers. When basal values of lymphocyte subsets were examined in a population of recreational MDMA users participating in different clinical trials, alterations in several immunological parameters were observed. The absolute number of lymphocytes, in particular T lymphocytes and CD4 T-helper cell subsets, showed a trend toward reduced values, although cell counts were within normal limits. By contrast, NK cells in MDMA consumers were reduced to one-third of those from healthy persons. A statistically significant decrease in affected immune parameters was recorded during a 2-year observation period in a subgroup of recreational MDMA users. These permanent alterations in immunologic homeostasis may result in impairment of general health and subsequent increased susceptibility to infection and immune-related disorders.

KEYWORDS: 3,4-methylenedioxymethamphetamine (MDMA); immune dysfunction; lymphocytes; natural killer (NK) cells; ecstasy

Address for correspondence: R. de la Torre, Institut Municipal d'Investigació Mèdica (IMIM), Doctor Aiguader 80, E-08003 Barcelona, Spain. Voice: +34 93 2211009; fax: +34 93 2213237. rtorre@imim.es

Ann. N.Y. Acad. Sci. 965: 421–433 (2002). © 2002 New York Academy of Sciences.

INTRODUCTION

Immunomodulating activity of MDMA (3,4-methylenedioxymethamphetamine, "ecstasy") after single-dose administration has recently been assessed in various animal models and in humans.[1] In particular, administration of MDMA in rats produces a rapid and sustained suppression of induced lymphocyte proliferation and a significant decrease in circulating lymphocytes.[2,3] In humans, a single dose of 100 mg MDMA caused a decrease in CD4 T-helper cells, a simultaneous increase in natural killer (NK) cells, and a decrease in functional responsiveness of lymphocytes to mitogenic stimulation. The correlation of MDMA pharmacokinetics and MDMA-induced cortisol secretion kinetics with the profile of MDMA-induced immune disregulation suggested a possible implication of the central nervous system in the impairment of immunological status.[4] Subsequent investigations showed that acute MDMA produced a large increase of immunosuppressive cytokines and an imbalance toward antiinflammatory response.[5] In any case, although a critical period during which immunocompetence was highly impaired was evidenced, the immune function showed a trend toward baseline levels 24 hours after a single MDMA administration.

Studies concerning patterns of MDMA use by consumers, however, show that recreational use of MDMA includes repeated drug administration (bingeing) by "stacking" (i.e., taking several tablets at one time) or "boosting" (i.e., taking several tablets but at intervals over a period of time such as an evening or even several days).[6] These circumstances could probably extend the period following MDMA administration during which immunocompetence is highly impaired. Furthermore, MDMA is consumed either alone or in combination with other drugs, such as ethanol, cannabis, and cocaine, which also are known to induce immune function alterations.[7-11] Hence, such effects have to be combined with those elicited by MDMA. Thus, more pronounced and long-lasting immunological changes may result from the aforementioned MDMA consumption patterns with potentially enhanced susceptibility to infection and immune-related disorders.

In this paper, experimental data on cell-mediated immune response in volunteers administered repeated doses of MDMA at different time intervals are reviewed. The impact of MDMA metabolism by cytochrome P 450 2D6 (CYP2D6) isoenzyme (debrisoquine 4-hydroxylase) on MDMA immunomodulatory effects is discussed. Data regarding immune baseline parameters in MDMA recreational users participating in different clinical trials during a two-year interval were also reviewed as a preliminary approach to midterm effects of MDMA immunotoxicity.*m*

STUDIES IN CONTROLLED SETTINGS: CLINICAL TRIALS OF REPEATED MDMA ADMINISTRATION

Cell-mediated immune response after the administration of two repeated doses of 100 mg MDMA at 4-hour and 24-hour intervals was evaluated in two randomized, double-blind and crossover clinical trials conducted in 18 healthy male MDMA consumers. Total leukocyte counts, blood lymphocyte subsets, and lymphocyte proliferative response to mitogenic stimulation, as well as cortisol and MDMA plasma concentrations, were investigated.[12] Subjects were phenotyped for CYP2D6 activity using dextromethorphan as a drug probe. The destromethorphan/dextrorphan ratio was used to classify subjects as poor or extensive metabolizers.[13] All the subjects but one turned out to be extensive metabolizers.

MDMA administration produced a time-dependent decrease in the number of CD4 T-helper cells, a decrease in the functional responsiveness of lymphocytes to mitogenic stimulation, and a simultaneous increase in natural killer cells as already described in single-dose studies. In the case of two 100-mg MDMA doses given 4 hours apart to eight volunteers who were extensive metabolizers, immune alterations produced by the first dose were strengthened by the second one. In fact, the first 100-mg dose produced alterations in immune parameters, which peaked at 1.5 hours from the start of the treatment, when C_{max} of MDMA was attained in plasma. A mean 30% decrease in CD4 proportion from baseline, a mean reduction of lymphoproliferative response to PHA stimulation of 68%, and a mean 103% peak increase of NK

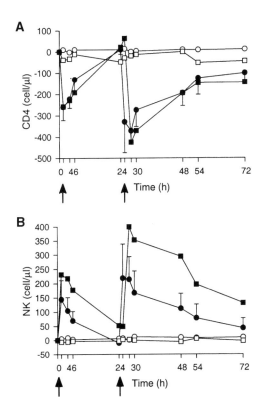

FIGURE 1. Time-course of CD4 T-helper cells (**A**) and NK cells (**B**) after the administration of two doses of 100 mg MDMA with a 24-hour interval in nine extensive metabolizers (● for MDMA administration and ○ for placebo) and one poor metabolizer (■ for MDMA administration and □ for placebo). *Arrows* below the abscissa indicate the administration of 100 mg MDMA. Values have been normalized by subtracting to experimental values the corresponding basal value of each treatment condition.

cells from the initial value were observed. At 1.5 hours after the administration of the second MDMA dose (5.5 hours after the beginning of the experiment) CD4 T cells and lymphocyte proliferative response to PHA showed a mean 40% and 87% decrease from basal values, respectively, compared with placebo. In contrast, the increase in NK cells showed a 141% rise from baseline values. A mean 20% peak rise was observed in cortisol concentrations at 2 hours after both the first and second MDMA dose. At 24 hours after the first administration, statistically significant residual effects were observed for all the altered immune parameters, in contrast with recovered homeostasis of immune function observed after MDMA single dose.[1]

In the second clinical trial, two 100-mg doses of MDMA were given 24 hours apart to nine extensive-metabolizer volunteers and one poor-metabolizer volunteer. In extensive metabolizers, the first dose produced alterations in immune parameters of the same magnitude and time course as those observed in previous studies.[1,4] All variables returned to baseline values within 24 hours. However, the second dose caused immunological changes significantly greater than those induced by the first pharmacological challenge (TABLE 1).

The magnitude of alterations induced by MDMA when comparing those observed after the first administration and two consecutive doses may be exemplified by comparing area under the curve $(AUC)_{24-48 h}$ versus $AUC_{0-24 h}$ of CD4 T-helper and NK cell kinetics (TABLE 1 and FIG. 1). Average increases for the second dose were threefold for CD4 T-helper cells and three and a half times for NK cells. It can also be noted that MDMA AUC also increased, on average, 49%. Conversely, peak values of cortisol concentration at 1.5 hours after the first and the second MDMA dose were not different.

Regarding the poor-metabolizer volunteer, he showed MDMA AUCs higher than those from extensive metabolizers after both the first and second MDMA doses (60% greater in AUC for both time intervals compared with extensive metabolizers), with a statistically significant difference after the second drug administration (TABLE 1). Nevertheless, this effect apparently did not influence the rise in cortisol and the decrease in CD4 T-helper cells, which were similar to those from extensive metabolizers after both the first and second MDMA doses. In contrast, NK cell kinetics showed a statistically significant increase in comparison with those of extensive metabolizers after both the first and second MDMA administration (FIG. 1). Peak effects of immune response appeared to show a delayed onset (TABLE 1). Similarly to the other volunteers, the poor metabolizer presented a 41% increase in MDMA AUC after the second drug dose, whereas altered immune parameters changed more than twofold.

Results obtained in clinical trials of double MDMA administration confirm the findings postulated in single-dose protocols; that is, MDMA administration induces changes in peripheral blood lymphocyte redistribution.[12] It is possible that some cell subsets (such as circulating CD4 T-helper cells) migrate to certain compartments to be protected from potential deleterious effects of MDMA. At the same time, other cell subpopulations (NK cells) may migrate from the immune compartment, like an adaptive compensatory response. This fact can be interpreted as an immunosuppressive action, since cells are removed from the primary site of action with a subsequent reduction in their cytotoxic effect.[14] This hypothesis is supported by the decrease in the functional responsiveness of lymphocytes to mitogenic stimulation observed after single and repeated MDMA administration.[1,12] Furthermore, in animal models,

TABLE 1. Area under the curve, maximal effect, and time of peak concentration for lymphocyte subsets, MDMA, and cortisol kinetics in extensive versus poor metabolizers after the administration of two repeated doses of 100 mg MDMA at 24-h intervals

		Extensive metabolizer ($n = 9$) mean values	Poor metabolizer ($n = 1$)
CD4 T-helper cells	$AUC_{0-24 h}$, cell·h·ml^{-1}	−2248.8	−2748.1
	$AUC_{24-48 h}$, cell·h·ml^{-1}	−5980.2	−6270.1
	$E_{max\ 0-24 h}$, cell·ml^{-1}	−266.7	−257.3
	$E_{max\ 24-48 h}$, cell·ml^{-1}	−389.3	−424.0
	$t_{max\ 0-24 h}$, hours	1.5	1.5
	$t_{max\ 24-48 h}$, hours	25.5	28.0
NK cells	$AUC_{0-24 h}$, cell·h·ml^{-1}	1120.4	3187.9[*]
	$AUC_{24-48 h}$, cell·h·ml^{-1}	3577.6	7209.3[*]
	$E_{max\ 0-24 h}$, cell·ml^{-1}	145.9	231.3
	$E_{max\ 24-48 h}$, cell·ml^{-1}	241.5	399.5
	$t_{max\ 0-24 h}$, hours	1.5	1.5
	$t_{max\ 24-48 h}$, hours	25.5	28
MDMA plasma levels	$AUC_{0-24 h}$, ng·h·ml^{-1}	1914.3	3096.2
	AUC_{24-48h}, ng·h·ml^{-1}	2767.4	4363.9[*]
	$C_{max\ 0-24 h}$, ng·ml^{-1}	173.0	233.1
	$C_{max\ 24-48 h}$, ng·ml^{-1}	223.3	327.2[*]
	$t_{max\ 0-24 h}$, hours	1.5	1.5
	$t_{max\ 24-48 h}$, hours	25.5	25.5
Cortisol plasma levels	$AUC_{0-6 h}$, μg·h·ml^{-1}	25.0	31.2
	$AUC_{24-30 h}$, μg·h·ml^{-1}	23.9	16.7
	$C_{max\ 0-6 h}$, μg·ml^{-1}	13.4	15.2
	$C_{max\ 24-30 h}$, μg·ml^{-1}	13.9	17.7
	$t_{max\ 0-6 h}$, hours	1.5	1.5
	$t_{max\ 24-30 h}$, hours	25.5	25.5

NOTE: Results from all variables were transformed to differences from baseline. Plasma cortisol was only measured in the 6 hours after each drug administration.

ABBREVIATIONS: AUC: area under the concentration–time curve calculated by the trapezoidal rule; E_{max}: peak effect as maximum absolute change from baseline values; C_{max}: peak plasma concentration; t_{max}: time of peak effect or peak plasma concentration.

*$p < 0.05$ using Student's *t* test to disciminate one single value from a mean.

MDMA induces the release of stress challenge-related neurotransmitters such as serotonin, norepinephrine, and dopamine.[15] It is possible that an increase in stress hormones and neurotransmitters may be involved in switching immune cells from the blood and various immune tissues. Interestingly, the same immune reactions were observed in the rapid response to several acute psychological and physical stressors in human volunteers. In fact, volunteers exposed to acute psychological stress showed a significant elevation in the percentage of NK cells and a fall in the CD4 cell percentages as early as 4 min after the start of challenge.[16] In addition, a study showed a number of lymphocytes reduced in blood but increased in several immune tissues as a result of acute stress or acute administration of glucocorticoids.[17]

Nevertheless, immune response to a second MDMA dose did not show a parallel course with cortisol or MDMA plasma concentrations They were either longer lasting compared with the first dose and/or otherwise disproportionate.

These findings are consistent with those of Connor et al.,[3] who observed a reduction in functional activity of lymphocytes in rats after MDMA administration even in the absence of corticosterone secretion. Therefore, it can be postulated that both in animal models and in human beings, MDMA-induced immune dysfunction may be also mediated by a glucocorticoid-independent mechanism directly involving the sympathetic nervous system (SNS).[18] Alternatively, the possibility that some kind of immune memory mechanism could also play a role cannot be discarded. Phenotypic analysis of blood-naive and activated/memory CD4 T cells after one and two administrations of MDMA could reveal important differences in the concentration of lymphocyte subsets, and it could justify the alteration of the mechanisms responsible for maintaining the systemic balance between functional subsets of peripheral lymphocytes.[18,19]

The accumulation of MDMA in the body of the poor metabolizer seemed to induce immune alterations higher than those observed in the extensive metabolizers. In any case, the increase was marginal in the case of CD4 cells; whereas, for the NK cells of the poor metabolizer, both $AUC_{0-24 h}$ and $AUC_{24-48 h}$ were more than doubled compared to the other volunteers. The fact is that NK cells are the cells of the innate immune response, which provides the first line of defense against infectious agents,[20] offering an immediate response to the aggression against immune homeostasis.[21] Conversely, CD4 T helper cells are immunoregulatory cells, which in the case of host offence, migrate to lymphoid tissues to generate effector lymphokine responses.[22] Thus, it may be postulated that the NK activation response is more affected by MDMA kinetics than the CD4 regulatory response, which seems to show a "ceiling effect." By contrast, NK cells do not own memory subsets. For the same reason, even if CD4 cell response in a poor metabolizer is only minimally increased, it is possible that this fact could be attributed only to a single CD4 subset, which could be highly modified.

Repeated administration of single oral doses of 100 mg MDMA at 4-hour and 24-hour intervals extended the critical period in which immunocompetence is highly impaired. The greater immunomodulating effects observed after the second dose suggest that MDMA-induced changes in immune function may have significant consequences for the ability of the immune system to respond to potential or ongoing immune challenge, because it can occur that appropriate leukocytes may not be present at the right time in the right place. Furthermore, it can be postulated that repeated aggression against immune homeostasis with continuous peripheral blood lymphocyte recirculation could collapse the whole cell-mediated immune surveillance. These hypotheses prompted the revision of basal values of cell-mediated immune parameters in habitual MDMA users and a two-year follow-up of immune function in a selected number of those consumers.

STUDIES IN NONCONTROLLED SETTINGS: BASAL CELL-MEDIATED IMMUNE RESPONSE IN MDMA RECREATIONAL USERS

Basal values of lymphocyte subsets were examined in a population of recreational users of MDMA who participated in different clinical trials that have been carried out at the Pharmacology Unit of our center over a two-year period. Elegibility criteria required the recreational use of MDMA on at least five occasions. Exclusion criteria included consumption of more than 20 cigarettes per day and more than 50 g ethanol/day (6 units/day). A total of 30 volunteers were observed. The participants had a mean age of 24.0 years (range: 20–36 years), mean weight of 67.9 kg (range: 56.5–86.0 kg), and a mean height of 175.4 cm (range: 167.0–189.0 cm). All the subjects declared that they were MDMA consumers. A history of drug and alcohol abuse was recorded for each volunteer. All of them were habitual users of cannabis with previous experience with cocaine and/or methamphetamine consumption. None had a history of drug abuse or dependence according to DSM-IV criteria (except for nicotine dependence) nor showed any adverse medical or psychiatric reaction after MDMA consumption. Subjects were requested to abstain from consumption of any drug of abuse during the clinical trials, and urine drug testing was performed before each experimental session for opioids, cocaine, cannabis, and amphetamines.

At the first visit, each participant underwent a general physical examination, routine laboratory tests, urinalysis, and a 12-lead electrocardiogram. Furthermore, total leukocyte counts and blood lymphocyte subsets were investigated following a method described elsewhere.[12] Cell-mediated immune response was checked during the clinical trial sessions, and none of the participants showed statistically significant changes or modifications (ANOVA for repeated measures) during the four sessions of the trial. Furthermore, the cell-mediated immune response of six MDMA consumers (range of consumption on 5 to 50 occasions) out of 30 participants in different trials could be checked three times during the two-year period and compared to that of a control group of eight healthy volunteers, matched for age and physical characteristics, who did not consume any kind of drug of abuse. The two populations were examined for immune parameters by the same laboratory using identical techniques.[12]

TABLE 2. A comparison of lymphocyte subpopulations in healthy Spanish blood donors and healthy recreational MDMA users participating in clinical trials

Population	Blood donors ($n = 24$)		Recreational MDMA users ($n = 30$)	
	Mean ± SD	Median	Mean ± SD	Median
Total lymphocytes (cell/µl)	2199.7 ± 918.4	2061.0	2022.9 ± 391.2	1864.0
T lymphocytes (cell/µl)	1694.4 ± 664.0	1525.5	1577.0 ± 311.0	1441.3
CD4 T cells (cell/µl)	1004.6 ± 443.8	936.5	977.4 ± 240.0	919.0
CD8 T cells (cell/µl)	559.6 ± 270.1	551.5	588.4 ± 146.6	570.4
B lymphocytes (cell/µl)	233.2 ± 134.9	191.0	241.4 ± 102.7	215.9
NK (cell/µl)	246.6 ± 180.3	217.0	89.4 ± 68.7**	70.7

**$p < 0.001$ in relation to NK from blood donors.

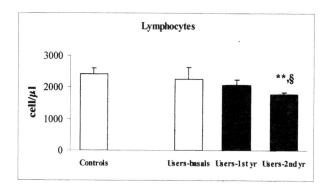

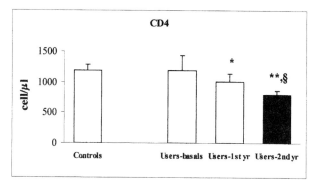

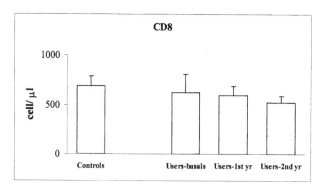

FIGURE 2A. Time-course of total number of lymphocytes, CD4 T-helper cells, and CD8 T-suppressor cells in six MDMA consumers and eight healthy volunteers during a two-year period. Data are expressed as mean and standard deviation (*bars*). Statistical significance was obtained using a one-way analysis of variance (ANOVA). If any significant change was found, post hoc multiple comparisons were performed using the Tukey's test. Statistically significant differences between MDMA users and healthy controls are indicated with filled columns ($p < 0.05$), between MDMA users checked at different years with asterisks (*$p < 0.05$; **$p < 0.01$) in relation to users' basals and with section mark ($^{\S}p < 0.05$) in relation to users' first year.

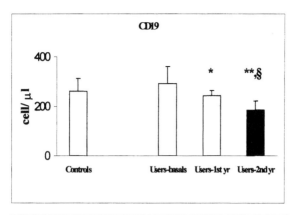

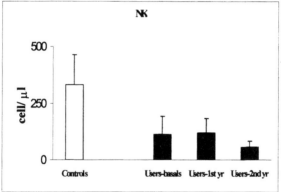

FIGURE 2B. Time-course of CD-19 B lymphocytes and NK cells in six MDMA consumers and eight healthy volunteers during a two-year period. Data are expressed as mean and standard deviation (*bars*). Statistically significant differences between MDMA users and healthy controls are indicated with filled columns, between MDMA users checked at different years with asterisks (*$p < 0.05$; **$p < 0.01$) in relation to users (basals) and with section mark ($\S p < 0.05$) in relation to users (first year).

Apparent alterations in several immunological parameters were observed in the 30 healthy recreational consumers of MDMA (TABLE 2). The absolute number of lymphocytes and absolute number of T cells and CD4 T-helper cells showed a decreasing trend if compared to mean values obtained in a Spanish population of blood donors having the same age range, although counts from recreational users fell within normal population ranges.[23] Conversely, NK cells in drug abusers were reduced to one-third of those from healthy persons. In addition to that observation, a progressive impairment of cell-mediated immune response was observed in the subgroup of six MDMA users followed for two subsequent years (FIG. 2).

Indeed, if comparing the six users with the eight healthy controls, at first observation (users-basals), MDMA consumers presented the immunological parameters tested, but for NK cells, similar to those from nonconsumers. One year after the first observation, the total number of lymphocytes decreased ($p < 0.05$), and at the end of second year the total number of lymphocytes, CD4 T-helper cells, CD19 (B lymphocytes), and NK cells all resulted in statistically significantly lower values. Furthermore, if considering only the time as a factor in the six MDMA users, a statistical impairment in the two following years was still observed, apart from NK cells, which were one-third of the values found in the eight controls and remained so during the two years of observation.

Results regarding basal cell-mediated immune response in MDMA recreational users seem to confirm the hypothesis that repeated challenge to immune homeostasis by MDMA consumption can affect cell-mediated immune response. The major impact is observed in case of NK cells. Evidently, as aforementioned, the high and temporary increase in NK cell number following acute MDMA administration could be an immune-compensatory response to alteration in the number and function of T helper cells. This adaptive or maladaptive response potentially could result in a net cost to the body when immune homeostasis is repeatedly challenged by use of MDMA. Therefore, it is not surprising that a large reduction of these cells, which in a normal population account for approximately 10–20% of peripheral blood lymphocytes,[24] to less than 5% is observed in recreational users of MDMA under baseline conditions. Furthermore, a positive correlation with a history of abuse seems evident, although the small sample size does not allow definitive conclusions.

Several clinical studies show that persons with a reduced number and/or function of NK cells may experience a higher risk of bacterial and viral infections.[25,26] In addition, recent experimental studies in mice selectively lacking NK cells demonstrated a critical role of these cells in defense against cytomegalovirus and herpes virus infections and resistance to tumor cells.[24] In addition, other immune parameters, such as total number of lymphocytes and CD4 T-helper cells, already involved in acute response to MDMA administration, and also in number of CD19 B lymphocytes, which did not appear implicated in acute response, were affected by chronic MDMA consumption.

These observations, together with all the evidence regarding acute effects of MDMA administration (single and repeated doses) on cell-mediated immune response, allow us to develop a pharmacological hypothesis for MDMA action on the immune surveillance system. Recreational use of MDMA has been associated with elevated scores of self-reported measures of depression and former chronic ecstasy users reported higher levels of depression than matched nonconsumer controls.[27] On the other hand, depressed mood has been associated with reduced NK cell activity, inversely correlated with the intensity of depression and reversable by means of serotonin-selective reuptake inhibitors (SSRIs).[28] Indeed, serotoninergic pathways in the central nervous system are related to psychiatric disorders such as depression.[29] In vitro studies indicate that serotonin regulates T-cell and NK-cell function and that it may be absolutely required for T-cell blastogenesis through its action on 5-HT_{1A} receptors.[30] The same receptors are involved in stimulation of T cells and mitogen-activated B-cell proliferation. Hence, serotonin itself and SSRIs, such as paroxetine or fluoxetine, are able to stimulate NK-cell activity in depressed patients exhibiting low activity at baseline. Furthermore, the administration of fluoxetine was associated with an alteration of leukocyte trafficking in primates;[31] and the 5-HT_{1A}

receptor agonist ipsapirone, which is given to depressed patients, led to a significant reduction of peripheral CD4 cells.[32]

The observations reported here are similar to those of our studies on acute and chronic effect of MDMA administration. In fact, MDMA consumers not under the direct effect of the drug present, at baseline levels present a situation of immunocompetence matching that of the depression mode. By contrast, acute effects of MDMA mimics the enhancing effects of serotonin and SSRI administration in depressed patients. It has to be said that even if direct determinations of neurotransmitters and/or their metabolites in biological fluids after MDMA administration had been never reported in humans, in animal models the release of stress neurotransmitters such as serotonin, norepinephrine, and dopamine was demonstrated after MDMA dose.[15]

The hypotheses illustrated here are supported by observations on *in vitro* cytokines release by SSRIs. Indeed, suppressed production of IL-2 and IFNγ by stimulated T lymphocytes and suppressed production of IL-1β and TNFα by stimulated monocytes by citalopram, fluoxetine, and sertraline[33] is in agreement with what is reported in our previous study after MDMA administration in healthy consumers.[5]

The clinical impact of immunomodulatory effects of MDMA consumption is still difficult to evaluate, especially when considering the type of consumers and patterns of abuse. In general, this phenomenon involves young people, well educated—most being students and employees—that consume ecstasy mainly on a weekend basis.[34] Hence, it can be acknowledged that risk of infection is certainly low, given the cohort considered. On the other hand, however, it has been reported that adolescents are the population at higher risk for acquiring transmitted diseases and that health problems, including depression and low self-esteem, may play an important role in the development and maintenance of high-risk sexual behavior.[35] In addition to this, MDMA abuse has been recently associated with high-risk sexual behavior among men who have sex with homosexual and bisexual men.[36] Therefore, the point is that MDMA-induced immune effects can enhance the susceptibility to infectious diseases, which can be a major health problem in case of association with high-risk sexual behavior. Nevertheless, a limitation in such observations is that they cannot be solely linked to MDMA consumption, because MDMA consumers included in the study are concurrent misusers of other substances. Neither can a definitive conclusion be drawn about the trend toward a progressive two-year impairment of the immune function in the MDMA consumers. Indeed, the observation was retrospective and included a small number of individuals, limiting the possibility of performing any kind of correlation between MDMA consumption and rate of impairment.

There are several reports on the impact of substances like nicotine, cannabinoids, or cocaine on the immune system, suggesting that under acute conditions they are able to induce profound alterations, whereas in chronic consumers results are more contradictory.[37] In addition, the impact on the immune system of other dance-scene drugs (like γ-hydroxybutyric acid [GHB] or ketamine) frequently ingested by the same MDMA users is still unknown. Even in the case of the hypothesis of lack of direct cause and effect between MDMA and immunologic impairment, however, it can be said that MDMA consumption in eventual association with other drugs of abuse could lead to pronounced immunological changes with enhanced susceptibility to infectious diseases and immunocorrelated pathologic conditions. Indeed, recently some cases of meningococcal meningitis were correlated with MDMA abuse,[38] and cocaine, which displays a common pattern of immune function alteration with MDMA, was suggested to be linked with a higher risk of infectious diseases including AIDS.[11]

ACKNOWLEDGMENTS

These studies were financially supported by Grants FIS 98/0181 and FIS 00/077, Department of Social Affairs (Italy), and intramural funding from Istituto Superiore di Sanità (Rome, Italy). We thank Marta Pulido, M.D., for editing the manuscript.

REFERENCES

1. PACIFICI, R. *et al.* 2000. Immunomodulating activity of MDMA. Ann. N.Y. Acad. Sci. **914:** 215–224.
2. CONNOR, T.J. *et al.* 1998. Acute 3,4-methylenedioxymethamphetamine (MDMA) administration produces a rapid and sustained suppression of immune function in the rat. Immunopharmacology **38:** 253–260.
3. CONNOR, T.J., M.G. MCNAMARA, J.P. KELLY & B.E. LEONARD. 1999. 3,4-Methylene-dioxymethamphetamine (MDMA; ecstasy) produces dose-dependent neurochemical, endocrine and immune changes in rat. Hum. Psychopharmacol. Clin. Exp. **14:** 95–104.
4. PACIFICI, R. *et al.* 1999. Immunomodulating properties of MDMA alone and in combination with alcohol: a pilot study. Life Sci. **65:** PL309–PL316.
5. PACIFICI, R. *et al.* 2001. Acute effects of MDMA alone and in combination with ethanol on the immune system in humans. J. Pharmacol. Exp. Ther. **296:** 207–215.
6. HAMMERSLEY, R., J. DITTON, I. SMITH & E. SHORT. 1999. Patterns of ecstasy use by drug users. Br. J. Criminol. **39:** 625–647.
7. TOPP, L. *et al.* 1999. Ecstasy use in Australia: patterns of use and associated harm. Drug Alcohol Depen. **55:** 105–115.
8. WINSTOCK, A.R., P. GRIFFITHS & D. STEWARD. 2001. Drugs and the dance music scene: a survey of current drug use patterns among a sample of dance music anthusiasts in the UK. Drug Alcohol Depend. **64:** 9–17.
9. SZABO, G. 1999. Consequences of alcohol consumption on host defence. Alcohol Alcohol. **34:** 830–841.
10. KLEIN, T.W., H. FRIEDMAN & S. SPECTER. 1998. Marijuana, immunity and infection. J. Neuroimmunol. **83:** 102–115.
11. PELLEGRINO, T. & B.M. BAYER. 1998. In vivo effects of cocaine on immune cell function. J. Neuroimmunol. **83:** 139–147.
12. PACIFICI, R. *et al.* 2001. Effects of repeated doses of MDMA ("ecstasy") on cell-mediated immune response in humans. Life Sci. **24:** 2931–2941.
13. SCHMID, B., J. BIRCHER, R. PREISIG & A. KÜPFER. 1985. Polymorphic dextromethorphan metabolism: co-segregation of oxidative o-demethylation with debrisoquin hydroxylation. Clin. Pharmacol. Ther. **38:** 618–624.
14. FRIEDMAN, E.M. & M.R. IRWIN. 1997. Modulation of immune cell function by the autonomic nervous system. Pharmacol. Ther. **74:** 27–38.
15. ROTHMAN, R.B. *et al.* 2001. Amphetamine-type central nervous system stimulants release norepinephrine more potently than they release dopamine and serotonin. Synapse **39:** 32–41.
16. BREZNITZ, S. *et al.* 1998. Experimental induction and termination of acute psychological stress in human volunteers: effects on immunological neuroendocrine, cardiovascular and psychological parameters. Brain Behav. Immunol. **12:** 34–52.
17. DHABHAR, F.S., A.H. MILLER, B.S. MCEWEN & R.L. SPENCER. 1995. Effects of stress on immune cell distribution. Dynamics and hormonal mechanisms. J. Immunol. **154:** 5511–5527.

18. Young, A.J., W.L. Marston & L. Dudler. 2000. Subset-specific regulation of the lymphatic exit of recirculating lymphocytes in vivo. J. Immunol. **165:** 3168–3174.
19. Stupack, D.G., S.Y. Cho & R.L. Klemke. 2000. Molecular signaling mechanisms of cell migration and invasion. Immunol. Res. **21:** 83–88.
20. Kim, S. *et al.* 2000. In vivo natural killer cell activities revealed by natural killer cell-deficient mice. Proc. Natl. Acad. Sci. USA **97:** 2731–2736.
21. Lanier, L.L. 2000. The origin and function of natural killer cells. Clin. Immunol. **95:** S14–S18.
22. Jenkins, M.K. *et al.* 2001. In vivo activation of antigen-specific CD4 T cells. Annu. Rev. Immunol. **19:** 23–45.
23. Larrea, L. *et al.* 1998. Subpopolaciiones linfocitarias en donantes de sangre. Sangre **43:** 380–384.
24. Moretta, L. *et al.* 2001. Human natural killer cell function and receptors. Curr. Opin. Pharmacol. **1:** 387–391.
25. Ogata, K. *et al.* 2001. Association between natural killer cell activity and infection in immunologically normal elderly people. Clin. Exp. Immunol. **124:** 392–397.
26. Brown, M.G. *et al.* 2001. Vital involvement of a natural killer cell activation receptor in resistance to viral infection. Science **292:** 934–937.
27. Macinnes, N., S.L. Handley & G.F. Harding. 2001. Former chronic methylene-dioxymethamphetamine (MDMA or ecstasy) users report mild depressive symptoms. J. Psychopharmacol. **15:** 181–186.
28. Frank, M.G. *et al.* 1999. Antidepressants augment natural killer cell activity: in vivo and in vitro. Neuropsychobiology **39:** 18–24.
29. Mizruchin, A. *et al.* 1999. Comparison of the effects of dopaminergic and serotoninergic activity in the CNSS on the activity of the immune system. J. Neuroimmunol. **101:** 201–204.
30. Serafeim, A. & J. Gordon. 2001. The immune system gets nervous. Curr. Opin. Pharmacol. **1:** 398–403.
31. Coe, C.L., F.Y. Hou & A.S. Clarke. 1996. Fluoxetine treatment alters leukocyte trafficking in the intrathecal compartment of the young primate. Biol. Psychiatry **40:** 361–367.
32. Hennig, J., H. Becker & P. Netter. 1996. 5-HT agonist-induced changes in peripheral immune cells in healthy volunteers: the impact of personality. Behav. Brain Res. **73:** 359–363.
33. Maes, M. 2001. The immunoregulatory effects of antidepressants. Hum. Psychopharmacol. Clin. Exp. **16:** 95–103.
34. Topp, L. *et al.* 1999. Ecstasy use in Australia : patters of use and associated harm. Drug Alcohol Depend. **55:** 105–115.
35. Shrier, L.A., S.K. Harris, M. Sternberg & W.R. Beardslee. 2001. Association of depression, self-esteem, and substance use with sexual risk among adolescents. Prev. Med. **33:** 179–189.
36. Klitzman, R.L., H.G. Pope, Jr. & J.I. Hudson. 2000. MDMA ("ecstasy") abuse and high-risk sexual behaviours among 169 gay and bisexual men. Am. J. Psychiatry **157:** 1162–1164.
37. Prasad, N. *et al.* 1994. "Ecstasy" and meningococcal meningitis. Infect. Dis. Clin. Pract. **3:** 122–123.

Methylphenidate-Evoked Potentiation of Extracellular Dopamine in the Brain of Adolescents with Premature Birth

Correlation with Attentional Deficit

PEDRO ROSA NETO, HANS LOU, PAUL CUMMING, OLE PRYDS, AND ALBERT GJEDDE

PET Center, Århus Kommunehospital, Nørrebrogade 44, Århus, Denmark

ABSTRACT: Perinatal anoxia/ischemia or premature birth increases the risk of developing attention deficit/hyperactivity disorder (ADHD). Brain imaging studies of idopathic ADHD reveal elevated dopamine transporter density in striatum of patients, predicting abnormal response to a challenge with methylphenidate in this population. We hypothesized that the severity of attention deficit in adolescents should correlate with the sensitivity to psychostimulant-evoked dopamine release. To test this hypothesis, we investigated six adolescent subjects (mean age 14.2 ± 2.4 yr) with documented birth trauma and/or low birth weight and a diagnosis of ADHD. Using positron emission tomography (PET), we measured the relative binding of [^{11}C]raclopride to dopamine receptors in striatum, first in the baseline condition and again after methylphenidate challenge at a therapeutic dose for ADHD (0.3 mg/kg, p.o.) in order to map the altered dopamine release evoked by the psychostimulant challenge. Neuropsychological measurements of impulsivity and inattention were also performed. We found a positive correlation between commission errors and the methylphenidate-evoked decrease in [^{11}C]raclopride binding, thought to reflect the balance of dopamine release and reuptake. The greater the decline in the [^{11}C]raclopride binding, the greater the ability of methylphenidate to block the reuptake of dopamine. As the ability to block the reuptake depends on the relative dopamine concentration, the result suggests that the impulsivity in these adolescents is associated with abnormally low extracellular dopamine concentration.

KEYWORDS: premature birth; attention deficit/hyperactivity disorder; dopamine; D2; receptors; raclopride

INTRODUCTION

Attention deficit hyperactivity disorder (ADHD) is a common behavioral disorder in childhood that is characterized by inattention, hyperactivity, and impulsivity, with a prevalence approaching 5%.[1] ADHD is a common sequela of preterm birth or

Address for correspondence: Pedro Rosa Neto, M.D., PET Center, Århus Kommunehospital, Nørrebrogade 44, Århus, Denmark.
pedro@pet.auh.dk

Ann. N.Y. Acad. Sci. 965: 434–439 (2002). © 2002 New York Academy of Sciences.

perinatal anoxia, frequently in association with MRI brain lesions.[2] Irrespective of the etiology, the majority of ADHD patients benefit from treatment with methylphenidate,[3] a drug that blocks monoamine neurotransmitter transporters in the plasma membrane. This clinical observation has lead to the hypothesis that a defect in catecholaminergic neurotransmission contributes to some clinical aspects of ADHD.[4] Thus, receptor images of the brain show an increased density of dopamine transporters (DAT) in the basal ganglia of adult patients with idiopathic ADHD.[3,6] There is also a positive correlation between clinical improvement and reduction of the density of DAT in the basal ganglia after a course of treatment with methylphenidate.[7] These abnormalities may underlie the high rate of comorbidity of ADHD and substance-related disorders. We hypothesize that the excess DAT contributes to a functional depletion of dopamine, which is corrected by the combined effects of methylphenidate blockade. Because the acute effect of psychostimulants on dopamine transmission in patients with attention deficit has not been documented, we tested the hypothesis by qualitative estimation of extracellular dopamine levels from methylphenidate's ability to block the binding of a dopamine receptor antagonist.

The binding of benzamide radioligands to dopamine $D_{2,3}$ receptors in human brain is reduced by competition from endogenous dopamine. Consequently, pharmacological challenges that block dopamine uptake decrease the availability of dopamine receptors for radioligand binding.[8] Thus, a high therapeutic dose of methylphenidate (0.8 mg/kg) decreased the binding of [^{11}C]raclopride in striatum of normal human volunteers by 9 to 20%.[9] A somewhat lower dose of methylphenidate (0.25 mg/kg) blocked 50% of the [^{11}C]methylphenidate binding to DAT in the striatum of healthy volunteers.[10] Thus, it is likely that premature birth perturbs the development of dopamine systems, resulting in the behavioral syndrome of ADHD, and that the severity of attentional deficit correlates with the potentiation of dopamine overflow after psychostimulant challenges. In order to test the above hypothesis, we first measured the stability and reproducibility of [^{11}C]raclopride uptake in brain of a group of adolescents with premature birth. The effects of *de novo* challenge with methylphenidate on [^{11}C]raclopride binding were mapped and correlated with individual measurements of impulsivity and inattention.

METHODS

Patient Recruitment

This study was approved by the Copenhagen County Committee on Human Research Ethics. Written informed consent and assent were obtained from all subjects and parents after complete description of the study. Drug naïve patients ($n = 8$) with a documented history of premature birth (27–34 weeks of gestational age[2]) were recruited from the John F. Kennedy Institute, Department of Pediatric Neurology, Glostrup, Denmark. The mean age was 14.2 ± 2.4 yr. A pediatric neurologist (H.L) and a child psychologist conducted the neuropsychological evaluations. Attention deficit and impulsivity were measured by the frequency of omission and commission errors, respectively, using the TOVA battery. All six subjects were given a clinical diagnosis of ADHD.

PET Scanning

Subjects were familiarized with the environment of the PET Centre. A catheter was inserted in the anterocubital vein of the nondominant hand for administration of [^{11}C]raclopride. At 12:00 P.M., patients received the first injection of 175 MBq [^{11}C]raclopride. One-half hour later, the patients were asked to recline on the scanning bed and were positioned with their head in the aperture of the ECAT EXACT HR+ (CTI/Siemens) whole-body tomograph. The emission recording consisted of three frames of five minutes' duration, each in 3D acquisition mode, followed by a five-minute transmission scan with the Ga^{2+} rotating rod source. Emission frames were reconstructed using filtered back-projection and Gaussian filtration, resulting in a final isotropic resolution of 7 mm.

Two hours after the first scan, the six subjects had a second [^{11}C]raclopride scan identical to the first, but initiated 30 minutes after an oral dose of methylphenidate (0.3 mg/kg, p.o.). Four subjects had previously been evaluated with [^{11}C]raclopride in the baseline condition. Baseline results from these subjects were used to estimate the test–retest stability of the method in this population.

Image Analysis

Images of the average tissue radioactivity during the 15-minute recording sequence were used to define anatomically the reference region (cerebellum). The striatum volume was defined by exclusion of voxels that contained less than 50% of the peak radioactivity of the striatum. These volumes were then applied to the dynamic emission images in order to extract the radioactivity concentrations in the last frame. Images of the ratio of radioactivity in striatal voxels to the average radioactivity concentration in cerebelum (S/C) were calculated and then manually resampled into a standard stereotaxic space using the program Register.[10] Reproducibility of the S/C ratio in the test–retest experiment was estimated using intraclass correlation. The effect of methylphenidate challenge was assessed by t statistical maps that were generated using SPM99, using two conditions and one scan per condition.

Results

There were no significant differences between the two baseline scans; the intraclass correlation was 0.5. Methylphenidate evoked significant decreases in [^{11}C]raclopride binding with peak significance in the putamen (right, t = 8.5; left, t = 7.0) (see FIG. 1). The effect of methylphenidate on the binding ratio is summarized in TABLE 1. The treatment decreased the mean ratio in striatum by 7.5%. No correlations were observed between S/C ratios of [^{11}C]raclopride in the baseline condition and the individual neuropsychological test scores. There was a positive correlation, however, between the magnitude of the change in [^{11}C]raclopride S/C ratios elicited by the methylphenidate challenge and the number of commission errors in the Go/No-go test (right side, r = 0.80, p = 0.02; left side, r = 0.97 p = 0.002). A similar trend was observed in the scores for omission errors (right side, r = 0.72, p = 0.06; left side, r = 0.59 p = 0.16).

TABLE 1. Effect of methylphenidate challenge on the [¹¹C]raclopride ratio in adolescents with premature birth

ROI	Baseline	Challenge	% Change
Left striatum	5.1 ± 0.4	4.7 ± 0.4*	7.8
Right striatum	5.1 ± 0.4	4.7 ± 0.5**	7.3

Mean $\pm$ SD of striatum cerebellum ratios at 60 min. *$p < 0.005$; **$p < 0.002$ in paired t-test.

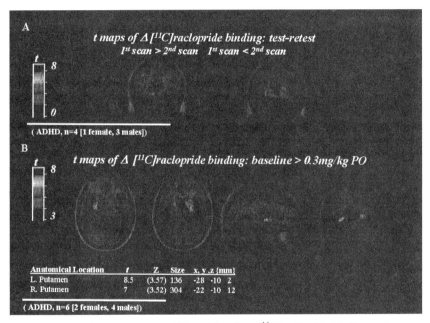

FIGURE 1. (**A**) Test–retest stability of baseline [¹¹C]raclopride binding ratios measured one year apart is represented by SPM maps superimposed on an average MRI. No significant differences were observed between the two scans. The scale indicates t statistic scores. (**B**) Differences between [¹¹C]raclopride binding ratios measured in the baseline resting state and during acute methylphenidate challenge. The [¹¹C]raclopride–SPM maps showed significant clusters in both striata, with peaks in the right and left putamen.

DISCUSSION

[¹¹C]Raclopride uptake ratios (S/C) had good stability and reproducibility in the present study group. The magnitude of the baseline ratio was close to that obtained in healthy adult volunteers.[12] The methylphenidate challenge elicited a significant reduction in the [¹¹C]raclopride binding ratio in the adolescents with premature birth, an effect somewhat lower than most reports in healthy adult volunteers.[13–16] This discrepancy might be attributed to age differences or to differences in the time delay between methylphenidate administration and PET recordings. We are currently investigating the methylphenidate response in a group of age-matched controls. The [^{11}C]raclopride uptake ratio, at steady state, is related to the binding potential, which reflects the binding of a drug relative to the unbound drug. The decline of the binding potential indicates the competition between the endogenous ligand, the tracer, and the inhibitor. We calculate that, depending on the dose of methylphenidate, the extracellular dopamine level is as much as four times greater for the least affected patients compared to the most affected.

The frontal-striatal pathway involved in stimulus suppression is sensitive to dopamine modulation.[17,18] Perturbation of this pathway, resulting in abnormal dopamine release, may account for the long-term behavioral consequences of low birth weight. In the present study there was a positive correlation between the reduction of [^{11}C]raclopride binding and the extent of impulsivity, as defined by commission errors during the Go/No-go test. This result shows that the extent of impulsivity in adolescents with premature birth is associated with increased responsiveness of the dopamine system to a psychostimulant challenge. Similarly, functional MR images of the brain engaged in a response inhibition task show that methylphenidate improves performance and increases blood flow in the striatum of ADHD patients.[17] Together, these findings suggest that rectification of low extracellular dopamine may underlie the therapeutic effect of methylphenidate on impulsivity. This result corroborates the hypothesis that the comorbidity of ADHD and substance-related disorder may reflect attempts at self-medication.

REFERENCES

1. ASSOCIATION, A.P. 1994. Diagnostic and Statistical Manual of Mental Disorders. 4th ed. American Psychiatric Association. Washington, DC.
2. KRAGELOH-MANN, I. et al. 1999. Brain lesions in preterms: origin, consequences and compensation. Acta Paediatr. **88:** 897–908.
3. SANTOSH, P.J. & E. TAYLOR. 2000. Stimulant drugs. Eur. Child. Adolesc. Psychiatry **9**(Suppl. 1): 127–143.
4. DRESEL, S. et al. 2000. Attention deficit hyperactivity disorder: binding of [99Tc]TRO-DAT-1 to the dopamine transporter before and after methylphenidate treatment. Eur. J. Nucl. Med. **27**(10): 1518–1524.
5. DOUGHERTY, D.D. et al. 1999. Dopamine transporter density in patients with attention deficit hyperactivity disorder. Lancet **354**(9196): 2132–2133.
6. KRAUSE, K.H. et al. 2000. Increased striatal dopamine transporter in adult patients with attention deficit hyperactivity disorder: effects of methylphenidate as measured by single photon emission computed tomography. Neurosci. Lett. **285**(2): 107–110.
7. LARUELLE, M. 2000. Imaging synaptic neurotransmission with in vivo binding competition techniques: a critical review. J. Cereb. Blood Flow Metab. **20**(3): 423–451.
8. VOLKOW, N.D. et al. 2001. Therapeutic doses of oral methylphenidate significantly increase extracellular dopamine in the human brain. J. Neurosci. **21**(2): RC121.
9. WIENHARD, K. et al. 1994. The ECAT EXACT HR: performance of a new high resolution positron scanner. J. Comput. Assist. Tomogr. **18**(1): 110–118.
10. MACDONALD, D. 1996. Program for Registration of Images (REGISTER) McConnell Brain Imaging Center, Montreal Neurological Institute, Montreal, Quebec.
11. SCHLOSSER, R. et al. 1998. Long-term stability of neurotransmitter activity investigated with ^{11}C-raclopride PET. Synapse **28**(1): 66–70.
12. RINNE, J.O. et al. 1993. Decrease in human striatal dopamine D2 receptor density with age: a PET study with [^{11}C]raclopride. J. Cereb. Blood Flow Metab. **13**(2): 310–314.

13. ANTONINI, A. *et al.* 1993. Effect of age on D2 dopamine receptors in normal human brain measured by positron emission tomography and ^{11}C-raclopride. Arch. Neurol. **50**(5): 474–480.
14. VOLKOW, N.D. *et al.* 2000. Association between age-related decline in brain dopamine activity and impairment in frontal and cingulate metabolism. Am. J. Psychiatry **157**(1): 75–80.
15. WANG, G.J. *et al.* 1999. Reproducibility of repeated measures of endogenous dopamine competition with [^{11}C]raclopride in the human brain in response to methylphenidate. J. Nucl. Med. **40**(8): 1285–1291.
16. VAIDYA, C.J. *et al.* 1998. Selective effects of methylphenidate in attention deficit hyperactivity disorder: a functional magnetic resonance study. Proc. Natl. Acad. Sci. USA **95**(24): 14494–14499.
17. RUBIA, K. *et al.* 1999. Hypofrontality in attention deficit hyperactivity disorder during higher-order motor control: a study with functional MRI. Am. J. Psychiatry **156**(6): 891–896.
18. RUBIA, K. *et al.* 2001. Neuropsychological analyses of impulsiveness in childhood hyperactivity. Br. J. Psychiatry **179**: 138–143.

The Competition Between Endogenous Dopamine and Radioligands for Specific Binding to Dopamine Receptors

PAUL CUMMING,[a] DEAN F. WONG,[b] ROBERT F. DANNALS,[b] NIC GILLINGS,[a] JOHN HILTON,[b] URSULA SCHEFFEL,[b] AND ALBERT GJEDDE[a]

[a]PET Center, Århus University Hospitals, Århus, Denmark

[b]Radiology Department, Johns Hopkins Medical Institutions, Baltimore, Maryland, USA

ABSTRACT: The ternary complex model of G-protein–linkage to receptors holds that agonists increase the affinity of the receptors for the G protein. Consequently, an agonist can exert the greatest inhibition of the binding of radioligands which are also agonists. We hypothesized that competition from endogenous dopamine in striatum of living mice should thus have a greater effect on the binding of the $D_{2,3}$ agonist N-[^{3}H]propylnorapomorphine ([^{3}H]NPA), than on the binding of the $D_{2,3}$ antagonist [^{11}C]raclopride in living brain. The binding potential ($p_{B(0)}$), defined as the ratio of bound-to-unbound ligand after reserpine treatment, was measured in mouse striatum for [^{11}C]raclopride ($p_{B(0)}^{RACC}$ = 8.5), and for [^{3}H]NPA ($p_{B(0)}^{NPA}$ = 5.3). Relative to these baseline values after dopamine depletion, saline-treatment decreased the p_B of [^{3}H]NPA by one-half, while the p_B of [^{11}C]raclopride declined by only one-third. Amphetamine decreased the p_B of [^{3}H]NPA to a greater extent than that of [^{11}C]raclopride. The apparent inhibition constant of endogenous dopamine depended on the dopamine occupancy and declined to a value 1.66 times greater for [^{3}H]NPA than for [^{11}C]raclopride at its highest occupancies. Thus, the agonist binding was more sensitive than antagonist binding to competition from endogenous dopamine. Dopamine agonist ligands may be especially useful for PET studies of dopamine receptor occupancy by endogenous synaptic dopamine. Analysis of the effect of dopamine occupancy on the inhibition of agonist indicated a limited supply of G protein, with a maximum ternary complex fraction of 40% of maximum antagonist binding capacity.

KEYWORDS: dopamine; receptors; D_2; affinity; agonist; [^{11}C]raclopride; N-[^{3}H]propylnorapomorphine; amphetamine; reserpine

INTRODUCTION

Dopamine $D_{2,3}$ antagonist binding sites can be detected with [^{11}C]raclopride and other benzamide radioligands for positron emission tomography (PET) or single photon emission computed tomography (SPECT) studies of living brain. The bind-

Address for correspondence: Paul Cumming, Ph.D., PET Center, Århus University Hospitals, Nørrebrogade 44, Århus, Denmark.
paul@pet.auh.dk

Ann. N.Y. Acad. Sci. 965: 440–450 (2002). © 2002 New York Academy of Sciences.

ing of exogenous radioligands to dopamine receptors *in vivo* is normally reduced by competition from endogenous dopamine. Consequently, pharmacological depletion of dopamine increases the availability of dopamine receptors in brain of rodent,[1,2] non-human primate,[3] and human.[4] Conversely, stimulation of dopamine release with amphetamine, or blockade of dopamine transport with cocaine, causes further displacement of benzamide radioligands from specific D_2 binding sites in striatum of living rat,[1] baboon,[5,6] and human.[7,8] Thus, altered synaptic dopamine concentrations can be measured *in vivo*.

The pharmacodynamic response to G-protein–mediated neurotransmission occurs in proportion to the quantity of ternary agonist-receptor-G-protein complex,[9] as defined by DeLean *et al.*[10] and Samama *et al.*[11] In this scenario, the affinity of G-protein–coupled receptors for the agonist is low when the receptor is dissociated from its G protein and high on interaction with the GTP-free form of the protein (GTP-shift; Jiang *et al.*[12] This property of dopamine binding sites affects the interpretation of PET studies of dopamine release.[13] An extension of the ternary complex model of del Castillo and Katz[14] expresses the quantity of bound agonist as

$$B_a = B_{\max}\left(\frac{C_a}{K'_a}\right)\bigg/\left(1 + \frac{C_a}{K'_a}\right), \tag{1}$$

where the subscript a refers to the specific agonist, the term B_a to the quantity of the receptor-agonist complex which is not coupled to G protein, K_a to the basal affinity to the agonist, and K'_a to the receptor affinity as modified by G-protein binding,

$$K'_a = K_a\bigg/\left(1 + \frac{C_g}{K_g}\right) = \frac{K_a}{1 + \chi_g}, \tag{2}$$

where C_g is the G-protein concentration, χ_g is the concentration of G protein relative to its affinity for the ternary complex, and K_g the receptors' affinity to the G protein.

The formation of the ternary complex results in a biphasic displacement of antagonist radioligands by dopamine, with components at nM (D_2^{High}) and µM concentrations (D_2^{Low}).[15,16] The characteristic interaction between receptor agonists and G proteins predicts that the inhibitory constant of dopamine toward an agonist is lower than the inhibitory constant toward an antagonist. We tested this prediction by comparing the dopamine inhibitory constant toward the agonist N-[^{3}H]propylapomorphine ([^{3}H]NPA) and the antagonist [^{11}C]raclopride in striatum of living mice.

METHODS

Male mice ($n = 126$) of the CD1 strain (Charles River Laboratories, Wilmington, MA) weighing 25–28 g were used in these experiments, which were approved by the research ethics committee of Johns Hopkins Medical Institutions. In experiment 1, groups of 18 mice were pretreated with intraperitoneal injections of 200 µL saline vehicle, quinagolide (CV 205,502, Novartis) at a dose of 1 or 10 mg/kg, i.p., or amphetamine sulfate (Sigma Chemicals, St. Louis, MO) at a dose of 10 mg/kg, i.p., administered 10 min before the radiotracer injections. In experiment 2, groups of 18 mice were pretreated with saline, or reserpine (5 mg/kg, i.p.) 20 h before tracer injection supplemented with α-methyl-*p*-tyrosine methyl ester (AMPT, 100 mg/kg, i.p., Sigma) 1 h before tracer injections, or nicotine (100 μg/kg, s.c.) 3 min before tracer injection.

Mice were immobilized for bolus injection to a tail vein of 200 μL saline containing 0.1 MBq *N*-[³H]propylnorapomorphine ([³H]NPA, New England Nuclear, specific activity 2 GBq/μmol) and 7 MBq [¹¹C]raclopride (specific activity 200 GBq/μmol at time of delivery) synthesized by the method of Ehrin *et al.*,[17] at the Johns Hopkins GE PET Trace cyclotron facility. Mice were killed at 5, 10, 20, 30, 45, and 60 min after tracer injection, with triplicate determinations.

Brains were rapidly removed and the cerebellar hemispheres and corpora striata dissected. After weighing, left striatum and cerebellar hemispheres were transferred into plastic vials for immediate measurement of gamma emissions using a γ-counter (LKB 1285). Right striata and cerebellar hemispheres were transferred to 20 mL glass liquid scintillation vials to which was added 1 mL of organic base (Solvable, Packard, Downers Grove, IL). After dissolving overnight at 40°C, 10 mL of liquid scintillation "cocktail" (Formula 989, Packard, Downers Grove, IL) was added to each vial, and the tritium concentration measured using a β-counter (Tricarb, Packard Instruments, Downers Grove, IL). Radioactivities were calculated as percentage injected dose per gram of tissue. Using the cerebellum radioactivities as the inputs, the binding potentials of [¹¹C]raclopride and [³H]NPA in mouse striatum were calculated in triplicate by the reference-region method of Lammertsma,[18] in the baseline condition and in the drug-treatment conditions.

The occupancy of dopamine was calculated from the decline of the binding potential from the dopamine-depleted baseline obtained with reserpine plus AMPT, according to the equation,

$$p_{B(I)} = (1 - \sigma)\, p_{B(0)}, \tag{3}$$

where σ is the occupancy of dopamine, $p_{B(I)}$ the binding potential of the ligand in the presence of dopamine, and $p_{B(0)}$ the binding potential in the absence of dopamine. This plot has an ordinate intercept of zero and a slope of $1 - \sigma$. However, in the case of the relatively increased affinity and binding potential of an agonist ligand, the binding potential of the ligand in the presence of the inhibiting agonist was fitted by the equation,

$$p_{B(I)} = (1 - e^{-\alpha\, p_{B(0)}})\, p_{B(0)}, \tag{4}$$

where α varies with the endogenous inhibitor concentration relative to its apparent inhibitory constant and the product $\alpha\, p_{B(0)}$ is a normalization for any difference of inherent binding affinity or density of available receptors between an antagonist and an agonist in the absence of endogenous competition. Equation 5 follows rearrangement of equations 3 and 4 such that

$$\sigma = \frac{\Delta p_B}{p_{B(0)}} = e^{-\alpha p_{B(0)}} \tag{5}$$

for any ligand because, by definition, $\sigma \rightarrow e^{-1/\chi}$ for $\chi \rightarrow \infty$, when the occupancy of the endogenous inhibitor is the following function of the normalized inhibitor concentration,

$$\sigma_a = \frac{\chi_a}{1 + \chi_a}, \tag{6}$$

where χ_a is the concentration of the endogenous agonist inhibitor relative to its apparent affinity ($\chi_a = C_a/K_a'$) such that

$$\chi_a = \frac{p_{B(0)}}{p_{B(I)}} - 1 = \frac{1}{e^{\alpha p_{B(0)}} - 1}. \tag{7}$$

Equation 7 was used to determine the normalized dopamine concentrations inhibiting the binding of the antagonist and agonist ligands. The change of affinity responsible for this difference was computed as

$$r_K = 1 + \frac{C_g}{K_g} = \frac{K_a}{K_a'} = 1 + \chi_g = \frac{\chi_a^{NPA}}{\chi_a^{RAC}} = \frac{e^{\alpha p_{B(0)}^{RAC}} - 1}{e^{\alpha p_{B(0)}^{NPA}} - 1}, \tag{8}$$

where C_g/K_g is the concentration of G protein relative to its affinity for the receptors, and χ_a^{NPA} and χ_a^{RAC} are the apparent normalized concentrations of the endogenous agonist inhibitor measured with an agonist and an antagonist radioligand, respectively.

RESULTS

Typical time-radioactivity curves for [^{3}H]NPA and [^{11}C]raclopride in striatum of groups of six mice treated with reserpine (FIG. 1A), saline (FIG. 1B), amphetamine (FIG. 1C), and the high dose of quinagolide (FIG. 1D) are illustrated. The continuous lines are the results of fitting of the cerebellar time-radioactivity input curves to the concentrations measured in striatum for the estimation of binding potential (p_B) in striatum. The mean p_B under the several conditions are summarized in FIGURE 2A. In the dopamine-depleted baseline, $p_{B(0)}$, the mean $\pm$ SD values were 5.30 ± 0.77 for [^{3}H]NPA and 8.42 ± 1.62 for [^{11}C]raclopride. In two replications of the normal or saline-treated condition, the p_B of [^{3}H]NPA were reduced by 52%, whereas the p_B of [^{11}C]raclopride was reduced by 30%. Amphetamine reduced the p_B of [^{3}H]NPA by 73%, and the p_B of [^{11}C]raclopride by 47%. The low dose of quinagolide decreased the p_B of [^{3}H]NPA by 77%, and the p_B of [^{11}C]raclopride by 63%, but the high dose decreased both p_B measurements by about 94%. Nicotine challenge increased the p_B of [^{3}H]NPA by 10%, but did not alter the p_B of [^{11}C]raclopride.

From these changes of p_B, relative to $p_{B(0)}$, the receptor occupancies, σ_a, were calculated according to equation 6 and plotted as a function of the concentration of dopamine relative to its affinity, χ_a (FIG. 2C), calculated from equation 7. This relationship obeyed the Michaelis-Menten formulation, indicating the presence of a sin-

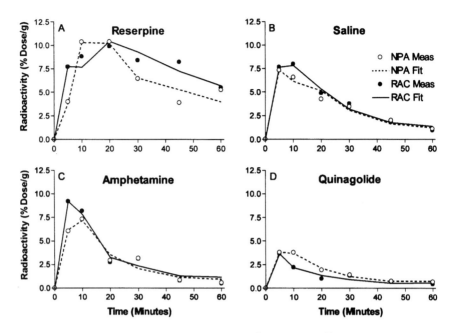

FIGURE 1. Radioactivity concentrations for [³H]NPA and [¹¹C]raclopride in mouse striatum during 60 minutes after intravenous injection of a single bolus containing 0.1 MBq [³H]NPA and 7 MBq [¹¹C]raclopride to groups of six mice that had been pretreated with (**A**) reserpine (5 mg/kg, i.p.) 20 h prior to tracer followed by AMPT (100 mg/kg) one hour prior to tracers, (**B**) saline vehicle (200 μL, i.p.), (**C**) amphetamine (10 mg/kg, i.p.) 10 min prior to tracers, and (**D**) quinagolide (10 mg/kg, i.p.) 10 min prior to the tracer administration. Radioactivity concentrations are calculated as the percentage of total injected dose per mg tissue. Lines are the results of fitting a two-compartment model to the radioactivities assuming reversible specific binding in striatum and zero specific binding in the reference tissue, cerebellum.

gle class of binding sites. In each pharmacological condition, the occupancy was higher for [³H]NPA, than for [¹¹C]raclopride. The resulting pairs of σ_a versus χ_a (Fig. 2C), show that values of χ_a^{NPA} were higher than values of χ_a^{RAC}. Figure 2D and 2E show the ratio between the antagonist and agonist affinities fitted to a second-order polynomial, which approaches a slope of 1.66 ± 0.11 (SE) at infinity of χ_a^{NPA}, indicating that the affinity of dopamine receptors toward an agonist approaches a value of 1.66-fold that of the receptors toward an antagonist. Another way of expressing the same result is to state that the C_g/K_g ratio (χ_g) declines to a ratio close to 0.66 for large values of $\chi_a^{agonist}$.

Figure 3A and 3B show the relationship between the concentration and occupancy of dopamine and the concentration and occupancy of the G protein, showing the decline of the estimated GTP-free G-protein concentration of elevated concentrations and occupancies of the endogenous agonist competitor.

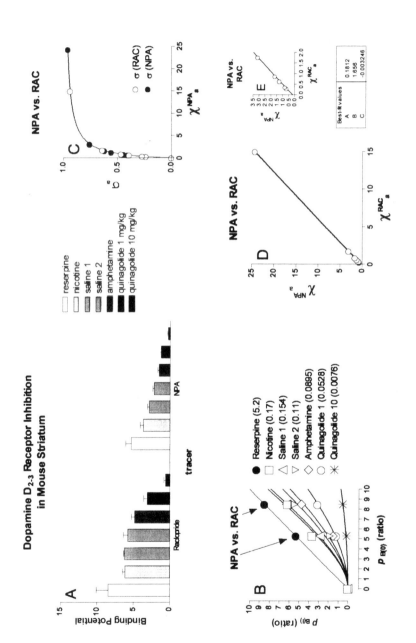

FIGURE 2. *See following page for legend.*

DISCUSSION

In the present study, the p_B of $[^{11}C]$raclopride in striatum was close to the ratio of radioactivity in striatum to that in cerebellum (less 1) at 30 min after $[^3H]$raclopride injection.[19] Likewise, the estimates of p_B for $[^3H]$NPA in mouse striatum were consistent with earlier reports of the binding of $[^3H]$NPA in rodent striatum during one hour of tracer circulation.[20,21] The apomorphines, like raclopride, do not distinguish between D_2 and D_3 receptors.[22] The differential sensitivity of NPA and raclopride to competition from dopamine is not evident from the earlier *in vivo* analyses performed in separate groups of mice. In the present study, we used the dynamic time-radioactivity curves measured in brain during 60 min of dual tracer circulation to calculate both p_B in striatum at equilibrium.

The 6-hydroxybenzoquinoline quinagolide is a dopamine agonist binding to D_2-like receptors in rat brain with an apparent affinty of 0.6 nM.[23] In the present study, the low dose of quinagolide was slightly more effective at displacing $[^3H]$NPA than $[^{11}C]$raclopride, but the two ligands were not discriminated by the high dose of quinagolide. Quinagolide, like the apomorphine derivatives, may also be a partial agonist, accounting for the ability of a low dose of quinagolide to differentiate only partially between the two radioligands.

Partial depletion of dopamine increases the availability of binding sites for $[^{11}C]$raclopride and other benzamide radioligands in human brain. The extent of this increase was greater in patients with schizophrenia than in healthy volunteers,[4] a finding which was interpreted to reveal the presence of elevated basal occupancy in schizophrenia. However, the partial dopamine depletion increased the availability of D_2 antagonist binding sites by less than 20%, even in the schizophrenic subjects. In contrast, the present study and earlier results in experimental animals[3,19,24] indicate basal occupancy of antagonist bindings sites of about 40%. Since complete dopamine depletions are not obtained in human PET studies, differences in p_B could be attributed to differential lability of the extacellular dopamine in addition to differences in basal occupancy. The present results show that a radiolabeled dopamine agonist is highly sensitive to changes in extracellular dopamine concentrations, and may thus be more suited than antagonists for detecting pathophysiological changes in occupan-

---

FIGURE 2. Binding potentials of $[^{11}C]$raclopride and $[^3H]$NPA in mouse striatum of mice after several pharmacological treatments, and the estimation of occupancy by dopamine, the putative endogenous agonist inhibitor, under the same condition. **Panel A:** Binding potentials of (*left*) $[^{11}C]$raclopride and (*right*) $[^3H]$NPA in mouse striatum at 20 h after reserpine treatment, and after acute treatements with nicotine (0.1 mg/kg, s.c.), saline (200 μL, i.p., two separate experiments), amphetamine (1 mg/kg, i.p.), or quinagolide (1 or 10 mg/kg). **Panel B:** Binding potentials in presence of endogenous agonist inhibitor released by treatments versus endogenous-agonist-inhibitor-depleted binding potentials measured after reserpine and AMPT treatment. Curves represent regression by Eq. (4) with corresponding estimates of α listed in legend. **Panel C:** Occupancies of endogenous agonist inhibitor determined with antagonist (RAC, *open circles*) and agonist (NPA, *filled circles*) radioligand according to Eqs. (6) and (7), indicating greater estimates of occupancy with agonist (NPA) ligand. **Panel D:** Antagonist ligand-determined occupancies of endogenous agonist inhibitor versus agonist ligand-determined endogenous agonist inhibitor, indicating second-order polynomial relationship. **Panel E:** Lower occupancies plotted at higher magnification.

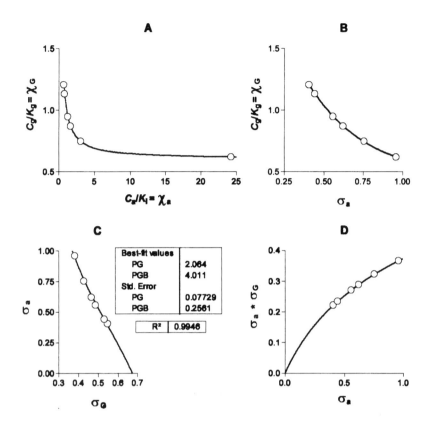

FIGURE 3. Binding potentials of G protein versus binding potentials of endogenous agonist inhibitor. **Panel A:** Normalized concentration of G protein (χ_g) versus normalized concentration of endogenous agonist inhibitor (χ_a^{NPA}) determined with agonist radioligand (NPA) according to Eq. (7). **Panel B:** Normalized concentration of G protein (χ_g) versus binding potential of endogenous agonist inhibitor σ_a^{NPA} determined with agonist radioligand. **Panel C:** Binding potential of GTP-free G protein (σ_g) versus binding potential of endogenous agonist inhibitor (σ_a^{NPA}) determined with agonist radioligand. Curve represents regression by Eq. (15), yielding estimates of total normalized concentration (χ_G) and binding potential (p_B) of G protein. **Panel D:** Ternary complex fraction of total binding capacity ($\sigma_g\sigma_a^{agonist}$) versus occupancy of endogenous agonist inhibitor ($\sigma_a^{agonist}$), indicating maximum achievable activation of receptor (40%).

cy of receptors in human brain. The present findings with [³H]NPA in living mouse suggest that ¹¹C-labeled NPA[25,26] is a good candidate for PET investigations of basal occupancy of dopamine receptors by endogenous dopamine in living human subjects.

Interaction with G Protein

The outcome of the study is consistent with the hypothesis that dopamine or an exogenous agonist competitor occupies a greater fraction of dopamine receptors when the occupancy is measured with an agonist radioligand than when measured with an antagonist radioligand. We based the hypothesis on the claim that an agonist radioligand undergoes the same GTP-shift of affinity enjoyed by dopamine or an exogenous agonist competitor. The theory of the GTP-shift of affinity yields the prediction that the ratio between the antagonist and agonist affinities depends on the ratio between the concentration of the G protein, which forms the ternary complex together with the receptor and its bound agonist. In the present study, this ratio was found to decline with increasing agonist concentrations, suggesting that the G-protein concentration is not so large as to render the unbound G-protein concentration essentially independent of the binding. Thus,

$$B_g = B_{max} \, \sigma_g \, \sigma_a, \tag{9}$$

where B_g is the difference between the total mass of G protein and the mass of unbound GTP-free G protein, and σ_g and σ_a are the occupancies of the GTP-free G protein and agonist, respectively. It follows that

$$B_g = (C_G - C_g) \, V_d, \tag{10}$$

where C_G is the concentration of total GTP-free G protein such that

$$(C_G - C_g)/V_d = B_{max} \, \sigma_g \, \sigma_a, \tag{11}$$

which rearranges to

$$\frac{C_g}{K_g} - \chi_g = \frac{B_{max}}{K_g V_d} \sigma_g \sigma_a, \tag{12}$$

where χ_g is the normalized concentration of GTP-free G protein available for binding. The equation further rearranges to,

$$\chi_G - \frac{\sigma_g}{1 - \sigma_g} = p_{B(0)}^G \sigma_g \sigma_a, \tag{13}$$

where χ_G is the normalized concentration (C_G/K_g) of total GTP-free G protein, and $p_{B(0)}^G$ is the baseline binding potential of the G protein. The equation was solved for the agonist occupancy,

$$\sigma_a = \frac{\chi_G}{p_{B(0)}^G \sigma_g} - \frac{1}{p_{B(0)}^G (1 - \sigma_g)}, \tag{14}$$

and subsequently fitted to the experimentally observed relationship between σ_a and σ_g, as shown in FIGURE 3C, yielding the estimates for χ_G and $p_{B(0)}^G$.

The inherent affinities of the receptors toward G protein and agonist are of the same order of magnitude (4.0 versus 5.3). They also show that the mass of available G protein is only half of the mass of receptors (2.1 versus 4.0).

The product of the occupancies of G protein and agonist defines the fraction of the total number of receptors in the ternary configuration. FIGURE 3D shows that this fraction reaches only 40% of the receptors at total agonist occupancy, indicating that no more than 40% of the receptors can be fully activated. We speculate that the remaining 60% of binding sites constitute the receptor reserve. Furthermore, changes in the abundance of G protein ($G_{i/o}$) may be implicated in the phenomenon of sensitization of dopamine receptors following chronic reserpine treatment[27] or 6-hydroxydopamine lesions of the dopamine pathway.[28]

ACKNOWLEDGMENTS

Our research was supported by MRC (Denmark) grants 9701888 and 9802563 and by the USPHS (NIH) Research Grants RO1 MH42821, RO1 DA11080, RO1 AA12839, RO1 NS38927, ROI SA 09482, and K24 DA00412. The authors thank Bisma El-Humadi and Paige Rauseo for expert technical assistance, and acknowledge the generous gift of quinagolide from Novartis.

REFERENCES

1. YOUNG, L.T. *et al.* 1991. Effects of endogenous dopamine on kinetics of [^{3}H]N-methyl-spiperone and [^{3}H]raclopride binding in the rat brain. Synapse **9:** 188–194.
2. INOUE, O. *et al.* 1991. Difference in *in vivo* receptor binding between [^{3}H]N-methyl-spiperone and [^{3}H]raclopride in reserpine-treated mouse brain. J. Neural Transm. **85:** 1–10.
3. GINOVART, N., L. FARDE, C. HALLDIN & C.G. SWAHN. 1997. Effect of reserpine-induced depletion of synaptic dopamine on [^{11}C]raclopride binding to D_2-dopamine receptors in the monkey brain. Synapse **35:** 321–325.
4. ABI-DARGHAM, A. *et al.* 2000. From the cover: increased basal occupancy of D_2 receptors by dopamine in schizophrenia. Proc. Natl. Acad. Sci. USA **97:** 8104–8109.
5. DEWEY, S.L. *et al.* 1993. Striatal binding of the PET ligand ^{11}C-raclopride is altered by drugs that modify synaptic dopamine levels. Synapse **13:** 350–356.
6. CARSON, R.E. *et al.* 1997. Quantification of amphetamine-induced changes in [^{11}C]raclopride binding with continous infusion. J. Cereb. Blood Flow Metab. **17:** 437–447.
7. SCHLAEPFER, T.E. *et al.* 1997. PET study of competition between intravenous cocaine and [^{11}C]raclopride at dopamine receptors in human brain. Am. J. Psychiatry **154:** 1209–1213.
8. LARUELLE, M. *et al.* 1997. Microdialysis and SPECT measurement of amphetamine-induced dopamine release in non-human primates. Synapse **5:** 1–14.
9. BURSTEIN, E.S., T.A. SPALDING & M.R. BRANN. 1997. Pharmacology of muscarinic receptor subtypes constitutively activated by G proteins. Mol. Pharmacol. **51:** 312–319.
10. DE LEAN, A., J.M. STADEL & R.J. LEFKOWITZ. 1980. A ternary complex model explains the agonist-specific binding properties of the adenylate cyclase-coupled beta-adrenergic receptor. J. Biol. Chem. **255:** 7108–7117.
11. SAMAMA, P., S. COTECCHIA, T. COSTA & R.J. LEFKOWITZ. 1993. A mutation-induced activated state of the beta 2-adrenergic receptor. Extending the ternary complex model. J. Biol. Chem. **268:** 4625–4636.
12. JIANG, M. *et al.* 2001. Most central nervous system D_2 dopamine receptors are coupled to their effectors by Go. Proc. Natl. Acad. Sci. USA **98:** 3577–3582.
13. GJEDDE, A. & D.F. WONG. 2001. Quantification of neuroreceptors in living human brain V: Endogenous neurotransmitter inhibition of haloperidol binding in psychosis. J. Cereb. Blood Flow Metab. **21:** 982–994.
14. DEL CASTILLO, J. & B. KATZ. 1957. Interaction at the endplate receptors between different choline derivatives. Proc. R. Soc. London B. **146:** 369–381.

15. CRESSE, I. & D.R. SIBLEY. 1979. Radioligand binding studies: Evidence for multiple dopamine receptors. Commun. Psychopharmacol. **3:** 385.
16. BATTAGLIA, G. & M. TITELER. 1982. [^{3}H]N-Propylapomorphine and [^{3}H]spiperone binding in brain indicate two states of the D_2-dopamine receptor. Eur. J. Pharmacol. **81:** 493–498.
17. EHRIN, E. *et al.* 1987. Synthesis of [methoxy-^{3}H]- and [methoxy-^{11}C]-labelled raclopride, a specific dopamine-D_2 receptor ligand. J. Labelled Comp. Radiopharm. **24:** 931–939.
18. LAMMERTSMA, A.A. *et al.* 1996. Comparison of methods for analysis of clinical [^{11}C]raclopride studies. J. Cereb. Blood Flow Metab. **16:** 42–52.
19. ROSS, S.B. & D.M. JACKSON. 1989. Kinetic properties of the accumulation of ^{3}H-raclopride in the mouse brain *in vivo*. Naunyn-Schmiedeberg's Arch. Pharmacol. **340:** 6–12.
20. HALL, M.D., P. JENNER & C.D. MARSDEN. 1983. Differential labelling of dopamine receptors in rat brain *in vivo*: comparison of [^{3}H]piribedil, [^{3}H]S 3608, and [^{3}H]N,n-propylnorapomorphine. Eur. J. Pharmacol. **87:** 85–94.
21. VAN DER WERF, J.F., J.B. SEBENS, W. VAALBURG & J. KORF. 1983. *In vivo* binding of N-n-propylnorapomorphine in the rat brain: regional localization, quantification in striatum and lack of correlation with dopamine metabolism. Eur. J. Pharmacol. **87:** 259–270.
22. LEVANT, B. 1997. The dopamine D_3 receptor: neurobiology and potential clinical relevance. Pharmacol. Rev. **49:** 221–252.
23. CHARUCHINDA, C., P. SUPAVILAI, M. KAROBATH & J.M. PALACIOS. 1987. Dopamine D_2 receptors in the rat brain: autoradiographic visualization using a high affinity selective agonist ligand. J. Neurosci. **7:** 1352–1360.
24. ROSS, S.B. & D.M. JACKSON. 1989. Kinetic properties of the *in vivo* accumulation of ^{3}H-(-)-N-*n*-propylnorapomorphine in mouse brain. Naunyn-Schmiedeberg's Arch. Pharmacol. **340:** 13–20.
25. HWANG, D.R., L.S. KEGELES & M. LARUELLE. 2000. N-[^{11}C]propyl-norapomorphine: a positron-labelled dopamine agonist for PET imaging of D_2 receptors. Nucl. Med. Biol. **27:** 533–539.
26. GILLINGS, N. & P. CUMMING. 2000. Synthesis of (R)-[1-^{11}C]propylnorapomorphine. 7th International Symposium on the Synthesis of Isotopes and Isotopically Labelled Compounds. Dresden, June 18–22.
27. BUTKERAIT, P. & E. FRIEDMAN. 1993. Repeated reserpine increases striatal dopamine receptor and guanine nucleotide binding protein RNA. J. Neurochem. **60:** 566–571.
28. TENN, C.C. & L.P. NILES. 1997. Sensitization of G protein-coupled benzodiazepine receptors in the striatum of 6-hydroxydopamine-lesioned rats. J. Neurochem. **69:** 1920–1926.

Repeated Administration of Gamma-Hydroxybutyric Acid (GHB) to Mice

Assessment of the Sedative and Rewarding Effects of GHB

YOSSEF ITZHAK[a] AND SYED F. ALI[b]

[a]Department of Psychiatry and Behavioral Science, University of Miami School of Medicine, Miami, Florida 33136, USA
[b]Neurochemistry Laboratory, Division of Neurotoxicology, National Center for Toxicological Research/FDA, Jefferson, Arkansas 72079, USA

ABSTRACT: Because of the sedative/hypnotic and euphoric effects of gamma-hydroxybutyric acid (GHB), the recreational use of the drug has increased significantly. In the current study we investigated the sedative and rewarding effects of GHB in Swiss Webster mice. Although the acute administration of GHB (200 mg/kg) caused marked hypolocomotion, repeated administration of the drug for 6 or 14 days produced tolerance to this effect. In addition, the administration of GHB 300 mg/kg to naive mice caused catalepsy, which dissipated in mice pre-exposed to GHB (200 mg/kg). Consequently, after repeated treatment with GHB, tolerance developed to both the hypolocomotion and cataleptic effects of the drug. The administration of GHB or its precursor gamma-butyrolactone for 14 days increased the striatal content of dopamine. The sedative effects of GHB may be due to hypodopaminergic activity from inhibition of dopamine release and a subsequent increase in the intraneuronal dopamine level. The rewarding effect of GHB was assessed in the conditioned place preference paradigm. Mice treated repeatedly with 250 mg/kg for 7 days developed conditioned preference for the GHB-paired compartment of the cage, suggesting that the GHB cue is rewarding. The development of tolerance to the sedative effects of GHB coupled with the rewarding properties of the drug support the abuse potential of GHB. Further studies are necessary to determine the mechanism underlying the development of tolerance to GHB and the rewarding effect of the drug.

KEYWORDS: gamma-hydroxybuturic acid; GHB; brain; drug abuse; hypolocomotion; reward

INTRODUCTION

Gamma-hydroxybutyric acid (GHB) is an endogenous substance generated in mammalian brain from the metabolism of gamma-aminobutyric acid

Address for correspondence: Yossef Itzhak, Ph.D., Department of Psychiatry & Behavioral Sciences, 1011 NW 15 Street, Gautier Bldg. Room 503, University of Miami School of Medicine, Miami, FL 33136. Voice: 305-243-4635; fax: 305-243-2771.
yitzhak@med.miami.edu

Ann. N.Y. Acad. Sci. 965: 451–460 (2002). © 2002 New York Academy of Sciences.

(GABA).[28,29,34] Besides the distribution of GHB in peripheral organs (kidney, heart, and skeletal muscles), evidence suggests that in the brain GHB has the properties of a neurotransmitter/neuromodulator.[23] GHB has a mechanism for biosynthesis, release, uptake, transport, turnover, and degradation,[38] and it is highly localized in the brain membrane synaptosomal fraction.[24,32,37] High-affinity GHB binding sites revealed the properties of G-protein coupled receptors [33] and are present in the hippocampus, cortex, thalamus, hypothalamus as well as the dopaminergic region such as the substantia nigra and the striatum.[15,17]

In humans, at a low dose GHB has an anxiolytic effect; at an intermediate dose it increases rapid-eye movement (REM) and deep low-wave sleep. GHB has been effective in treating narcolepsy.[30,31] Experimentally, GHB has been used as a model for petit mal epilepsy, because it causes generalized absence seizures in rats.[1,2] At a high dose, GHB has been used as a general anesthetic.[18] Other therapeutic properties have been attributed to GHB; evidence suggests that GHB may be useful in the treatment of (a) alcohol withdrawal and dependence and (b) opiates withdrawal.[12]

During the 1980s GHB and its precursor gamma-butyrolactone (GBL) were sold in health food stores as food supplements. Recently, recreational use of GHB has been reported in many major cities throughout the United States. Users report the feeling of "high" and the pleasurable effects besides its sedative effect. The combination of feeling high and sedation is probably what makes GHB so popular among drug users.[3,36] An overdose of GHB can occur rapidly and usually produces dizziness, drowsiness, nausea, and visual disturbances. A larger dose may lead to unconsciousness, seizures, severe respiratory depression, and coma.[7,20,35] A recent report from the Community Epidemiology Work Group (CEWG; June 13–16, 2000) warns about the growing epidemic of GHB abuse among other "club drugs" such as MDMA ("ecstasy"), methamphetamine, ketamine, and LSD. As a result, the drug was recently placed in Schedule I of the Controlled Substances Act (March 13, 2000).

The present study was undertaken to investigate whether repeated administration of GHB to mice produces (a) tolerance to the sedative/hypolocomotion effects of the drug and (b) conditioned place preference (CPP), a paradigm that evaluates the rewarding/abuse potential effects of the drug.

MATERIAL AND METHODS

Locomotor Activity and Catalepsy

To determine the dose-response of GHB on locomotor activity, male Swiss Webster mice (6–8 weeks old) were administered (i.p.) various doses of GHB (0, 100, 200, and 300 mg/kg). Locomotor activity was recorded by infrared beam interrupts (Opto-Varmix Mini, Columbus Instruments, Columbus, OH), as we described previously.[22] To investigate the effect of repeated administration of GHB, mice received daily injections of GHB (200 mg/kg) for 14 days. The animal's response to the drug was recorded on days 1, 6, and 14. In a second experiment, mice were pretreated with GHB (200 mg/kg) for 14 days, and on day 15 naive mice and the GHB-pretreated mice were challenged with GHB 300 mg/kg. The cataleptic response was measured by the Bar Test. The forepaws of the mouse were placed on a bar 4 cm above the floor, and the elapsed time was measured.

Conditioned Place Preference

Conditioned place preference (CPP) experiments were performed as we described previously.[22] Briefly, male C57BL/6 mice (8 weeks old) were administered (i.p.) GHB either 125 or 250 mg/kg every other day for 7 days and were confined for 30 minutes to the least preferred compartment (white) of a tow-compartment cage. Saline injections were also given every other day for 7 days, and animals were confined to the preferred compartment (black) for 30 minutes. On the test day (day 16), each mouse had free access to both compartments of the cage, and the time spent in each compartment was recorded for 20 minutes.

Striatal Dopamine Concentration

Male Swiss Webster mice were treated with saline, GHB, or GBL (200 mg/kg each) for 14 days. Animals were sacrificed after 48 hours, and striatal tissue was prepared for determination of the dopamine concentration by HPLC combined with electrochemical detection, as we described previously.[21]

Statistical Analysis

Results were analyzed by one-way ANOVA followed by the posthoc Neuman-Keuls test.

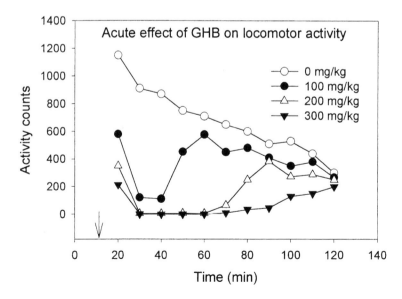

FIGURE 1. Effect of various doses of GHB on Swiss Webster mice locomotor activity. *Arrow on the left* indicates the time injections were delivered (10 minutes after habituation). Each *symbol* represents the average counts of 7–10 mice.

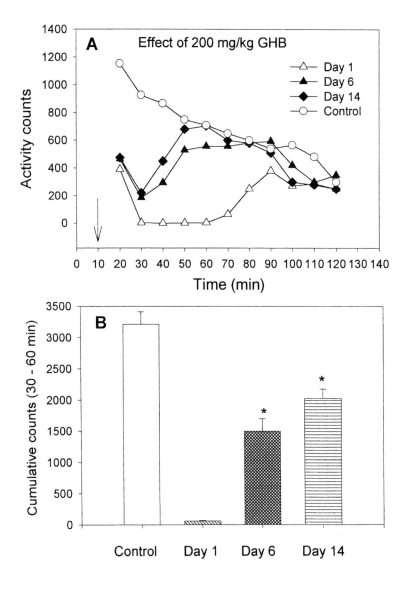

FIGURE 2. Tolerance to GHB-induced hypolocomotion. Swiss Webster mice ($n = 10$) were administered GHB (200 mg/kg) for 14 days, and locomotor activity was measured on days 1, 6, and 14. (**A**) Time course of drug effect on days 1, 6, and 14. (**B**) Total cumulative counts for a 40-minute period. Activity counts on days 6 and 14 were significantly higher than those on day 1 (*$p < 0.01$), suggesting the development of tolerance.

RESULTS

GHB (100–300 mg/kg) induced dose-dependent inhibition of locomotor activity (FIG. 1). The sedative effect occurred 10 minutes after drug administration. Depending on the dosage, animals recovered within 60 to 120 minutes. Results in FIGURE 2 show the effect of repeated administration of GHB 200 mg/kg on mice locomotion. On the first day, GHB had a pronounced sedative effect that lasted about 90 minutes. On days 6 and 14 the hypolocomotion effect of GHB was less prominent, and full recovery of locomotion was achieved within 50–60 minutes. FIGURE 2B depicts the significant differences between the responses on days 1 and 6 and those on days 1 and 14. The results suggest the development of tolerance to the sedative effect of GHB.

In a second experiment, mice were treated with GHB (200 mg/kg) for 14 days, and on day 15 they were challenged with 300 mg/kg GHB. FIGURE 3A shows again the different response of naive and GHB-pretreated mice to challenge injection of GHB. The rapid recovery of the GHB-pretreated mice suggests the development of tolerance to the hypolocomotion effect of the drug. FIGURE 3B shows the development of tolerance to the cataleptic effect of GHB. Although 300 mg/kg GHB caused marked catalepsy in naive mice (time spent on the bar 48 ± 10 seconds), the drug had no significant cataleptic effect on GHB-pretreated mice.

The rewarding effect of GHB was assessed in the CPP paradigm. FIGURE 4 indicates that whereas the low dose of GHB (125 mg/kg) did not produce place preference, the higher dose (250 mg/kg) produced significant preference for the GHB-paired compartment. This finding suggests that GHB had a rewarding effect in mice.

The concentration of striatal content of dopamine was measured in mice treated for 14 days with 200 mg/kg GHB or GBL. Results in FIGURE 5 indicate that repeated administration of GHB or GBL produced a significant increase in tissue content of dopamine.

DISCUSSION

The development of tolerance to the sedative effects of GHB is not well characterized. Repeated injections of GBL to ICR mice were reported to produce tolerance to the hypolocomotion effect of GHB.[13] The same investigators found that chronic treatment with GBL (in drinking solution) caused a decrease in [^{3}H]GABA binding in the cortex, striatum, and cerebellum of CD-1 mice.[14] In the present study we found that GHB produced dose-dependent inhibition of locomotion in Swiss Webster mice. Repeated administration of the intermediate dose of GHB (200 mg/kg) caused a time-dependent tolerance to the inhibitory effect of GHB. Six and 14 days of repeated drug administration led to tolerance to the sedative effect of GHB compared to the acute response on day 1 (FIG. 2B). The high dose of GHB (300 mg/kg) caused marked catalepsy in naive mice. However, mice that were treated with 200 mg/kg GHB for 14 days were resistant to the cataleptic effect of GHB (FIG. 3B), suggesting the development of tolerance to GHB-induced catalepsy.

The sedation and akinesia produced by GHB may be due to hypodopaminergic activity, similar to the effects of dopamine receptor antagonists.[10,16] Chronic treatment of rats with the GHB precursor GBL caused a marked decrease in the firing rates of A9 dopamine cells, a finding that was considered a model for dopamine hy-

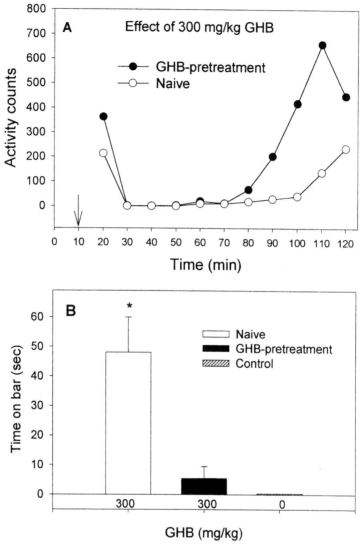

FIGURE 3. Tolerance to GHB-induced hypolocomotion and catalepsy. Swiss Webster mice were treated with GHB (200 mg/kg) for 14 days. On day 15, naive mice ($n = 10$) and GHB-treated mice ($n = 10$) were challenged with 300 mg/kg GHB. (**A**) The differences between the hypolocomotion in the two groups is shown. Recovery of GHB-pretreated mice was faster than that of naive mice, resulting in a significant difference between the two groups (*$p < 0.02$). (**B**) Depiction of the cataleptic response as determined by the bar test in which the forepaws of the mouse are placed on a bar 4 cm above the floor. Whereas control animals spent less than 1 second on the bar, naive mice challenged with GHB (300 mg/kg) spent 48 ± 8 seconds, and the GHB-pretreated mice spent only 5 ± 4 seconds on the bar. The significant difference between naive and GHB-pretreated mice (*$p < 0.05$) suggests the development of tolerance to GHB-induced catalepsy.

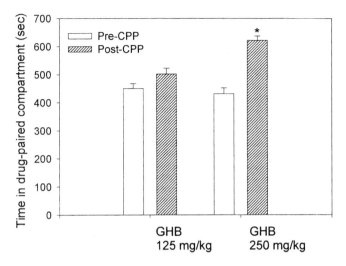

FIGURE 4. GHB-induced conditioned place preference (CPP). C57BL/6 mice ($n = 7$ per group) were administered either 125 or 250 mg/kg GHB every other day for 7 days and were confined to the least preferred compartment (*white*) of the cage. Saline injections were also given every other day for 7 days in the preferred compartment (*black*). On the test day, mice had free access to both compartments, and the time spent in each compartment was recorded for 20 minutes. Results are presented as mean ± SEM time spent in the drug-paired compartment before and after conditioning. Whereas the dose of 125 mg/kg did not produce CPP, 250 mg/kg produced significant CPP (*$p < 0.05$).

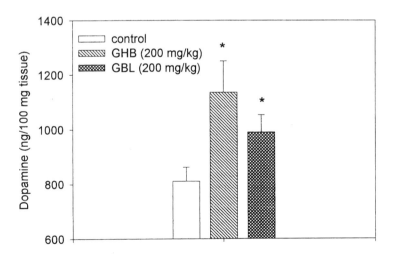

FIGURE 5. Effect of GHB and GBL on striatal dopamine level. Swiss Webster mice were administered saline, GHB (200 mg/kg), or GBL (200 mg/kg) for 14 days and sacrificed 24 hours after the last injection. Striatal tissue was processed for determination of dopamine concentration by HPLC. GHB and GBL caused increases of 40 and 22%, respectively, in dopamine concentration. *$p < 0.05$ compared to control value.

poactivity.[27] Also, in the awake rat, a high dose of GHB caused inhibition of the firing rate of dopaminergic cells in the nigrostriatal system, which led to inhibition of basal dopamine release in mesolimbic pathways. In turn, this led to an increase in intraneuronal dopamine synthesis.[6,10] Accordingly, the increase in tissue content of dopamine after repeated administration of GHB or its precursor GBL (FIG. 5) may be due to inhibition of dopamine release and an increase in intraneuronal synthesis of dopamine.

Several studies suggest that GHB has rewarding properties in animals. For instance, mice were able to acquire GHB self-administration,[9,25] and in rats, the discriminative stimulus effect of GHB was completely blocked by the GHB antagonist NCS 382.[4] Furthermore, GHB produced conditioned place preference in rats, suggesting that the GHB cue, like the cocaine cue, is sufficiently rewarding to produce place-conditioned response.[9,26] In the present study we demonstrated that the intermediate dose of GHB (250 mg/kg) produced significant CPP in C57BL/6 mice (FIG. 4). Although it is uncertain if a "true" addiction develops in humans abusing GHB, several cases of withdrawal symptoms of GHB have been reported.[5,8,11,19] These include anxiety, insomnia, muscular cramps, and tremor, symptoms that developed 1–6 hours after the last dose of GHB. The initial symptoms progressed to severe delirium and autonomic instability 5–15 days after GHB discontinuation.[8]

In summary, the development of tolerance to the sedative effects of GHB coupled with the rewarding properties of the drug support the abuse potential of GHB. Further studies are necessary to determine the mechanism underlying the development of tolerance to GHB and the rewarding effect of the drug.

ACKNOWLEDGMENTS

This work was supported by Award RO1DA08584 and DA12867 from the National Institute on Drug Abuse.

REFERENCES

1. BANERJEE, P.K. & O.C. SNEAD, III. 1992. Involvement of excitatory amino acid mechanisms in gamma-hydroxybutyrate model of generalized absence seizures in rats. Neuropharmacology **31:** 1009–1119.
2. BERNASCONI, R. et al. 1992. Experimental absence seizures: potential role of gamma-hydroxybutyric acid and GABA$_B$ receptors. J. Neural Transm. Suppl. **35:** 155–177.
3. BOYCE, S.H., K. PADGHAM, L.D. MILLER & J. STEVENSON. 2000. Gamma hydroxybutyric acid (GHB): an increasing trend in drug abuse. Eur. J. Emerg. Med. **7:** 177–181.
4. COLOMBO, G. et al. 1995. Blockade of the discriminative stimulus effects of gamma-hydroxybutyric acid (GHB) by the GHB receptor antagonist NCS-382. Physiol. Behav. **58:** 587–590.
5. CRAIG, K., H.F. GOMEZ, J.L. MCMANUS & T.C. BANIA. 2000. Severe gamma-hydroxybutyrate withdrawal: a case report and literature review. J. Emerg. Med. **18:** 65–70.
6. DI CHIARA, G. 1995. The role of dopamine in drug abuse viewed from the perspective of its role in motivation. Drug Alcohol Depend. **38:** 95–137.
7. DYER, J.E. 1991. Gamma-hydroxybutyrate: a health-food product producing coma and seizure-like activity. Am. J. Emerg. Med. **9:** 321–324.
8. DYER, J.E., B. ROTH & B.A. HYMA. 2001. Gamma-hydroxybutyrate withdrawal syndrome. Ann. Emerg. Med. **37:** 147–153.

9. FATTORE, L., M.C. MARTELLOTTA, G. COSSU & W. FRATTA. 2000. Gamma-hydroxybutyric acid: an evaluation of its rewarding properties in rats and mice. Alcohol 20: 247–256.
10. FEIGENBAUM, J.J. & S.G. HOWARD. 1996. Does gamma-hydroxybutyrate inhibit or stimulate central dopamine release? Int. J. Neurosci. 88: 53–69.
11. GALLOWAY, G.P. et al. 1997. Gamma-hydroxybutyrate: an emerging drug of abuse that causes physical dependence. Addiction 92: 89–96.
12. GALLOWAY, G.P. et al. 2000. Abuse and therapeutic potential of gamma-hydroxybutyric acid. Alcohol 20: 263–269.
13. GIANUTSOS, G. & K.E. MOORE. 1978. Tolerance to the effects of baclofen and gamma-butyrolactone on locomotor activity and dopaminergic neurons in the mouse. J. Pharmacol. Exp. Ther. 207: 859–869.
14. GIANUTSOS, G & P.D. SUZDAK. 1984. Evidence for down-regulation of GABA receptors following long-term gamma-butyrolactone. Naunyn. Schmiedeberg's Arch. Pharmacol. 328: 62–68.
15. HECHLER, V., S. GOBAILLE & M. MAITRE. 1992. Selective distribution pattern of gamma-hydroxybutyrate receptors in rat forebrain and midbrain are revealed by quantitative autoradiography. Brain Res. 572: 345–348.
16. HECHLER, V. et al. 1993. Gamma-hydroxybutyrate ligands possess antidopaminergic and neuroleptic-like activity. J. Pharmacol. Exp. Ther. 264: 1406–1414.
17. HECHLER, V. et al. 1987. Regional distribution of high affinity gamma-[^{3}H]-hydroxybutyrate binding sites determined by quantitative autoradiography. J. Neurochem. 49: 1025–1032.
18. HENDERSON, R.S. & C.M. HOLMES. 1976. Reversal of the anesthetic action of sodium gamma-hydroxybutyrate. Anaesth. Intensive Care 4: 351–354.
19. HERNANDEZ, M., C.H. MCDANIEL, C.D. COSTANZA & O.J. HERNANDEZ. 1998. GHB-induced delirium: a case report and review of literature on gamma-hydroxybutyric acid. Am. J. Drug Alcohol Abuse 24: 179–183.
20. INGELS, M., C. RANGAN, J. BELLEZO & R.F. CLARK. 2000. Coma and respiratory depression following the ingestion of GHB and its precursors: three cases. J. Emerg. Med. 19: 47–50.
21. ITZHAK, Y. & S.F. ALI. 1996. The neuronal nitric oxide synthase inhibitor, 7-nitroindazole, protects against methamphetamine-induced neurotoxicity in vivo. J. Neurochem. 67: 1770–1773.
22. ITZHAK, Y. & J.L. MARTIN. 2000. Blockade of alcohol-induced locomotor sensitization and conditioned place preference in DBA mice by 7-nitroindazole. Brain Res. 858: 402–407.
23. MAITRE, M. et al. 2000. Gamma-hydroxybutyric acid as a signaling molecule in brain. Alcohol 20: 277–283.
24. MAITRE, M., J.F. RUMIGNY, C.D. CASH & P. MANDEL. 1983. Subcellular distribution of gamma-hydroxybutyrate binding sites in rat brain. Principal localization in synaptosomal fraction. Biochem. Biophys. Res. Commun. 110: 262–265
25. MARTELLOTTA, M.C. et al. 1998. Intravenous self-administration of gamma-hydroxybutyric acid in drug-naive mice. Eur. Neuropsychopharmacol. 8: 293–296.
26. MARTELLOTTA, M.C., L. FATTORE, G. COSSU & W. FRATTA. 1997. Rewarding properties of gamma-hydroxybutyric acid: an evaluation through place preference paradigm. Psychopharmacology 132: 1–5.
27. NOWYCKY, M.C. & R.H. ROTH. 1979. Chronic gamma-butyrolactone (GBL) treatment: a potential model of dopamine hypoactivity. Naunyn Schmiedeberg's Arch. Pharmacol. 309: 247–254.
28. ROTH, R.H. & J. GIARMAN. 1970. Natural occurrence of gamma-hydroxybutyrate in mammalian brain. Biochem. Pharmacol. 346: 331–337.
29. RUMIGNY, J.F., M. MAITRE, C.D. CASH & P. MANDEL. 1980. Specific and non-specific succinic semialdehyde reductases from rat brain: isolation and properties. FEBS Lett. 117: 111–116.
30. SCRIMA, L. 1992. Gamma-hydroxybutyrate (GHB) treated narcolepsy patients continue to report cataplexy controlled for up to five years. Sleep Res. 21: 262.

31. SCRIMA, L. *et al.* 1990. The effect of gamma-hydroxybutyrate on sleep of narcolepsy patients: a double-blind study. Sleep **13:** 479–490.
32. SNEAD, O.C., III. 1987. Gamma-hydroxybutyric acid in subcellular fractions of rat brain. J. Neurochem. **41:** 869–872.
33. SNEAD, O.C., III. 2000. Evidence for a G protein-coupled gamma-hydroxybutyric acid receptor. J. Neurochem. **75:** 1986–1996.
34. SNEAD, O.C., III, R. FURNER & C.C. LIU. 1989. *In vivo* conversion of gamma-aminobutyric acid and 1,4-butanediol to gamma-hydroxybutyric acid in rat brain. Biochem. Pharmacol. **38:** 4375–4380.
35. STEELE, M.T. & W.A. WATSON. 1995. Acute poisoning from gamma-hydroxybutyrate (GHB). Mo. Med. **92:** 354–357.
36. TUNNICLIFF, G. 1997. Site of action of gamma-hydroxybutyrate (GHB)—a neuroactive drug with abuse potential. J. Toxicol. Clin. Toxicol. **35:** 581–590.
37. VAYER, P. *et al.* 1988. Gamma-hydroxybutyrate distribution and turnover rates in discrete brain regions of the rat. Neurochem. Int. **12:** 53–59.
38. VAYER, P., P. MANDEL & M. MAITRE. 1987. Gamma-hydroxybutyrate: a possible neurotransmitter. Life Sci. **41:** 1547–1557.

Enzyme and Receptor Antagonists for Preventing Toxicity from the Gamma-Hydroxybutyric Acid Precursor 1,4-Butanediol in CD-1 Mice

LAWRENCE S. QUANG, [a,b,c] MALHAR C. DESAI,[c] JAMES C. KRANER,[d] MICHAEL W. SHANNON,[a,b,c] ALAN D. WOOLF,[b,c] AND TIMOTHY J. MAHER[c]

[a]Division of Emergency Medicine, Children's Hospital Boston, Harvard Medical School, Boston, Massachusetts 02115, USA

[b]Program in Clinical Pharmacology/Toxicology, Children's Hospital Boston, Harvard Medical School, Boston, Massachusetts 02115, USA

[c]Department of Pharmaceutical Sciences, Massachusetts College of Pharmacy and Health Sciences, Boston, Massachusetts 02115, USA

[d]American Institute of Toxicology (AIT) Laboratories, Indianapolis, Indiana 46241, USA

ABSTRACT: 1,4-Butanediol (1,4-BD), the diol alcohol precursor of gamma-hydroxybutyric acid (GHB), undergoes *in vivo* enzymatic biotransformation to GHB by alcohol dehydrogenase (ADH) and aldehyde dehydrogenase. The subsequent metabolite, GHB, is pharmacologically active at $GABA_B$ and GHB receptors. GHB can be metabolized *in vivo* to gamma-aminobutyric acid (GABA) and *trans*-4-hydroxycrotonic acid (T-HCA), which are also pharmacologically active at $GABA_B$ receptors and GHB receptors, respectively. Therefore, we speculate that 1,4-BD overdose toxicity can be prevented or attenuated with the ADH enzyme inhibitor 4-methylpyrazole (4-MP) as well as with CGP-35348 and NCS-382, novel high-affinity receptor antagonists of $GABA_B$ receptors and GHB receptors, respectively. In our murine model of acute 1,4-BD overdose, pretreatment of CD-1 mice with 4-MP significantly attenuated increases in blood GHB concentrations and prevented loss of the righting reflex and failure of the rotarod test. Also, pretreatment with CGP-35348 and its combination with NCS-382 significantly decreased the duration of failure for the rotarod test and the percentage of animals failing the rotarod test, respectively. However, pretreatment of CD-1 mice with NCS-382 alone produced prolonged failure of the rotarod test, an unexpected synergistic effect with 1,4-BD and presumably GHB, which has not previously been demonstrated.

KEYWORDS: 1,4-butanediol; gamma-hydroxybutyric acid; 4-methylpyrazole; NCS-382; CGP-35348; gamma-aminobutyric acid; trans-4-hydroxycrotonic acid; $GABA_B$ receptor; GHB receptor; alcohol dehydrogenase

Address for correspondence: Lawrence S. Quang, M.D., Division of Emergency Medicine, Children's Hospital Boston, 300 Longwood Ave., Boston, MA 02115. Voice: 617-355-5189; fax: 617-738-0032.

lawrence.quang@tch.harvard.edu.

Ann. N.Y. Acad. Sci. 965: 461–472 (2002). © 2002 New York Academy of Sciences.

INTRODUCTION

Gamma-hydroxybutyric acid (GHB) and its precursor 1,4-butanediol (1,4-BD) are illicit drugs of abuse that have been gaining widespread popularity for their purported effects as soporifics, euphoriants, natural psychedelics, muscle builders, "growth hormone releasers," weight loss aids, sexual enhancers, and chemical submission ("date rape") drugs.[1–5] Abuse of GHB and its precursors has accounted for >7100 overdoses and law enforcement encounters in 45 states, 65 GHB-related deaths, 30 GHB-related sexual assaults, and 150 clandestine GHB laboratories discovered since 1990.[6] The Community Epidemiology Work Group (CEWG) of the National Institute on Drug Abuse (NIDA) recently reported that GHB abuse is on the rise in 9 of the 21 CEWG areas, and emergency department encounters with GHB more than doubled from 1282 in 1998 to 3178 in 1999.[7] Poison control centers also recently reported that GHB precursors, such as 1,4-BD, have been responsible for up to 71% of persons with GHB-related intoxication since 2000.[7,8]

Overdoses with these drugs have resulted in life-threatening symptoms of CNS depression, coma, respiratory depression, apnea, bradycardia, hypotension, seizure as well as death.[1–5,9–15] Currently, a universally accepted antidote does not exist for

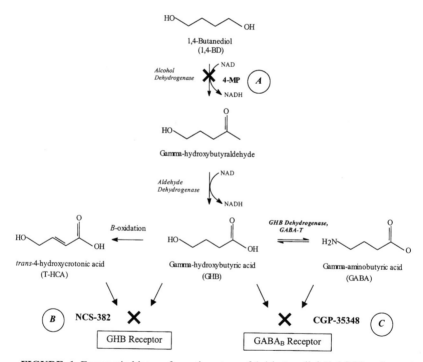

FIGURE 1. Enzymatic biotransformation steps of 1,4-butanediol (1,4-BD) and receptor sites for its metabolites gamma-hydroxybutyric acid (GHB), gamma-aminobutyric acid (GABA), and *trans*-4-hydroxycrotonic acid (T-HCA), as well as proposed sites for enzymatic inhibition with 4-MP (**A**) and receptor antagonism with NCS-382 (**B**) and CGP-35348 (**C**).

GHB or its precursor 1,4-BD. Without an antidote, patients with these overdoses often require endotracheal intubation and mechanical ventilation for respiratory failure as well as other intensive care supportive measures.[1–5,9–15] However, the enzymatic biotransformation of 1,4-BD to GHB as well as the receptor sites shared by 1,4-BD and GHB offer several potential sites for pharmacologic reversal agents. 1,4-BD, the dihydroxy precursor of GHB, undergoes *in vivo* enzymatic biotransformation to gamma-hydroxybutyraldehyde by alcohol dehydrogenase (ADH), which undergoes oxidation to GHB by aldehyde dehydrogenase or auto-oxidation.[16–22] GHB is pharmacologically active at GABA$_B$ receptors and high affinity GHB-specific receptors and subsequently undergoes metabolism to succinic semialdehyde (SSA) by NADP-dependent GHB dehydrogenase.[23] SSA is then oxidized in the Kreb's cycle or it is converted to GABA by mitochondrial GABA-transaminase (GABA-T) and released in neuronal circuits expressing mainly GABA$_B$ receptors.[23] Alternatively, GHB can be converted via β oxidation to *trans*-4-hydroxycrotonic acid (T-HCA), which has a greater affinity for GHB-specific receptors than does GHB itself.[23]

Because 1,4-BD is believed to be pharmacologically active after its ADH-mediated conversion to GHB, we hypothesize that the ADH inhibitor 4-methylpyrazole (4-MP) can block the ADH-mediated biotransformation of 1,4-BD to its toxic metabolite GHB and prevent toxicity (FIG. 1A).[24] Mechanistically, 4-MP would only be useful for acute 1,4-BD overdoses. Because GHB metabolism does not involve ADH, an alternative reversal agent for GHB would be a receptor antagonist. We also hypothesize that the GHB receptor antagonist NCS-382 can block toxicity related to 1,4-BD and its metabolites GHB and T-HCA (FIG. 1B) and that the GABA$_B$ receptor antagonist CGP-35348 can block toxicity related to 1,4-BD and its metabolites GHB and GABA (FIG. 1C).[23,25] In this paper we present preliminary findings of studies with 4-MP, CGP-35348, and NCS-382 in a murine model of acute 1,4-BD overdose that we previously developed.[26]

MATERIAL AND METHODS

Study Design

This investigation was a controlled trial of 4-MP, CGP-35348, and NCS-382 as pretreatment blocking agents in a murine model of acute 1,4-BD overdose. Study methods were in accordance with the National Institutes of Health (NIH) guidelines for animal use and were approved by the Institutional Animal Care and Use Committee (IACUC) of our institutions.

Material

Male CD-1 mice weighing 20–30 g were obtained from Charles River Labs (Wilmington, MA). All animals were housed in a climate-controlled facility with 12-hour alternating light and dark cycles and acclimated to our facility for at least 3 days. All animals had *ad libitum* access to food (Purina 5001) and tap water. The highest available purity of the chemicals 1,4-BD (99+%) and 4-MP (99%) was obtained from the Sigma-Aldrich Chemical Supply Company (St. Louis, MO). CGP-35348 and NCS-382 were obtained from Tocris Cookson, Inc. (Ballwin, MO). The test compounds 1,4-BD, 4-MP, and CGP-35348 were dissolved in distilled, deionized water at a concentration of 10 mg/mL. Control injections for 4-MP and CGP-35348 consisted of the distilled, deionized water vehicle. NCS-382 was dissolved in a 60:40 vehicle of deionized, distilled water and DMSO; the control injection for NCS-382 consisted of the 60:40 deionized, distilled water and DMSO vehicle.

Study Protocol

Outcome measures for 1,4-BD toxicity were the righting reflex and the rotorod test, both of which are well-established laboratory assessments that can demonstrate neurologic deficits produced by pharmacologic agents. The righting reflex tests the ability of the animal to regain an upright posture within 10 seconds of being placed supine. The rotarod test assesses the ability of the animal to log roll for 10 seconds on a 1-inch-diameter rod revolving at 6 revolutions per minute. Animals were given two consecutive attempts to demonstrate the righting reflex and perform the rotorod test before failure was documented.

Previous dose-response studies with CD-1 mice in our laboratory had determined that the righting reflex and the rotarod test are inhibited by 1,4-BD at a toxic dose-50 (TD_{50}) of 585 mg/kg and 163 mg/kg, respectively.[26] Hence, a 1,4-BD dose of 600 mg/kg was used to produce toxic manifestations in study animals for both the righting reflex and the rotarod test. A 1,4-BD dose of 300 mg/kg was used to produce toxic manifestations in those experiments in which the rotarod test only was used. Previous dose-response studies in our laboratory had also determined that pretreatment of CD-1 mice with 25 mg/kg of 4-MP prior to 1,4-BD can preserve their righting reflex and their ability to perform the rotarod test.[27] CGP-35348 and NCS-382 were both administered at 200 mg/kg, which was within the dose range used by previous investigators (12.5–800 mg/kg). The route of administration for all drugs was intraperitoneal (ip) injection.

Blood specimens were collected following decapitation and promptly stored in Eppendorf tubes at −80°C. On completion of the experiment, all blood specimens were sent on dry ice to a laboratory for subsequent chemical analysis. Blood 1,4-BD and GHB quantitative assays were done by gas chromatography/mass spectrometry (GC/MS) methods described by Kraner et al.[15] Bovine adult serum and all reagents were purchased from the Sigma Chemical Supply Company (St. Louis, MO). Solvents were VWR HPLC/ACS grade. Calibration standards and controls were prepared in bovine adult serum. Sample calibration standards (5–100 μg/mL) and controls were extracted from 200 μL aliquots of bovine adult serum. Working standards were prepared from 1 mg/mL stocks of GHB and BD. Concentrations above the linear range were established by dilution. Preparation was performed using UCT SPE cartridge ZSGHB020 with a method obtained from UCT for the analysis of GHB. This method was modified to allow for the analysis of 1,4-butanediol.

A 1-μL aliquot of the derivatized sample was injected onto a Hewlett-Packard (HP) 5890 Series II GC attached to a mass selective detector (HP5971) with a HP7673 autosampler. Data were collected on an HP Enhanced Chem Station (G1701BA). The capillary column was a 15-m Phenomenex ZB-1 (0.25-mm i.d. and 0.25-μm film thickness) using helium as a carrier gas. The injector and detector temperatures were maintained at 160°C and 300°C, respectively. The temperature program was initially set at 50°C for 1 minute and increased to 80°C at 10°C/min, then held for 2 minutes. The temperature was then increased to 180°C at a rate of 20°C/min, and held for 2 minutes. The total run time was 13 minutes. Samples were injected to the splitless mode, and the purge was turned on (split mode) after 0.5 minute. Analysis was accomplished by selected ion monitoring of ions in a window between 4.00 minutes and 7.30 minutes at m/z 219, 220, 221 for 1,4-butanediol and 223, 224, 225 for 1,4-butanediol-d4. Between 7.30 and 13.00 minutes monitoring was performed at m/z 233, 234, and 235 for GHB and 239, 240, 241 for GHB-d3. The dwell times were set to 50 ms per ion. The detection limit of these assays for both 1,4-BD and GHB was 20 μg/mL.

Four controlled murine experiments comprised this study. In experiment 1, 20 mice were pretreated with 4-MP 25 mg/kg ip ($n = 10$) or deionized, distilled water ($n = 10$). Five minutes later, all mice were administered 1,4-BD 600 mg/kg ip. Sixty minutes later, all mice were tested for the righting reflex and rotarod test and were sacrificed for subsequent 1,4-BD and GHB blood determinations. In experiment 2, 10 mice were pretreated with CGP-35348 200 mg/kg ($n = 5$) or deionized, distilled water. Ten minutes later, both groups were administered 1,4-BD 300 mg/kg ip. A third group of mice ($n = 5$) was administered only CGP-35348. Mice in all groups were subsequently evaluated for toxicity with the rotarod test every 10 minutes until recovery. In experiment 3, 10 mice were pretreated with NCS-382 200 mg/kg ip ($n = 5$) or deionized, distilled water ($n = 5$). Ten minutes later, both groups were administered 1,4-BD 300 mg/kg ip. A third group of mice ($n = 5$) was administered only NCS-382. Mice in all groups were subsequently evaluated for toxicity with the rotarod test every 10 minutes until recovery. In experiment 4, 10 mice were pretreated with a combination of NCS-382 and CGP-35348 ($n = 5$) or deionized, distilled water ($n = 5$). Ten minutes later, both groups were administered 1,4-BD 300 mg/kg ip. A third group of mice ($n = 5$) was administered only the combination of NCS-382 and CGP-35348. Mice in all groups were subsequently evaluated for toxicity with the rotarod test every 10 minutes until recovery.

Data Analysis

In experiment 1, data for 1,4-BD and GHB blood concentrations were expressed as the mean (μg/mL) ± standard error measurement (SEM) and were compared with the unpaired Student's *t* test. Data for the righting reflex and rotarod are expressed as the percentage of animals exhibiting the righting reflex and passing the rotarod test. Comparison of these data between the pretreatment and control groups was done with the two-tailed Fisher's exact test. In experiments 2–4, data for all groups at each 10-minute observation period are expressed as the percentage of mice failing the rotarod test. The percentage of pretreated mice failing the rotarod test at each 10-minute observation period was compared with that of control mice by the two-tailed Fisher exact test. In all experiments, statistical significance was set at an alpha of 0.05.

RESULTS

In experiment 1, the mean blood concentration of 1,4-BD was 396.7 ± 12.6 μg/mL and <20 μg/mL for 4-MP pretreated and control mice, respectively ($p < 0.05$). Conversely, the mean blood concentration of GHB was <20 μg/mL and 321.4 ±

TABLE 1. Effects of 4-MP pretreatment versus controls on 1,4-BD and GHB blood concentrations, righting reflex, and rotarod test performance

	4-MP Pretreatment	Controls	p
1,4-BD concentration (μg/mL)[a]	396.7 ± 12.6	<20	<0.05
GHB concentration (μg/mL)	<20	321.4 ± 18.3	<0.05
Righting reflex[b]	100	0	<0.05
Rotarod test[b]	100	0	<0.05

[a]Data for 1,4-BD and GHB blood concentrations are expressed as mean (μg/mL) ± standard error measurement (SEM).

[b]Data for righting reflex and rotarod are expressed as the percentage of animals exhibiting the righting reflex and passing the rotarod test.

18.3 μg/mL for 4-MP pretreated and control mice, respectively ($p < 0.05$). All mice pretreated with 4-MP maintained their righting reflex and passed the rotarod test, whereas 0% of their controls maintained their righting reflex and passed the rotarod test ($p < 0.05$) (TABLE 1).

In experiment 2, all control mice initially failed the rotarod test and required 170 minutes for recovery. Conversely, all mice pretreated with CGP-35348 initially failed the rotarod test, but recovered it by 70 minutes ($p < 0.05$ between 80 and 130 minutes). The duration of 1,4-BD toxicity for the rotarod test was decreased by 58% with CGP-35348 pretreatment. CGP-35348 alone did not affect the rotarod test (FIG. 2). In experiment 3, all control mice initially failed the rotarod test and required 170 minutes for recovery. However, all mice pretreated with NCS-382 had a prolonged course for failure of the rotarod test that extended up to 360 minutes ($p < 0.05$ between 170 and 210 minutes). The duration of 1,4-BD toxicity for the rotarod test was increased by 212% with NCS-382 pretreatment. NCS-382 alone did not affect the rotarod test (FIG. 3). In experiment 4, no significant difference in the duration of 1,4-BD toxicity for the rotarod test was observed between mice pretreated with a combination of NCS-382 and CGP-35348 and control mice. However, the percentage of animals that failed the rotarod test as a result of 1,4-BD intoxication decreased from 100% of control mice to 40% of mice pretreated with the combination of NCS-382 and CGP-35348 ($p = 0.17$). The combination of NCS-382 and CGP-35348 alone did not affect the rotarod test (FIG. 4).

DISCUSSION

The use of a competitive enzyme inhibitor to block specifically the metabolism of 1,4-BD to GHB by ADH was successfully demonstrated with pyrazole and various substituted derivatives of pyrazole.[19,28,29] However, subsequent investigators demonstrated that pyrazole and its principal metabolite, 4-hydroxypyrazole, cause significant hepatotoxicity and nephrotoxicity, thereby precluding its clinical utility.[30–32] Derivatives of pyrazole incorporating nucleophilic group monosubstitutions in the 4-position of the pyrazole ring were subsequently shown to exhibit even greater potency for ADH blockade. Among these, 4-iodopyrazole and 4-bromopyrazole

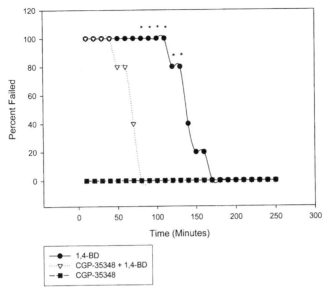

FIGURE 2. Effect of CGP-35348 pretreatment on the rotarod test versus controls (*$p <$ 0.05 between pretreated and control mice).

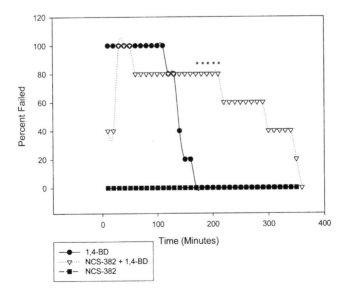

FIGURE 3. Effect of NCS-382 pretreatment on the rotarod test versus controls (*$p < 0.05$ between pretreated and control mice).

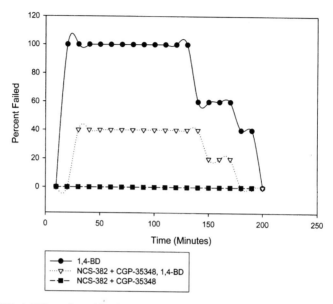

FIGURE 4. Effect of combined NCS-382 and CGP-35348 pretreatment on the rotarod test versus controls.

were the most effective.[33,34] However, in our laboratory, we chose to investigate 4-MP as a potential blocking agent for ADH-mediated 1,4-BD enzymatic biotransformation to GHB. Because 4-MP has an affinity for ADH that is 8000 times greater than that of ethanol and is currently approved by the FDA as an ADH inhibitor for ethylene glycol and methanol poisoning, it had the greatest potential among the pyrazole derivatives for immediate clinical application in 1,4-BD poisoning.[35,36]

In previous investigations, our laboratory had determined that pretreatment of CD-1 mice with 4-MP (25 mg/kg ip) produces a significant rightward shift in the dose-response curves of 1,4-BD for the righting reflex and the rotarod test.[27] In that study, 4-MP increased the TD_{50} of 1,4-BD 10-fold for the righting reflex from 585 mg/kg (95% CI, 484-707 mg/kg) in control mice to 5550 mg/kg (95% CI, 5353–5756 mg/kg) in pretreated mice ($Z > 20$, $p < 0.001$).[27] Pretreatment with 4-MP also increased the TD_{50} of 1,4-BD 30-fold for the rotarod test from 163 mg/kg (95% CI, 136–196 mg/kg) in control mice to 4900 mg/kg (95% CI, 4812–4989 mg/kg) in pretreated mice ($Z > 20$, $p < 0.001$).[27] Although 4-MP significantly decreased 1,4-BD toxicity for both the righting reflex and the rotarod test when administered as pretreatment in this study, we could only presume that the mechanism was by competitive inhibition of ADH biotransformation of 1,4-BD to GHB. The lack of corroborating blood concentrations of 1,4-BD and GHB was the chief limitation that did not permit our study to define the exact mechanism of 4-MP.

In the present study, we addressed the previous study's limitation by incorporating blood 1,4-BD and GHB concentrations with neurobehavioral outcome measures in a similar study of 4-MP pretreatment. The blood quantitative data of this study support the theory that ADH substrate specificity for 4-MP is greater than that for

1,4-BD, leading to competitive inhibition of ADH. As a result, mice pretreated with 4-MP had decreased GHB blood concentrations and increased 1,4-BD blood concentrations. As the parent compound, 1,4-BD did not result in toxicity when its biotransformation to GHB was inhibited by 4-MP. The mechanism of this inhibition may involve the formation of an inactive ternary complex by the bonding of 4-MP to the 4-carbon of the pyridium ring of NAD^+, at or near the substrate binding site of ADH.[33] Conversely, in control mice, the resultant elevated GHB blood concentrations resulted in failure of both the righting reflex and the rotarod test.

Mechanistically, 4-MP would only be useful for reversal of toxicity from 1,4-BD, not its metabolites GHB, GABA, and T-HCA. Because the pharmacologic actions and metabolism of GHB, GABA, and T-HCA are independent of ADH, an alternative reversal agent for them would be a receptor antagonist. The effects of GHB and GABA at $GABA_B$ receptors as well as the effects of GHB and T-HCA at GHB receptors could potentially be blocked with CGP-35348 and NCS-382, respectively. Receptor binding assays have shown that CGP-35348 is a centrally active and selective $GABA_B$ receptor antagonist with an inhibitory concentration-50 (IC_{50}) of 34 µM.[25] Electrophysiologic *in vitro* studies with CGP-35348 confirmed that it antagonized rat[25] and guinea pig[37] neuronal membrane hyperpolarization produced by $GABA_B$ agonists and antagonized the increase in intracellular Ca^{2+} concentration produced by GHB stimulation of $GABA_B$ receptors in cultured mouse cerebellar granule cells.[38]

We present data in an *in vivo* murine model of acute 1,4-BD overdose demonstrating that CGP-35348 can decrease toxicity related to 1,4-BD biotransformation to GHB. By antagonizing $GABA_B$ receptors, CGP-35348 decreased the duration of 1,4-BD/GHB toxicity for the rotarod test by 58% in pretreated mice versus controls. A similar finding of CGP-35348 therapeutic benefit for chronic GHB intoxication was recently reported by the investigations of Gibson *et al.* on succinic semialdehyde dehydrogenase (SSADH) deficiency or 4-hydroxybutyric aciduria. In this rare inborn error of metabolism, GABA catabolism is shunted toward GHB formation, leading to elevated GHB concentrations in physiologic fluids and a clinical phenotype resembling acute GHB intoxication.[39–41] Gibson *et al.* recently developed a knockout mouse model of SSADH deficiency in C57/129 murine strains (−/−).[42,43] Exhibiting clinical (hypotonia, ataxia, hyporeflexia, seizures/EEG abnormalities, and somnolence) and laboratory (elevated blood, urine, and CSF GHB concentrations) phenotypic features of SSADH deficiency, (−/−) mice systematically developed generalized seizures and died from status epilepticus on postnatal days 17–20.[42,43] However, CGP-35348 administered in drinking water at a dose of 100 mg/kg/day to (−/−) mice resulted in significant improvement in life span. Whereas untreated (−/−) mice died from status epilepticus at the "critical period" of 17–20 days, treated (−/−) mice had 90.9% survival beyond 62 days (with several mice surviving to 111 days).[42,43] Thus, CGP-35348 might be an effective reversal agent for both acute and chronic toxicity from 1,4-BD and its metabolites GHB and GABA.

As an antagonist of high affinity GHB-specific receptors, NCS-382 would be expected to block GHB and T-HCA from interacting with this receptor. Activation of this receptor by GHB has been extensively demonstrated in animals to induce EEG and behavioral changes that resemble absence seizures,[44–46] produce reinforcing effects,[47] and induce sedation, sleep, and catalepsy.[48] However, NCS-382 attenuated epileptiform EEG spike and wave discharges,[44–46] completely antagonized the reinforcing effects of GHB,[47] and diminished the sedative, anesthetic, and cataleptic effects of GHB in a dose-dependent manner with respect to the grasping test, swimming test, chimney test, and cork test.[48] The dosing range of NCS-382 in these studies was 12.5–800 mg/kg ip. In our study, NCS-382 pretreatment was administered within this range at a dose of 200 mg/kg ip, but produced apparent synergistic toxicity with 1,4-BD.

To our knowledge, this is the first study to demonstrate that the GHB receptor antagonist NCS-382 can have deleterious effects when combined with 1,4-BD and presumably GHB. In our animal model of acute overdose with the GHB precursor 1,4-BD, NCS-382 more than doubled the duration of rotarod failure in pretreated mice versus control mice. There are two possible explanations for this unexpected observation. T-HCA, the metabolite of GHB via β-oxidation, has demonstrated a greater affinity for the GHB receptor than has GHB itself.[23,49,50] Perhaps this T-HCA affinity for the GHB receptor might also be greater than the receptor antagonist NCS-382. Additionally, perhaps NCS-382 antagonism of GHB receptors results in a metabolic shunt of GHB back to succinic semialdehyde (SSA) by NADP-dependent GHB dehydrogenase. While a proportion of SSA would then be oxidized in the Kreb's cycle, some SSA could alternatively be converted to GABA by GABA transaminase. In overdose situations, this could potentially result in a significant increase in the total brain GABA pool, leading to toxicity. This theory is supported by the results of experiment 4, in which the pretreatment combination of NCS-382 *and* CGP-35348 prior to 1,4-BD overdose decreased the percentage of animals that failed the rotarod test from 100% in control mice to 40% in pretreated mice and decreased the duration of toxicity by about 50% compared to NCS-382 pretreatment alone prior to 1,4-BD overdose.

In conclusion, we demonstrated in murine pilot studies that one enzyme and two receptors may be potential sites for pharmacologic intervention with reversal agents for acute overdoses with GHB and its precursor 1,4-BD. 4-MP pretreatment effectively blocked ADH enzymatic biotransformation of 1,4-BD to GHB, which prevented toxic manifestations. Pretreatment with CGP-35348 and its combination with NCS-382 also decreased toxicity related to 1,4-BD and GHB, presumably by antagonizing GABA_B and GHB receptors, respectively. These enzyme and receptor antagonists warrant further investigation as potential antidotes for these increasingly reported, life-threatening drugs of abuse.

ACKNOWLEDGMENTS

This research was supported by National Institute on Drug Abuse Grant 1 R03 DA15951-01, National Institutes of Health Grant 1 T32 HD40128-01, and an unrestricted research grant from Orphan Medical Inc.

REFERENCES

1. QUANG, L.S. & M.W. SHANNON. 2000. Gamma-hydroxybutyrate, gamma-butyrolactone, and 1,4-butanediol: a case report and review of the literature. Pediatr. Emerg. Care **16:** 435–440.
2. ZVOSEC, D.L. *et al.* 2001. Adverse events, including death, associated with the use of 1,4-butanediol. N. Engl. J. Med. **344:** 87–94.

3. CENTERS FOR DISEASE CONTROL. 1990. Multistate outbreak of poisonings associated with illicit use of gamma hydroxybutyrate. MMWR **39:** 861–863.
4. CENTERS FOR DISEASE CONTROL. 1997. Gamma hydroxybutyrate use–New York and Texas, 1995–1996. MMWR **46:** 281–283.
5. FOOD AND DRUG ADMINISTRATION. MEDWATCH–More on GBL, GHB, BD [electronic source]. Http://www.fda.gov/medwatch/SAFETY/1999/gblghb.htm. Accessed 4/16/01.
6. DRUG ENFORCEMENT AGENCY. Gamma-hydroxybutyrate (GHB) [electronic source]. Http://www.usdoj.gov/dea/pubs/cngrtest/ct990311.htm. Accessed 4/16/01.
7. COMMUNITY EPIDEMIOLOGY WORK GROUP: Epidemiologic trends in drug abuse advance report, June 2001 (electronic source). Http://www.nida.nih.gov/CEWG/AdvancedRep/601ADV/601adv.html. Accessed 8/12/01.
8. DOYON, S. 2000. Gammahydroxybutyrate and analogues. Toxalert **17:** 1–3.
9. LI, J., S.A. STOKES & A. WOECKENER. 1998. A tale of novel intoxication: a review of the effects of gamma-hydroxybutyric acid with recommendations for management. Ann. Emerg. Med. **31:** 729–736.
10. LI, J., S.A. STOKES A. WOECKENER. 1998. A tale of novel intoxication: seven cases of gamma-hydroxybutyric acid overdose. Ann. Emerg. Med. **31:** 723–728.
11. CHIN, R.L. *et al.* 1998. Clinical course of gamma-hydroxybutyrate overdose. Ann. Emerg. Med. **31:** 716–722.
12. CHIN, M.Y., R.A. KREUTZER & J.E. DYER. 1992. Acute poisoning from gamma-hydroxybutyrate in California. West. J. Med. **156:** 380–384.
13. DYER, J.E. 1991. Gamma-hydroxybutyrate: a health food product producing coma and seizure-like activity. Am. J. Emerg. Med. **9:** 321–324.
14. DYER, J.E., M.J. GALBO & K.M. ANDREWS. 1999. 1,4-butanediol "pine needle oil": overdose mimics toxic profile of GHB. J. Toxicol. Clin. Toxicol. **35:** 554.
15. KRANER, J., J. PLASSARD & D. MCCOY. 2000. Fatal overdose from ingestion of 1,4-butanediol, a GHB precursor. J. Toxicol. Clin. Toxicol. **38:** 534.
16. SPRINCE, H., J.A. JOSEPHS & C.R. WILPIZESKI. 1966. Neuropharmacological effects of 1,4-butanediol and related congeners compared with those of gamma-hydroxybutyrate and gamma-butyrolactone. Life Sci. **5:** 2041–2052.
17. ROTH, R.H. & N.J. GIARMAN. 1968. Evidence that central nervous system depression by 1,4-butanediol is mediated through a metabolite, gamma-hydroxybutyrate. Biochem. Pharmacol. **17:** 735–739.
18. PIETRUSZKO, R., K. VOIGTLANDER & D. LESTER. 1978. Alcohol dehydrogenase from human and horse liver–substrate specificity with diols. Biochem. Pharmacol. **27:** 1296–1297.
19. BESSMAN, S.P. & E.R.B. MCCABE. 1978. 1,4-Butanediol: a substrate for rat liver and horse liver alcohol dehydrogenases. Biochem. Pharmacol. **27:** 1296–1297.
20. MAXWELL, R. & R.H. ROTH. 1972. Conversion of 1,4-butanediol to gamma-hydroxybutyric acid in rat brain and in peripheral tissue. Biochem. Pharmacol. **21:** 1521–1533.
21. POLDRUGO, F. & O.C. SNEAD. 1984. 1,4-Butanediol, gamma-hydroxybutyric acid, and ethanol: relationship and interaction. Neuropharmacology **23:** 109–113.
22. SNEAD, O.C., R. FURNER & C.C. LIU. 1989. *In vivo* conversion of gamma-aminobutyric acid and 1,4-butanediol to gamma-hydroxbutyric acid in rat brain: studies using stable isotopes. Biochem. Pharmacol. **38:** 4375–4380.
23. MAITRE, M. 1997. The gamma-hydroxybutyrate signalling system in brain: organization and functional implications. Prog. Neurobiol. **51:** 337–361.
24. SHANNON, M.S. 1998. Fomepizole: a new antidote. Pediatr. Emerg. Care **14:** 170–172.
25. OLPE, H.R. *et al.* 1990. CGP 35348: a centrally active blocker of GABAB receptors. Eur. J. Pharmacol. **187:** 27–38.
26. QUANG, L., T. MAHER, M. SHANNON & A. WOOLF. 2000. Determination of 1,4-butanediol toxic dose-50 in CD-1 mice. J. Toxicol. Clin. Toxicol. **38:** 533.
27. QUANG, L., T. MAHER, M. SHANNON & A. WOOLF. 2000. Pretreatment of CD-1 mice with 4-methylpyrazole (4-MP) blocks 1,4-butanediol (BD) toxicity. J. Toxicol. Clin. Toxicol. **38:** 527.
28. TABENER, P.V., J.T. RICK & G.A. KERKUT. 1972. Metabolic factors involved in the interaction between pyrazole and butane-1,4-diol and 4-hydroxybutyric acid. Life Sci. **11:** 335–341.

29. POLDRUGO, F. & O.C. SNEAD. 1986. 1,4 Butanediol and ethanol compete for degradation in rat brain and liver *in vitro*. Alcohol **3:** 367–370.
30. GOLDSTEIN, D.B. & N. PAL. 1971. Comparison of pyrazole and 4-brompyrazole as inhibitors of alcohol dehydrogenases: their potency, toxicity and duration of action in mice. J. Pharmacol. Exp. Ther. **178:** 199–203.
31. MACDONALD, E., E. IHALAINEN & J.P. PISPA. 1981. Pharmacological and toxicological properties of 4-hydroxypyrazole, a metabolite of pyrazole. Acta Pharmacol. Toxicol. (Copenh). **48**(5): 418–423.
32. WILSON, W.L. & N.G. BOTTIGLIERI. 1962. Phase I studies with pyrazole. Cancer Chemother. Rep. **21:** 137–141.
33. LI, T.K. & H. THEORELL. 1969. Human liver alcohol dehydrogenase: inhibition by pyrazole and pyrazole analogs. Acta Chem. Scand. **23**(3): 892–902.
34. THEORELL, H. & T. YONETANI. 1969. On the effects of some heterocyclic compounds on the enzymic activity of liver alcohol dehydrogenase. Acta Chem. Scand. **23:** 255–260.
35. BRENT, J. *et al.* 1999. Fomepizole for the treatment of ethylene glycol poisoning. Methylpyrazole for toxic alcohols study group. N. Engl. J. Med. **340:** 832–838.
36. BRENT, J. *et al.* 2001. Methylpyrazole for toxic alcohols study group. Fomepizole for the treatment of methanol poisoning. N. Engl. J. Med. **344:** 424–429.
37. WAGNER, E.J., M.A. BOSCH, M.J. KELLY & O.K. RONNEKLEIV. 1999. A powerful GABA(B) receptor-mediated inhibition of GABAergic neurons in arcuate nucleus. Neuroreport **10:** 2681–2687.
38. ITO, Y. *et al.* 1995. Gamma-hydroxybutyric acid increases intracellular Ca^{2+} concentration and nuclear cyclic AMP-responsive element- and activator protein 1 DNA-binding activities through GABAB receptor in cultured cerebellar granule cells. J. Neurochem. **65:** 75–83.
39. JAKOBS, C. *et al.* 1981. Urinary excretion of gamma-hydroxybutyric acid in a patient with neurologic abnormalities. The probability of a new inborn error of metabolism. Clin. Chim. Acta **111:** 169–178.
40. JAKOBS, C. *et al.* 1984. 4-Hydroxybutyric aciduria: a new inborn error of metabolism. II. Biochemical findings. J. Inher. Metab. Dis. 7(Suppl. 1): 92–94.
41. GIBSON, K.M. *et al.* 1997. The clinical phenotype of succinic semialdehyde dehydrogenase deficiency (4-hydroxybutyric aciduria): case reports of 23 new patients. Pediatrics **99:** 567–574.
42. GIBSON, K.M. *et al.* 2000. Pharmacologic rescue of lethal seizures in a murine knockout model of succinic semialdehyde dehydrogenase (SSADH) deficiency. J. Inherited Metab. Dis. **23** (Suppl. 1): 110.
43. TAYLOR, M.J. *et al.* 2000. Pharmacologic rescue of lethal seizures in a murine knockout model of succinic semialdehyde dehydrogenase (SSADH) deficiency. Am. J. Hum. Genet. **67** (Suppl. 2): 39.
44. GODSCHALK, M., M.R. DZOLZIC & I.L. BONTA. 1976. Antagonism of gamma-hydroxybutyrate induced hypersynchronism in the EEG of the rat by anti petit mal drugs. Neurosci. Lett. **3:** 145–150.
45. DEPAULIS, A. *et al.* 1988. Effects of gamma-hydroxybutyrate and gamma-butyrolactone derivatives on spontaneous generalized non-convulsive seizures in the rat. Neuropharmacology **27:** 683–689.
46. AIZAWA, M., Y. ITO & H. FUKUDA. 1997. Roles of gamma-aminobutyric acid B (GABA B) and gamma-hydroxybutyric acid receptors in hippocampal long-term potentiation and pathogenesis of absence seizures. Biol. Pharmaceut. Bull. **20:** 1066–1070.
47. MARTELLOTTA, M.C. *et al.* 1998. Intravenous self-administration of gamma-hydroxybutyric acid in drug-naïve mice. Eur. Neuropsychopharmacol. **8:** 293–296.
48. SCHMIDT, C. *et al.* 1991. Anti-sedative and anti-cataleptic properties of NCS-382, a gamma-hydroxybutyrate receptor antagonist. Eur. J. Pharmacol. **203:** 393–397.
49. BOURGIGNON, J.J. *et al.* 1988. Analogues of gamma-hydroxybutyric acid. Synthesis and binding studies. J. Med. Chem. **31:** 893–897.
50. HECHLER, V., M. SCHMITT, J.J. BOURGIGNON & M. MAITRE. 1990. Trans-gamma-hydroxycrotonic acid binding sites in brain: evidence for a subpopulation of gamma-hydroxybutyrate sites. Neurosci. Lett. **110:** 204–209.

Cell Signaling as a Target and Underlying Mechanism for Neurobehavioral Teratogenesis

JOSEPH YANAI,[a,b] ORI VATURY,[b] AND THEODORE A. SLOTKIN[a]

[a]*Department of Pharmacology and Cancer Biology, Duke University Medical Center, Durham, North Carolina 27710, USA*

[b]*The Ross Laboratory for Studies in Neural Birth Defects, Department of Anatomy and Cell Biology, The Hebrew University-Hadassah Medical School, Box 12272, 91010 Jerusalem, Israel*

ABSTRACT: A wide variety of drugs and chemicals elicit neurobehavioral teratogenesis. Surprisingly, however, despite the obvious differences among unrelated compounds, the behavioral outcomes often display striking similarities, such as cognitive and attentional deficits. Recent studies of drugs of abuse (heroin, nicotine, barbiturates) and environmental toxins (environmental tobacco smoke, pesticides, metals) suggest that, regardless of the originating mechanism for perturbation of brain development, disparate neuroteratogens converge downstream on common families of alterations, characterized by changes in the expression and/or activity of the cell-signaling molecules that are essential to neuronal differentiation and synaptic communication. Identification of these common targets may help in the design of pharmacologic interventions that, administered in adulthood, can reverse the impact of exposure to neurobehavioral teratogens.

KEYWORDS: acetylcholine; adenylyl cyclase; β-adrenergic receptors; brain development; chlorpyrifos; cholinergic receptors; cyclic AMP; heroin; muscarinic receptors; nicotine protein kinase C (PKC)

Numerous drugs and chemicals are neurobehavioral teratogens, and the search for underlying mechanisms is complicated by the fact that these substances affect multiple brain regions and neurotransmitter pathways, resulting in a panoply of neurochemical and behavioral changes. The fact that neurotransmitters themselves are trophic factors that control brain cell replication and differentiation, as well as architectural organization of brain circuits,[1–3] means that any disruption of cell-to-cell communication during critical periods of brain development can potentially elicit long-term disruption of synaptic function. Curiously, despite this complexity, common threads emerge in the outcomes of exposures to disparate compounds: learning

Address for correspondence: Dr. Joseph Yanai, The Ross Laboratory for Studies in Neural Birth Defects, Department of Anatomy and Cell Biology, The Hebrew University-Hadassah Medical School, Box 12272, 91010 Jerusalem, Israel. Voice: 972-2-675-8439; fax: 972-2-675-8443.

yanai@md.huji.ac.il

Ann. N.Y. Acad. Sci. 965: 473–478 (2002). © 2002 New York Academy of Sciences.

disabilities, attentional disorders, conduct disorders, and cognitive dysfunction. This suggests that, regardless of originating mechanism, different neuroteratogens may eventually converge on a common set of end pathways to produce their adverse effects. Over the past few years, we established a model for evaluating region- and innervation-specific neurobehavioral teratogenesis by focusing on behaviors that require the participation of known neurotransmitter circuits in a specified region, namely the septohippocampal cholinergic pathway. This particular pathway appears to be especially vulnerable to perinatal insult, either because it is extremely plastic (and hence responsive to changes in input during critical developmental periods), or because it receives multiple inputs, so that perturbations elsewhere in the brain ultimately have an impact on its function. As described below, we have conducted extensive comparisons of the effects of otherwise unrelated compounds and have found similarities of mechanism and outcome for heroin, phenobarbital, nicotine, environmental tobacco smoke, and one of the most commonly used pesticides, chlorpyrifos. Moreover, the effects are shared by other teratogens, notably ethanol.[4]

HEROIN AND PHENOBARBITAL: TARGETING OF PROTEIN KINASE C

Exposure of mice to either heroin or phenobarbital during mid- to late gestation elicits marked deficits in hippocampus-related behaviors, including the eight-arm and Morris mazes and spontaneous alternations.[5–8] Biochemical studies confirm that these treatments elicit major changes in cholinergic synaptic function within the hippocampus. First, we found an increase in the number of high-affinity choline transporter sites assessed with the specific radioligand hemicholinium-3 (HC-3).[6,9,10] Autoradiographic studies confirmed that the changes involve the behaviorally relevant subregion, hippocampal CA1.[11] The activity of the choline transporter is rate-limiting in acetylcholine synthesis and is responsive to the rate of neural firing,[12–14] so upregulation of the transporter implies hyperactivation of cholinergic inputs. In turn, this suggests that the primary site of heroin- or phenobarbital-induced defects is downstream, at the level of postsynaptic signal transduction. Further support for this interpretation comes from our observation that acetylcholine release is increased in the drug-exposed groups.[15] Defective postsynaptic signaling could involve changes either in the expression/function of cholinergic receptors or in the cell signaling cascades controlled by the receptors. It is therefore critical that we found *upregulation* of muscarinic receptors in offspring exposed prenatally to heroin or phenobarbital.[7,16] A similar upregulation was found in the initial steps linking the receptors to cellular function, G-protein activation, and carbachol-induced inositol phosphate formation.[6,9,17] Nevertheless, when we looked farther downstream in the signaling pathway, at the activation of protein kinase C (PKC), we found complete desensitization of the receptor-mediated response, in association with a global elevation of basal membrane-bound PKC activity.[9,10,15,17] It is thus apparent that the basic defect arises at the level of a specific downstream signaling element, PKC. Given the elevation of basal PKC activity, there is most likely a "ceiling" effect at which PKC cannot be increased any further above the already-elevated basal levels, thus obtunding receptor-mediated responses. In keeping with this view, we found that the deficit in PKC responses, when examined for within-animal correlations, was highly predictive of the disruption of septohippocampal cholinergic synaptic markers and behaviors.[5,9,10,17,18]

If defective signaling through PKC is responsible for the neurochemical and behavioral deficits seen after prenatal exposure to heroin or phenobarbital, then once the animals reach adulthood, interventions that target PKC should be able to elicit functional reversal of neurobehavioral teratogenesis. Indeed, when we transplanted embryonic cholinergic septal cells into the impaired hippocampus, we reversed the desensitization of PKC and consequently abolished the presynaptic hyperactivity, the receptor upregulation, and the behavioral deficits.[6,10,17] This effect was specific to cholinergic cells, as grafting of noradrenergic cells had no effect.[6,10,17,19] Again, the dominant role played by PKC was demonstrable using within-animal correlations of behavior and biochemistry:[6,10] reversal of behavioral effects was highly correlated with the restoration of PKC activity and less so with the changes in markers upstream from this step.

Our results thus point to a specific signaling protein downstream from presynaptic input and from postsynaptic cholinergic receptors as the primary site for neurobehavioral teratogenesis by otherwise unrelated developmental disruptors. These effects are likely to be shared by such disparate teratogens as lead,[20,21] methylmercury,[22] copper,[23] ethanol,[24] nicotine,[25] and chlorpyrifos.[26] The most promising common thread is the relative expression of the various PKC isoforms that participate differentially in cell signaling, issues that we are currently pursuing with the heroin model and with other models of prenatal exposure to drugs of abuse and environmental toxins.

SIGNALING TARGETS OTHER THAN PKC: ADENYLYL CYCLASE

The fact that heroin, phenobarbital, heavy metals, ethanol, nicotine, and other neuroteratogens all share a common target, the signaling molecule PKC, means that the adverse effects seen for the impact on cholinergic systems is actually heterologous. Because PKC is a common endpoint for multiple signaling pathways, alterations in the expression and function of PKC isoforms is likely to compromise a wide variety of neural inputs, not just those involving cholinergic pathways. If signaling proteins downstream from the receptors are a common target for neurobehavioral teratogenesis, then it is likely that such changes also are not limited to PKC. We have conducted extensive studies on another signaling protein, adenylyl cyclase (AC). Like PKC, AC, through its generation of cyclic AMP and regulation of protein kinase A, provides a common final pathway for the integration of numerous neurotransmitter and hormonal inputs. In our earlier work with environmental exposures to various drugs and chemicals, we identified AC as a major target for lasting changes in regulation of synaptic function;[27–31] just as was found for PKC, these other agents typically affected the expression of the signaling protein itself.

Using the prenatal heroin exposure model, we found postnatal elevations of AC activity that lasted into adulthood.[32] The effect was most robust with stimulants that activate AC directly (forskolin, Mn^{2+}), indicating increased expression of AC itself; we also identified shifts in catalytic properties suggestive of a change in the AC isoform. Superimposed on the overall induction of AC, there were deficits in the responses to stimulants working through G proteins or G-protein-coupled receptors, indicating loss of response to stimulants acting upstream from AC. Accordingly, this pattern is virtually identical to what we found for effects of unrelated neuroteratogens on PKC. Moreover, effects on the regulation of AC activity were seen not only in the hippocampus, but also in brain regions with widely disparate maturational timetables. These effects also occurred in regions, like the cerebellum, that are sparse in cholinergic input. These results suggest that a common family of mechanisms may underlie the common endpoints seen with disparate neuroteratogens, and, further, that PKC is not the only such target. Given the global alterations, neurobehavioral teratogenesis by compounds like heroin will not be limited to septohippocampal cholinergic projections, nor even to hippocampal behaviors, so that although these are clearly affected by heroin,[6,8–10] they are likely to represent the tip of the iceberg. Additionally, just as with PKC, the effects on AC expression and/or function appear to be a common feature of apparently unrelated neuroteratogens, including heroin,[32] pesticides,[29] glucocorticoids,[28] nicotine,[27,33] and environmental tobacco smoke.[31,34] It is highly unlikely that such diverse compounds act by the same exact originating mechanism within the fetal brain, or that they share the same spectrum of effects on maternal hormone levels or in eliciting generalized maternal toxicity. Rather, they are likely to converge on the common sets of downstream events that ultimately lead to abnormalities of cell signaling. As just one example, nicotine, cocaine, the pesticide chlorpyrifos, and opiates all evoke inhibition of neural cell replication and differentiation and can promote apoptosis.[3,35–40] In this way, a common pattern of cellular alterations may underlie neurobehavioral dysfunction attributable to a wide variety of prenatal insults, in turn disrupting the function of multiple neurotransmitter pathways, leading ultimately to a shared medley of behavioral disturbances. Understanding these cellular mechanisms may then lead to pharmacotherapies designed to restore neurobehavioral function in adulthood.

ACKNOWLEDGMENTS

This work was supported by US Public Health Service Grants HD40820, DA14247, DA6670, ES10356, ES10387, and HD09713, and by grants from the Israeli Anti Drug Authority and the North Carolina–Israel Partnership.

REFERENCES

1. WHITAKER-AZMITIA, P.M. 1991. Role of serotonin and other neurotransmitter receptors in brain development: basis for developmental pharmacology. Pharmacol. Rev. **43:** 553–561.
2. HOHMANN, C.F. & J. BERGER-SWEENEY. 1998. Cholinergic regulation of cortical development and plasticity: new twists to an old story. Perspect. Dev. Neurobiol. **5:** 401–425.
3. SLOTKIN, T.A. 1998. Fetal nicotine or cocaine exposure: which one is worse? J. Pharmacol. Exp. Ther. **285:** 931–945.
4. PICK, C.G. et al. 1993. Hippocampal cholinergic alterations and related behavioral deficits after early exposure to ethanol. Int. J. Dev. Neurosci. **11:** 379–385.
5. PICK, C.G. & J. YANAI. 1984. Long term reduction in spontaneous alternations after early exposure to phenobarbital. Int. J. Dev. Neurosci. **2:** 223–228.
6. STEINGART, R.A. et al. 2000. Neural grafting reverses prenatal drug-induced alterations in hippocampal PKC and related behavioral deficits. Dev. Brain Res. **125:** 9–19.

7. ROGEL-FUCHS, Y., M.E. NEWMAN, D. TROMBKA & E.A. ZAHALKA. 1992. Hippocampal cholinergic alterations and related behavioral deficits after early exposure to phenobarbital. Brain Res. Bull. **29:** 1–6.
8. YANAI, J. *et al.* 1992. Alterations in septohippocampal cholinergic innervation and related behavior after early exposure to heroin and phencyclidine. Dev. Brain Res. **69:** 207–214.
9. STEINGART, R.A. *et al.* 1998. Pre- and postsynaptic alterations in the septohippocampal cholinergic innervations after prenatal exposure to drugs. Brain Res. Bull. **46:** 203–209.
10. STEINGART, R.A. *et al.* 2000. Neurobehavioral damage to cholinergic systems caused by prenatal exposure to heroin or phenobarbital: cellular mechanisms and the reversal of deficits by neural grafting. Dev. Brain Res. **122:** 125–133.
11. YANAI, J., J. BARG, T.A. SLOTKIN & O. VATURY. 2001. Prenatal heroin-induced hippocampal behavioral deficits and global cholinergic hyperactivity: studies on the role of choline transporter. Proc. Int. Soc. Addict. Med. 52.
12. KRISTOFIKOVÁ, Z., E. FALES, E. MAJER & J. KLASCHKA. 1995. [^{3}H]Hemicholinium-3 binding sites in postmortem brains of human patients with Alzheimer's disease and multi-infarct dementia. Exp. Gerontol. **30:** 125–136.
13. SIMON, J.R., S. ATWEH & M.J. KUHAR. 1976. Sodium-dependent high affinity choline uptake: a regulatory step in the synthesis of acetylcholine. J. Neurochem. **26:** 909–922.
14. ZAHALKA, E. *et al.* 1993. Differential development of cholinergic nerve terminal markers in rat brain regions: implications for nerve terminal density, impulse activity and specific gene expression. Brain Res. **601:** 221–229.
15. ABU-ROUMI, M., M.E. NEWMAN & J. YANAI. 1996. Inositol phosphate formation in mice prenatally exposed to drugs: relation to muscarinic receptors and postreceptor effects. Brain Res. Bull. **40:** 183–186.
16. YANAI, J., C.G. PICK, Y. ROGEL-FUCHS & E.A. ZAHALKA. 1992. Alterations in hippocampal cholinergic receptors and hippocampal behaviors after early exposure to nicotine. Brain Res. Bull. **29:** 363–368.
17. ROGEL-FUCHS, Y., E. ZAHALKA & J. YANAI. 1994. Reversal of early phenobarbital-induced cholinergic and related behavioral deficits by neuronal grafting. Brain Res. Bull. **33:** 273–279.
18. PICK, C.G. & J. YANAI. 1985. Long-term reduction in eight-arm maze performance after early exposure to phenobarbital. **3:** 223–227.
19. YANAI, J. & C.G. PICK. 1988. Neuron transplantation reverses phenobarbital-induced behavioral birth defects in mice. Int. J. Dev. Neurosci. **6:** 409–416.
20. HUSSAIN, R.J., P.J. PARSONS & D.O. CARPENTER. 2000. Effects of lead on long-term potentiation in hippocampal CA3 vary with age. Dev. Brain Res. **121:** 243–252.
21. CHEN, H.H. *et al.* 1997. Developmental lead exposure and two-way active avoidance training alter the distribution of protein kinase C activity in the rat hippocampus. Neurochem. Res. **22:** 1119–1125.
22. HAYKAL-COATES, N., T.J. SHAFER, W.R. MUNDY & S. BARONE. 1998. Effects of gestational methylmercury exposure on immunoreactivity of specific isoforms of PKC and enzyme activity during postnatal development of the rat brain. Dev. Brain Res. **109:** 33–49.
23. JOHNSON, W.T. & J.R. PROHASKA. 2000. Gender influences the effect of perinatal copper deficiency on cerebellar PKC gamma content. Biofactors **11:** 163–169.
24. PERRONE-BIZZOZERO, N.I. *et al.* 1998. Prenatal ethanol exposure decreases GAP-43 phosphorylation and protein kinase C activity in the hippocampus of adult rat offspring. J. Neurochem. **71:** 2104–2111.
25. HASAN, S.U., N. SIMAKAJORNBOON, Y. MACKINNON & D. GOZAL. 2001. Prenatal cigarette smoke exposure selectively alters protein kinase C and nitric oxide synthase expression within the neonatal rat brainstem. Neurosci. Lett. **301:** 135–138.
26. BUZNIKOV, G.A. *et al.* 2001. An invertebrate model of the developmental neurotoxicity of insecticides: effects of chlorpyrifos and dieldrin in sea urchin embryos and larvae. Environ. Health Perspect. **109:** 651–661.
27. SLOTKIN, T.A., E.C. MCCOOK, S.E. LAPPI & F.J. SEIDLER. 1992. Altered development of basal and forskolin-stimulated adenylate cyclase activity in brain regions of rats exposed to nicotine prenatally. Dev. Brain Res. **68:** 233–239.

28. SLOTKIN, T.A. *et al.* 1994. Glucocorticoids enhance intracellular signaling via adenylate cyclase at three distinct loci in the fetus: a mechanism for heterologous teratogenic sensitization? Toxicol. Appl. Pharmacol. **127:** 64–75.
29. SONG, X. *et al.* 1997. Cellular mechanisms for developmental toxicity of chlorpyrifos: targeting the adenylyl cyclase signaling cascade. Toxicol. Appl. Pharmacol. **145:** 158–174.
30. ZEIDERS, J.L., F.J. SEIDLER & T.A. SLOTKIN. 1999. Agonist-induced sensitization of β-adrenoceptor signaling in neonatal rat heart: expression and catalytic activity of adenylyl cyclase. J. Pharmacol. Exp. Ther. **291:** 503–510.
31. SLOTKIN, T.A. *et al.* 2001. Perinatal exposure to environmental tobacco smoke induces adenylyl cyclase and alters receptor-mediated signaling in brain and heart of neonatal rats. Brain Res. **898:** 73–81.
32. SLOTKIN, T.A., F.J. SEIDLER & J. YANAI. 2001. Heroin neuroteratogenicity: targeting adenylyl cyclase as an underlying biochemical mechanism. Dev. Brain Res. **132:** 75–85.
33. SLOTKIN, T.A., H.A. NAVARRO, E.C. MCCOOK & F.J. SEIDLER. 1990. Fetal nicotine exposure produces postnatal up-regulation of adenylate cyclase activity in peripheral tissues. Life Sci. **47:** 1561–1567.
34. SLOTKIN, T.A., K.E. PINKERTON & F.J. SEIDLER. 2000. Perinatal exposure to environmental tobacco smoke alters cell signaling in a primate model: autonomic receptors and the control of adenylyl cyclase activity in heart and lung. Dev. Brain Res. **124:** 53–58.
35. SLOTKIN, T.A. 1999. Developmental cholinotoxicants: nicotine and chlorpyrifos. Environ. Health Perspect. **107**(Suppl. 1)**:** 71–80.
36. NASSOGNE, M.C., J. LOUAHED, P. EVRARD & P.J. COURTOY. 1997. Cocaine induces apoptosis in cortical neurons of fetal mice. J. Neurochem. **68:** 2442–2450.
37. ROY, T.S., J.E. ANDREWS, F.J. SEIDLER & T.A. SLOTKIN. 1998. Nicotine evokes cell death in embryonic rat brain during neurulation. J. Pharmacol. Exp. Ther. **287:** 1135–1144.
38. BERGER, F., F.H. GAGE & S. VIJAYARAGHAVAN. 1998. Nicotinic receptor-induced apoptotic cell death of hippocampal progenitor cells. J. Neurosci. **18:** 6871–6881.
39. ZAGON, I.S. & P.J. MCLAUGHLIN. 1992. Maternal exposure to opioids and the developing nervous system: laboratory findings. *In* Maternal Substance Abuse and the Developing Nervous System, I.S. Zagon and T.A. Slotkin, Eds.: 241–282. Academic Press. San Diego.
40. HAUSER, K.F. *et al.* 2000. Opioids intrinsically inhibit the genesis of mouse cerebellar granule neuron precursors in vitro: differential impact of mu and delta receptor activation on proliferation and neurite elongation. Eur. J. Neurosci. **12:** 1281–1293.

Nitric Oxide Production and Nitric Oxide Synthase Expression in Platelets from Heroin Abusers before and after Ultrarapid Detoxification

ANA BATISTA,[a] TICE MACEDO,[a] PAULA TAVARES,[a]
CARLOS FONTES RIBEIRO,[a] JOÃO RELVAS,[b] PIEDADE GOMES,[c]
CARLOS RAMALHEIRA,[b] ISABEL BOTTO,[b] LUISA VALE,[b] LUÍS FERREIRA,[b]
ORLANDO GÜETE,[b] AND GUADALUPE RUIZ[b]

[a]Institute of Pharmacology and Experimental Therapeutics, Faculty of Medicine, University of Coimbra, 3004-504, Coimbra, Portugal

[b]Department of Psychiatry, Coimbra University Hospital, 3049 Coimbra, Portugal

[c]Department of Anesthesiology, Coimbra University Hospital, 3049 Coimbra, Portugal

ABSTRACT: Prolonged heroin abuse has been associated with neurotoxicity. Thus, the involvement of nitric oxide (NO) in heroin-induced dopaminergic neurotoxicity could be a reasonable explanation for heroin-induced changes in brain. Enzymatically derived NO has been implicated in numerous physiological and pathological processes in the brain. Whereas during development NO participates in growing and maturation processes, excess NO production in the adult in response to inflammation, injury, or trauma, participates in both cell death and repair. The expression and activity of the inducible isoform of NO synthase (iNOS) play a pivotal role in sustained and elevated NO release. Recent evidence suggests that neurons can respond to proinflammatory stimuli and take part in brain inflammation. The effect of heroin abuse on platelet NO production and on expression of iNOS in drug addicts submitted to an ultrarapid detoxification was studied. The NO production was estimated from the nitrite concentration, and nitric oxide synthase was determined by Western blotting analysis. Results showed no difference in nitrite content of resting platelets between heroin abuser and control groups. However, after platelet stimulation, heroin abusers showed significantly lower nitrite values. The Western blotting analysis reinforced these results. After ultrarapid detoxification, platelet nitrite production in heroin abusers showed no differences compared to control subjects. Our results suggest that heroin consumption decreases the iNOS synthase expression and platelet NO production. Detoxification treatment restores these changes.

KEYWORDS: neurotoxicity; nitric oxide; nitric oxide synthase; platelets; heroin; ultrarapid detoxification

Address for correspondence: Tice Macedo, Institute of Pharmacology and Experimental Therapeutics, Faculty of Medicine, University of Coimbra, Rua Larga, 3004-504, Coimbra, Portugal. Voice: +351-239-857720; fax: +351-239-823236.
tice@ci.uc.pt

Ann. N.Y. Acad. Sci. 965: 479–486 (2002). © 2002 New York Academy of Sciences.

INTRODUCTION

Reinforcing properties of drugs of abuse have been partly ascribed to an increase in extracellular dopamine (DA) levels in the mesolimbic system, as observed in animal models.[1] In addition, deamination of DA by monoamine oxidase-B with generation of reactive oxygen species may damage dopaminergic neurons.[2] Other neurotransmitters than DA have been implicated as well.[3] Moreover, damage due to excess glutamate, which changes the permeability of cells to Ca^{2+} by acting at N-methyl-D-aspartate (NMDA) receptors, is regarded as a major mechanism of neurodegeneration that occurs during severe hypoxia or ischemia.[4,5] Calcium influx, promoted by the activation of NMDA receptors, induces the stimulation of nitric oxide synthase (NOS),[6] thus increasing cellular oxidation reactions through the formation of peroxynitrite, which is believed to be the major mediator of NO cytotoxic effects.[7,8] In drug addiction, a similar neuronal damage may occur because mesolimbic DA neurons receive rich glutaminergic inputs from both the neocortex and the subthalamic nucleus. Although there is no clear evidence that human drug addicts suffer from similar neurotoxic pathways, it is reasonable to conceive it.

The human platelet has been proposed as a peripheral model for the study of dopamine neurons of the central nervous system, because it stores, releases, and metabolizes DA like a dopamine neuronal cell.[9] Furthermore, it synthesizes NO and reactive oxygen species, allowing the *ex vivo* study of the NO system and oxidative stress. Abnormal platelet NOS expression, either inducible NOS (iNOS) or constitutive NOS (cNOS), and abnormal NO production by drug addicts may have several resulting effects. Also, alteration of NO levels may unbalance the release of other platelet-derived factors, contributing to endothelial and vascular dysfunction.

The aim of this work was to verify the effects of heroin consumption in parameters such as production of NO and expression of iNOS in human platelets. We have taken the platelet as a neuronal model, with the goal of using the results to make inferences about neurotoxicity mechanisms.

MATERIALS AND METHODS

Subjects and Blood Sampling

Venous blood samples were obtained from 16 heroin addicts (14 males and 2 females; mean age 31 ± 8, range 18 to 46 years) attending an ultrarapid detoxification therapy with opioid receptor antagonists naloxone and naltrexone (FIG. 1).[10–12] Mean heroin abuse duration was 11 ± 7, range 4 to 23 years, while mean daily consumption was 1.12 ± 0.5, range 0.25 to 3 g. The study was approved by the Ethics Committee of Coimbra University Hospital, and the samples collected with informed consent. Blood work was done twice, before (time T1) and shortly after (time T2) detoxification treatment, always between the 10:00 A.M. and 12:30 P.M. period. A control group of 17 healthy volunteers (12 males and 5 females; mean age 30 ± 11, range 20 to 56 years) was sampled in a similar fashion.

Blood (10 mL) was collected into tubes containing 3.8% ACD as anticoagulant, and within 1 h centrifuged at $160 \times g$ to separate platelet-rich plasma (PRP) from the

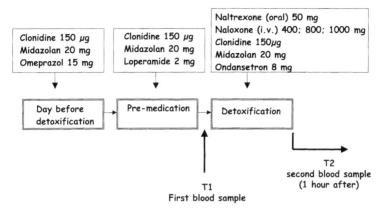

FIGURE 1. Schematic representation of standard ultrarapid opioid detoxification protocol. Blood samples were collected at time T1, before the beginning of therapy, and at time T2, immediately after completion.

erythrocyte fraction. Platelets were further isolated from PRP by centrifugation at $730 \times g$. Samples were used for NO estimation and for determination of iNOS expression.

NO Production

Isolated platelets were resuspended in physiological saline buffer containing 145 mM NaCl, 5 mM KCl, 1 mM $MgSO_4.7H_2O$, 10 mM D-glucose, plus 10 mM HEPES adjusted to pH 7.40; and incubated in the presence or absence of an iNOS stimulus with interleukin-1-β (IL1-β) (4 ng/mL) (Roche) plus bacterial lipopolysaccharide (LPS) (200 μg/mL) (Sigma) at 37°C for 2 h.

Nitric oxide production was evaluated from the determination of stable end-products nitrite and nitrate. The total nitrite amount was quantified by the Griess diazotization reaction,[13] following the reduction of nitrate to nitrite by treating the samples with 20 mU/mL nitrate reductase (Sigma) in the presence of 1.44 mM NADH (Sigma), at 37°C for 1 h.[14] Total nitrite amount was expressed as the sum of extracellular and intraplatelet nitrite contents, determined in the supernatants before and after lysing cells, respectively.

iNOS Expression

Platelets were lysed by incubation with buffer containing 140 mM NaCl, 15 mM EDTA, 20 mM Tris, 2 mM PMSF, 10% glycerol, 1% NP40, 0.1% Triton X-100, pH 8.0, at 4°C for 15 min. Supernatants were stored at –70°C until experimental procedures were undertaken. Proteins (80 μg/lane) were size-fractionated electrophoretically in a 8% polyacrilamide gel. Prestained molecular weight marker standards (Bio-Rad) were run in parallel. After completion, proteins were transferred to nitrocellulose membranes (Schleicher & Schuell) and blocked overnight at 4°C. Membranes were incubated with primary polyclonal antibody against iNOS

(Transduction Laboratories) at 1:10,000 dilution for 1 h. Goat anti-rabbit antibody conjugated to horseradish peroxidase (Bio-Rad) was used as a secondary antibody at a 1:3,000 dilution, for another 1-h incubation period. Specific protein bands were detected by enhanced chemiluminescence (ECL) (Amersham) on special autoradiography film (Amersham).

Statistics

Statistically significant differences with respect to control values were analyzed by one-way analysis of variance and Sheffé's multiple-comparisons test. Significant differences were set at $p < 0.05$.

RESULTS AND DISCUSSION

Results in FIGURE 2 show the basal levels of platelet NO, as given by the nitrate/nitrite concentration, determined in control group and heroin group at time T1 and time T2 of detoxification treatment. Experiments were conducted in the absence of calcium in the medium. Since platelets have both constitutive and inducible NOS isoforms,[15] this feature restricts the functioning of the constitutive Ca^{2+}/calmodulin-dependent enzyme, and allows to study the inducible synthase. Basal NO concentration was significantly lower in drug addicts than in control subjects. However, after iNOS stimulation with IL1-β plus LPS, NO was still significantly lower during the influence of heroin; it increased, however, to control levels after naloxone/naltrexone administration.

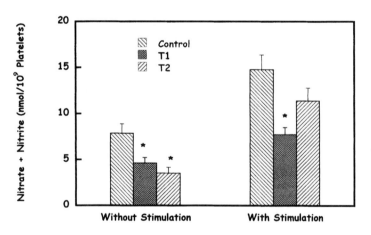

P<0.05 related to control

FIGURE 2. NO production by platelets of healthy subjects and of heroin addicts submitted to detoxification with naloxone/naltrexone. Times T1 and T2 refer to determinations made prior and after treatment, respectively. Induction of iNOS was achieved with IL1-β (4 ng/mL) plus LPS (200 μg/mL). Results are expressed as mean ± SEM of NO nmol per 10^9 platelets; *$p < 0.05$, significantly different from control group.

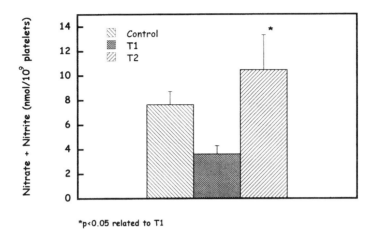

*p<0.05 related to T1

FIGURE 3. Production of NO due to induction of platelet iNOS with IL1-β (4 ng/mL) plus LPS (200 µg/mL). Times T1 and T2 refer to determinations made prior and after heroin detoxification, respectively. Results are expressed as mean ± SEM of NO nmol per 10^9 platelets; *$p < 0.05$, significantly different from T1 group.

The net NO production, relative to the induction of iNOS, was estimated by subtracting data obtained in the absence of stimulus from data collected under stimulation. As depicted in FIGURE 3, there was a trend to decreased NO production under heroin consumption but a significant NO increase after drug withdrawal. This result was further stressed by expressing variation in NO levels in terms of percentage, as shown in FIGURE 4. Following detoxification, a strong increase in iNOS activity was observed.

To examine whether the small NO production, observed following iNOS stimulation in samples from subjects under the effect of heroin, was due to lower expression of the enzyme or to expression of a dysfunctional enzyme, Western blotting analysis of iNOS from T1 blood samples was performed. The results of this experiment are shown in FIGURE 5. Immunoblotting revealed a band corresponding to iNOS with estimated molecular weight of approximately 200 kDa, which is in agreement with earlier reports on the isolation and characterization of the platelet-inducibe NOS isoform.[15] Densitometry analysis of the bands confirmed a lower expression of iNOS in heroin addicts compared to normal subjects.

Overall, data from the present study suggest that heroin consumption decreases both the iNOS synthase expression and platelet NO production, and that detoxification with opioid antagonists restores these changes. These results are in very good agreement with those reported by Lysle and How,[16] who found that heroin administration to rats induced a pronounced reduction of iNOS expression in the spleen, lung, and liver, along with a reduction in NO plasma levels. Furthermore, naltrexone was observed to inhibit the heroin-induced effects. Also, data agree with those reported by Sullivan *et al.*,[17] who observed an increase in NO formation during morphine withdrawal in rats. However, it differs from those reported by Zhou *et al.*,[18]

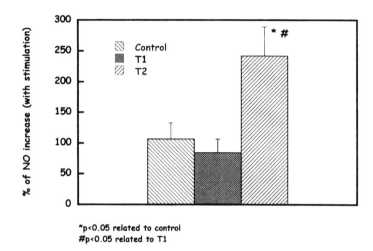

FIGURE 4. Percentage of increase of NO production after stimulation of iNOS activity with IL1-β (4 ng/mL) plus LPS (200 μg/mL). Times T1 and T2 refer to determinations made prior and after heroin detoxification, respectively. Data are expressed as mean ± SEM of percentage of NO increase relative to basal conditions; *$p < 0.05$ and #$p < 0.05$, significantly different from control and T1 groups, respectively.

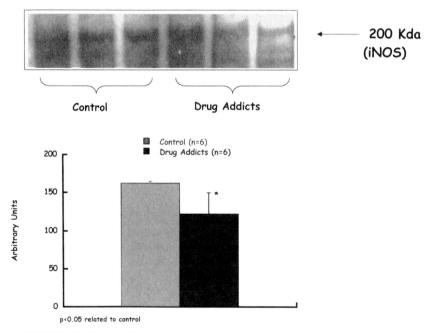

FIGURE 5. Western blotting analysis of iNOS extracted from platelets of control and heroin addicts subjects. *Inset graph* represents relative band intensities. Data are expressed as mean ± SEM of arbitrary density units; *$p < 0.05$, significantly different from control group.

who verified an increase in human NO plasma levels with prolonged heroin abuse and increased drug daily consumption.

When conceiving this study, we aimed to address whether a link would exist between dopaminergic neurotoxicity and prolonged heroin abuse. The hypothesis relating NO to neurodegeneration relied on the fact that DA neurons, through promoting glutamate/Ca^{2+} influx pathways, would unbalance NOS normal regulation, raising NO levels, thus triggering a cascade of cytotoxic effects. Our data, however, suggest that heroin abuse decreases both iNOS expression and NO production. One first pertinent question is whether any of the substances administered along with naloxone and naltrexone has effects on the platelet NO metabolism. If so, results are conditioned by its use during detoxification. Second, only a small amount of literature is available regarding human studies and heroin, the bulk of it concerning animal studies using morphine. Whether humans/experimental animals and heroin/morphine exert similar effects on NO is yet to be determined.

The progressive nature of drug addiction coupled with the slow and protacted degeneration of mesolimbic neurons may present an opportunity for therapeutic intervention. Accessing the NO platelet pathway was a first attempt to provide insights into the neuronal pathway. We feel this is an important open field requiring further investigation. We intend to extend future studies to the effects of heroin and morphine on animal and cellular lines models, as well as to the monitoring of other significant molecules, such as peroxynitrite and 3-nitrotyrosine.

REFERENCES

1. DI CHIARA, G. & A. IMPERATO. 1988. Drugs abused by humans preferentially increase synaptic dopamine concentrations in the mesolimbic system of freely moving rats. Proc. Natl. Acad. Sci. USA **85:** 5274–5278.
2. OLANOW, C.W., P. JENNER & D. BROOKS. 1998. Dopamine agonists and neuroprotection in Parkinson's disease. Ann. Neurol. **44:** S167–S174.
3. WESTWOOD, S.C. & G.R. HANSON. 1999. Effects of stimulants of abuse on extrapyramidal and limbic neuropeptide Y systems. J. Pharmacol. Exp. Ther. **288:** 1160–1166.
4. CHLEIDE, E. *et al.* 1991. Biochemistry of hypoxic damage in brain cells—roles of energy metabolism, glutamate and calcium ion. Neuroscience **17:** 375–390.
5. BECKMAN, J.S. 1990. The double-edged role of nitric oxide in brain function and superoxide-mediated injury. J. Dev. Physiol. **15:** 53–59.
6. GARTHWAITE, J. 1991. Glutamate, nitric oxide, and cell-cell signaling in the nervous system. Trends Neurosci. **14:** 60–67.
7. KOPPENOL, W.H. *et al.* 1992. Peroxynitrite: a cloaked oxidant from superoxide and nitric oxide. Chem. Res. Toxicol. **5:** 834–842.
8. RADI, R., J.S. BECKMAN, K.M. BUSH & B.A. FREEMAN. 1991. Peroxynitrite oxidation of sulfhydryls. The cytotoxic potential of superoxide and nitric oxide. J. Biol. Chem. **266:** 4244–4250.
9. DEAN, B. & D.L. COPOLOV. 1989. Dopamine uptake by platelets is selective, temperature dependent and not influenced by the dopamine-D1 or dopamine-D2 receptor. Life Sci. **45:** 401–411.
10. ELIZAGÁRATE, E. *et al.* 1998. Antagonización rápida de opiáceos: eficácia en una muestra de 91 pacientes. Psiquiatr. Com. **2:** 1–13.
11. SEOANE, A. *et al.* 1997. Efficacy and safety of two new methods of rapid intravenous detoxification in heroin addicts previously treated without success. Br. J. Psychiatry **171:** 340–345.

12. LOIMER, N. *et al.* 1991. Technique for greatly shortening the transition from methadone to naltrexone maintenance of patients addicted to opiates. Am. J. Psychiatry **148:** 933–935.
13. GREEN, L.C. *et al.* 1982. Analysis of nitrate, nitrite and [^{15}N]nitrate in biological fluids. Anal. Biochem. **126:** 131–136.
14. CHEN, L.Y., M.N. SOLAFRANCA & J.L. METHA. 1997. Cyclooxigenase inhibition decreases nitric oxide synthase activity in human platelets. Am. J. Physiol. **42:** 1854–1859.
15. CHEN, L.Y. & J.L. METHA. 1996. Further evidence for the presence of constitutive and inducible nitric oxide synthase isoforms in human platelets. J. Cardiovas. Pharmacol. **27:** 154–158.
16. LYSLE, D.T. & T. HOW. 2000. Heroin modulates the expression of inducible nitric oxide synthase. Immunopharmacology **46:** 181–192.
17. SULLIVAN, M.E. *et al.* 2000. Suppression of acute and chronic opioid withdrawal by a selective soluble guanylyl cyclase inhibitor. Brain Res. **859:** 45–56.
18. ZHOU, J.F. *et al.* 2000. Heroin abuse and nitric oxide, oxidation, peroxidation, lipoperoxidation. Biomed. Environ. Sci. **13:** 131–139.

Toxic Effects of Opioid and Stimulant Drugs on Undifferentiated PC12 Cells

M.T. OLIVEIRA,[a] A.C. REGO,[a] M.T. MORGADINHO,[b] T.R.A. MACEDO,[b] AND C.R. OLIVEIRA[a]

[a]Institute of Biochemistry, Faculty of Medicine and Center for Neuroscience and Cell Biology of Coimbra, University of Coimbra, 3004-504 Coimbra, Portugal

[b]Institute of Pharmacology and Experimental Therapeutics, Faculty of Medicine, University of Coimbra, 3004-504 Coimbra, Portugal

ABSTRACT: Cell death and reactive oxygen species production have been suggested to be involved in neurodegeneration induced by the drugs of abuse. In this study we analyze the toxicity of the following drugs of abuse: heroin, morphine, d-amphetamine, and cocaine in undifferentiated PC12 cells, used as dopaminergic neuronal models. Our data show that opioid drugs (heroin and morphine) are more toxic than stimulant drugs (d-amphetamine and cocaine). Toxic effects induced by heroin are associated with a decrease in intracellular dopamine, an increase in DOPAC levels, and the formation of ROS, whereas toxic effects induced by amphetamine are associated with a decrease in intracellular dopamine and in ATP/ADP levels. In contrast with cocaine, both amphetamine and heroin induced features of apoptosis. The data suggest that the death of cultured PC12 cells induced by the drugs of abuse is correlated with a decrease in intracellular dopamine levels, which can be associated with an increased dopamine turnover and oxidative cell injury.

KEYWORDS: amphetamine; cocaine; dopamine; heroin; morphine; PC12 cells

INTRODUCTION

Drug addiction is associated with a repeated use of a drug or a combination of drugs. The dopaminergic system has been identified as a critical and shared pathway involved in drug reward, and the drugs prone to abuse have been shown to elevate synaptic dopamine levels in this pathway.[1] Dopamine can be oxidized by MAO_B in humans, giving rise to DOPAC and H_2O_2.[2] Although not a free radical because it does not contain unpaired electrons, H_2O_2 can interact with transition metal ions and produce the highly toxic hydroxyl radical ($^{\bullet}OH$) via the Fenton-Haber Weiss reaction. Therefore, reactive oxygen species (ROS) have been frequently associated with neuronal cell death due to damage to carbohydrates, amino acids, phospholipids, and nucleic acids. Moreover, the rise in H_2O_2 levels can be followed by a decrease in the

Address for correspondence: M.T. Oliveira, Institute of Biochemistry, Faculty of Medicine and Center for Neuroscience and Cell Biology of Coimbra, University of Coimbra, 3004-504 Coimbra, Portugal. Voice: 351 239 820190; fax: 351 239 822776.

mteroliv@cnc.cj.uc.pt

Ann. N.Y. Acad. Sci. 965: 487–496 (2002). © 2002 New York Academy of Sciences.

levels of reduced glutathione (GSH), which can lead to the inhibition of mitochondrial respiratory chain activity and, subsequently, to cell death.[3] In addition, dopamine has been shown to induce cell death by apoptosis in several cell types,[4–6] and to inhibit mitochondrial respiration.[7]

In the present study, using PC12 cells as models of dopaminergic neurons,[8,9] we explored the effects of toxic concentrations of some opioid and stimulant drugs of abuse—namely, amphetamine, heroin, and cocaine—that are known to cause severe health problems in the Portuguese population. The data highly suggest that toxic effects induced by the drugs of abuse *in vitro* are associated with a decrease in intracellular dopamine levels, probably related with an enhanced dopamine turnover and oxidative stress.

METHODS

Culture of Undifferentiated PC12 Cells

PC12 cells[10] were cultured in 75 cm^2 flasks, in RPMI 1640 medium supplemented with 10% (v/v) horse serum, 5% (v/v) bovine serum, 50 U/mL penicillin, and 50 mg/mL streptomycin. Cultures were maintained at 37°C in a humidified incubator containing 95% air and 5% CO_2, and passed twice a week. The cells were plated on poly-L-lysine–coated multiwells at a density of 50,000 cells/cm^2 for MTT studies or at a density of 160,000 cells/cm^2 for other studies. For the analysis of chromatin condensation, the cells were incubated in suspension at 180,000 cells/mL. The cells were further incubated with the drugs of abuse, morphine, heroin, cocaine and amphetamine, for 24, 48 or 96 h.

Analysis of Cell Viability

The integrity of the plasma membrane of PC12 cells was determined by monitoring the leakage of lactate dehydrogenase (LDH), by following the rate of conversion of NADH to NAD$^+$ at 340 nm, according to Bergmeyer and Brent.[11] LDH release into the extracellular medium was expressed as a comparison to the release observed in control conditions. Cell viability was also measured using the 3-(4,5-dimethyl-thiazol-2-yl)-2,5-diphenyltetrazolium bromide (MTT) reduction assay at 570 nm.[12] The capacity of treated cells in reducing the tetrazolium salt was expressed as a percentage of absorbance in control cells.

Measurement of ATP/ADP Levels

Intracellular adenine nucleotides, ATP and ADP, were determined after cell extraction with 0.3 M perchloric acid (0–4°C). The cells were centrifuged at 15,800 g for 10 min, and the pellet was solubilized with 1 M NaOH for total protein analysis using the Sedmak method.[13] The supernatants were neutralized with 10 M KOH in 5 M Tris, and centrifuged at 15,800 g for 10 min. The resulting supernatants, stored at –80°C, were assayed for ATP and ADP determination by separation in a reverse-phase HPLC, as described previously.[14]

Analysis of Chromatin Condensation

Analysis of neuronal cell death by necrosis and/or apoptosis was assessed using the fluorescent probes SYTO-13 (Molecular Probes) and PI (propidium iodide). SYTO-13 labels RNA and DNA in living cells with an UV-excited green emission. Propidium iodide is excluded from viable cells, with an UV-excited red emission. The cells were loaded for 3 min with a solution of sodium medium (in mM): 140 NaCl, 5 KCl, 1 $MgCl_2$, 1 NaH_2PO_4, 1.5 $CaCl_2$, 5.6 glucose, 20 HEPES (pH 7.4), containing 4 µM SYTO-13 and 4 µg/mL PI. The cells were visualized by confocal microscopy.

Measurement of Intracellular Dopamine and DOPAC Levels

The levels of intracellular dopamine and DOPAC were determined after cell extraction with 0.1 M perchloric acid (0–4°C). The cells were centrifuged at 15,800 g for 10 min, and the pellet was solubilized with 1 M NaOH for total protein analysis using the Sedmak method.[13] The resulting supernatants, stored at –80°C, were assayed for dopamine and DOPAC analysis by liquid chromatography with electrochemical detection, as described previously.[15]

Analysis of Intracellular Production of ROS

The cells were loaded with the membrane-permeant $DCFH_2$-DA (2′,7′-dichlodi-hydrofluorescein–diacetate, 20 µM), which allows the detection of intracellular reactive oxygen species (ROS) after the cleavage of diacetate by cytosolic esterases. In the presence of intracellular peroxides, $DCFH_2$ is oxidized to the fluorescent dichlorofluorescein (DCF). The increase in cell fluorescence was measured during 10 min, at 37°C, with excitation at 502 nm and emission at 550 nm, using a SPEX Fluorolog spectrometer. The changes in fluorescence were calculated in arbitrary units in relation to the initial values.

Statistical Analysis

Data are the means ± SEM from at least two experiments, performed in duplicate or triplicate. Statistical analysis was performed by the one-way ANOVA test (p <0.05 was considered significant).

RESULTS

FIGURE 1 shows the changes in cell viability induced by the opioid (heroin and morphine) and stimulant (cocaine and amphetamine) drugs, as evaluated by the MTT assay. All the drugs of abuse induced a dose-dependent decrease in cell viability after four days of exposure. Nevertheless, the opioids were shown to be more toxic to PC12 cells than the stimulant drugs, as determined by the analysis of the IC_{50} values: $IC_{50} \sim 10^{-4.2}$ (*street* heroin) < $IC_{50} \sim 10^{-3.3}$ (heroin) < $IC_{50} \sim 10^{-3.2}$ (morphine) $IC_{50} \sim 10^{-2.9}$ (*d*-amphetamine) < $IC_{50} \sim 10^{-2.5}$ (cocaine). Interestingly, *street* heroin was shown to be the most toxic of the drugs tested (FIG. 1), probably due to the presence of toxic contaminants.

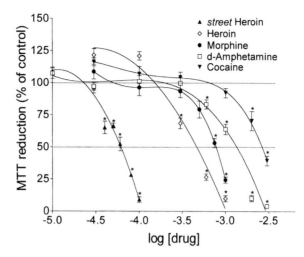

FIGURE 1. Dose-response curves of cytotoxic effects induced by the drugs of abuse. PC12 cells were incubated with increasing concentrations of *street* heroin, heroin, morphine, amphetamine, or cocaine for four days, and the toxic effects were evaluated by the MTT reduction assay. Data are the means ± SEM of 3–5 experiments performed in triplicate. Statistical significance: [*]P <0.001 as compared to the control.

The toxic effects of the drugs were further examined by following the leakage of LDH to the extracellular medium (FIG. 2), a known test that evaluates the changes in cell membrane integrity. Concentrations of the drugs close to the IC_{50} values were used. The drugs amphetamine, heroin, and cocaine were chosen because they are known to cause severe health problems in the Portuguese population. The results show that exposure to concentrations up to 600 µM heroin, 3 mM cocaine, or 2 mM amphetamine for four days does not significantly alter the integrity of the plasma membrane of PC12 cells, as compared to the controls, in the absence of the drugs of abuse (FIG. 2).

Analysis of the ratio ATP/ADP is a good indicator of the metabolic status of the cells. Although the exposure to cocaine or heroin did not significantly change this ratio, amphetamine induced a significant decrease (by about 45%) in intracellular ATP/ADP levels (FIG. 3).

Apoptotic cell death has been shown to play an important role in the pathogenesis of several diseases in the central nervous system (CNS). However, the role of apoptosis in the toxic effect of drugs of abuse, heroin, amphetamine, and cocaine, in dopaminergic cells has not been fully addressed. Accordingly, we have also analyzed the condensation of chromatin, a characteristic feature of apoptosis, by using the SYTO-13/PI assay. As a positive control, serum withdrawal for 48 h induced a pronounced condensation of the chromatin in PC12 cells, as observed by the labeling with SYTO-13. Similar features of apoptosis were observed in cells incubated in the presence of heroin or amphetamine, but not in the presence of cocaine (FIG. 4). Interestingly, only a very small percentage of cells incubated in serum-free medium

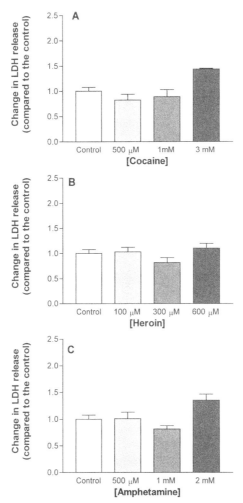

FIGURE 2. Evaluation of membrane integrity upon exposure of the cells to different concentrations of the drugs of abuse. Membrane integrity was measured by LDH release, after exposure of the cells for four days to (A) cocaine (500 μM, 1 mM, and 3 mM); (B) heroin (100 μM, 300 μM, and 600 μM); or (C) amphetamine (500 μM, 1 mM, and 2 mM). Data are the means ± SEM of two experiments performed in triplicate.

were shown to be labeled with PI, a nonpermeable fluorescent dye and a marker of necrotic cells.

Because the drugs of abuse interfere with the uptake systems (cocaine[16]), or the synaptic vesicle accumulation of dopamine (amphetamine[17] and cocaine[16]), which can induce changes in dopamine neuronal content, we have used the PC12 cells as models of dopaminergic neurons[8,9] to determine the changes in intracellular dopamine levels upon incubation with heroin, amphetamine, or cocaine (FIG. 5). Exposure

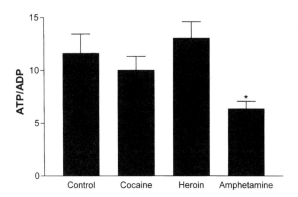

FIGURE 3. Intracellular ATP/ADP levels in PC12 cells incubated with 3 mM cocaine, 300 μM heroin, or 1 mM amphetamine for four days. Data are the means ± SEM of four experiments performed in triplicate. Statistical significance: *P <0.05 as compared to the control.

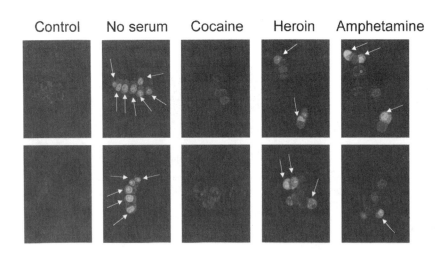

FIGURE 4. Analysis of chromatin condensation in PC12 cells exposed to the drugs of abuse. SYTO-13 and propidium iodide (PI) were used to evaluate apoptotic cell death upon exposure to cocaine (3 mM), heroin (300 μM), or amphetamine (1 mM) for 48 h. The cells were incubated in the absence of serum for 48 h (*no serum*). All PC12 cells shown in the pictures are labeled with SYTO-13 (green fluorescence). Only a small percentage of cells incubated with medium without serum were found to be labeled with PI (red fluorescence). The arrows indicate PC12 cells showing chromatin condensation.

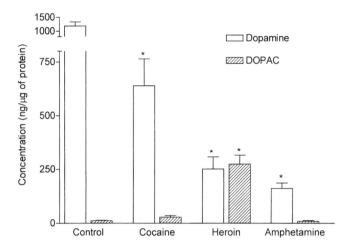

FIGURE 5. Intracellular dopamine and DOPAC levels upon exposure to the drugs of abuse. The cells were incubated with cocaine (3 mM), heroin (300 μM) or amphetamine (1 mM) for four days. Data are the means ± SEM of four experiments performed in triplicate. Statistical significance: $^*p < 0.05$, as compared to the respective control.

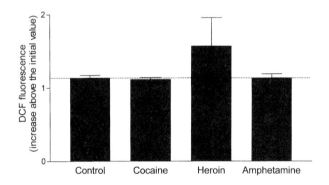

FIGURE 6. Analysis of ROS formation in cells incubated with the drugs of abuse. The oxidation of the probe $DCFH_2$ (20 μM) to DCF was followed in cells incubated with 3 mM cocaine, 300 μM heroin, or 1 mM amphetamine for 24 h. Data are the means ± SEM of three experiments performed in triplicate.

to cocaine decreased the dopamine levels by about 40%, whereas exposure to heroin and amphetamine largely decreased dopamine levels, by about 80%. In addition, an increase in intracellular DOPAC levels, suggesting an enhanced turnover of dopamine by MAO, followed the decrement in dopamine upon incubation with heroin. These data also suggested an increased formation of intracellular peroxides. Therefore, we measured the intracellular oxidation of $DCFH_2$ (Fig. 6). Although not statistically significant, the results show an increase in intracellular peroxides in the presence of heroin, as compared to control conditions. Changes in basal DCF fluorescence were not observed after the incubation with cocaine or amphetamine. These data indicate that an increased formation of intracellular peroxides may follow the increase in intracellular DOPAC resulting from dopamine metabolization upon exposure to heroin.

DISCUSSION

In this study we show that cell death induced by the drugs of abuse involves a decrease in intracellular dopamine content in cultured undifferentiated PC12 cells, without major changes in membrane integrity, suggesting an alteration in dopamine metabolic pathways and/or an increase in extracellular dopamine accumulation.

Cytotoxic effects induced by cocaine were not very evident in PC12 cells, as demonstrated by the maintenance of MTT reduction or ATP/ADP levels, the nonappearance of apoptotic features or the small decrease in intracellular dopamine, in contrast with heroin or amphetamine. Nevertheless, cocaine was previously shown to induce cell death by apoptosis in several cell types, including fetal mouse cortical neurons,[18] fetal rat myocardial cells,[19,20] bovine coronary artery endothelial cells,[21,22] or in rat testes.[23] Moreover, cocaine, and in particular its N-oxidative metabolites, were shown to depress mitochondrial respiration.[24]

Cytotoxic effects induced by heroin were associated with a large decrease in intracellular dopamine, an increase in DOPAC levels, and an apparent, nonstatistical increase in intracellular ROS production. In addition, toxic effects induced by amphetamine in PC12 cells were associated with a decrease in intracellular dopamine and a decrease in ATP/ADP levels, suggesting a certain degree of metabolic dysfunction. Interestingly, both amphetamine and heroin induced chromatin condensation, a feature of apoptotic cell death, which is in agreement with previous studies showing the induction of apoptotic cell death by heroin[25] and amphetamine.[26] Furthermore, although our data show an attenuation of ATP production and the appearance of apoptotic features upon exposure to amphetamine, recent data reported by Lotharius and O'Malley[27] support the idea that amphetamine-induced toxicity in dopaminergic neurons involves production of ROS, although neither protein oxidation, ATP decrement, mitochondrial dysfunction, nor cell death was observed.

In conclusion, toxic effects of amphetamine and heroin in undifferentiated PC12 cells are associated with the induction of apoptotic cell death, which may be due to a metabolic dysfunction induced by amphetamine or an increase in dopamine metabolization and production of ROS induced by heroin. As for cocaine, further experimental approaches are needed to clarify the cytotoxic mechanisms. The results reported in this study are compatible with the hypothesis that dopamine plays a major role in reinforcing the toxic effects of the drugs of abuse.

REFERENCES

1. Di Chiara, G. & A. Imperato. 1988. Drugs abused by humans preferentially increase synaptic dopamine concentrations in the mesolimbic system of freely moving rats. Proc. Natl. Acad. Sci. USA 85: 5274–5278.

2. OLANOW, C.W. & W.G. TATTON. 1999. Etiology and pathogenesis of Parkinson's disease. Annu. Rev. Neurosci. **22:** 123–144.
3. CADET, J.L. & C. BRANNOCK. 1998. Free radicals and the pathobiology of brain dopamine systems. Neurochem. Int. **32:** 117–131.
4. LUO, Y. *et al.* 1998. Dopamine induces apoptosis through an oxidation-involved SAPK/JNK activation pathway. J. Biol. Chem. **273:** 3756–3764.
5. LUO, Y. *et al.* 1999. Intrastriatal dopamine injection induces apoptosis through oxidation-involved activation of transcription factors AP-1 and NF-kappaB in rats. Mol. Pharmacol. **56:** 254–264.
6. LEE, H.J. *et al.* 2001. Antiapoptotic role of NF-kappaB in the auto-oxidized dopamine-induced apoptosis of PC12 cells. J. Neurochem. **76:** 602–609.
7. BEN-SHACHAR, D., R. ZUK & Y. GLINKA. 1995. Dopamine neurotoxicity: inhibition of mitochondrial respiration. J. Neurochem. **64:** 718–723.
8. TAKASHIMA, A. & T. KOIKE. 1985. Relationship between dopamine content and its secretion in PC12 cells as a function of cell growth. Biochim. Biophys. Acta **847:** 101–107.
9. SHAFER, T.J. & W.D. ATCHISON. 1991. Transmitter, ion channel and receptor properties of pheochromocytoma (PC12) cells: a model for neurotoxicological studies. Neurotoxicology **12:** 473–492.
10. GREENE, L.A. & A.S. TISCHLER. 1976. Establishment of a noradrenergic clonal line of rat adrenal pheochromocytoma cells which respond to nerve growth factor. Proc. Natl. Acad. Sci. USA **73:** 2424–2428.
11. BERGMEYER, H.U. & E. BERNT. 1974. Lactate dehydrogenase UV assay with pyruvate and NADH. *In* Methods in Enzymatic Analysis, Vol. 2: 574–579. Academic Press. New York.
12. MOSMANN, T. 1983. Rapid colorimetric assay for cellular growth and survival: application to proliferation and cytotoxicity assays. J. Immunol. Methods **65:** 55–63.
13. SEDMAK, J.J. & S.E. GROSSBERG. 1977. A rapid, sensitive, and versatile assay for protein using coomassie brilliant blue G250. Anal. Biochem. **79:** 544–552.
14. FOWLER, J.C. 1993. Changes in extracellular adenosine levels and population spike amplitude during graded hypoxia in the rat hippocampal slice. Naunyn Schmiedebergs Arch. Pharmacol. **347:** 73–78.
15. MORGADINHO, M.T., C.A. FONTES RIBEIRO & T.R.A. MACEDO. 1999. Presynaptic dopamine receptors involved in the inhibition of noradrenaline and dopamine release in the human gastric and uterine arteries. Fund. Clin. Pharmacol. **13:** 662–670.
16. BROWN, J.M., G.R. HANSON & A.E. FLECKENSTEIN. 2001. Regulation of the vesicular monoamine transporter-2: a novel mechanism for cocaine and other psychostimulants. J. Pharmacol. Exp. Ther. **296:** 762–767.
17. JONES, S.R., R.R. GAINETDINOV, R.M. WIGHTMAN & M.G. CARON. 1998. Mechanisms of amphetamine action revealed in mice lacking the dopamine transporter. J. Neurosci. **18:** 1979–1986.
18. NASSOGNE, M.C., J. LOUAHED, P. EVRARD & P.J. COURTOY. 1997. Cocaine induces apoptosis in cortical neurons of fetal mice. J. Neurochem. **68:** 2442–2450.
19. XIAO, Y., J. HE, R.D. GILBERT & L. ZHANG. 2000. Cocaine induces apoptosis in fetal myocardial cells through a mitochondria-dependent pathway. J. Pharmacol. Exp. Ther. **292:** 8–14
20. ZHANG, L., Y. XIAO & J. HE. 1999. Cocaine and apoptosis in myocardial cells. Anat. Rec. **257:** 208–216.
21. HE, J., Y. XIAO, C.A. CASIANO & L. ZHANG. 2000. Role of mitochondrial cytochrome c in cocaine-induced apoptosis in coronary artery endothelial cells. J. Pharmacol. Exp. Ther. **295:** 896–903.
22. HE, J., Y. XIAO & L. ZHANG. 2001. Cocaine-mediated apoptosis in bovine coronary artery endothelial cells: role of nitric oxide J. Pharmacol. Exp. Ther. **298:** 180–187.
23. LI, H. *et al.* 1999. Cocaine induced apoptosis in rat testes. J. Urol. **162:** 213–216.
24. BOESS, F., F.M. NDIKUM-MOFFOR, U.A. BOELSTERLI & S.M. ROBERTS. 2000. Effects of cocaine and its oxidative metabolites on mitochondrial respiration and generation of reactive oxygen species. Biochem. Pharmacol. **60:** 615–623.

25. FECHO, K. & D.T. LYSLE. 2000. Heroin-induced alterations in leukocyte numbers and apoptosis in the rat spleen. Cell Immunol. **202:** 113–123.
26. STUMM, G. *et al.* 1999. Amphetamines induce apoptosis and regulation of bcl-x splice variants in neocortical neurons. FASEB J. **13:** 1065–1072.
27. LOTHARIUS, J. & K.L. O'MALLEY. 2001. Role of mitochondrial dysfunction and dopamine-dependent oxidative stress in amphetamine-induced toxicity. Ann. Neurol. **49:** 79–89.

Recombinant μ-δ Receptor as a Marker of Opiate Abuse

SVETLANA A. DAMBINOVA AND GALINA A. IZYKENOVA

Laboratory of Molecular Neurobiology, Institute of the Human Brain, Russian Academy of Sciences, St. Petersburg 197376, Russia

ABSTRACT: The brain is particularly vulnerable to drugs of abuse changing the neuroreceptor functions. Opiates interact and overstimulate heterogeneous opioid receptors leading to their desensitization, internalization, and activation of recombinant opioid receptor. The molecular properties of rat and human brain recombinant μ-δ receptor were compared with those of purified μ- and δ-receptors. cDNA coding the unique fragment of recombinant μ-δ receptor was isolated and sequenced. We hypothesized that recombinant μ-δ receptor may be a hallmark of opiate abuse. Peptide fragments of the μ- (MOR), δ- (DOR), and recombinant μ-δ- (MDOR) receptors were used as antigens to assess the presence of autoantibodies in the blood of rats that self-administered heroin and cocaine, as well as drug abusers. Significant steady elevation of MDOR autoantibodies were measured in sera of rats that self-administered heroin compared to that for cocaine and vehicle animals. The appearance and increased level of MDOR autoantibodies in opiate abusers correlated with severity of the disorder and duration of drug exposure.

KEYWORDS: receptor heterogeneity; recombinant μ-δ receptor; cDNA; autoantibodies; self-administration; opiate abusers

INTRODUCTION

The mechanisms of molecular and cellular adaptation are initiated with repeated administration of opioids and result in short-term as well as protracted changes defining tolerance, sensitization, and dependence. Tolerance describes diminishing sensitivity to opioid drugs such that higher doses are required to gain the desired effect; sensitization describes the opposite.[1] Dependence, which is often used to define the addiction, is a physiological state caused by chronic drug exposure and leads to withdrawal symptoms when drug use is discontinued.

There is clear evidence that the expression of tolerance in individual neurons occurs with the specificity of changes in responsiveness and temporal development.

Address for correspondence: Svetlana Dambinova, D.Sci., Ph.D., Visiting Professor, of Emory University, Atlanta, GA. Voice: 1(404) 325 8734; fax: 1(404) 633 9494.
sdambin@emory.edu

Ann. N.Y. Acad. Sci. 965: 497–514 (2002). © 2002 New York Academy of Sciences.

Homologous desensitization is highly specific to opioids, and develops rapidly following receptor occupation with or without internalization.[1] Another somewhat slower (hours) form of homologous tolerance depends on changes in the adenylyl cyclase cascade.[2] The third heterologous form develops even more slowly (days) and has been suggested to be due to a partial depolarization resulting from down-regulation of the sodium pump.[3]

Mechanisms of opiate dependence are based on positive and negative reinforcing effects of opioids and are defined by withdrawal. Long-lived molecular adaptations in specific brain regions cause the major aspect of addiction. Although opioids activate the mesolimbic brain reward pathways, they produce compensatory adaptations, for example, acting on opioid receptors in locus ceruleus that control somatic functions and thereby produce physical dependence.[1,2]

Opioids and opiates exert their effects after binding to specific receptors located throughout the central and peripheral nervous systems. Pharmacological approaches have suggested that the μ-receptor, for which morphine has the highest affinity, serves as a principle site for morphine actions in inducing behavioral reward,[4] locomotion,[5] analgesia,[6] tolerance,[2] and physical dependence.[1] There is growing evidence implicating the involvement of δ-receptors in the reinforcing actions of opiates. Delta-2 but not δ_1-receptors appear to be involved in the dependence-producing effects of morphine in mouse.[7,8] Under certain conditions, δ_2 agonists and antagonists can modulate μ-mediated antinociceptive potency which may represent action at a μ-δ_2 receptor complex.[9]

We hypothesized that chronic opiate treatment increases the synthesis of opioid receptors in the brain reflecting neuroadaptation.[10] Abnormal gene expression of opioid receptors leads to their metabolic damage, followed by removal via the blood–brain barrier of the product of nerve-cell degradation. The immune system recognizes these products as foreign antigens and responds by generation of autoantibodies[11] serving as a tracer of opioid receptor synthesis-degradation alterations underlying the tolerance/dependence mechanisms. We supposed the presence in the brain of a new pharmacological receptor subtype—recombinant μ-δ receptor—which could be a biomarker of opioid dependence.

The first evidence concerning the existence of a new recombinant opioid receptor is presented here. The recombinant μ-δ receptor (rMDOR) was purified from rat and human brain. It was demonstrated that rMDOR pharmacological, immunochemical, and functional characteristics are similar to those for μ- and δ-receptors isolated from hybrid cells. The unique cDNA coding the fragment recombinant receptor has been isolated and compared with known opioid receptor sequences. We hypothesized that recombinant μ-δ receptor may be a hallmark of opiate addiction. Specific peptide fragments of N-terminal sequences of the rMDOR, μ- (MOR), and δ- (DOR) receptors were designed, synthesized, and used as antigens to assess the presence of autoantibodies in the blood of rats that self-administered heroin and cocaine, as well as opiate abusers.

This overview focuses on the opioid neuroreceptor system and its participation in molecular heterogeneity of adaptive changes in synaptic function induced by opioids. Current research describes the possible role of rMDOR autoantibodies as a tracer of opioid dependence in neurochemical mechanisms of opioid tolerance/dependence.

NEUROCHEMICAL MECHANISMS OF ADAPTATION TO OPIATES AND OPIOID RECEPTORS

Usually exogenic chemical stimuli are much stronger than endogenous ones and have a prolonged effect when exposed. Repeated opiate administration activates natural mechanisms of adaptations in neurons of locus ceruleus, VTA, and periaqueductal grey that lead to long-lived changes and opposing processes of development of tolerance and dependence.[1]

Tolerance involves a number of distinct cellular and neural processes including desensitization, phosphorylation, and internalization. It was demonstrated that agonist binding to a receptor promotes a conformational change that results in heterotrimeric G-protein activation and dissociation from the receptor.[3] Free G protein β/γ-subunits facilitate translocation of G-protein-coupled receptor kinase to the membrane where they phosphorylate the COOH-terminal region.[1] The phosphorylated receptor subsequently binds with high affinity to the regulatory proteins called β-arrestin, which prevents association of inactive G proteins with the receptor and initiates internalization.[1,2] Receptor phosphorylation appears to be a critical event for internalization but not for desensitization to occur. Many of the details of this scheme have been confirmed for the μ-receptor, but a number of contentious issues remain.

It has long been recognized that internalization is not required for desensitization to occur, but when it does, the process necessarily affects sensitivity to agonists by removing surface receptors. Pak et al.[12] demonstrated that μ-receptor desensitization was associated with a loss of binding sites on the plasma membrane. It was shown that δ- and κ-receptor trafficking occurred to and from the plasma membrane under a certain opiate stimulus. These receptors were found in plasma membranes and vesicular compartments.[13] Receptors situated in vesicular compartments and membranes may be newly synthesized as well as recycled.

The cascade of cellular events, as presented above, following opioid binding to receptor may explain homologous tolerance, but from that position it is very difficult to describe physiological dependence. Multiple phenomena of opioid dependence suggest the existence of various neurochemical mechanisms.[3] It has been recognized that opioids alter spontaneous activity of the neuronal membrane following decreased excitability. Because this altered state of excitability is responsible both for subsensitivity to inhibitory substances and supersensitivity to excitatory substances, this mechanism is a clear example of one that can explain both tolerance and physical dependence.[1,3]

The actions of opioids in any biological system are a combination of multiple independent components acting together. The first source of diversity is the receptor where at least three major types of opioid receptors (μ-, δ-, and κ-) mediate the response to exogenous or endogenous opioid ligands.[14] Each of these receptors is a member of the superfamily of G-protein-coupled receptors characterized by seven transmembrane-spanning tertiary structures.

Highly selective ligands and antibodies make it possible to define receptor binding characteristics and anatomical distributions. Each major opioid receptor has a unique anatomical distribution in brain limbic structures generally found in perisynaptic areas, rather than in subsynaptic sites.[19,20] Mu receptors are found in dense patches in the nucleus accumbens, with greatest density being detected in the rostral and medial aspects.[19] Delta receptors are also dense in the nucleus accumbens relative to other structures, but are not localized in patches and are somewhat less abundant compared to m receptors.

There is disagreement regarding the exact classification of the opioid receptor subtypes, suggesting the possibility of other subtypes as multiple μ-,[15] δ-,[7] and μ-δ complex[16] receptors. The cloning of each of the three major opioid receptors has done little to support further expansion of opioid receptors classification.[8,9,15] About 60% sequence homology was shown between the μ-, δ-, and κ-receptors.[14] There are reports of alternative splice variants, although it is not clear at what level they are expressed or if they can be distinguished pharmacologically.[17,18] Functional studies using selective agonists and antagonists have revealed substantial parallels between μ- and δ-receptors and dramatic contrasts between μ/δ- and the κ-receptors.

It is obvious that not all the opioid receptors have been cloned yet. A rich array of natural and synthetic opioid ligands are supposed to regulate a number of receptors having different structures and second messengers as defined for other neurotransmitter receptors. Therefore, this issue remains an open one.

Different ligands may produce divergent allosteric changes in a given opioid receptor, leading to different efficiencies or resulting in coupling to different combinations of signaling pathways, and to various rates of receptor internalization. These changes in turn may lead to unique patterns of altered gene expression of target proteins that could in turn differentially modify behavior. Some questions arise: is the existence of a new recombinant receptor type possible? If it is, what role may it play in development of opioid dependence?

CHARACTERIZATION OF RECOMBINANT μ-δ RECEPTOR

Considerable data concerning opioid receptor cloning and characterization are demonstrated in the current literature,[14] with the problem of the heterogeneity and existence of recombinant types of opioid receptors open to be explored. Despite the significant volume of data on opiates and their receptors, knowledge of the neurobiology and neurochemistry underlying compulsive opiate use is still rather limited.

To investigate the role of opiate binding proteins (OBP) in drug abuse pathogenesis we isolated these membrane proteins from rat[21,22] and human[10,23,24] brains by affinity chromatography and preparative electrophoresis. Fractions of synaptic membranes from whole rat brain (without cerebellum) or human cortex were isolated by differential centrifugation.[21] Opiate-binding proteins from the synaptic membrane fraction were purified by affinity chromatography on solid matrix containing β-endorphin[22] or the novel opioid peptide dalargin (Tyr-D-Ala-Gly-Phe-Leu-Arg). Dalargin is the [Leu5]-enkephalin analogue synthesized in the Scientific Cardiological Center (Moscow, Russia) and was shown to be the agonist of μ- and δ-receptors.[25,26]

The electrophoresis of total OBP_r isolated from rat brain revealed three protein bands with molecular weights of 29, 45, 66 kDa, and those of M_r 29, 65 for OBP_h were purified from human synaptic membranes.[24] The electrophoretic point for both OBP_r and OBP_h was pI 5.4. The major component of human and rat OBP with M_r

TABLE 1. Constants of ^{3}H-naloxone-specific binding to the synaptic membranes and opiate binding proteins

^{3}H-naloxone specific binding constants	Synaptic membranes		Solubilized synaptic membranes		Opiate binding proteins, Mr 65-66 kD	
	Rat	Human	Rat	Human	Rat	Human
Kd (nM)	1.2 ± 0.5	19.0 ± 2.5	17 ± 2.1	22.3 ± 3.2	21.2 ± 5.1	42.0 ± 7.0
B_{max} (pmol/mg of protein)	2.7 ± 0.4	4.5 ± 1.2	1.8 ± 0.7	41.6 ± 4.8	181 ± 34	153 ± 27

65–66 kDa was purified by use of one of the following approaches: preparative electrophoresis, high-performance liquid chromatography (HPLC) on a TSK-3000 column, or immunoaffinity chromatography on a column containing immobilized polyclonal antibodies raised against OBP$_r$.[22] Separated by HPLC or electrophoresis, the main protein fraction 65–66 kDa from both origins specifically bound ^{3}H-naloxone and was found to have common immunoactive determinants to bind to polyclonal antibodies IZ17 (IgG) raised against OBP$_r$.[24,27] Schiff reagent staining of total OBP indicated the presence of glycoside fragment and pointed out the glycoprotein nature of isolated proteins.[21,22] It was found that the OBP with M$_r$ 29 from both origins is a result of proteolytic degradation of the 65–66 kDa protein, which also possessed [^{3}H]DAGO ([Tyr-D-Ala-Gly-Methyl-Phe-Glyol]-enkephalin) binding activity inhibited by DADLE (D-Ala2-D-Leu5-enkephalin).

The OBP fragment of 45 kDa has been isolated from rat total OBP fraction by use of DAGO elution from dalargin-sepharose.[21] Protein 45 kDa specifically bound μ-agonists and demonstrated phosphatase activity[28] associated with μ-opioid receptor.[29]

Isolated proteins by specific binding with radiolabeled agonists and antagonists of opiate receptors were characterized.[22] The analysis of ^{3}H-naloxone binding to the rat and human synaptic membranes demonstrated the existence of one binding site with corresponding constants.[22,24] Digitonin-solubilized protein fractions of synaptic membranes and OBP with M$_r$ 65–66 kDa specifically bound μ-antagonist with close parameters (TABLE 1).

The competitive binding of opioid agonists and antagonists with binding sites of OBP$_h$, purified by HPLC, appeared to exist mostly of μ- and δ-receptors (TABLE 2). The pharmacological profile of ^{3}H-DAGO specific binding to solubilized proteins was generally the same as that for membrane-bound sites (one binding site). High-affinity binding of isolated OBP$_h$ to specific ligands of μ- and δ-receptors was observed: DAMGO, morphine, DPDPE[10] (TABLE 2).

The next stage of OBP characterization dealt with immunochemical identification of opioid receptor fragments using polyclonal antibodies to subunits of the receptors. Polyclonal antibodies were raised against total OBP$_r$ by rabbit immunization using standard protocol.[30] Polyclonal antibodies IZ17, producing immunoglobulins G1, were developed in preparative quantities and used for identification of OBP purified by HPLC from both origins. Polyclonal antibodies inhibited the ^{3}H-DAGO and ^{3}H-naloxone specific binding to OBP$_h$.[10] Polyclonal antibodies IZ17 at concentrations 10^{-6}–10^{-10} irreversibly blocked evoked potential in electroreceptors of *Ampullae lorenzini* of the skate *Raja clavata* (research results of Dr. I. Rizhova, Pavlov Institute of Physiology, St. Petersburg, Russia).

TABLE 2. Results of competitive of ^{3}H-DAGO-specific binding to the opiate binding proteins (M$_r$ 65-66 kD) isolated from human synaptic membranes

| Agonist or antagonist | Ki, µM | | |
	Specific binding	Total binding	Inhibition of ^{3}H-DAMGO binding
DAMGO	0.35	0.67	0.82
Morphine	1.57	2.80	2.05
Naloxone	1.34	2.90	1.55
DPDPE	1.57	3.99	1.02
Ethylketocyclazocine	>1,00	5.20	>1,000

Polyclonal antibodies IZ17 bound only 66- and 29-kDa components of human synaptic membranes.[22] Immunocytochemical and colloidal gold-labeled anti-OBP IZ17 were used for determination of OBP localization in rat thalamus.[27] Maximal concentrations of OBP-like immunoreactivity were found in synaptic terminals of opiate-receptive neuronal axons and, to a lesser extent, in the soma of the cells.[27]

In order to compare purified OBP$_r$ and OBP$_h$ with opioid receptors, µ-receptor from plasmatic membranes of mMOR-CHO cells and δ-receptor from hybrid NG108-15 neuroblastoma x glioma cells[31,32] were isolated and solubilized by digitonin. The affinity chromatography on a dalargin-sepharose 4B column allowed to purify these receptors. SDS-electrophoresis of purified receptors showed similar protein bands with molecular weight 65–66 kDa.[33,34] Western blot analyses of purified receptors and OBP from both origins, with commercial antibodies to µ- and δ-receptors (Chemicon, CA) as well as IZ17, revealed protein bands with M$_r$ 66 kDa.[34] These results clearly indicated the existence of common antigenic fragments on the surface of all isolated receptors including OBP. This receptor fragment was isolated by preparative electrophoresis in nondenatured conditions. The isolated receptor reacted with serum samples from patients with opiate dependence in Western blot assay. Antibodies (IgG) purified from pooled blood serum of those patients specifically stained the fraction 66 kDa of OBP.

Thus, all the above-described research data concerning purified OBP convinced us that these opiate-binding proteins could be the recombinant µ-δ receptor (rMDOR). It was necessary to determine the cDNA coding the immunoactive fragment of rMDOR responsible for the appearance of the autoantibodies in order to recognize precisely which receptor subtype is involved in the immune response.[11]

It is known that genes encoding neurotransmitter receptors belong, as a rule, to rare sequences. In such cases the cDNA search and cloning method of Young and Davis is recommended.[35] It resides in protein-encoding sequences isolated from the recombinant RNA or DNA library by polyclonal antibodies raised to receptor fragments. The system is based upon the vector λgt11, which incorporates the alien DNA fragment in *lac Z* bacterial gene. Thus, in *E. coli* cells, the hybrid protein involving beta-galactosidase (lac Z product) and allele DNA product are synthesized. The immunoscreening of 10^6 clones in human brain cDNA library by Western blot using polyclonal antibodies IZ17 and total IgG, isolated from patients with opioid dependence, revealed one recombinant phage λ-OBP clone with a positive immunological signal.[10]

The λ-OBP DNA analysis showed the existence of a 1.2 kb cDNA insert. This means that the isolated sequence length is only a part of the cDNA coding the synthesis of OBP. For the cDNA restriction map construction, the EcoR1 fragment of the λ-OBP clone was transferred in M13mp11 vector. This fragment was isolated from the agarose gel after the DNA was treated by radiolabeled EcoR1, then by a number of restrictase kits. The results of the treatment were analyzed by PAAG electrophoresis. This analysis revealed three unique sites within the fragments: Pst1, BamH1, and Psal.[10]

We determined the 5′-3′ cDNA orientation by analyzing λ-OBP DNA with Kpn1, BamH1, and EcoR1 restrictases. The partial cDNA sequence allowed us to map more accurately the position of the BamH1 and Pst1 restriction sites. Eco R1-Pst1, Pst1-BamH1, and BamH1-EcoR1 DNA fragments were then transferred in M13mp10 and M13mp11 vectors to attain EcoR1-Pst1. The Pst1 site was found to be located 130th in from the 5′-end; the BamH1 110th in from the 3′-end of nucleotide pairs.

The isolated cDNA coding human μ-δ recombinant receptor was transcribed to mRNA and amplified by PCR. The Northern blot of ^{35}S-methionine–labeled products of the OBP mRNA expression was performed by use of IZ17 and blood sera from patients with opiate dependence.

After cDNA nucleotide sequence determination (720 bp), the open reading frame for polypeptide with M_r 23 kDa consisting of 183 amino acid residues was found.[10] A computer analysis of the known nucleotide sequence banks revealed the existence of 43–45% homology of our polypeptide to N-terminal domains of both MOR and DOR.

A specific MDOR peptide (21 amino acids) corresponding to rMDOR receptor N-terminus sequence was designed on the basis of protein sequences obtained using the computer analysis GCG program (Madison, WI) for prediction of antigenic determinants in the protein structure based on the profile of hydrophobicity[36] and antigenicity.[37] Receptor rMDOR and antigenic peptide MDOR were immobilized on matrix and used to assess the presence of autoantibodies.

PARTICIPATION OF OPIOID RECEPTOR IN EXPERIMENTAL TOLERANCE AND DEPENDENCE

Humans and experimental animals can develop profound tolerance to opioids over a period of several days to weeks of escalating chronic treatment. There are a number of various experimental models of animal exposure to opioids producing the complex behavior normally associated with tolerance and dependence in humans.

Usually short-term nonspecific tolerance is produced in mice or rat by multiple i.p. injections with ascending doses of drugs and occurs at day 4–5 of the experiment.[3] The long-term nonspecific tolerance is produced by, for example, morphine pellet implantation which occurs at day 6-7 after pellet implantation. The qualitative evaluation of nonspecific tolerance in both models is performed on the basis of subsensitivity to inhibitory agents and supersensitivity to excitatory agents.[3]

The acquisition of intravenous drug-reinforced behavior occurs rapidly. Usually with opioids the number of infusions self-administered by an animal ranges from very few and continues to increase to a maximum number over several weeks. There are three methods to systematically, objectively, and quantitatively describe this transition behavior when intravenous drug delivery is dependent on an operant response.[38]

The simplest method is to expose animals to a drug for a fixed amount of time each day; acquisition of drug self-administration is said to occur when responding initiates pass through an erratic escalating phase, then stabilize at a steady daily rate that is considerably higher than responding in a vehicle group (e.g., saline), or drop to few responses when the drug is changed on saline (saline extensions).[39] This type of analysis can be used to study the effects of session length, medication pretreatments, etc.

A second method that has often been used is similar except that one or two pre-injections are given by the experimenter at the start of session, and latency to acquisition of drug behavior is also measured. Acquisition is defined by comparing the upper limit of 99% confidence intervals for responses on the drug-reinforced lever and a second nonreinforced lever. When these confidence intervals are no longer overlapping, acquisition has occurred.

A third method is an adaptation of an autoshaping procedure by pairing a stimulus (key light and/or sound) associated with automatic reinforcer delivery. During the self-administration session, the retractable lever remains extended, and drug infusions are contingent on lever pressing under a fixed-ratio schedule. The combination of all three methods and variations of session duration, number, concentration, time and manner of drug component availability (ascending or descending), and fixed or progressive ratio schedule are defined by researcher.[39] There is a wide range of factors that account for either the acceleration of or the decrease in acquisition of drug self-administration, such as environmental conditions, pharmacological variables, and individual differences.[38]

Animal self-administration studies have provided a laboratory model for drug use in humans and have been used extensively to study the reinforcing properties of drugs. Infusions of heroin and morphine can be readily used to maintain responding in rats.[39] It is accepted that μ-receptors drive the initial steps of the addictive side effects of opioids. Receptor-alkylating μ-opioid agonists β-funaltrexamine administrated i.c.v. and μ-opioid antagonists injected into nucleus accumbens and VTA attenuated heroin self-administration in rats.[39] The i.c.v. injections into mice of antibodies generated against the second extracellular loop of the μ-receptor or the first 16 amino acids of its N-terminus have also been shown to reduce the expression of multiple symptoms of withdrawal.[7] Repeated i.c.v. administration of oligonucleotides to μ-receptor, before starting chronic morphine, promoted a significant reduction of naloxone-precipitated withdrawal symptoms.[39]

Test of chronic morphine action in knockout mice expressed half of wild-type μ-receptor displays attenuated locomotion, reduced morphine self-administration, and intact tolerance.[40] They demonstrate full physical dependence following five days of morphine self-administration, whereas transgenic knockout mice without μ-opioid receptors showed the lack of morphine-induced tolerance and dependence.[40] From other sites the results of pharmacogenomic research of individual morphine response to genetic differences, such as single nucleotide polymorphism in μ-, δ- or κ-opioid receptors, clearly showed that no polymorphism that correlates with differences in opioid tolerance.[41]

There is a growing body of evidence implicating the involvement of δ-receptors in the reinforcing actions of opiates. The δ-selective antagonist naltridole-5′-isothiocyanate has been reported to attenuate heroin self-administration[42] and inhibited the development of physical dependence on chronic morphine.[7]

We hypothesized that abuse of opiates may result in the desensitization and breakdown of opioid receptors producing antigenic peptide fragments that the immune system recognizes as exogenous antigens, resulting in the production of autoantibodies to the μ- and δ-opioid receptor subunits.

Our preliminary experiments involved mice models of acute and chronic morphine administrations, which showed the appearance of increased levels of rMDOR autoantibodies (51% of control) in blood samples from chronically treated animals in comparison to control.[10,24] There were no changes of autoantibodies in the blood of mice with acute tolerance following 8 days of i.p. morphine injections (ascending doses of 10–80 µg/kg, 1–3 times daily). These results supposed that the appearance of rMDOR autoantibodies may be involved in chronic effects of opiates.

The investigation of μ-, δ-, and recombinant μ-δ receptor involvement in molecular mechanisms of chronic drug effects was performed using the known models of heroin and cocaine self-administration.[39,42] Following implantation of jugular catheters, animals (F-344 rats, 90–150 days old, Harlan, Indianapolis, IN) were trained to self-administer a range of doses of cocaine (0.125, 0.25, and 0.5 mg/infusion) or heroin (4.5, 9, 18 µg/infusion) and saline (vehicle) during 3.5-h sessions five days per week under a FR 2 schedule.[39] The dose of drug is varied by delivering different volumes of the drug solution (i.e., 50, 100, or 200 µL of 90 µg/mL of heroin). The doses are made available in ascending order with each dose available for 1 h with

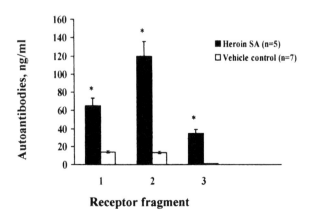

FIGURE 1. The concentrations of μ- (*bar 1*), δ- (*bar 2*), and recombinant **μ-δ** receptor (*bar 3*) autoantibodies in blood sera of rats self-administered heroin (80 sessions) compared with naive animals. Each bar represents the condition mean (± SEM) of autoantibody detections from five heroin rats and seven naive rats. *$p < 0.05$ versus autoantibodies levels for naive animals.

components separated by 10-min time-out periods. Responding was considered stable when the number of infusions at each dose of drug for each five successive days did not vary by more than 10% of the mean.

Experiments to assess the presence of autoantibodies to purified rMDOR, μ- and δ-receptors in the blood of rats self-administering heroin ($n = 5$) and vehicle animals ($n = 7$) have been completed (FIG. 1). In followed experiments, specific peptides MOR (17 amino acids) and DOR (18 amino acids) corresponding to N-terminal sequences of μ- and δ-receptors were designed additionally to compare with MDOR peptide. The antigenic peptides design, based on rodent and human protein sequences of N-terminal fragments of μ- and δ-receptors from the National Center for Biotechnology Information, NIH; the European Molecular Laboratory; and the National Biomedical Research Foundation data banks were performed using GCG program (Madison, WI) and hydrophobicity[36]/antigenicity[37] of protein structures. The antigenic peptides were synthesized, immobilized on matrix, and also used to assess the presence of autoantibodies in ELISA technique.[43]

The baseline level of autoantibodies was 13.0 ± 0.3 ng/mL for MOR and DOR peptides, and 0.7 ± 0.05 ng/mL for MDOR peptide was detected in the sera of the vehicle controls ($n = 5$). Statistically significant increases in autoantibody amounts were measured for peptides MOR (40%), DOR (251%), and MDOR (123%) in serum of animals self-administering heroin ($n = 6$) compared to vehicle controls.[44] These data suggested potential differential relationships among these receptor subtypes to produce autoantibodies in the blood of animals self-administering heroin. No changes in the levels of receptor autoantibodies have been detected in the blood of rats self-administering cocaine ($n = 7$) in comparison to vehicle animals self-administering saline.[44]

The immunoreactivity of μ- and δ-receptors and rMDOR subunits in the striatum of rats self-administering heroin have been detected by Western blot using commercial antibodies and IZ17. Rats self-administering heroin, but not cocaine, exhibited strong rMDOR immunoreactivities in striatum at the end of the first week of chronic treatment compared with that for vehicle-treated rats. However, the rMDOR subunit immunoreactivity decreased significantly by the 50th session of heroin self-administration.

Monitoring of peptide autoantibodies showed the uncommon accumulation profiles for different receptor fragments in blood samples from rats self-administering heroin (FIG. 2B). The concentrations of autoantibodies to MDOR peptide increased on day 10 of heroin self-administration in comparison to that for naive animals. Autoantibodies reached the maximum by the 15th session of the experiment and was accompanied by the stabilization of chronic drug consumption (FIG. 2C). The same time concentrations of autoantibodies for MOR and DOR peptides increased sufficiently by the 25th and 15th sessions, respectively, with maximal appearance at the 35th session of heroin self-administration (FIG. 2A). It was noticed that autoantibodies to MDOR peptide remained elevated to the end of experiment, while those for MOR and DOR peptides decreased to normal levels by the 50th session of observations. We did not detect sufficient changes in the dynamics of autoantibodies to all peptides in the blood of rats that self-administered cocaine (0.5 mg/infusion, FR2, 3-h session, $n = 7$).[44]

On the basis of experimental research, we supposed that the MDOR fragment of recombinant μ-δ receptors may serve as a biomarker of desensitization transition to sensitization and may be used for diagnosis of opiate dependence, while the appearance of MOR and DOR may reflect the stable pathological state of opiate dependence. In subsequent experiments the MDOR peptide was used for the assessment of autoantibody concentrations in blood sera of drug abusers and healthy controls.

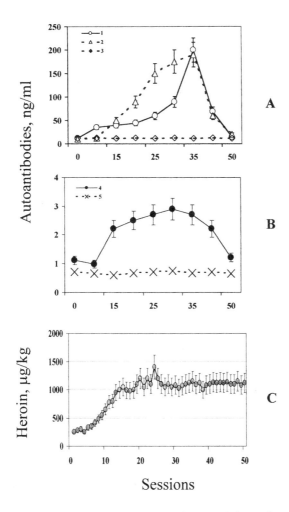

FIGURE 2. Monitoring and assessment of accumulations of autoantibodies to (**A**) MOR (*1, open circles*) and DOR (*2, open triangles*) peptides in blood of rats that self-administered heroin (*n* = 6) or vehicle (*n* = 5) animals (*3, diamonds*); (**B**) to MDOR peptide (*4, filled circles*) in blood of rats that self-administered heroin or vehicle animals (*5, cross hatches*); and (**C**) total drug intake during heroin self-administration (*n* = 6). Duration of the session was 3 h (FR2) with heroin dose 18 µg/infusion. Each point represents the condition mean (± SEM).

AUTOANTIBODIES TO μ-δ RECEPTOR IN DIAGNOSIS
OF OPIATE ADDICTION

The participation of opioid receptors in the pathogenesis of opioid abuse and dependence has been demonstrated, but clinical experience is scarce. There are a number of laboratory tests that detect the presence of drugs in hair,[45] blood,[46] and other biological fluids and tissues.[47,48] Routine urine toxicology and forensic tests are often positive for opioid drugs in individuals with opioid dependence. Urine tests remain positive for most opioids for 12–36 h after administration. Longer-acting opioids (e.g., methadone and LAAM) can be identified in urine for several days. Therefore, toxicological laboratory analysis identifies drugs without evaluation of the physiological state of the drug user. Such tests cannot be used for identification of the risk group and control of progress of treatment.

There are attempts to assess consequences of drug use on the basis of supersensitivity of heroin addicts to apomorphine[49] or naloxone.[50] The latter approach allows to define the physical dependence by measurement of pupil dilation. The method was reported about 81% reliable in diagnosing opiate addicts during the first examination. Thus, there is no laboratory test for dependence, diagnostic differentiation of use, or abuse; dependence is operationally defined in the Diagnostic and Statistical Manual of Mental Disorders, Fourth Edition (DSM-IV-TR) to be reliable and valid.[51]

On the basis of our experimental research we proposed a method for the diagnosis of opiate dependence by detection of autoantibodies to recombinant μ-δ receptor in the blood of drug users.[10,24] Patients ($n = 58$) admitted to the Narcology Clinic of Leningrad District (Russia) during 1998–1999, as well as 35 patients observed during 1999–2000 in the Clinic of the Human Brain Institute (St. Petersburg, Russia), were subdivided according to symptoms defined in the DSM-IV-TR.[51] All patients used opioids including opium, morphine, and heroin from 3 months to 7 years. The blood serum samples from these patients in sex- and age-matched groups (men, 21.5 ± 5.5 years old) and medical histories were kindly provided by Dr. V. Vostrikov and Dr. Y. Poliakov. Patients with physical dependence received nonspecific detoxication and maintenance therapy including anti-pain medication, anti-sedatives and anti-depressants.

Clinical evaluation of each patient resulted in four groups: (1) occasional opioid users , beginners who had experience using opiates 1–3 times ($n = 7$); (2) opioid abusers ($n = 13$); (3) those with opioid dependence ($n = 58$); (4) patients with early partial remission ($n = 15$). Healthy volunteers (men, age 25.0 ± 5.0 years), who never had used hypnotics, sedatives, or other drugs, and neurologic patients (men, 30 ± 5.0 years) were divided into in two control groups. The laboratory blood test detecting MDOR autoantibodies was performed under the approval of the Human Research Ethics Committee.

The level of MDOR autoantibodies in the serum of healthy volunteers was 1.7 ± 0.2 ng/mL (TABLE 3). Sufficiently elevated levels of MDOR autoantibodies (4.6 ± 0.7 ng/mL) in the sera of all observed opiate users in comparison to controls were detected. The highest concentration of MDOR autoantibodies was measured in the blood of patients with opioid dependence accompanied by withdrawal symptoms.

The comparison of blood test results and clinical observations showed the correlation between the level of autoantibodies and severity of the disorder. The concentration of MDOR autoantibodies increased in group 1 < group 2 < group 3 ($p < 0.01$).

TABLE 3. MDOR autoantibodies distribution in the blood of observed groups of individuals

Groups of patients	N	MDOR autoantibodies ng/mL	Patients			
			MDOR autoantibodies <2 ng/mL		MDOR autoantibodies >2 ng/mL	
			N	Percent	N	Percent
Healthy volunteers	30	1.7 ± 0.2	29	96.7	1	3.3
Patients with neuro-logical disorders	24	1.8 ± 0.1	20	83.8	4	16.7
1 group (occasional opioid users)	7	2.7 ± 0.3	3	42.8	4	57.2
2 group (occasional opioid dependence)	13	3.8 ± 0.4*	4	30.8	9	69.2
3 group (opioid dependence	58	5.6 ± 0.5**†	8	13.8	50	86.2
4 group (early partial remission)	15	4.1 ± 0.3*	0	0	15	100

*$p < 0.01$ for MDOR autoantibodies in 2 and 4 groups versus that for healthy volunteers.
**$p < 0.001$ for MDOR autoantibodies in 3 group versus that for healthy voluteeers.
†$p < 0.001$ for MDOR autoantibodies in 3 group versus that for patients with neuro-logical disorders; $p < 0.01$ for that between 2 and 3 groups (Student's test).

Statistically significant levels of autoantibodies elevated above that of the control (>2 ng/mL) were detected in 86.2% of cases of opioid-dependent users, in 69.2 % of drug abusers, and in 57.2% of beginners, whereas only 3.3% of healthy volunteers and 16.7% of patients with neurologic disorders had MDOR autoantibodies higher than control (TABLE 3).

We observed insignificant elevation of MDOR autoantibodies from 5.6 ± 0.5 ng/mL to 6.1 ± 0.5 ng/mL in the blood of patients with opioid dependence under opioid withdrawal conditions. The slight decrease in the level of autoantibodies from 6.1 ± 0.5 ng/mL to 5.1 ± 0.6 ng/mL in blood of physically dependent patients was ana-lyzed during 40 days of hospitalization without improvement of major clinical symptoms.

Statistically significant attenuation of MDOR autoantibodies was detected in blood of patients with early partial remission who used opium, but not heroin (TABLE 3). The levels of autoantibodies lower than 3 ng/mL were determined in 21% patients during the first month of remission and in 40% of those after 3–8 months of volun-tary drug withdrawal. The decrease in concentration of MDOR autoantibodies was accompanied by improved patients' physiological state and emotionally negative to positive mood alteration. However, the amounts of MDOR autoantibodies remained above control level, maintaining opportunity for relapse.

We found different profiles of MDOR autoantibody accumulation for heroin and opium addicts from the duration of drug use (TABLE 4). High levels of MDOR au-toantibodies in the blood of opium addicts were analyzed within 6 months of injec-

TABLE 4. Dependence of MDOR autoantibodies from disease duration

Drug abusers	N	MDOR autoantibodies in years, ng/mL			
		3–6 months	1 year	3 years	5–7 years
Opiate	47	3.9 ± 0.3	4.5 ± 0.5	3.2 ± 0.2	3.3 ± 0.4
Heroin	11	1.8 ± 0.2	6.5 ± 0.4	6.1 ± 0.7	—

tions, with stabilization of those increased levels at the end of the first year without many changes in the following 5–7 years. In contrast, within half a year of inhalation heroin addicts had approximately control levels of MDOR autoantibodies, which drastically (6 times) increased to the end of the first year and remained high for three years of use.

The results obtained in clinical research support our hypothesis that rMDOR autoantibodies are the tracers of opioid dependence development and reflect the severity of the disorder, depend on type of opiate used, and correlate with duration of drug exposure. rMDOR may serve as a marker for objective evaluation of patient state.

CONCLUSION

Many expensive and disturbing social problems can be traced directly to drug dependence. Recent studies[52,53] estimated the high costs of drug dependence for society in crime, lost work productivity, foster care, and other social problems. These expensive effects of drugs on all social systems have been important in shaping the public view that drug dependence is primarily a social problem that requires interdiction and law enforcement rather than a health problem that requires objective diagnosis, prevention, and treatment. Unfortunately, this opinion is apparently shared by many physicians. A survey[54] of general practice physicians indicated that most believed no available medical or health care interventions would be "appropriate or effective in treating addiction." In fact, 40% to 60 % of patients treated for alcohol or other drug dependence return to active substance use within one year following treatment discharge. From the other hand, it was confirmed that drug dependence is more like a chronic illness such as diabetes, hypertension, and asthma, which are widely believed to have effective diagnoses and treatments, although they are not yet curable.

The objective evaluation of the patient's state and particularly the condition of his brain under drug impairment are important for a better treatment cure. These problems would be solved if the appropriate biomarkers reflecting the pathologic mechanisms of dependence are available for monitoring in laboratory tests. One such biomarker may be heterogenous opioid receptors—actual targets of exogenous and endogenous drugs.

The effect of various opioid ligands depends on receptor heterogeneity by which allosteric alterations may lead to unique patterns of altered gene expression of target receptor that could have peculiar functions appeared in modification of behavior.

The right choice of ligand possesses the stable peptide structure, abilities of endogenous opioids, and equal action on μ- and δ-receptors, used for receptor purification, should allow isolation of a new type of recombinant opioid receptor. Such an opioid peptide—dalargin—was elaborated for that purpose.

Data concerning the existence of recombinant μ-δ receptor were presented in this research. It was shown that rMDOR shares the complex of μ- and δ-receptors' properties to bind agonists and antagonists, to have similar but lesser density compared to μ- and δ-receptors' densities in limbic structures of normal rat brain. The fragment of this receptor is coded by the unique cDNA insert of 1.2 kb and has molecular weight of 23 kDa. rMDOR belongs to hydrophobic lipoproteins formed by the membrane receptor family. The irreversible inhibition of evoked potential from single neuron by polyclonal antibodies raised against rMDOR demonstrated that the receptor may conduct the effect of opiates to attenuate the membrane excitability.[3] We also observed the withdrawal symptoms in rabbits followed 3-4 weeks of immunization by rMDOR to produce antibodies. Symptoms progressed and correlated to increased concentration of rMDOR antibodies in the animal's blood. This fact convinced us that the rMDOR may be a marker of dependence.

Experimental research involving the model of heroin self-administration showed high MDOR sensitivity to reveal autoantibodies in the blood of animals exposed to heroin. The fast accumulation of MDOR autoantibodies in the blood of rats coincided with increased striatum immunoreactivity indirectly reflected the increase of rMDOR gene expression, and followed stabilization in heroin acquisition. We supposed that MDOR autoantibodies may trace the tolerance to dependence transition. In spite of MOR and DOR peptides designed to correspond to similar positions in receptors as MDOR peptide has, they demonstrated distinct functions, detected autoantibodies in experimental rats later, and with somewhat lower sensitivity. Because μ- and δ-receptors drive the addictive effects of opiates,[7,39,40,42] it is highly possible that autoantibodies to them may mark the actual dependence on the molecular level when physiological symptoms have not yet appeared.

The laboratory test detecting MDOR autoantibodies in blood of opiate abusers and addicts demonstrated their correlation with severity of drug use, dependence degree, and type of drug (short- or long-acting). For short-acting opiate heroin, the correlation of MDOR autoantibodies with duration of drug exposure was found. The different profiles of autoantibodies accumulation were determined for those who used opium and heroin. This laboratory test showed high reliability (86%) in revealing opiate addicts. Moreover, we identified the risk group on dependence within occasional drug users and drug abusers when withdrawal symptoms did not yet appear. The early remission period in drug addicts followed a significant decrease of autoantibodies and improvement in emotional and physiological state. However, in the latter cases, concentrations of MDOR autoantibodies still remained higher than control levels of healthy volunteers, maintaining possibility for relapse.

Thus, results of experimental and clinical research supported our hypothesis that MDOR autoantibodies are the tracer of opiate neuroreceptors damage, and naturally existing recombinant μ-δ receptor is a biomarker of opiate abuse due to molecular alterations of gene expressions. The following research concerning rMDOR mRNA expression changes in experimental and human drug abuse studies would make it possible obtain the additional evidence.

ACKNOWLEDGMENTS

The animal research reported in this manuscript was conducted in accordance with the Guide for the Care and Use of Laboratory Animals as adopted and promulgated by the National Institutes of Health (NIH). The authors would like to thank Dr. S. Childers, Wake Forest University School of Medicine (Winston-Salem, NC), for kindly supplying us cell cultures, and Dr. E. Zvartau, St. Petersburg's Medical University (St. Petersburg, Russia), Drs. T. Martin and J. Smith, Wake Forest University School of Medicine, for help in part of the animal research. The authors appreciate Dr. Y. Poliakov, Clinic of the Institute of the Human Brain (St. Petersburg, Russia) and V. Vostrikov, Head of Narcology Clinic (Leningrad District, Russia) for assistance in part of the clinical research. The research of animal investigations was in part supported by the Fogarty Foundation, NIH.

REFERENCES

1. WILLIAMS, J.T., M.D.J. CHRISTIE & O.MANZONI. 2001. Cellular and synaptic adaptations mediating opioid dependence. Pharmacol. Rev. **81:** 299–343.
2. NESTLER, E.J. & D. LANDSMAN. 2001. Learning about addiction from the genome. Nature **409:** 834–835
3. TAYLOR, D.A. & W.W. FLEMING. 2001. Unifying perspectives of the mechanisms underlying the development of tolerance and physical dependence to opioids. J. Pharmacol. Exp. Ther. **297:**11–18.
4. WISE, R.A. 1998. Drug-activation of brain reward pathways. Drug Alcohol Depend. **51:** 13–22.
5. STEVENS, K.E., G.A. MICKLEY & L.J. McDERMOTT. 1986. Brain areas involved in production of morphine-induced locomotor hyperactivity of the C57B1/6J mouse. Pharmacol.Biochem. Behav. **24:** 1739–1747.
6. PORRECA, F. & T.F. BURKS. 1993. Supraspinal opioid receptors in antinociception. *In* Opioids II. Handbook of Experimental Pharmacology. A. Herz, Ed.: 21–52. Springer-Verlag. Berlin.
7. SANCHEZ-BLAZQUEZ, P., A. GARCIA-ESPANA & J.GARZON. 1997. Antisense oligodeoxynucleotides to opioid μ and δ receptors reduced morphine dependence in mice: role of δ-2 opioid receptors. J. Pharmacol. Exp. Ther. **280:**1423–1431.
8. MIYAMOTO, Y., P.S. PORTOGHESE & A.E. TAKEMORI. 1993. Involvement of delta-2 opioid receptors in the development of morphine dependence in mice. J. Pharmacol. Exp. Ther. **264:** 1141–1145.
9. VANDERAH, T.W., K.D. WILD, A.E. TAKEMORI, *et al.* 1993. Modulation of morphine antinociception by swim-stress in the mouse: involvement of supraspinal opioid delta-2 receptors. J. Pharmacol. Exp. Ther. **267:** 449–455.
10. DAMBINOVA, S.A. & G.A. IZYKENOVA, inventors. 1998. Japanese patent 2,782,695. Date of application: May 8, 1994.
11. DAMBINOVA, S.A. 1989. Neuroreceptors of Glutamate. 149 pp. Nauka. Leningrad [Russian].
12. PAK, Y., A. KOUVELAS, M.A. SCHEIDELER, *et al.* 1996. Agonist-induced functional desensitization of the mu-opioid receptor is mediated by loss of membrane receptors rather than uncoupling from G protein. Mol. Pharmacol. **50:** 1214–1222.
13. SHUSTER, S.J., M. RIEDL, X. LI, *et al.* 1999. Stimulus-dependent translocation of kappa opioid receptors to the plasma membrane. J. Neurosci. **19:** 2658–2664.
14. AKIL, H., C. OWENS, H. GUTSTEIN, *et al.* 1998. Endogenous opioids: overview and current issues. Drug Alcohol Depend. **51:** 127–140.
15. PASTERNAK, G.W. 2001. Insights into mu opioid pharmacology. The role of mu opioid receptor subtypes. Life Sci. **68:** 2213–2219.

16. ROTHMAN, R.B., J.A. DANKS, M. HERKENHAM, et al. 1985. Evidence that the δ-selective alkylating agent, FIT, alters the μ-noncompetitive opiate δ binding site. Neuropeptides **6:** 227–237.
17. GAVERIAUX-RUFF, C., J. PELUSO, K. BEFORT, et al. 1997. Detection of opioid receptor mRNA by RT-PCR reveals alternative splicing for the delta and kappa opioid receptors. Mol. Brain Res. **48:** 298–304.
18. PAN, Y.X., J. XU, E.A. BOLAN, et al. 2000. Isolation and expression of a novel alternatively spliced mu opioid receptor isoform, MOR-1F. FEBS Lett. **466:** 337–340.
19. MANSOUR, A., C.A. FOX, H. AKIL, et al. 1995. Opioid receptor mRNA expresion in the rat CNS: anatomical and functional implications. TINS **18:** 22–28.
20. SVINGOS, A.L., M. GARSON, E.E.O. COLAGO & V.M. PICKEL. 2001. Mu-opioid receptors in the ventral tegmental area are targeted to presynaptically and directly modulate mesocortical projection neurons. Synapse **41:** 221–229.
21. IZYKENOVA, G.A. & N.P. TARANOVA. 1992. Dalargin binding proteins of rat brain synaptic membranes: isolation, characterization, and comparison with opiate receptors. Biochemistry **57:** 663–670 [Russian].
22. IZYKENOVA, G.A. 1992. Opiate binding proteins of rat brain synaptic membranes: isolation and characterization. Ph.D. thesis, Russian Commonwealth University, Moscow.
23. IZYKENOVA, G.A. & S.A. DAMBINOVA. 1994. Dalargin binding proteins—components of the brain opioid receptors [abstr.]. J. Neurochem. **63:** S55B.
24. IZYKENOVA, G.A., V.V. SIRENKO & S.A. DAMBINOVA. 1995. Immunodiagnostics of drug addiction. Problemi Narcologii **1:** 45–49 [Russian].
25. PENCHEVA, N., C. IVANCHEVA, E. DIMITROV, et al. 1995. Dalargin and [Cys-(O₂NH₂)]² analogues of enkephalins and their selectivity for mu opioid receptors. Gen. Pharmacol. **26:** 799–808.
26. PENCHEVA, N., A. BOCHEVA, E. DIMITROV, et al. 1996. [Cys-(O₂NH₂)]² enkephalin analogues and dalargin: selectivity for delta-opioid receptors. Eur. J. Pharmacol. **304:** 99–108.
27. IZYKENOVA, G.A., Y.V. BOBRYSHEV & S.A. DAMBINOVA. 1993. Immunochemical localization of brain opiate receptors. Russian Biochem. Soc. Meeting (Abstr.) (Zvenigorod, Russia).: 17–18 [Russian]. Russian Biochemistry Society, Moscow.
28. TARANOVA, N.P., G.A. IZYKENOVA & N.L. IZVARINA. 1991. Characterization of opiate receptors isolated from synaptic membranes. Biol.Membr. **8:** 1170–1171 [Russian].
29. ROY, S., N.M. LEE & H.H. LOH. 1986. Mu-opioid receptor is associated with phosphatase activity. Biochem. Biophys. Res. Commun. **140:** 660–665.
30. WARR, G.W. 1982. Purifications of antibodies. In Antibody as a Tool. J.J. Marchalonis & G.W. Warr, Eds.: 59–96. John Wiley & Sons Ltd. London.
31. BREIVOGEL, C.S., D.E. SELLEY & S.R. CHILDERS. 1997. Acute and chronic effects of opioids on delta and mu receptor activation of G-proteins in NG108-15 and SK-N-SH cell membranes. J. Neurochem. **68:** 1462–1472.
32. SELLEY, D.E., Q.LIU & S.R.CHILDERS. 1998. Signal transduction correlates of mu opioid agonist intrinsic efficacy: receptor-stimulated [³⁵S]GTPγS binding in mMOR-CHO cells and rat thalamus. J. Pharmacol. Exp. Ther. **285:** 496–505.
33. IZYKENOVA, G.A., J.E. SMITH & S.A. DAMBINOVA. 1997. Development of new rapid and sensitive tests for diagnosis and treatment control of drug abuse and for screening drugs in peripheral fluids. CPDD Ann. Meeting, Nashville, TN.: 32.
34. IZYKENOVA, G.A. & S.A. DAMBINOVA. 1998. The role of mu-delta opiate neuroreceptors in diagnostics of drug abuse [abstr.]. J. Neurochem. **71:** S30D.
35. WINNACKER, E.L. 1987. From Genes to Clones: Introduction to Gene Technology. John Wiley & Sons Ltd. London. 635 pp.
36. HOPP, T.P. & K.R. WOODS.1981. Prediction of protein antigenic determinants from amino acid sequences. Proc.Natl. Acad. Sci. USA **6:** 3824–3828.
37. WELLING, G.W., W.J. WEIJER, R. VAN DER ZEE & S.WELLING-WESTER. 1985. Prediction of sequential antigenic region in proteins. FEBS Lett. **188:** 215–218.
38. CAMPBELL, U.C. & M.E. CARROLL. 2000. Acquisition of drug self-administration: environmental and pharmacological interventions. Exp. Clin. Psychopharmacol. **8:** 312–325.

39. MARTIN, T.J., M.G. DE MONTIS, S.A. KIM, *et al.* 1998. Effect of beta-funaltrexamine on dose-effect curves for heroin self-administration in rats: comparison with alteration of ^{3}[H]DAMGO binding to rat brain sections. Drug Alcohol Depend. **52:** 135–147.
40. SORA, I., G. ELMER, M. FUNADA, *et al.* 2001. Mu opiate receptor gene dose effects on different morphine actions: evidence for differential *in vivo* mu receptor reserve. Neuropsychopharmacol. **25:** 41–54.
41. GANT, T.M., P. RIBA & N.M. LEE. 2001. Morphine tolerance in mice is independent of polymorphisms in opioid receptor sequences. Brain Res. Bull. **55:** 59–63.
42. MARTIN, T.J., S.A. KIM, D.G. CANNON, *et al.* 2000. Antagonism of delta (2)-opioid recepors by naltrindole-5′-isothiocyanate attenuates heroin self-administration but not antinociception in rats. J. Pharmacol. Exp. Ther. **294:** 975–982.
43. NGO, T.T. & H.M. LENOFF. 1980. A sensitive and versatile chromatographic assay for peroxidase and peroxidase-coupled reaction. Anal. Biochem. **105:** 389–397.
44. IZYKENOVA, G.A. & J.E. SMITH. 2000. Identification of autoantibodies to peptide candidate for opiate receptors in peripheral fluids and brain. CPDD Meeting, San Juan, Puerto Rico.: 72
45. PATTERSON, S., N. MCLACHLAN-TROUP, R. CORDERO, *et al.* 2001. Qualitative screening for drugs of abuse in hair using GC-MC. J. Anal. Toxicol. **25:** 203–208.
46. KELLER, T., A. SCHNEIDER, R. DIRBHOFER, *et al.* 2000. Fluorescence polarization immunoassay for the detection of drugs of abuse in human whole blood. Med. Sci. Law **40:** 258–262.
47. SPECK, I.M., J. HALLABACH, W.G. GUDER, *et al.* 1999. Opiate detection in saliva and urine—a prospective comparison by gas chromatography-mass spectrometry. J. Toxicol. **37:** 441–445.
48. MOODY, D.E. & M.L. CHEEVER. 2001. Evaluation of immunoassays for semiquantitative detection of cocaine and metabolites or heroin and metabolites in extracts of sweat patches. J. Anal. Toxicol. **25:**190–197.
49. CASAS, M., J. GUARDIA, G. PRAT & J. TRUJOLS. 1995. The apomorphine test in heroin addicts. Addiction **90:** 831–835.
50. GHODSE, A.H., J.L. GREAVES & D. LYNCH. 1999. Evaluation of the opioid addiction test in an out-patient drug dependency unit. Br. J. Psychiatry **175:** 158–162.
51. DSM-IV-TR. 2000. Diagnostic and statistical manual of mental disorders. Fourth edit., text revision. Washington, DC, American Psychiatric Association.: 191–283.
52. Behind Bars: Substance Abuse and America's Prison Population. 1998. National Center for Addiction and Substance Abuse at Columbia University. New York.
53. PJATNIZKAYA, I.N. 1998. Addictions. 544 pp. Meditzina [Russian]. Moscow.
54. WEISNER, C.M. & L. SCHMIDT. 1993. Alcohol and drug problems among diverse health and social service populations. Am. J. Public Health **83:** 824–829.

Neonatal Exposure to Cocaine

Altered Dopamine Levels in the Amygdala and Behavioral Outcomes in the Developing Rat

TERESA SUMMAVIELLE,[a,b] ANA MAGALHÃES,[a,b] IVONE CASTRO-VALE,[a,c] LILIANA DE SOUSA,[a,b] AND MARIA AMÉLIA TAVARES[a,c]

[a]*Institute of Molecular and Cell Biology (IBMC), University of Porto, Portugal*

[b]*Institute of Biomedical Sciences Abel Salazar, University of Porto, Portugal*

[c]*Institute of Anatomy, Medical School of University of Porto, Portugal*

ABSTRACT: The amygdala is a brain region that is known to be implicated in the development of behavioral sensitization to cocaine. This area is often related to conditioned associations, stress responses, and anxiety; and these behaviors are usually posited to be due to altered dopamine levels. This study aimed to evaluate the effects of neonatal exposure to cocaine on the levels of neurotransmitters in the amygdala of developing rats and to relate these levels with open-field observations, mainly rearing behavior, that is regarded to reflect emotional components. Male and female Wistar rats were given 15 mg of cocaine hydrochloride/kg body weight, subcutaneously, in two daily doses, from postnatal day 1 (PND1) to PND30. Controls were given 0.9% saline. Open-field activity was registered on PND14, 21, and 30 in three sessions of 15 min each. In PND30, rats were decapitated, and the amygdala dissected from both brain hemispheres and processed for determination of dopamine (DA) and metabolites by high-performance liquid chromatography with electrochemical detection (HPLC-EC). Results show that in PND14 and 21 all registered activity behaviors were increased in male and female cocaine-exposed animals. In PND30, there was a significant decrease in rearing and in global activity in the group exposed to cocaine, and DA levels were significantly decreased in the amygdala of the same group. No differences were found between the left and right amygdala. These results suggest that chronic neonatal cocaine administration leads to depletion of DA levels in the amygdala, which is consistent with previous findings. Furthermore, the lower levels of DA are associated with decreased rearing behavior, which may indicate emotional depression. These results can help to clarify the role of amygdala in cocaine-induced behavioral sensitization in the developing rat.

KEYWORDS: cocaine; neonatal; dopamine; amygdala; rat; development; behavior; open-field activity; rearing; chronic exposure

Address for correspondence: Teresa Summavielle, Neurobehavior Unit, IBMC, Rua do Campo Alegre 823, 4150-180 Porto, Portugal. Voice: 351226074945; fax: 351226099157. tsummavi@ibmc.up.pt

Ann. N.Y. Acad. Sci. 965: 515–521 (2002). © 2002 New York Academy of Sciences.

INTRODUCTION

The amygdala is a limbic structure that integrates positive and aversive emotional information mediating behavioral reactions.[1] Several studies point to the essential role of the amygdala in the acquisition of both emotional and motor-conditioned responses.[2,3] Establishment and eventual storage of long-term emotionally conditioned memories are probably associated with the amygdala's role in connecting environmental events to reinforcing stimuli.[4] The amygdala participates in the conditioning of autonomic fear responses through its projections to the hypothalamus, which in turn projects to brainstem areas and spinal premotor neurons of the autonomic nervous system;[5,6] thus, another hypothesis concerning the role of the amygdala is that it can exert a modulatory influence on memory processes occurring in other brain regions.[7,8] Large amygdala lesions have been found to reduce open-field activity, a behavior that may be seen as indicative of reduced fear.[9]

The involvement of the amygdala in the processes underlying addictive behavior seems to be quite specific, as this structure appears to be involved in cue-controlled cocaine-seeking behavior, reinstatement of cocaine self-administration, and conditioned reinforcement.[10] Conditioned associations, stress responses, and anxiety behaviors are usually related to altered dopamine (DA) levels.[4] One technique for assessment of the functional maturation of the neurotransmitter systems is to examine the ontogenetic pattern of behavioral effects induced by psychoactive drugs; relating information from behavioral approaches to that obtained from neurochemical and neuroanatomical studies can be very useful in elucidating developmental processes.[11]

This study aimed at evaluating the effects in the amygdala of neonatal exposure to cocaine in the developing rat by assessing the concentrations of DA and its metabolites and relating these to open-field behavioral observations, essentially rearing behavior (regarded to reflect emotional components[12]) and global activity.

MATERIALS AND METHODS

Animal Model

Rats used in this study were male offspring born from nulliparous Wistar females purchased from the Colony of the Gulbenkian Institute of Science, Oeiras, Portugal. They were bred at the Institute of Molecular and Cell Biology, University of Porto. Institutional guidelines regarding animal experimentation were followed. At the onset of breeding, females were placed with males from 8:00 P.M. to 8:00 A.M. Pregnant females had *ad libitum* access to food and water. All litters were standardized to eight pups (4 males and 4 females). Rats in the cocaine (CO) group were given subcutaneous injections of cocaine hydrochloride (Sigma Chemical Co., St. Louis, MO) in a daily dose of 15 mg/kg body weight in 0.9% saline from the day after birth (postnatal day 1 or PND1) to PND30. Each daily dose was divided into two equal parts, given at 8:30 to 9:00 A.M. and 6:00 to 8:00 P.M. Controls (C) received saline (0.9%), subcutaneously, with the same experimental protocol.

Neurotransmitter Determinations

Rats obtained from different litters were decapitated on PND30, and the amygdala dissected (according to the atlas by Palkovits and Brownstein[13]) from both brain hemispheres. The right and left amygdala were frozen and stored at −80°C until used for determinations. Concentrations of DA, 3,4-dihydroxyphenylacetic acid (DOPAC), and homovanillic acid (HVA) were quantified by a modified method[14] of high-performance liquid chromatography with electrochemical detection (HPLC/EC) in a Gilson Medical Electronics system (Pump 307, Electrochemical Detector 142, Autoinjector 234, and 712 HPLC Controller Software version 1.30). Dissected amygdala were weighed and diluted in 300 µl of 0.2 N perchloric acid. Tissue was disrupted and centrifuged (15,000 g; 7 min), supernatant was filtered through Costar microcentrifuge filter (0.2 µm), and 50 µl were injected onto the HPLC/EC system for separation of DA and metabolites. The ratio of the DA metabolites (DOPAC + HVA) to DA was determined for each animal and used as an index of dopamine turnover rates.

Behavioral Determinations

Open-field activity was registered in 20 males and 20 females per experimental group, on PND14, 21, and 30, in three sessions of 15 min each. The open-field test took place 5 hours after the first daily injection and was performed in a Cromotrack apparatus from San Diego Instruments. The following parameters were determined: rearing behavior and center and peripheral activity. The sum of all these behaviors was considered as global activity. The open-field arena was thoroughly cleaned before each test, and a period of two minutes was provided for adaptation before starting the counts.

Data Analysis

Differences in rearing behavior were analyzed by Student's *t* test, and a two-way ANOVA (within-subjects design) was used to determine differences in global activity results among control and cocaine-treated rats for global activity results. Monoamine data were assessed by a two-way MANOVA, and when statistical differences were detected, multiple comparisons were made using the Scheffé test. All statistics were carried out at the significance level of 5%, using the software Statistica 5.5A (StatSoft Inc., 1995).

RESULTS

Cocaine exposure induced an initial increase in global activity in PND14 and in PND21 when compared to the saline-control group, whereas in PND30 a decrease in global activity was registered for the cocaine-exposed group (FIG. 1), these differences being statistically significant over the three tested ages ($F(2,156) = 11.32$; $p < 0.0001$). There were no significant differences due to gender in global activity. Simultaneously, in PND30 it was possible to observe a significant ($t(78) = 2.37$; $p < 0.05$) decrease in the rearing behavior (FIG. 2) in the cocaine-exposed group when compared to the control group.

TABLE 1. Concentrations of dopamine and DOPAC and DOPAC/dopamine ratio in the amygdala of PND30 cocaine-exposed rats and respective controls

Group	Gender	Dopamine	DOPAC	DOPAC/dopamine
Control	Female ($n = 4$)	38.2 (3.3)[a]	17.0 (0.6)	0.45 (0.03)[c]
	Male ($n = 10$)	34.4 (2.4)[b]	17.1 (0.5)	0.51 (0.02)
Cocaine	Female ($n = 12$)	24.8 (1.4)[a]	17.0 (0.6)	0.70 (0.03)[c]
	Male ($n = 7$)	25.3 (2.0)[b]	15.3 (0.5)	0.62 (0.03)

NOTE: Values represent mean (SEM) expressed as ng/100 mg wet weight of tissue. Values in the same column with the same letter are significantly different: [a]($p < 0.01$); [b]($p < 0.05$); and [c]($p < 0.005$).

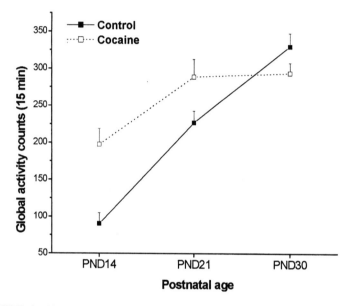

FIGURE 1. Global activity in the open field in PND14, 21, and 30 rats. Values represent means plus SEM of three consecutive daily sessions expressed in counts per 15 min. Rats were neonatally exposed to cocaine (15 mg/kg per day) or to saline (control). The cocaine-exposed group significantly differs from controls in all tested ages ($F(2,156) = 11.32$; $p < 0.0001$).

Concomitantly with the decrease in global activity and rearing behavior, DA concentration (TABLE 1) was significantly lower on PND30 for both females ($t(16) = -3.15$; $p < 0.01$) and males ($t(15) = 2.39$; $p < 0.05$) neonatally exposed to cocaine, whereas for DOPAC no differences were found. HVA was only detected in a reduced number of samples (10 out of 34), and therefore results could not be presented. No differences in catecholaminergic contents were found due to hemisphere laterality of amygdala.

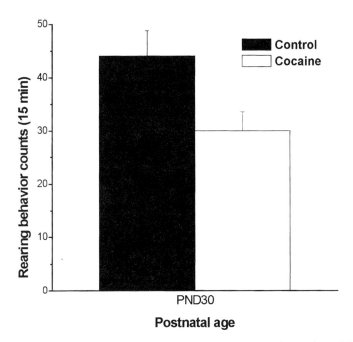

FIGURE 2. Rearing behavior in the open field, measured as the number of times the animals reared on their hind legs in a 15-min period. Values represent means plus SEM of counts obtained in the first daily session. Results for the cocaine-exposed group are significantly different from controls ($t(78) = 2.37; p < 0.05$).

DISCUSSION

The rat behavioral response to novelty is typically characterized, not only from horizontal locomotion, but also mostly from vertical activation, that is, from rearing behavior. This type of response is considered to reflect not merely exploratory activity, but also emotionality.[12] In previous studies, patterns of high rearing behavior in a novel open field were related to higher levels of DA.[12]

The amygdala has a rich distribution of D_2-type DA receptors that are potentially blocked in the presence of cocaine, inhibiting DA neural activity.[15] Chronic exposure to cocaine during the neonatal period is likely to disrupt the normal development of the central nervous system, and therefore to alter catecholaminergic neurotransmission. In this study, results show that chronic neonatal cocaine administration increased global activity in PND14 and 21 compared with the saline group. Nevertheless, in PND30 a significant decrease in global activity could be observed, as well as a significant decrease in rearing behavior in the first session of open field, which represents a stressful and fear-inducing situation. These decreases in global activity and rearing were consistent with the depletion of DA content in amygdala that was also observed at the same postnatal age (PND30). These patterns of behavior were observed for both male and female rats, and differences due to gender were not detected. Our results are in accordance with previous reports that associated inhibition of DA neural activity with a reduction in emotional conditioned and fear responses.[4,16,17] Moreover, the fact that the initial increase in activity is later replaced by a state of decreased activity is coherent with the generally accepted mechanism for long-term feedback regulation of DA in chronic cocaine exposure (for review, see Hammer[18]). Determining the concentrations of DA and its metabolites in PND14 and 21 rats neonatally exposed to cocaine would be useful to further complete this study.

Taken together, these findings provide evidence of a state of possible emotional depression (in PND30 rats) that could be an outcome of the neonatal exposure to cocaine and that could be helpful in clarifying the role of amygdala in cocaine-induced behavioral sensitization.

CONCLUSIONS

Neonatal cocaine exposure induced a decrease in global activity and in rearing behavior in PND30 rats. At the same postnatal age, DA concentration in the amygdala was lower in the same group, evidencing a possible state of depression for these animals. Taking these findings together, chronic neonatal cocaine exposure seems to effectively lead to neurochemical changes in the amygdala, resulting in altered associated behaviors.

ACKNOWLEDGMENTS

This work was supported by Project PRAXIS PSAU/C/SAU/8/96 and Programa de Financiamento Plurianual (IBMC). Teresa Summavielle received the grant from PRAXIS BD/14742/97 and Ana Magalhães received the grant from PRAXIS/BD/20075/99.

REFERENCES

1. BEGGS, M.J. et al. 1999. Learning and Memory: Basic Mechanisms. In Fundamental Neuroscience. Michael J. Zigmond, et al., Eds.: 1411–1455. Academic Press. San Diego, CA.
2. MINTZ, M. & Y. WANG-NINIO. 2001. Two-stage theory of conditioning: involvement of the cerebellum and the amygdala. Brain Res. **897:** 150–156.
3. LeDoux, J. 2000. The amygdala and emotion a view through fear. In The Amygdala. John P. Aggleton, Ed.: 289–310. Oxford University Press. Oxford.
4. GREBA, Q., A. GIFKINS & L. KOKKINIDIS. 2001. Inhibition of amygdaloid dopamine D2 receptors impairs emotional learning measured with fear-potentiated startle. Brain Res. **899:** 218–226.
5. ANTONIADIS, E.A. & R.J. McDONALD. 2001. Amygdala, hippocampus, and unconditioned fear. Exp. Brain Res. **138:** 200–209.
6. McGAUGH, J.L., B. FERRY, A. VAZDARJANOVA & B. ROOZENDAAL. 2000. Amygdala: role in modulation of memory storage. In The Amygdala. John P. Aggleton, Ed.: 391–424. Oxford University Press. Oxford.
7. PACKARD, M.G. & L.A. TEATHER. 1998. Amygdala modulation of multiple memory systems: Hippocampus and caudate-putamen. Neurobiol. Learn. Mem. **69:** 163–203.

8. DAVIS, M. 2000. The role of amygdala in conditioned and unconditioned fear and anxiety. *In* The Amygdala. John P. Aggleton, Ed.: 213–288. Oxford University Press. Oxford.
9. GROSSMAN, S.P., L. GROSSMAN & L. WALSH. 1975. Functional organization of the rat amygdala with respect to avoidance behavior. J. Comp. Physiol. Psychol. **88:** 829–850.
10. EVERITT, B.J. *et al.* 2000. Differential involvement of amygdala subsystems in appetitive conditioning and drug addiction. *In* The Amygdala. John P. Aggleton, Ed.: 353–390. Oxford University Press. Oxford.
11. SPEAR, L.P. & J. BRICK. 1979. Cocaine-induced behavior in the developing rat. Behav. Neural. Biol. **26:** 401–415.
12. THIEL, C.M., C.P. MULLER, J.P. HUSTON & R.K.W. SCHWARTING. 1999. High versus low reactivity to a novel environment: behavioral, pharmacological and neurochemical assessments. Neuroscience **93:** 243–251.
13. PALKOVITS, M. & M.J. BROWNSTEIN. 1988. Maps and Guide to Microdissection of the Rat Brain. Elsevier. New York. p. 223.
14. ALI, S.F., S.N. DAVID & G.D. NEWPORT. 1993. Age-related susceptibility of MPTP-induced neurotoxicity in mice. Neurotoxicology **14:** 29–34.
15. SEIDLER, F.J., S.W. TEMPLE, E.C. MCCOOK & T.A. SLOTKIN. 1995. Cocaine inhibits central noradrenergic and dopaminergic activity during the critical development period in which catecholamines influence cell development. Dev. Brain Res. **85:** 48–53.
16. MUNRO, L.J. & L. KOKKINIDIS. 1997. Infusion of quinpirole and muscimol into the ventral tegmental area inhibits fear-potentiated startle: implications for the role of dopamine in fear expression. Brain Res.**746:** 231–238.
17. NADER, K. & J.E. LEDOUX. 1999. Inhibition of the mesoamygdala dopaminergic pathway impairs the retrieval of conditioned fear associations. Behav. Neurosci. **113:** 891–901.
18. HAMMER, R.P. The Neurobiology of Cocaine: Cellular and Molecular Mechanisms: 272. CRC Press. Boca Raton, FL.

Structural and Functional Cellular Alterations Underlying the Toxicity of Methamphetamine in Rat Retina and Prefrontal Cortex

CRISTINA PRUDÊNCIO,[a] BRUNO ABRANTES,[a] ISABEL LOPES,[b] AND MARIA AMÉLIA TAVARES[a,b]

[a]Instituto de Investigação em Ciências da Vida e da Saúde, Escola de Ciências da Saúde, Universidade do Minho, Braga, Portugal

[b]Instituto de Anatomia, Faculdade de Medicina da Universidade do Porto, Portugal

ABSTRACT: The consumption of illicit drugs is an increasing problem in contemporary societies, and is one of the major causes of death and illness all over the world. Methamphetamine is among the drugs more widely used. Although evidence for a role of reactive species—especially reactive oxygen species (ROS) and apoptotic events—has been shown, the mechanism(s) underlying the cellular toxicity induced by this drug is not yet fully identified. In this context the elucidation of the cytotoxic effects induced by methamphetamine in rat frontal cortex and retina, which compromise cell viability and ultimately result in cell death, can further contribute to the understanding of its mechanism of action. This knowledge may provide new insights into the development of new therapeutic approaches to prevent or ameliorate deleterious alterations of the nervous system. The use of epifluorescence microscopy associated with different fluorescent probes, markers of structural and/or functional cell parameters, can be used as a powerful tool to carry out those studies, in particular, the viability probes propidium iodide (PI) to assess plasma membrane integrity and fluorescein diacetate (FDA), which can monitor intracellular esterase activity and/or pH. In a preliminary study, the kinetic assessment of cellular changes induced by different drug concentrations (0, 1.2, 3, and 6 mM) allowed detection of dose-dependent alterations that are observed earlier in the retina. In fact, in the retina it was possible to monitor alterations (at 4 h of incubation) both in plasma membrane integrity and in esterase activity and/or pH for the lowest drug concentration (1.2 mM). In the prefrontal cortex these changes were only visible for drug concentrations ≥3 mM. This work is a novel approach to the mechanisms of action of illicit drugs in the central nervous system and will provide the foundations and guidelines for further investigations in the context of tolerance, dependence, and addiction.

KEYWORDS: methamphetamine; neurotoxicity; retina; prefrontal cortex; mechanism of action

Address for correspondence: Maria Amélia Tavares, Instituto de Anatomia, Faculdade de Medicina do Porto, Alameda Hernâni Monteiro 4200-319, Porto, Portugal. Voice: 351225096808; fax: 351225505640.
anatclin@med.up.pt

Ann. N.Y. Acad. Sci. 965: 522–528 (2002). © 2002 New York Academy of Sciences.

INTRODUCTION

Methamphetamine is an illicit drug that is abused all over the world. Its effects upon the central nervous system (CNS) have been extensively studied both in developing and adult animals.[1,2] An important insight into these effects has been provided using morphometric and neurochemical determinations in a well-controlled animal model.[3,4] However, the mechanisms underlying these effects were not assessed on previous investigations. Methamphetamine neurotoxicity includes dopamine and serotonin depletion as well as their metabolites and uptake sites, a decrease in tyrosine hydroxylase and tryptophan hydroxylase activities, a depolarization of mitochondria, and a slight decrease in ATP production.[5] Moreover, subchronic methamphetamine exposure results in the induction of oscillations in intracellular calcium concentration of ventral tegmental area dopamine neurons, which might be related to psychostimulant effects, such as dependence on the sensitization to methamphetamine.[6] The mechanism(s) underlying the cellular toxicity induced by methamphetamine seems to include induction of reactive oxygen species (ROS) and some apoptotic events, but the general mechanism is not yet fully identified.[7–15] Moreover, little is known about the mechanisms underlying the effects of drugs of abuse on developing neural circuitry.[7]

In the present work we present a preliminary study that aims to contribute to the elucidation of the cytotoxic effects induced by methamphetamine in the rat CNS, and possibly to further contribute to the understanding of its mechanism of action. The technique used was double staining with the fluorescent probes fluorescein diacetate (FDA) and propidium iodide (PI), markers of structural and/or functional cell parameters,[16,17] in association with epifluorescence microscopy.

In further studies we aim to compare the response obtained in development and in fully mature nervous systems in order to further elucidate the effects on different vulnerable periods of the neural circuitry.

MATERIAL AND METHODS

Tissue Samples and Methamphetamine Treatment

After decapitation of adult Wistar rats the retina and the prefrontal cortex were dissected and transferred to Eppendorf tubes. The cells were washed (500 µL) with solution 1 (KCl, 40 mg; NaCl, 680 mg; $NaH_2PO_4.2H_2O$, 1.5 mg; D-glucose, 350 mg; phenol red, 1.0 mg; $MgSO_4$ (anhydrous), 1.81 mg; BSA, 300 mg; $NaHCO_3$, 200 mg in 100 mL distilled water), and trypsinized (trypsin, 1 mg in 10 mL solution 1) for 10 min at 37°C. Following this treatment the cells were centrifuged and resuspended (500 µL) in the presence of the trypsin inhibitor (trypsin inhibitor soybean, 5.0 mg; $MgSO_4$ (anhydrous), 1.42 mg in 7.5 mL solution 1), and subjected to gentle mechanical trituration. The cells were then passed through a Pasteur pipette followed by a micropipette tip and finally centrifuged (800 rpm, 5 min at 4°C) and resuspended in 1 mL of solution 1. The cellular concentration was determined using a Neubauer chamber and when necessary was corrected to 2×10^6 cell/mL. In order to incubate the cells with methamphetamine (0, 1.2, 3, and 6 mM final concentration), four Eppendorf tubes with 250 µL of cell suspension were prepared. For each drug concentration and at each time of drug incubation (0, 4, 8, 24, and 48 h) the cells were collected (40 µL), centrifuged (800 rpm, 5 min at 4°C), and resuspended in PBS (10 µL) for the staining protocol described below.

Staining Protocol

A fluorescein diacetate (FDA) working solution (0.0125 µg/mL) was prepared daily from a stock solution by dilution in PBS (0.1 M, pH 7.0). The FDA stock solution was prepared in DMSO (5 µg/mL) and kept at –20°C. The working solution (0.3 µg/mL) of propidium iodide (PI) was prepared from a stock solution (50 µg/mL) also by diluting in PBS. Both working solutions were kept in ice and in the dark until use.

For the staining protocol, 10 µL of working solution of FDA and 10 µL of working solution of PI were added to 10 µL of cell suspension and incubated for 10 min at room temperature in the dark. FDA is a hydrophobic, nonpolar and nonfluorescent compound that is able to cross the plasma membrane (FIG. 1A), is hydrolyzed to acetate and fluorescein by nonspecific esterases in the cytoplasm. The cell will present a green fluorescence if the plasma membrane remains intact and fluorescein is retained. Fluorescein fluorescence is also pH dependent; it is higher with higher pH. On the other hand, PI is hydrophilic and only cells with a compromised plasma membrane (FIG. 1B) are able to stain red. Therefore viable, nonaltered cells were

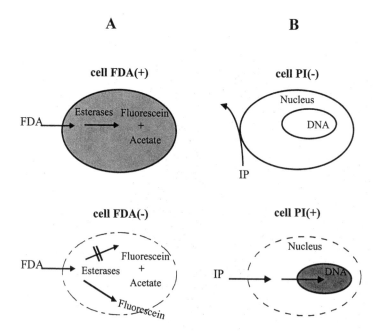

FIGURE 1. Staining mechanism of **A,** fluorescein diacetate (FDA); of **B,** propidium iodide (PI). Nonaltered cells were designated as FDA+ and PI– and stained green; altered cells were designated FDA– and PI+ and stained red.

designated as FDA+ and PI– and stained green; on the other hand, altered cells (death or dying) were designated FDA– and PI+ and stained red.

The cells were then counted in an epifluorescence microscope under simultaneous white light transmitted and blue light epi-illumination with a total magnification of 400×. Preparations were observed with a Zeiss Axioskop HBO 100 fluorescence microscope and digital images collected through a SPOT 2 camera. For each sample, in a total of 200 cells, the number of cells was counted (%) discriminating between the ones that stained red, green, or did not stain.

RESULTS

Rat cells either from the retina or from the prefrontal cortex injured by the presence of methamphetamine (1.2, 3, and 6 mM) were studied by epifluorescence microscopy using the staining procedures previously optimized.[16] As expected, with FDA and PI double staining, there was a progressive decrease in the percentage of cells exhibiting green fluorescence and a progressive increase in the percentage of cells exhibiting red fluorescence (FIG. 2). These results suggested an increase in the number of altered cells with the incubation time in the presence of the drug. The kinetic assessment of cellular changes induced by different drug concentrations (0, 1.2, 3, and 6 mM) allowed detection of dose-dependent alterations that were observed earlier in retina (FIG. 2C and 2D). In fact, in the retina it was possible to mon-

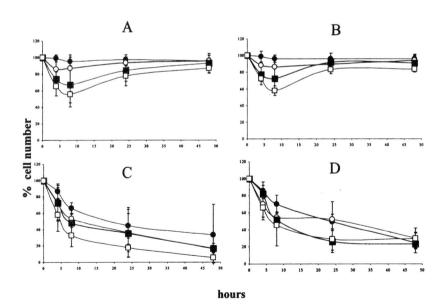

FIGURE 2. Relative number (% in order to time 0) of FDA+ (**A** and **C**) and PI– (**B** and **D**) prefrontal cortex (**A** and **B**) or retina (**C** and **D**) cells after incubation in the absence (*solid circles*) and in the presence of 1.2 (*open circles*), 3 (*solid squares*), and 6 (*open squares*) mM of methamphetamine.

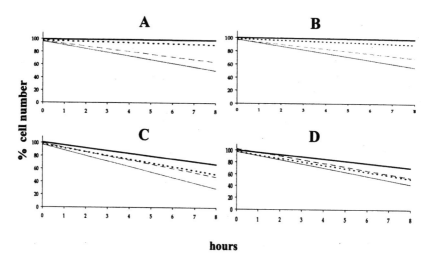

FIGURE 3. Linear plots for the first 8 h of drug incubation obtained from the curves presented in FIGURE 2. FDA+ (**A** and **C**) and PI– (**B** and **D**) prefrontal cortex (**A** and **B**) or retina (**C** and **D**) cells after incubation in the absence (—) and in the presence of 1.2 (· · ·), 3 (– – –), and 6 (—) mM of methamphetamine.

itor alterations (at 4 h of incubation) both in plasma membrane integrity and in esterase activity and/or intracellular pH for the lowest drug concentration (1.2 mM), whereas in the prefrontal cortex these changes were only visible for drug concentrations equal to or higher than 3 mM (FIG. 2A and 2B). For retina cell suspensions a decrease in nonaltered cells was observed along time even in the absence of the drug. Nevertheless, this effect was higher for higher drug concentrations indicating a dose-effect relationship. The prefrontal cortex cell suspensions exhibited a peculiar behavior. In fact, after a decrease in nonaltered cells for the first 8 h of incubation, a recovery was found in the percentage of nonaltered cells to values similar to that observed in the control. This was more accentuated in the higher concentrations of methamphetamine. In all the cases the percentage of FDA+ cells and PI– cells was very similar.

In order to elucidate the kinetics of the cellular changes induced by the drug, linear plots for the first 8 h of drug incubation were displayed (FIG. 3). These plots yielded a straight line of negative slope, which was designated as alteration constant (k_a). Both in the retina and the prefrontal cortex cells, the absolute values of k_a increased with methamphetamine concentration (TABLE 1), indicating a higher toxicity induced by the higher drug concentrations. The highest values of the ratio k_{aX}/k_{a0} (between the values of k_a for the different methamphetamine concentrations and those obtained for the control) presented for prefrontal cortex suggested a higher susceptibility to methamphetamine exhibited by this tissue when compared with retina. Consistently, as with the values obtained for the percentage of FDA+ cells and PI–, the values of k_a obtained with FDA and PI were also very similar.

TABLE 1. Values of the alteration constant (k_a) obtained (as slope) from the linear plots presented in FIGURE 3

MeTH (mM)	Cortex				Retina			
	FDA stained cells		PI stained cells		FDA stained cells		PI stained cells	
	k_a (h^{-1})	*k_{aX}/k_{a0}	k_a (h^{-1})	*k_{aX}/k_{a0}	k_a (h^{-1})	*k_{aX}/k_{a0}	k_a (h^{-1})	*k_{aX}/k_{a0}
0	−1.5	1.0	−0.85	1.0	−3.86	1.0	−3.34	1.0
1.2	−0.75	0.7	−1.06	1.2	−5.83	1.5	−5.71	1.7
3	−4.09	3.6	−3.47	4.1	−6.46	1.7	−6.04	1.8
6	−5.56	4.8	−5.25	6.2	−8.42	2.2	−6.83	2.0

*k_{aX}/k_{a0} is the ratio between the values of the alteration constant (k_a) for the different methamphetamine (MeTH) concentraions (k_{aX}) and those obtained for the control (k_{a0}).

DISCUSSION

This preliminary study allowed the detection of dose-dependent cellular changes induced by different methamphetamine concentrations both in the retina and the prefrontal cortex cells. These changes were observed earlier (at 4 h of incubation) in the retina and for a lower drug concentration (1.2 mM). Taking into account the mechanisms underlying the staining of the two probes[18–20] used in the kinetic approach and that the results were very similar with both, the results suggest that both probes are measuring plasma membrane integrity.[21,22] In fact, in retina cells at drug concentrations higher than 1.2 mM and in the prefrontal cortex cells at drug concentrations higher than 3 mM, the plasma membrane seems to have already lost its integrity, and at that state the leakage of FDA could be related to PI permeability. The observed decrease in nonaltered cells in retina cells incubated in the absence of the drug can be due to the tissue susceptibility to the experimental procedure, namely, enzymatic and mechanical treatment, necessary to obtain the cell suspension. In the prefrontal cortex, although detected for higher drug concentrations, the cellular alterations seem to be more severe than those observed for the retina. These results point to the prefrontal cortex as more susceptible to methamphetamine than the retina. In what concerns the peculiar behavior displayed by the prefrontal cortex cell suspensions, the recovery in the percentage of nonaltered cells might be related to the potentialities of drug tolerance exhibited in this brain area.

In conclusion, the use of epifluorescence microscopy as well as the use of different fluorescent probes constitutes a powerful analytical tool for the elucidation of mechanisms underlying the cytotoxic drug effects. In fact, depending on the probe (and on its mechanism of staining) this procedure allow the detection of early or late changes in the functional status of the cell and thus the order of appearance of cellular events associated with loss of cell viability induced by a lethal agent. In this context, we intend to extend this study to other probes in further studies.

REFERENCES

1. GOMES DA SILVA, J., M.C. SILVA & M.A. TAVARES. 1998. Developmental exposure to methamphetamine: a neonatal model in the rat. Ann. N.Y. Acad. Sci. **844:** 310–313.
2. GOMES-DA-SILVA, J. *et al.* 2000. Neonatal methamphetamine in the rat. Evidence for gender-specific differences upon tyrosine hydroxylase in the dopaminergic nigrostriatal system. Ann. N.Y. Acad. Sci. **914:** 431–438.
3. SILVA-ARAÚJO, A. *et al.* 1995. Effects of prenatal cocaine exposure in the photoreceptor cells of the rat retina. Mol. Neurobiol. **11:** 77–86.
4. TAVARES, M.A., M.C. SILVA, A. SILVA-ARAÚJO & M.R. XAVIER. 1996. Effects of prenatal exposure to ampmhetamine in the prefrontal cortex of the rat. An evaluation of growth, morphometric and neurochemical parameters. Int. J. Dev. Neurosci. **14:** 585–586.
5. LAU, J.W., S. SENOK & A. STADLIN. 2000. Methamphetamine-induced oxidative stress in cultured mouse astrocytes. Ann. N.Y. Acad. Sci. **914:** 146–156.
6. URAMURA, K., T. YADA, S. MUROYA & M. TAKIGAWA. 2000. Ca^{2+} oscillations in response to methamphetamine in dopamine neurons of the ventral tegmental area in rats subchronically treated with this drug. Ann. N.Y. Acad. Sci. **914:** 316–322.
7. FROST, D.O. & J.L. CADET. 2000. Effects of methamphetamine-induced neurotoxicity on the development of neural circuitry: a hypothesis. Brain Res. Rev. **34:**103–118.
8. CADET, J.L. & C. BRANNOCK. 1998. Free radicals and the pathobiology of brain dopamine systems. Neurochem. Int. **32:** 117–131.
9. CADET, J.L., S.V. ORDONEZ & J.V. ORDONEZ. 1997. Methamphetamine induces apoptosis in immortalized neural cells: protection by the proto-oncogene *bcl2*. Synapse **25:** 176–184.
10. HIRATA, H. & J.L. CADET. 1997. Methamphetamine-induced serotonin neurotoxicity is attenuated in p53-knockout mice. Brain Res. **768:** 345–348.
11. JAYANTHI, S., B. LADENHEIM, A.M. ANDREWS & J.L. CADET. 1999. Overexpression of human cooper/zinc superoxide dismutase in trangenic mice attenuates oxidative cause by methylenedioxymethamphetamine (ecstasy). Neuroscience **91:** 1484–1491.
12. SHENG, P., C. CERRUTI, S.F. ALI & J.L. CADET. 1996. Nitric oxide is a mediator of methamphetamine (MeTH)-induced neurotoxicity: *in vitro* evidence from primary cultures of mesencephalic cells. Ann. N.Y. Acad. Sci. **801:** 174–186.
13. SIMANTOV, R. & M. TAUBER. 1997. The abused drug MDMA ("ecstasy") induces programmed death of human serotonergic cells. FASEB J. **11:** 141–146.
14. STUMM, G., J. SCHLEGEL, T. SCHAFER, *et al.* 1999. Amphetamines induce apoptosis and regulation of bcl-x splice variants in neocortical neurons. FASEB J. **13:** 1065–1072.
15. YAMAMOTO, B.K. & W. ZHU. 1998. The effects of methamphetamine on the production of free radicals and oxidative stress. J. Pharmacol. Exp. Ther. **287:** 107–114.
16. PRUDÊNCIO, C., F. SANSONETTY & M. CÔRTE-REAL. 1998. Flow cytometric assessment of cell structural and functional changes induced by acetic acid in the yeasts *Zygosaccharomyces bailii* and *Saccharomyces cerevisiae*. Cytometry **31:** 307–313.
17. PRUDÊNCIO, C. *et al.* 2000. Rapid detection of efflux pumps and their relation with drug resistance in yeast cells. Cytometry **39:** 26–35.
18. ROTMAN, B. & B.W. PAPERMASTER. 1966. Membrane properties of living mammalian cells as studied by enzymatic hydrolysis of fluorogenic esters. Proc. Natl. Acad. Sci. USA **55:** 134–141.
19. ORMEROD, M.G. 1994. Flow Cytometry: A Practical Approach. Oxford University Press. New York.
20. GROGAN, W.M. & J.M. COLLINS. 1990. Guide to Flow Cytometry Methods. Dekker. New York.
21. JONES, R.P. 1987. Measures of yeast death and deactivation and their meaning. Pt. I. Process Biochem. **22:** 118–128.
22. JONES, R.P. 1987. Measures of yeast death and deactivation and their meaning. Part II. Process Biochem. **24:** 130–134.

Postnatal Cocaine Exposure: Effects on Behavior of Rats in Forced Swim Test

ANA MAGALHÃES,[a,b] MARIA AMÉLIA TAVARES,[a,c] AND LILIANA DE SOUSA[a,b]

[a]*Institute for Molecular and Cell Biology (IBMC), University of Porto, Portugal*

[b]*Institute for Biomedical Sciences Abel Salazar (ICBAS), University of Porto, Portugal*

[c]*Institute of Anatomy, Medical School of Porto, University of Porto, Portugal*

ABSTRACT: Exposure to cocaine in early periods of postnatal life has adverse effects on behavior, namely, it induces the display of anxiety and fear-like behaviors that are associated with stress and depression. This study examined the effects of early developmental cocaine exposure in several categories of behavior observed in forced swim test. Male and female Wistar rats were given 15 mg/kg of cocaine hydrochloride/body weight/day, subcutaneously, in two daily doses, from postnatal day (PND) 1 to PND27. Controls were saline injected in the same protocol. In PND26–PND27, rats were placed in a swimming pool during 5 min in two sessions. The categories of behavior studied in this work included horizontal and vertical rotation, vibrissae clean, head clean, fast and slow swim, struggling, floating, sliding, diving, head-diving, and wagging head. Results showed differences in the frequencies of several behavioral categories that allowed the discrimination of the behaviors that may constitute "behavioral despair" indicators, as well as which behaviors are most affected by cocaine exposure. Cocaine groups were less active and more immobile than controls. These results suggest that postnatal exposure to cocaine can produce depression-like effects and affect the ability of these animals to cope with stress situations.

KEYWORDS: cocaine; postnatal; behavior; forced swim test; Wistar rat

INTRODUCTION

Chronic exposure to cocaine during the early postnatal period has negative effects on emotional behaviors in humans and in rats. Experimental cocaine administration can produce anxiety-like behaviors,[1–4] defensive and escape behaviors,[2] immobility,[2] hyperresponsiveness,[5] and fear behaviors,[3] which characterize depressive states.

There is some evidence that cocaine exposure may provoke neurobehavioral alterations in response to environmental modifications, such as stressful situations. Overstreet *et al.*[6] observed that rats exposed to cocaine during the prenatal period were more immobile than were controls in forced swim test. However, other studies show

Address for correspondence: Liliana de Sousa, Ph.D., Institute for Molecular and Cell Biology (IBMC), Rua do Campo Alegre 823, 4150-180 Porto, Portugal. Voice: +351 22 6074945; fax: +351 22 6099157.

anam@ibmc.up.pt

Ann. N.Y. Acad. Sci. 965: 529–534 (2002). © 2002 New York Academy of Sciences.

that rats prenatally exposed to cocaine were less immobile in this stress situation.[5,7] An immobile response, indicative of an animal's inability to react to inescapable stress situations, has been interpreted as a sign of depression or a state of despair.[8–10]

The present study aims to evaluate the behavioral effects of neonatal cocaine exposure on the ability of immature developing rats to cope with stress situations.

MATERIALS AND METHODS

Animal Model

Rats used in this study were male offspring born from nulliparous Wistar females, purchased from the colony of the Gulbenkian Institute of Science, Oeiras, Portugal, and bred at the Institute for Molecular and Cell Biology, Porto. Institutional guidelines regarding animal experimentation were followed. In the day after birth (postnatal day 1, PND1) all litters were standardized to eight pups (4 males and 4 females), individually marked, and were randomly attributed to cocaine or control groups. Rats in the cocaine group were given subcutaneous injections of cocaine hydrochloride (Sigma Chemical Co., St. Louis, MO) in a dose of 15 mg/kg body weight/day in 0.9% saline from PND1 until PND27. The daily dose was divided into two equal parts, administered between 8:30 to 9:00 A.M. and 6:00 to 8:00 P.M. Controls received isovolumetric saline (0.9%), subcutaneously, with the same experimental protocol. Pups were weaned on PND21.

Behavioral Test: Forced Swim Test

The present study used the method described by Porsolt et al.[8] with some modifications. Briefly, a cylinder (54 cm high) was filled with 45 cm of water to prevent animals from touching the bottom with their tails; a wide diameter (47 cm) allowed the display of more behaviors. Water temperature was 24°C. Rats ($n = 48$; 24 treated with cocaine and 24 control) were evaluated in the forced swim test on PND26 and PND27. Rats were placed individually into the cylinder of water for 5 min, and 24 h later animals were placed in water for another 5 min. These sessions were video recorded by a camera (Sony DCR-TRV9E) set at 1 m above the cylinder. Data analysis was performed with Observer 4.0 (Noldus, Information Technology), and the behavioral categories in the swim cylinder were scored for frequencies.

Statistics

A 2×2 analysis of variance was performed on each behavioral category, using a within-subjects design. Independent variables were group (control and cocaine) and session (first and second). All statistics were carried out using the software statistics 5.5A (Statsoft Inc., 1995).

RESULTS

Analysis of the swimming sessions allowed to define the following behavioral categories: right-horizontal rotation (RHR), left-horizontal rotation (LHR), right-

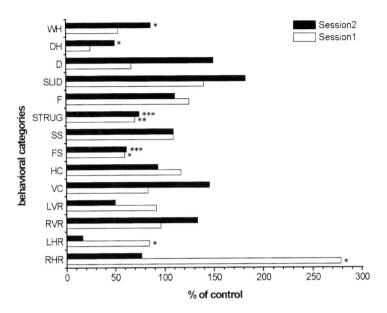

FIGURE 1. Effect of postnatal cocaine exposure upon registered behaviors. Values are expressed as percentage of control (*t* test for independent samples). Behavioral categories: right-horizontal rotation (RHR), left-horizontal rotation (LHR), right-vertical rotation (RVR), left-vertical rotation (LVR), vibrissae clean (VC), head clean (HC), fast swim (FS), slow swim (SW), struggling (STRUG), floating (F), sliding (SLID), diving head (DH), diving (D), and wagging head (WH). $^{***}p < 0.001$; $^{**}p < 0.01$; and $^{*}p < 0.05$.

vertical rotation (RVR), left-vertical rotation (LVR), vibrissae clean (VC), head clean (HC), fast swim (FS), slow swim (SW), struggling (STRUG), floating (F), sliding (SLID), diving head (DH), diving (D), and wagging head (WH).

FIGURE 1 shows the values in percentages of the variation of each behavioral category relative to the control group. The main effects for groups show that postnatally cocaine-exposed rats display fewer behaviors than controls in fast swimming [$F(1,46) = 20.46$, $p < 0.001$], in struggling [$F(1,46) = 19.95$, $p < 0.001$], and in diving head [$F(1,46) = 5.47$, $p = 0.02$].

The interaction effects between group and session show that fast swim is significantly more frequent in the first session than in the second of the two groups, but cocaine-exposed animals swam more than did controls in the second session [$F(1,46) = 4.94$, $p = 0.03$] (FIG. 2a), and right-horizontal rotation decreases in the second session for cocaine-exposed animals but not in controls [$F(1,46) = 6.92$, $p = 0.01$] (FIG. 2b).

DISCUSSION

Rats postnatally exposed to cocaine exhibit significantly lower frequency of fast swimming than do controls, suggesting that early developmental exposure to co-

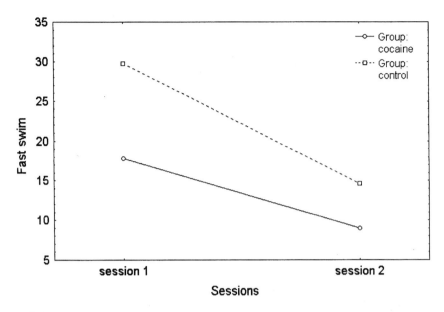

FIGURE 2a. Comparison of fast swim in postnatal cocaine exposure and control groups between the two sessions [$F(1,46) = 4.94$; $p < 0.05$].

caine decreases the persistence to search for an escape. The frequency of struggling behavior is significantly lower in the cocaine-exposed group than in the control group, suggesting that, in a stressful situation, cocaine-treated animals are less active and make fewer attempts to search for an escape. According to Armario et al.,[11] struggling behavior seems to be more directly related to attempts to escape than is swimming, and for these authors struggling behavior is a less subjective measure of antidepressant action than immobility.

In this study cocaine exposure during early postnatal development results in a decrease in general activity. This hypoactivity is one of the symptoms indicative of depression in animals subjected to an uncontrollable stress situation.[12] Results of this study are similar to those shown by Overstreet et al.,[6] that is, that prenatal exposure to cocaine increased immobility; the results are, however, contradictory to the findings of other studies in which the effect of prenatal cocaine is to decrease the immobility behavior of rats in forced swim test.[5,7] These differences in results of immobility behavior, after prenatal or postnatal cocaine exposure, may be related with the methodological differences in experimental procedures, with the amount of drug administered or/and related with the period of development in which the drug is administered.

Head diving may be associated with exploratory behaviors and is observed less in cocaine-exposed animals than in controls. The higher frequency of wagging head in controls may be related to the higher activity of the animals, which results in fur being frequently wet.

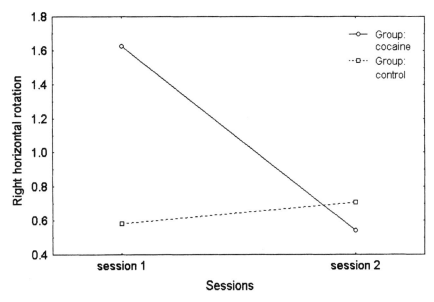

FIGURE 2b. Comparison of right-horizontal rotation in postnatal cocaine exposure and control groups between the two sessions [$F(1,46) = 6.92$; $p < 0.05$].

Rats postnatally exposed to cocaine present a significantly higher frequency of body horizontal rotation to the right in the first session, whereas in the second session left-horizontal rotation is significantly higher in controls. The present results suggest that postnatal cocaine exposure may affect brain laterality.

CONCLUSIONS

In the present study, rats postnatally exposed to cocaine generally display less activity and less exploration than do controls during forced swim test. Animals postnatally exposed to cocaine seem to give up earlier to find an escape from these stressful situations; they stay less active, which may reflect a state of despair.

Cocaine exposure during the first month of life appears to compromise the ability of young rats to adapt to a stressful situation (forced swim test).

ACKNOWLEDGMENTS

This work was supported by Project PRAXIS PSAU/C/SAU/8/96 and Programa de Financiamento Plurianual (IBMC). Ana Magalhães was recipient of the grant PRAXIS XXI/BD/20075/99.

REFERENCES

1. SPEAR, L.P. 1997. Neurobehavioral abnormalities following exposure to drugs of abuse during development. *In* Drug Addiction and its Treatment: Nexus of Neuroscience and Behavior. B.A. Johnson and J.D. Roache, Eds.: 233–255. Lippincott-Raven Publishers. Philadelphia, PA.
2. BLANCHARD, R.J. *et al.* 1998. Acute cocaine effects on stereotypy and defense: an ethoexperimental approach. Neurosci. Biobehav. Rev. **23:** 179–188.
3. BLANCHARD, D.C. & R.J. BLANCHARD. 1999. Cocaine potentiates defensive behaviors related to fear and anxiety. Neurosci. Biobehav. Rev. **23:** 981–991.
4. HEBERT, M.A., D.C. BLANCHARD & R.J. BLANCHARD. 1999. Intravenous cocaine precipitates panic-like flight response and lasting hyperdefensiveness in laboratory rats. Pharmacol. Biochem. Behav. **63:** 349–360.
5. BILITZKE, P.J. & M.W. CHURCH. 1992. Prenatal cocaine and alcohol exposure affect rat behavior in a stress test (the Porsolt swim test). Neurotoxicol. Teratol. **14:** 359–364.
6. Overstreet, D.H. *et al.* 2000. Enduring effects of prenatal cocaine administration on emotional behavior in rats. Physiol. Behav. **70:** 149–156.
7. MOLINA, V.A., J.M. WAGNER & L.P. SPEAR. 1994. The behavioral response to stress is altered in adult rats exposed prenatally to cocaine. Physiol. Behav. **55:** 941–945.
8. PORSOLT, R.D., M. LE PICHON & M. JALFRE. 1977. Depression: a new animal model sensitive to antidepressant treatments. Nature **266:** 730–732.
9. PORSOLT, R.D., G. ANTON, N. BLAVET & M. JALFRE. 1978. Behavioral despair in rats: a new model sensitive to antidepressant treatments. Eur. J. Pharmacol. **47:** 379–391.
10. WEISS, J.M., M.A. CIERPIAL & C.H.K. WEST. 1998. Selective breeding of rats for high and low motor activity in a swim test: toward a new animal model of depression. Pharmacol. Biochem. Behav. **61:** 49–66.
11. ARMARIO, A., A. GAVALDÀ & O. MARTÍ. 1988. Forced swimming test in rats: effect of desipramine administration and the period of exposure to the test on struggling behavior, swimming, immobility and defecation rate. Eur. J. Pharmacol. **158:** 207–212.
12. WILLNER, P. 1991. Animal models as simulations of depression. Trends Pharmacol. Sci. **12:** 131–136.

Index of Contributors